Recent Results in Cancer Research

Fortschritte der Krebsforschung

Progrès dans les recherches sur le cancer

47

Investigation and Stimulation of Immunity in Cancer Patients

Edited by

G. Mathé and R. Weiner

With 143 Figures

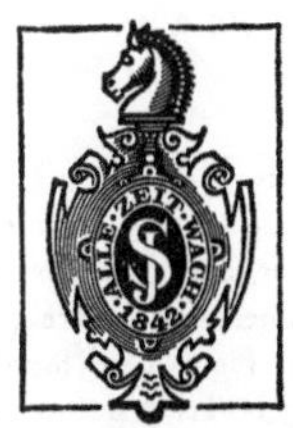

Springer-Verlag Berlin · Heidelberg · New York 1974

Proceedings of the CNRS Colloquium. Paris, June 21—22, 1972

GEORGES MATHÉ, Professor, Institut de Cancérologie et d'Immunogénétique,
Hôpital Paul-Brousse, F-94 Villejuif

ROY WEINER, M.D., Children's Cancer Research Foundation,
35 Binney Street, Boston, MA 02115/USA

Sponsored by the Swiss League against Cancer

Library of Congress Cataloging in Publication Data

Main entry under title:
Investigation and stimulation of immunity in cancer patients.
(Recent results in cancer research, 47)
"Proceedings of the CNRS colloquium, Paris, June 21—22, 1972 ... Sponsored by the Swiss League against Cancer."
Bibliography: p.
1. Cancer-Immunological aspects. I. Mathé, Georges, 1922— ed. II. Weiner, Roy S., ed. III. France. Centre national de la recherche scientifique. IV. Schweizerische Nationalliga für Krebsbekämpfung und Krebsforschung. V. Series.
RC261.R35 no. 47 [RC262] 616.9'94'008s [616.9'94'079] 74-10816

ISBN 978-3-642-49286-0 ISBN 978-3-642-49284-6 (eBook)
DOI 10.1007/978-3-642-49284-6

Softcover reprint of the hardcover 1st edition 1974

Contents

Introduction 1

First Part. Investigation of Immunity in Cancer Patients

1. Non Specific

MILLER, J. F. A. P.: Selective Activation of T Lymphocytes. Its Possible Application in the Immunomanipulation of Tumours 5

THOMAS, E. D., FASS, L., OCHS, H. D., MICKELSON, E. M., STORB, R., FEFER, A.: Immunological Reactivity of Human Recipients of Syngeneic and Allogeneic Marrow Grafts 12

SANTOS, G. W., MULLINS, G. M., BIAS, W. B., ANDERSON, P. N., GRAZIANO, K. D., KLEIN, D. L., BURKE, P. J.: Immunological Studies in Acute Leukemia 17

HERSH, E. M., FREIREICH, E. J., MCCREDIE, K. B., GUTTERMAN, J. U., BODEY, G. P., WHITECAR, J. P., MAVLIGIT, G., CHEEMA, A. R.: Primary and Secondary Immune Responses in the Evaluation of Immunocompetence and Prognosis in Cancer Patients 25

PINSKY, C. M., EL DOMEIRI, A., CARON, A. S., KNAPPER, W. H., OETTGEN, H. F.: Delayed-Hypersensitivity Reactions in Patients with Cancer 37

SCHNEIDER, M., MATHÉ, G., SCHWARZENBERG, L., POUILLART, P., WEINER, R., AMIEL, J. L., HAYAT, M., JASMIN, C., DE VASSAL, F.: Nonspecific Immune Responses in Hematosarcomas and Acute Leukemias 42

2. Specific

BARSKI, G., YOUN, J. K., LE FRANCOIS, D.: Kinetics of Specific Cell-Mediated Immune Response in Cancer-Bearing Hosts 54

LEWIS, M. G.: Technical and Interpretative Problems with Immunofluorescence 58

CLARK, D. A., NATHANSON, L.: Patterns of Cellular Immunity in Malignant Melanoma 67

WIDMER, M. B., SEGALL, M., BACH, F. H., BACH, M. L.: Lymphocyte-Defined Histocompatibility Differences as a Model for Tumor Antigens 79

MAVLIGIT, G. M., GUTTERMAN, J. U., MCBRIDE, CH. M., HERSH, M. E.: Cell-Mediated Immunity to Human Solid Tumors: *in vitro* Detection by Lymphocyte Blastogenic Responses to Cell-Associated and Solubilized Tumor Antigens 84

GUTTERMAN, J. U., HERSH, E. M., MAVLIGIT, G., FREIREICH, E. J., ROSSEN, R. D., BUTLER, W. T., MCCREDIE, K. B., BODEY, G. P., RODRIGUEZ, V.: Cell-Mediated and Humoral Immune Response to Acute Leukemia Cells and Soluble Leukemia Antigen-Relationship to Immunocompetence and Prognosis 97

LEVENTHAL, B. G., HALTERMAN, R. H., ROSENBERG, E. B., MCCOY, J. L., HERBERMAN, R. B.: Lymphocyte Cytotoxicity in Human Acute Leukemia . 113

CEROTTINI, J.-C.: Lymphocyte-Mediated Cytotoxicity and Tumor Immunity . 118

LECLERC, J. C., LEVY, J. P., GOMARD, E., PLATA, F., KOURILSKY, F. M.: Cell-Mediated Immunity in Allogeneic and Tumor-Systems: Nature of the Cells Involved in Killing Target Cells 122

REMOLD, H. G.: Inhibition of Leukocyte Migration in Man 127

LACOUR, F., LACOUR, J., SPIRA, A., BAYET, S.: Effect of Autologous Serum on *in vitro* Inhibition of Leukocyte Migration by Autochthonous Tumor Extracts from Human Patients 129

FREEMAN, C. B., WALKER, J. S., DAVIES, D., COCKING, H., HARRIS, R.: Serum Inhibitory Factors in Acute Leukemia 133

HERBERMAN, R. B.: Delayed Hypersensitivity Response toward Autochthonous Tumor Extracts 140

Second Part. Stimulation of Immunity and Cancer Immunity

1. Experimental

MATHÉ, G., KAMEL, M., DEZFULIAN, M., HALLE-PANNENKO, O., BOURUT, C.: Experimental Screening for "Systemic Adjuvants of Immunity" Applicable in Cancer Immunotherapy 149

CHEDID, L., LAMENSANS, A.: Experimental Screening of Systemic Adjuvants Extracted from Mycobacteria 166

PETIT, J. F., ADAM, A., CIORBARU, R., WIETZERBIN-FALSZPAN, J., LEDERER, E.: Chemical Structure of Mycobacterial Cell Walls 173

ADAM, A., CIORBARU, R., PETIT, J. F., LEDERER, E.: Water-Soluble, Immuno-Adjuvants form the Cell Wall of *Mycobacterium Smegmatis* 179

JACOBS, D., YASHPHE, D. J., ABRAHAM, C.: Stimulation of T Cell Activity by a Methanol-Extraction Residue (MER) of BCG 183

PARANT, M., CHEDID, L.: Biological Properties of Non-Toxic Water-Soluble Immunoadjuvants from Mycobacterial Cells 190

BONA, C., HEUCLIN, C., CHEDID, L.: Enhancement of Human Mixed-Lymphocyte Cultures by a Water-Soluble Adjuvant 196

LIACOPOULOS, P., BIRRIEN, J. L., BLEUX, C., COUDERC, J.: Early Recovery of the Immune Response of a Specifically Depleted Cell Population under the Influence of Water-Soluble Adjuvant 201

MIGLIORE-SAMOUR, D., JOLLÈS, P.: An Adjuvant-Active Water-Soluble Substance ("Polysaccharide-Peptidoglycan") from Mycobacterial Cells. Preparation by a Simple Extraction Technique 207

HIU, I. J.: MAAF: A Fully Water-Soluble Lipid-Free Fraction from BCG with Adjuvant and Antitumor Activity 213

ASSELINEAU, J., PORTELANCE, V.: Comparative Study of the Free Lipids of Eight BCG Daughter Strains 214

VILKAS, E., AMAR-NACASCH, C., MARKOVITS, J.: A Galactose Disaccharide from Immunoadjuvant Fractions of Mycobacterium Tuberculosis (Cell Wall and Wax D) 221

BENACERRAF, B.: Summary of Working Session on the Mechanism of Action of Immunological Adjuvants 224

ROSENTHAL, S. R.: BCG and the Lympho-Reticuloendothelial System 228

STIFFEL, C., MOUTON, D., BIOZZI, G.: Effect of Corynebacterium Parvum on Resistance to Experimental Leukemia in Relation to Genetic Modification of Immunoresponsiveness 239

MUNDER, P. G., MODOLELL, M.: The Influence of *Mycobacterium Bovis* and *Corynebacterium Parvum* on the Phospholipid Metabolism of Macrophages 244

GOREN, M. B., BROKL, O.: Separation and Purification of Cord Factor (6,6′-Dimycoloyl Trehalose) from Wax C or from Mycolic Acids 251

BEKIERKUNST, A.: Granuloma Induction and Stimulation of the Immune Response in Mice with Trehalose-6,6′-Dimycolate 259

HALPERN, B.: Corynebacterium Parvum: An Immunomodulator 262

WOODRUFF, M. F. A.: Nonspecific Effects of Corynebacteria on Systemic Immunity Responses 272

KOUZNETZOVA, B., BIZZINI, B., CHERMANN, J.-C., DEGRAND, F., PREVOT, A.-R., RAYNAUD, M.: Immunostimulating Activity of Whole Cells, Cell-Walls and Fractions of Anaerobic Corynebacteria 275

PILET, CH., LE GARREC, Y., TOUJAS, L., SABOLOVIC, D., MONTEIL, J. C., ROTHIER, F., MISHRA, U., GHEBREHIWET, B., GUELFI, J.: Nonspecific Stimulation by Inactivated or Ultrasonicated Brucella Abortus 294

TOUJAS, L., DAZORD, L., GUELFI, J.: Increase of Brucella-Induced Immunostimulation by Administration in Combination with a Specific Antiserum . 302

DONNER, M., VAILLIER, D.: Alterations in Immune Response to Experimental Murine Tumor-Associated Antigens Following Administration of BCG or Polysaccharide from *Proteus vulgaris* 308

BORTIN, M. M., RIMM, A. A., SALTZSTEIN, E. C., SHALABY, M. R., RODEY, G. E.: Cell-Mediated Immunity in AKR Mice Treated with Lentinan, a Fungal Polysaccharide 320

GRESSER, I.: The Antitumor Effects of Interferon 327

MARDINEY, M. R., CHESS, L., LEVY, C., SCHMUKLER, M., SMITH, K.: Use of Double-Stranded Synthetic Polynucleotides in Amplifying Immunologically Induced Lymphocyte Proliferation 330

BRAUN, W., SHIOZAWA, C.: Immunoenhancing and Antitumor Effects of Agents that Elevate Endogenous Cyclic AMP Levels 338

BALDWIN, R. W., PIMM, M. V.: BCG Immunotherapy of Pulmonary Deposits from Experimental Rat Tumours of Defined Immunogenicity 345

ZBAR, B.: Specific and Nonspecific Immunotherapy: Use of BCG 350

LACOUR, F., LACOUR, J., SPIRA, A.: Poly A. Poly U as an Adjunct to Surgery in the Treatment of Spontaneous Murine Mammary Adenocarcinoma . . . 352
BEKESI, J. G., HOLLAND, J. F.: Combined Chemotherapy and Immunotherapy of Transplantable and Spontaneous Murine Leukemia in DBA/2 and AKR Mice 357
SIMMONS, L. R., RIOS, A.: Modification of Immunogenicity in Experimental Immunotherapy and Prophylaxis 370
PRAGER, M. D., RIBBLE, R. J., MEHTA, J. M.: Aspects of the Immunology of the Tumor-Host Relationship and Responsiveness to Modified Lymphoma Cells 379
DORÉ, J. F., HADJIYANNAKIS, M. J., COUDERT, A., GUIBOUT, C., MARHOLEY, L., IMAI, K.: Use of Enzyme-Treated Cells in Immunotherapy of Leukemia . . 387
MATHÉ, G., HALLE-PANNENKO, O., BOURUT, C.: Active Immunotherapy of AKR Mouse Spontaneous Leukemia 389
BOONE, C. W.: Augmented Immunogenicity of Tumor Cell Homogenates Infected with Influenza Virus 394
MARTYRE, M.-C., HALLE-PANNENKO, O., JOLLES, P.: Characterization and Purification of Rauscher Leukemia-Associated Transplantation Antigens . . . 401
MARTYRE, M.-C., WEINER, R., HALLE-PANNENKO, O.: The *in vivo* Activity of Soluble Extracts Obtained from RC19 Leukemia: Effect of the Method of Extraction 405
BENJAMINI, E., SCIBIENSKI, R. T.: The Preferential Induction of Cell-Mediated Immunity and Some Preliminary Observations on its Application to Tumor Immunotherapy 408

2. Clinical

BLUMING, A., VOGEL, L., ZIEGLER, J. L.: Clinical Screening of Systemic Adjuvants of Immunity 415
ROSENTHAL, S. R., CRISPEN, R. G., THORNE, M. G., PIEKARSKI, N., RAISYS, N., RETTIG, P.: BCG Vaccination and Leukemia Mortality 421
MARDINEY, M. R., CHESS, L., BOCK, G. N., UNGARO, P. C., BUCHHOLZ, D. H.: Immunologic Effects of BCG in Patients with Malignant Melanoma . . . 426
MATHÉ, G., POUILLART, P., SCHWARZENBERG, L., WEINER, R., RAPPAPORT, H., HAYAT, M., DE VASSAL, F., AMIEL, J. L., SCHNEIDER, M., JASMIN, C., ROSENFELD, C.: Attempts at Immunotherapy of 100 Acute Lymphoid Leukemia Patients: Some Factors Influencing Results 434
POWLES, R., MCELMAIN, T. J., ALEXANDER, P., CROWTHER, D., FAIRLEY, G., PIKE, M.: Immunotherapy of Acute Myeloblastic Leukemia in Man . . . 449
SAUTER, C., LINDENMANN, J., GERBER, A., MARTZ, G.: Acute Myeloblastic Leukemia: Replication of Avian Influenza Virus in Human Myeloblasts and First Attempt at Clinical Application 455
MAGRATH, I. T., ZIEGLER, J. L., BLUMING, A. Z.: Preliminary Results of a Randomized Trial of BCG Immunotherapy in Burkitt's Lymphoma 461
PINES, A.: BCG Immunotherapy in the Treatment of Inoperable Carcinoma of the Lung 466

RÜMKE, P., BERNHEIM, J., V. D. VORM, D. H., VAN PEPERZEEL, H. A., LOOYSEN, R.: Effect of BCG Stimulation on the Growth Rate of Pulmonary Metastases in 3 Patients with Melanoma 470
BERNHEIM, J. J. L.: Immunotherapy of a Solid Tumor (Melanoma) with BCG: A Comment on the Risks of Enhancement 473
GUTTERMAN, J. U., MAVLIGIT, G., MCBRIDE, CH. M., FREI, E. III, HERSH, E. M.: BCG Stimulation of Immune Responsiveness in Patients with Malignant Melanoma 476
ISRAEL, L.: Clinical Results with Corynebacteria 486
MARCOVE, R. C.: A Clinical Trial of Autogenous Vaccines in the Treatment of Osteogenic Sarcoma 488
SOKAL, J. E., AUNGST, C. W.: Immunization with Cultured Cell-BCG Mixtures 496

Introduction

G. MATHÉ

Institut de Cancérologie et d'Immunogénétique (INSERM et Association Claude-Bernad), Hôpital Paul-Brousse and Institute Gustave-Roussy, Villejuif

20 years ago, the main, if not only object of the cancer therapist was to effect complete surgical exeresis or radiotherapeutic destruction of a local tumor, or to obtain, by means of chemotherapy, an "apparently complete regression" of a local or disseminated neoplasia.

Today it is realized that (a) at the time of the operation or radiotherapy, two patients in every three carrying an apparently localized tumor have a few cancer cells outside the area where the tumor seems localized; (b) when "apparently complete regression" or even an "apparently complete remission" is induced by chemotherapy, not all the neoplastic cells have been eradicated.

In both cases an imperceptible residual neoplasm persists, the growth of which will in due course make it perceptible again, giving rise to metastasis or to a systemic or localized relapse.

There is thus an urgent need for a new technique capable of killing the last cell or cells. Our experiments in mice on the effectiveness of active immunotherapy, which involves the manipulation of the immune machinery, have shown that this treatment is able to kill *all* the cells, down to the very last cell of a given leukemia, provided that the total number of cells does not exceed a few thousand [1, 2].

We proposed in 1964 to use active immunotherapy to eradicate the residual cells left by chemoradiotherapy in acute lymphoid leukemia (ALL). Seven of the 20 patients randomized in the immunotherapy group are still in remission today and have not presented with a relapse for periods varying from 7 to 10 years. On the other hand, all the controls relapsed within a few months. This is indeed a demonstration of the ability of immunotherapy to eradicate the last cells [3, 4].

The evidence is accumulating: our other trials on ALL [4, 5], our trial on leukemic (terminal) lymphosarcomas [5], those of POWLES in the U.K. [6] and of the South Eastern Group in the U.S.A. [7] on acute myeloid leukemia, Sokal's trials on chronic myeloid leukemia [8] and on non leukemic lymphomas [9], BLUMING'S trial [10], and the trial of GUTTERMAN, HERSCH, FREIREICH and FREI on melanoma [11], and now that of MARCOVE and SOUTHAM [12] on osteosarcoma demonstrate that immunotherapy acts on the imperceptible residual disease.

Another approach to active immunotherapy, called "local" because of the intratumor administration of the immunity-manipulating agents, has been tried with success by ZBAR and RAPP [13] in guinea pigs, and by MORTON *et al.* [14] in man.

Active immunotherapy [15], complementing the adoptive immunotherapy proposed by us in 1959 [16], and passive immunotherapy [17], is now the fourth method of treating cancer. The time is now ripe for it to be used in an attempt to eradicate the imperceptible residual disease left by the surgeon, the radiotherapist, or the chemotherapist.

For this treatment to succeed, progress must be made not only in the techniques and methods of active immunotherapy, but also in evaluating the immune status of the patient. And finally, there is still room for improvement in the logistics of treating cancer patients.

References

1. Mathe, G.: Immunothérapie active de la leucémie L 1210 appliquée après la greffe tumorale. Rev. Fr. Et. Clin. Biol. **13**, 881 (1968).
2. Mathe, G., Pouillart, P., Lapeyraque, F.: Active immunotherapy of L 1210 leukemia applied after the graft of tumour cells. Brit. J. Cancer **23**, 814 (1969).
3. Mathe, G., Amiel, J. L., Schwarzenberg, L., Schneider, M., Cattan, A., Schlumberger, J. R., Hayat, M., de Vassal, F.: Active immunotherapy for acute lymphoid leukemia. Lancet **1969 I**, 697.
4. Mathe, G., Schwarzenberg, L., Amiel, J. L., Pouillart, P., Hayat, M., de Vassal, F., Rosenfeld, C., Jasmin, C.: New experimental and clinical data on leukemia immunotherapy. Proc. Royal Soc. Med. 1974, in press.
5. Mathe, G., Pouillart, P., Schwarzenberg, L., Hayat, M., Amiel, J. L., de Vassal, F.: Leukaemic conversion of non-Hodgkin's malignant lymphomas. Brit. J. Cancer 1974, in press.
6. Powles, R., Kay, H. E. M., McElwain, T. J., Alexander, P., Crowther, D., Hamilton-Fairley, G., Pike, M.: Immunotherapy of acute myeloblastic leukaemia in man. In: Investigation and stimulation of immunity in cancer patients (G. Mathe and R. Weiner, Eds.). Berlin-Heidelberg-New York: Springer 1974.
7. Vogler, W. R., Chan, Y. K.: Effect of bacillus-Calmette Guérin (BCG) in prolongation of remissions in acute myeloblastic leukemia (AML). Proc. Amer. Ass. Cancer Res. **15**, 164 (1974). (Abstract no. 723.)
8. Sokal, J. E., Aungst, C. W.: Immunization with cultured cell-BCG mixtures. In: Investigation and stimulation of immunity in cancer patients (G. Mathe and R. Weiner, Eds.). Berlin-Heidelberg-New York: Springer 1974.
9. Sokal, J. E., Aungst, C. W., Snyderman, M.: Prolongation of remission in stage I and II lymphoma by BCG vaccination. Proc. Amer. Ass. Cancer Res. **15**, 13 (1974). (Abstract no. 51.)
10. Bluming, A. Z., Vogel, C. L., Ziegler, J. L., Mody, N., Kamya, G.: Immunological effects of BCG in patients with malignant melanoma. A comparison of two modes of administration. Ann. Intern. Med. **76**, 405 (1972).
11. Gutterman, J. U., McBride, C., Freireich, E. J., Mavligit, G., Frei, E. III, Hersh, E. M.: Active immunotherapy with BCG for recurrent malignant melanoma. Lancet **1973 I**, 1208.
12. Marcove, R. C., Southam, C. M., Levin, A. G., Huvors, A. G., Mike, V.: A clinical trial of autogenous vaccine in the treatment of osteogenic sarcoma. In: Investigation and stimulation of immunity in cancer patients (G. Mathe and R. Weiner, Eds.). Berlin-Heidelberg-New York: Springer 1974.
13. Zbar, B., Bernstein, I. D., Rapp, H. J.: Suppression of tumor growth at the site of infection with living bacillus Calmette-Guérin. J. Nat. Cancer Inst. **46**, 831 (1971).
14. Morton, D. L., Eilber, F. R., Malmgren, R. A., Wood, W. C.: Immunological factors which influence response to immunotherapy in malignant melanomas. Surgery **68**, 158 (1970).
15. Mathe, G.: Active immunotherapy. Adv. Cancer Res. **14**, 1 (1971).
16. Thompson, R. B., Mathe, G.: Adoptive immunotherapy in malignant disease. Transplant Rev. **9**, 54 (1972).
17. Motta, R.: Passive immunotherapy of leukemia and other cancers. Adv. Cancer Res. **14**, 161 (1971).

First Part

Investigation of Immunity in Cancer Patients

1. Non Specific

Selective Activation of T Lymphocytes. Its Possible Application in the Immunomanipulation of Tumours

J. F. A. P. Miller

The Walter and Eliza Hall Institute of Medical Research
Royal Melbourne Hospital, Victoria 3050, Australia

It is now well established that lymphocytes can interact with antigen to initiate immune responses and that they can be divided into two broad classes: thymus-derived or T cells and non-thymus-derived or (bone marrow-derived) B cells. T and B lymphocytes can be distinguished, not by their morphology, but by their functional properties and by the existence of certain specific markers.

B lymphocytes are antibody-forming cell precursors involved in humoral immunity. T lymphocytes do not secrete classical antibody molecules but play a role in cellular immunity — delayed type hypersensitivity, immunity to transplantation and tumour-specific transplantation antigens, and resistance to certain infections, notably viral and mycobacterial. They can become killer cells causing lysis of target cells with which they establish contact. T lymphocytes also collaborate with B lymphocytes in some humoral antibody responses. In these they act as "helper" cells facilitating, in some unknown way, the response of B cells to antigen.

T lymphocytes can be distinguished from B lymphocytes by the existence of certain characteristic "differentiation" antigens. Thus, for instance, the θ antigen is present on thymus lymphocytes and on T lymphocytes outside the thymus but is absent from B lymphocytes [18, 19]. B cells have a high density of immunoglobulin molecules on their surface in contrast to T cells which have a very low density of such molecules [15, 17]. B lymphocytes carry receptors for the Fc portion of some classes of antibody molecules. The bond between cell and antibody is weak but may be stabilized by adding the corresponding antigen. T cells do not possess such a receptor [1]. Furthermore, a subpopulation of B lymphocytes carry receptors for modified C3 capable of binding antibody-antigen-complement complexes (CRL) [4].

The markers which characterize T and B cells have been exploited to deplete various lymphocyte populations of T or B cells by *in vitro* methods. Thus, anti-θ serum eliminates most T cells [13, 18]. Rabbit anti-mouse kappa chain serum selectively eliminates only B cells [14], presumably because these have a much higher density of immunoglobulin molecules on their surface than do T cells. Lymphocyte populations incubated with antibody can be passaged through a column of beads coated with the corresponding antigen: B cells are retained on the columns (because of their receptor for antibody-antigen complexes) and T cells are free to emerge in the effluent [1]. Finally CRL which are allowed to form rosettes with erythrocytes, antibody and complement can be separated from non-CRL and from T lymphocytes by differential centrifugation [4].

Animals can be treated in various ways designed to augment or deplete their lymphocyte populations of T or B cells.

Depletion of T cells in intact adult mice can be achieved by thoracic duct drainage [6] or treatment with antilymphocyte serum [7] as these procedures eliminate mainly recirculating T lymphocytes. Mice having few or no T cells can be obtained by the technique of neonatal thymectomy [8] or adult thymectomy followed by total body irradiation and marrow protection [9]. The lymphoid population of such mice is composed predominantly of B cells. The nu nu strain of mice, in which the thymus fails to develop [16], is deprived of T cells and can thus be used to provide only B lymphocytes [21].

Table 1. Specific markers on T and B lymphocytes (Data compiled from [1, 11, 13, 14, 18])

Sources of lymphocytes	% cells killed by			% cells labelled with antibody-antigen complexes
	CBA anti-C 57 BL serum	anti-θ C 3 H serum	anti-kappa serum	
Normal CBA TDL	0	79	15	16
TDL from NTx CBA reconstituted with (CBA × C 57 BL)F_1 thymus cells	79	68	16	19
CBA T. TDL (for T. TDL see text)	0	90	0	0.3
nu nu TDL (TDL from athymic nu nu mice; nu + mice possess the θ C 3 H allele)	—	0	85	97

Mice can be treated in such a way that they contain a chimaeric population of lymphocytes in which the T and B cells bear stable unequivocal markers and occur in a proportion that can readily be determined. Thus, for instance, CBA mice can be thymectomized at birth and reconstituted to near normal immunological status, by injecting thymus lymphocytes from an F_1 hybrid donor such as (CBA × C57BL)F_1. The F_1 cells are genetically incapable of reacting against their host which is, itself, as a result of neonatal thymectomy, unable to reject F_1 cells. A chimaera is thus produced in which the thoracic duct lymphocyte (TDL) population is composed of T cells derived from the F_1 thymus inoculum and B cells from the neonatally thymectomized CBA host which has very few T cells of its own. Relatively pure populations of B cells can thus be obtained by treating the TDL with a CBA anti-C57BL serum and complement [13].

Depletion of B cells can be achieved in chickens by bursectomy [25] but is difficult to achieve in other animals in which the bursa equivalent has not been identified as a single (or even multifocal) organ. Mice can, however, be manipulated so that they produce pure populations of T lymphocytes. For this purpose, thymus cells are injected into heavily irradiated mice and subjected to an immunogenic stimulus. As a result, the cells become specifically activated and proliferate to produce a progeny of T cells which can be recovered by thoracic duct drainage (T. TDL) [20, 22] as will be described below.

The various means of enriching for T and B cells and the markers by which such cells can be distinguished are summarized in Table 1.

Selective Activation of Lymphocytes

5×10^7 thymus cells from CBA mice were injected intravenously into lethally irradiated (800 r) (CBA × C57BL) F_1 or (CBA × BALB/c) F_1 mice (CBA, C57BL and BALB/c differing from one another at the strong H2 locus). Intense cell proliferation was evident 3 days later in the white pulp of the spleen and cortex of the

Table 2. Characteristic properties of cells emerging from the thoracic duct of irradiated (CBA × C 57 BL)F_1 mice 4 days after injection of thymus cells

	Inoculum	
	10^8 CBA thymus cells	10^8 (CBA × C 57 BL)F_1 thymus cells
Average no. of cells collected in 24 hrs ($\times 10^{-6}$) ± SE	15.3 ± 0.5	2.0 ± 0.3
% of cells resistant to CBA anti C 57 BL serum	98	2
% of cells susceptible to anti θ C 3 H serum	96	—
% of cells susceptible to anti kappa serum	0	—
% of cells binding antibody antigen complexes	0.3	—
% of cells labelled with tritiated thymidine (± SE)	94.1 ± 0.4	19.3 ± 1.5
Average no. of labelled cells collected in 24 hrs ($\times 10^{-6}$)	14.9	0.38

lymph nodes. Autoradiographic studies indicated that the proliferating cells (labelled with tritiated thymidine) left the lymph nodes and spleen after 3—4 days via lymphatics and blood [23]. Thoracic duct cannulation was thus performed in the irradiated hybrid hosts 24 hrs after irradiation and injection of CBA thymus cells. The mice received 25 μCi tritiated thymidine every 12 hrs and the cell content of their lymph was examined at 12 hourly intervals [22]. Only few cells (2—4 million/12 hrs) emerged from the thoracic duct 1—3 days after irradiation and cell injection. After 3½ days, however, there appeared large numbers of pyroninophilic blasts, of which more than 95% had incorporated tritiated thymidine and were susceptible to lysis by anti-θ serum and complement but resistant to CBA anti-C57BL serum and complement (when the irradiated hosts were (CBA × C57BL) F_1 mice) (Table 2). These cells were also resistant to anti-kappa serum and less than 1 in 200 bound antibody-antigen complexes. Evidently, they were derived from the inoculated thymus cells, not from the irradiated hosts, and had all the characteristics of T cells. They were thus referred to as T. TDL. Very few cells emerged from the thoracic duct of irradiated recipients of syngeneic thymus cells after 3½ days post-irradiation.

Table 3. Effect of T. TDL on growth of DBA/2 mastocytoma cells in NTx CBA mice

Lymphocytes given	No. of mice in group	No. of lymphocytes	Survival time (days) of NTx CBA recipients of 10^6 mastocytoma cells	No. of mice surviving beyond 50 days
CBA thymus	10	5×10^7	20.1 (12—32)	0
	10	5×10^6	17.6 (11—18)	0
	10	5×10^5	14.1 (6—20)	0
CBA TDL	10	5×10^6	30.8 (12—49)	1
	10	5×10^5	20.8 (17—25)	0
	10	5×10^4	15.8 (11—20)	0
BALB/c activated	10	5×10^6	27.8 (24—41)	5
CBA T. TDL	10	5×10^5	18.8 (8—25)	4
	10	5×10^4	15.3 (13—18)	0
C 57 BL activated	10	5×10^6	10.1 (6—13)	0
CBA T. TDL	10	5×10^5	14.0 (12—18)	0
	10	5×10^4	12.3 (8—10)	0

Table 4. Cytotoxic effects of CBA T. TDL on DBA/2 mastocytoma cells *in vitro*

	Type of lymphocytes used *in vitro*					
	BALB/c-activated CBA T. TDL			C 57 BL-activated CBA T. TDL		
Lymphocyte: target cell ratio	100/1	50/1	25/1	100/1	50/1	25/1
% specific ^{51}Cr release by target cells 3 hrs	75	61	56	13	9	4
6 hrs	100	100	100	44	41	21
No of H 2 sites available to sensitized lymphocytes		9/9			5/8	
% inhibition by 1 : 10 CBA anti-BALB/c serum		90			100	
Sites covered by antibody/sites attacked by lymphocytes		9/9			9/5	

T. TDL were just as capable of recirculating as normal TDL when injected intravenously into syngeneic mice [22]. Striking specificity was evident in the ability of T. TDL to reject allogeneic skin grafts. Thus, when 10^7 C57BL-activated CBA T.TDL were injected into neonatally thymectomized (NTx) CBA mice grafted within 4 hrs with C57BL or BALB/c skin, the former grafts were rejected rapidly within 9 days or less whereas the latter survived indefinitely [24]. These data, and those given below, indicate that T. TDL have their immunological activities directed mostly, if not exclusively, against the antigens which initially provoked their formation.

Effect of Specifically Activated T Cells on Tumour Growth *in vivo* or *in vitro*

Intraperitoneal injection of from 5×10^5 to 5×10^6 BALB/c activated CBA T.TDL together with 10^6 DBA/2 mastocytoma cells into NTx CBA mice completely suppressed the growth of the tumour in 9 out of 20 mice. Similar numbers of C57BL-activated CBA T. TDL were entirely ineffective. The same dose of normal CBA TDL protected only 1 of 20 NTx mice (Table 3).

T. TDL were highly effective as killer cells *in vitro*. Complete lysis of ^{51}Cr labelled mastocytoma cells, as measured by the technique of Brunner *et al.* [2] occurred when the tumour cells were incubated *in vitro* with BALB/c-activated T. TDL. Lysis was specific since it was inhibited by CBA anti-BALB/c serum (in the absence of added complement). ^{51}Cr release was less, though still evident, when C57BL-activated CBA T. TDL were used (Table 4). This is presumably a reflection of the fact that, with respect to activation of CBA thymus cells by H2 antigens, the $H2^d$ allele (possessed by BALB/c and DBA/2) shares 5 antigenic determinants with the $H2^b$ allele (possessed by C57BL).

Conclusions

A method has been devised by which thymus cells can be "activated" against antigenic tumour cells. The thymus cells were injected into heavily irradiated hosts, which provided a source of antigens identical to those present on the tumour selected for study. The thymus cells proliferated and produced a progeny of circulating lymphocytes which were immunulogically competent and highly specialized in the sense that they could only react to the antigens which initially provoked their formation. They were highly effective in protecting T cell-deprived mice from the growth of inoculated tumour cells and in lysing the tumour cells *in vitro*. In previous work, it was shown that the spleens of irradiated F_1 recipients of parental thymus cells could be used as a source of killer cells *in vitro* [3, 12]. More recent studies have also indicated that cells in spleen may differentiate into killer cells when activated against histoincompatible, mitomycin C-treated spleen cells *in vitro* [26]. T. TDL, as a pure population of lymphocytes, offer distinctive advantages over cells obtained by these methods particularly with respect to their high viability (98%) and low degree of contamination by other cell types (0—5%).

The identification of markers on T and B lymphocytes and the establishment of various techniques by which pure populations of T and B cells can be obtained should help towards the task of selectively stimulating the function of T cells in tumour immunity. Although an allogeneic tumour was used in the present studies, it is felt that the same rules will apply to syngeneic tumours that differ from their host by the possession of certain tumour-specific antigens.

Many tumours, including human tumours, are "self-enhancing": the host can generate killer cells (T lymphocytes) but these are ineffective in limiting tumour development *in vivo* because of the production by the host's B lymphocytes of "blocking" antibodies which protect the tumour cells from the activity of the killer lymphocytes [5]. Inhibition of this tumour protecting mechanism would have great potential clinical applications. Methods of immunomanipulation must be devised by which the killer function of T lymphocytes is enhanced (e.g., by specific activation as mentioned above or by nonspecific activation with adjuvants such as poly-AU) whilst the activity of B lymphocytes in producing blocking antibody is depressed. We still do not have definite evidence to decide whether the blocking antibody responses of B cells require the facilitation of T helper cells, and whether T helper cells and T killer cells are derived from one and the same T cell precursor or whether they belong to separate lines of T cells.

The situation *in vivo* is certainly more complex as it has recently been shown that B lymphocytes can act as killer cells under defined conditions [10]. Thus, in the presence of anti-target antibody, but in the absence of complement, pure populations of B lymphocytes (derived from nonsensitized mice) can kill antibody-coated target cells *in vitro*. Presumably, the B lymphocytes, through their receptors for the Fc piece of immunoglobulin molecules, adhere to the target cells and, as a result of this intimate contact, target cell lysis occurs. There are certain indications which strongly suggest that B lymphocyte killing may occur *in vivo* via this mechanism. It is therefore urgent to obtain more detailed knowledge of the mechanism by which T and B lymphocytes respond to tumour-specific antigens before immunomanipulation can become a practical reality in clinical medicine.

Acknowledgements

The author is indebted to his colleagues Dr. JONATHAN SPRENT and Dr. ANTONY BASTEN for publishing, in this article, data obtained as a result of work performed with their collaboration. These investigations were supported by the National Health and Medical Research Council of Australia, the Australian Research Grants Committee and the Damon Runyon Fund for Cancer Research.

References

1. BASTEN, A., SPRENT, J., MILLER, J. F. A. P.: Receptor for antibody-antigen complexes used for separation of T cells from B cells. Nature New Biol. **235**, 178 (1971).
2. BRUNNER, K. T., MAUL, J., RUDOLF, H., CHAPUIS, B.: Studies of allograft immunity in mice. I. Induction, development and *in vitro* assay of cellular immunity. Immunology **18**, 501 (1970).
3. CEROTTINI, J. C., NORDIN, A. A., BRUNNER, K. T.: *In vitro* cytotoxic activity of thymus cells sensitized to alloantigens. Nature **227**, 72 (1970).
4. DUKOR, P., BIANCO, C., NUSSENZWEIG, V.: Bone marrow origin of Complement-Receptor-Lymphocytes. Europ. J. Immunol. **1**, 491 (1971).
5. HELLSTRÖM, K. E., HELLSTRÖM, I.: Immunological enhancement as studied by cell culture techniques. Ann. Rev. Microbiol. **24**, 373 (1970).
6. MCGREGOR, D. D., GOWANS, J. L.: The antibody response of rats deplated of lymphocytes by chronic drainage from the thoracic duct. J. exp. Med. **117**, 303 (1963).
7. MARTIN, W. J., MILLER, J. F. A. P.: Cell to cell interaction in the immune response. IV. Site of action of antilymphocyte globulin. J. exp. Med. **128**, 354 (1968).
8. MILLER, J. F. A. P.: Immunological function of the thymus. Lancet **1961 II**, 748.
9. MILLER, J. F. A. P.: Immunological significance of the thymus of the adult mouse. Nature **195**, 318 (1962).
10. MILLER, J. F. A. P., BASTEN, A.: Unpublished data, 1972.
11. MILLER, J. F. A. P., BASTEN, A., SPRENT, J., CHEERS, C.: Interaction between lymphocytes in immune responses. Cell. Immunol. **2**, 469 (1971).

12. Miller, J. F. A. P., Brunner, K. T., Sprent, J., Russel, P. J., Mitchell, G. F.: Thymus-derived cells as killer cells in cell-mediated immunity. In: Proc. of the IIIrd International Congress of the Transplantation Society. Transplant. Proc. **3**, 915 (1970).
13. Miller, J. F. A. P., Sprent, J.: Thymus-derived cells in mouse thoracic duct lymph. Nature New Biol. **230**, 267 (1971).
14. Miller, J. F. A. P., Sprent, J., Basten, A., Warner, N. L.: Selective cytotoxicity of anti-kappa serum for B-lymphocytes. Nature New Biol. **237**, 18 (1972).
15. Nossal, G. J. V., Warner, N. L., Lewis, H., Sprent, J.: Quantitative features of a sandwich radio-immunolabeling technique for lymphocyte surface receptors. J. exp. Med. **135**, 405 (1972).
16. Pantelouris, E. M.: Observations on the immunobiology of "nude" mice. Immunology **20**, 247 (1971).
17. Rabellino, F., Colon, S., Grey, H. M., Unanue, E. R.: Immunoglobulins on the surface of lymphocytes. I. Distribution and quantitation. J. exp. Med. **133**, 156 (1971).
18. Raff, M. C.: Theta antigen as a marker for thymus-derived lymphocytes. Nature **224**, 378 (1969).
19. Reif, A. E., Allen, J. M. V.: The AKR thymic antigen and its distribution in leukemias and nervous tissues. J. exp. Med. **120**, 413 (1964).
20. Sprent, J., Miller, J. F. A. P.: Activation of thymus cells by histocompatibility antigens. Nature New Biol. **234**, 195 (1971).
21. Sprent, J., Miller, J. F. A. P.: Thoracic duct lymphocytes from nude mice: migratory properties and lifespan. Europ. J. Immunol. **2**, 384 (1972).
22. Sprent, J., Miller, J. F. A. P.: The interaction of thymus lymphocytes with histoincompatible cells. II. Recirculating lymphocytes derived from antigen activated thymus cells. Cell. Immunol. **3**, 385 (1972).
23. Sprent, J., Miller, J. F. A. P.: The interaction of thymus lymphocytes with histoincompatible cells. I. Quantitation of the proliferative response of thymus cells. Cell. Immunol. **3**, 361 (1972).
24. Sprent, J., Miller, J. F. A. P.: The interaction of thymus lymphocytes with histoincompatible cells. III. Immunological characteristics of antigen activated thymus-derived recirculating lymphocytes. Cell. Immunol. **3**, 213 (1972).
25. Wagner, H., Feldmann, M.: Cell-mediated immune response *in vitro*. I. A new *in vitro* system for the generation of cell-mediated cytotoxic activity. Cell. Immunol. **3**, 405 (1972).
26. Warner, N. L.: The immunological role of the avian thymus and bursa of Fabricius. Folia Biologica **13**, 1 (1967).

Immunological Reactivity of Human Recipients of Syngeneic and Allogeneic Marrow Grafts*

E. D. Thomas,** L. Fass, H. D. Ochs, E. M. Mickelson, R. Storb, and A. Fefer***

Departments of Medicine and Pediatrics, University of Washington, School of Medicine, and the U. S. Public Health Service Hospital, Seattle, Washington

This report describes preliminary observations of immunological function on 7 patients with bone marrow grafts. Three patients with aplastic anemia were prepared for grafting with cyclophosphamide (CY) and received marrow from HL-A-matched siblings [7, 10]. Four patients with hematological malignancy were prepared for grafting with whole body irradiation; 2 of these patients received marrow from an identical twin [6], and 2 patients received marrow from an HL-A-matched sibling [8, 9]. Table 1 summarizes the clinical and hematological data in these patients. None of these patients had significant graft-versus-host (GVH) disease and none has, as yet, shown recurrence of disease. Thus, immunologic parameters could be studied in the absence of these 2 important variables.

Methods

The techniques of measuring immunoglobulins [2] and testing in mixed leukocyte culture [5] phage immunization [3], and DNCB skin testing [1], have been described in detail elsewhere. Normal antibody responses, expressed as K values, are 10 to 100 following primary and 200 to 2,000 following secondary immunization with bacteriophage θX 174.

Results

Table 2 summarizes the results. Measurement of immunoglobulin levels from 35 to 626 days after grafting showed, in general, levels of gamma G, gamma M and gamma A within the normal range. Peripheral blood lymphocyte levels were 600 to

* This work was supported by grants CA 10895 and CA 05231 from the National Cancer Institute and by contract PH 43-67-1435 from the National Institutes of Health, U. S. Public Health Service.

** Dr. Thomas is supported by Research Career Award 5 K 6 AI 02425 from the National Institute of Allergy and Infectious Diseases.

*** Dr. Fefer is a scholar of the Leukemia Society of America.

Table 1. Summary of clinical data of marrow graft recipients

Age	Sex	Donor sex	Relationship	Disease	Preparation for grafting	Marrow cells administered ($\times 10^8$/kg)	"Take"	GVH [c]	Survival (days)
16	M	F	HL-A identical	Aplastic anemia	CY [a]	1.8	Yes	0	> 400
13	M	F	HL-A identical	Aplastic anemia	CY [a]	2.9	Yes	+	> 323
23	M	M	HL-A identical	Aplastic anemia	CY [a]	2.3	Yes	0	> 218
10	M	F	HL-A identical	ALL	Irradiation [b]	4.2	Yes	±	> 665
7	F	M	HL-A identical	ALL	Irradiation [b]	7.1	Yes	0	> 173
19	M	M	Identical twin	Lymphosarcoma	Irradiation [b]	2.0	Yes	—	> 697
13	F	F	Identical twin	ALL	Irradiation [b]	2.9	Yes	—	> 193

[a] CY: Cyclophosphamide, 50 mg/kg on each of 4 days.
[b] Irradiation: 1000 rad midpoint tissue exposure from opposing ^{60}Co sources.
[c] GVH: Graft-versus-host disease; + = minimal, ++ = moderate, +++ = severe, ++++ = life threatening.

Table 2. Summary of immunological evaluation of marrow graft recipients

Case	Day[a]	DNCB results	Phage antibody (K values)		Immunoglobulins (mg/100 ml)			In vitro lymphocyte reactivity (ratio to control)		
			1°	2°	IgG	IgA	IgM	allogeneic cells	PHA	PHA of normal controls
1	28[b]	neg.[c]	0.01	0.0						
	80	neg.[c]						94	29	—
	151							64	1	62
	174				2200	105	85			
2	30[b]	neg.	0.0	0.08				2.5	6	26
	57							17.5	8	74
	100				975	105	180	10	6.8	75
	214				1500	200	115			
3	78				475	105	52			
	127[b]	neg.	0.20	2.24 (IgM)[d]						
	154				570	40	140			
	204				1800	40	94	185	33	23
4	51							148	268	425
	85[b]							67	147	12
	365[b]	neg.	1.86	0.73 (IgM)[d]	2000	300	100	23	43	35
	626[b]			1.58 (3°)	1500	250	180			
5	84[b]	neg.	0.12	0.96 (IgM)[d]						
	110				1400	61	100			
	166				1850	53	250	53	18	89
6	39							174		
	365[b]		53 (IgG)[d]	1120 (IgG)[d]	675	105	61	86	29	30
	678	pos.								
7	39[b]	neg.	3.3	199.6 (IgM)[d]		2240	200	60		
	179				1650	83	58	593	47	80

[a] Day post-grafting.

[b] Time after marrow transplant when primary (1°) phage injection was given. Secondary (2°) phage immunization was done 4 weeks later. Antibody titer was determined 2 weeks after immunization.

[c] Marrow donor was sensitized before transplantation. Recipient was tested 28 and 80 days post-grafting.

[d] Determined by chromatography on Sephadex G-200 columns.

3,500 per mm^3. 100 days after grafting and 2,000 to 5,500 after 200 days with no apparent difference between syngeneic and allogeneic recipients.

One recipient of syngeneic marrow tested at 1 year post-grafting showed good production of circulating antibody against phage antigen with the normal pattern of IgM after primary immunization and IgG after secondary immunization. The other recipient of syngeneic marrow, tested at day 39, showed production of IgM after secondary immunization. Recipients of allogenice grafts had not produced antibody to phage antigen when tested 28 to 365 days post-grafting. Case 4 received phage a third time 626 days after grafting and showed a very low response of 1.58 K.

Skin tests for *Candida*, mumps and PPD were negative in all patients tested before the marrow graft. One patient (Case 6) and his donor were both positive to *Candida* when first tested 2 years after the graft.

Reactivity to DNCB was not observed after attempted sensitization 35 days to 1 year following allogeneic grafting. One HL-A-matched donor was sensitized to DNCB before the marrow graft and challenge of the recipient 28 and 75 days after engraftment failed to demonstrate transfer of immunological memory. One identical twin was negative to DNCB on day 39 while another responded to DNCB when tested 2 years after grafting.

In vitro response of circulating (donor) lymphocytes of these patients was normal, with one exception, to allogeneic cells and to phytohemagglutinin (PHA) after methotrexate was discontinued. Reduced reactivity was observed in Case 2 while he was on methotrexate.

Discussion

We have recently described 50 canine recipients of allogeneic marrow grafts studied for immunologic reactivity between 20 days and 8 years after grafting [4]. For 4 to 8 weeks after grafting these animals were severely deficient with regard to the same parameters reported here in our human cases. After that time, recovery began so that almost all animals became normal by about 200 days after grafting. These measurements correlated well with the clinical observation that these animals are prone to infection in the first 1 to 3 months after grafting and that they then regain health and are able to live in an unprotected environment without increased susceptibility to infections.

The preliminary studies in the patients reported here suggest a much slower recovery of immunologic function in the recipient of allogeneic grafts. They appear to be deficient in both B and T lymphocytes. The finding that peripheral blood lymphocytes from the chimeras respond to allogeneic cells in the mixed leukocyte test is inconsistent with the results of *in vivo* tests and may indicate that the *in vitro* phenomenon requires fewer reacting cells.

A possible explanation of the more rapid recovery observed in the dogs is the fact that they received proportionately more marrow ($1.6 \pm 0.66 \times 10^9$ marrow cells per kg) than did the patients ($3.3 \pm 1.6 \times 10^8$ per kg). It should be noted that both the dogs and the patients received a short course of methotrexate after grafting in an effort to ameliorate GVH disease.

Immunologic recovery in the identical twins may reflect the favorable environment of a syngeneic graft or the absence of methotrexate post-grafting or both.

However, the twins also received additional donor lymphoid cells as a part of the attempted immunotherapy [6]. These cells may have contributed to the immunologic recovery.

Despite the laboratory evidence of immunologic deficiency, most of the patients appear to be doing reasonably well clinically. Patient 4 has had two major episodes of infection, a pneumococcal pneumonia 3 months after grafting and at Hemophilus *influenzae* meningitis 18 months after grafting, and has recovered satisfactorily. Patient 1 developed an interstitial pneumonitis 3 months after grafting, but recovered in 1 week. The other 5 patients have had no significant episodes of infection.

These observations have important implications with regard to the post-transplantation status of marrow graft recipients. Continued severe immunologic deficiency in patients receiving allogeneic grafts points out the necessity for protection against infection and for vigilance in early detection and treatment of infection. Further observation and follow-up of these patients should determine whether or not they will eventually recover immunologic capability. If not, it may be necessary to attempt to develop methods of correcting the immunologic defect by enrichment of the infused marrow with immunologically competent cells or by non-specific stimulation of immunity. Effective immunotherapy by marrow transplantation may depend on the development of methods for accelerating immunologic recovery.

References

1. BROWN, R. S., HAYNES, H. A., FOLEY, H. T., GODWIN, H. A., BERARD, C. W., CARBONE, P. P.: Hodgkin's disease. Immunologic, clinical and histologic features of 50 untreated patients. Ann. int. Med. **67**, 291 (1967).
2. FAHEY, J. L., MCKELVEY, E. M.: Quantitative determination of serum immunoglobulins in antibody-agar plates. J. Immunol. **94**, 34 (1965).
3. OCHS, H. D., DAVIS, S. D., WEDGWOOD, R. J.: Immunologic responses to bacteriophage ⌀X 174 in immunodeficiency disease. J. clin. Invest. **50**, 2559 (1971).
4. OCHS, H. D., STORB, R., GRAHAM, T. C., RUDOLPH, R. H., KOLB, H. J., SHIURBA, R. A., THOMAS, E. D.: Immune status of long-term canine irradiation chimeras. Blood **38**, 787 (1971) (Abstract).
5. RUDOLPH, R. H., MICKELSON, E., THOMAS, E. D.: Mixed leukocyte reactivity and leukemia: Study of identical siblings. J. clin. Invest. **49**, 2271 (1970).
6. RUDOLPH, R. H., FEFER, A., THOMAS, E. D., BUCKNER, C. D., CLIFT, R. A.: Isogeneic marrow grafts for hematologic malignancy. in man. Arch. intern. Med. **132**, 279 (1973).
7. STORB, R., EVANS, R. S., THOMAS, E. D., BUCKNER, C. D., CLIFT, R. A., FEFER, A., NEIMAN, P., WRIGHT, S. E.: Paroxysmal nocturnal hemoglobinuria and refractory marrow failure treated by marrow transplantation. Brit. J. Haemat. **24**, 741 (1973).
8. THOMAS, E. D., BUCKNER, C. D., RUDOLPH, R. H., FEFER, A., STORB, R., NEIMAN, P. E., BRYANT, J. I., CHARD, R. L., CLIFT, R. A., EPSTEIN, R. B., FIALKOW, P. J., FUNK, D. D., GIBLETT, E. R., LERNER K. G., REYNOLDS, F. A., SLICHTER, S.: Allogeneic marrow grafting for hematologic malignancy using HL-A matched donor-recipient sibling pairs. Blood **38**, 267 (1971).
9. THOMAS, E. D., BUCKNER, C. D., CLIFT, R. A., FASS, L., FEFER, A., GLUCKSBERG, H., JOHNSON, F. L., KANE, P. J., LERNER, K. G., NEIMAN, P. E., STORB, R.: Marrow grafting for aplastic anemia and for leukemia using HL-A matched donor-recipent sibling pairs. Exp. Haemat. **22**, 138 (1972).
10. THOMAS, E. D., BUCKNER, C. D., STORB, R., NEIMAN, P. E., FEFER, A., CLIFT, R. A., SLICHTER, S. J., FUNK, D. D., BRYANT, J. I., LERNER, K. G.: Aplastic anemia treated by marrow transplantation. Lancet **1972 I**, 284.

Immunological Studies in Acute Leukemia*

G. W. Santos, G. M. Mullins, W. B. Bias, P. N. Anderson, K. D. Graziano, D. L. Klein, and P. J. Burke

Divisions of Oncology and Medical Genetics, Department of Medicine, The Johns Hopkins University, and Oncology Service, Department of Medicine, Baltimore City Hospitals, Baltimore, Maryland, USA

Advances in chemotherapy and supportive care over the past several years have led to remarkable gains in the treatment of certain forms of acute leukemia. Acute leukemia, however, remains an incurable disease. The major emphasis in the management of this disease has been to employ intensive treatment with cytotoxic agents. These agents are designed to kill as many tumor cells as possible without causing irreparable damage to other vital cell systems, such as the bone marrow, gastrointestinal tract, liver, etc.

A number of observations have stimulated clinical scientists to modify and broaden their therapeutic strategies in acute leukemia. These findings include demonstration of tumor-specific antigens in animals and in man, increasing awareness of the importance of host immune responses to tumors in animals, documentation of the viral nature of certain animal tumors, and collection of suggestive evidence for a possible viral etiology for certain human tumors. The effect of cytotoxic agents upon immune function, the development of various anti-viral agents, and an increasing understanding of the principles of tumor immunology and immunotherapy have become of paramount interest to the clinician.

The present studies represent preliminary attempts to measure immunological responsiveness of patients and their family members to acute leukemia cells. It is hoped that the careful correlation of several *in vitro* tests of anti-tumor reactivity with the clinical course of the patient will increase our understanding of the nature of immune responsiveness in neoplasia. This should, in turn, lead to the design of clinical trials of immunotherapy based on a better rationale than is currently available.

Patient Population Studied

In general all patients were studied during the initial florid phase of acute leukemia (80—90% blasts in the peripheral blood) before receiving anti-leukemic therapy. A total of 30 patients and their families (17 parents and 75 siblings) comprised the material for these studies. There were 12 patients with acute myelogenous leukemia

* Supported in part by a National Cancer Institute Contract, PH-71-2109.

(AML) (6 female and 6 male) with a mean age of 57.8 years; 13 patients with acute myelomonocytic leukemia (AMMOL) (4 female and 9 male) with a mean age of 50.0 years; 1 male age 27 with acute progranulocytic leukemia (APGL); and 4 patients with acute lymphocytic leukemia (ALL) (1 female and 3 males) with a mean age of 27 years.

Materials and Methods

Skin Testing. Intradermal injections (0.1 ml) were given into the skin of the back on admission. Reactions were read at 24 and 48 h. Erythema and induration were measured in two perpendicular diameters. An area of induration 0.5 cm $\times$ 0.5 cm or greater was considered a positive response. The antigen battery used consisted of the following: intermediate strength purified protein derivative of tuberculin (PPD), 0.0001 mg or 5 T.U. per 0.1 ml; mumps skin test antigen; Varidase (streptokinase-streptodornase mixture), 40 units and 10 units, respectively; *Candida albicans* extract, 1 : 100 dilution of full strength antigen; *Trichophyton gypseum* extract, 1 : 30 dilution; and histoplasmin, 1 : 100 dilution. Skin testing with autologous tumor was performed by intradermal injection of a 0.1 ml suspension of 25 $\times$ 10^6 tumor cells (inactivated by incubation with mitomycin C, 75 µg per 10^6 cells at 37 °C for 60 min, washed and suspended in RPMI 1640 medium). Incubation of leukemic cells at various times up to 8 days, then 16 h-culture in tritiated thymidine, showed no growth or thymidine uptake at any time after mitomycin C treatment.

HL-A Typing and Testing for Cytotoxic Antibody. HL-A typing and testing for serum cytotoxic antibody activity were performed in triplicate cultures in Falcon plastic microtitre trays. One µl (10^6 cells per ml) of cell suspension (nylon column-purified lymphocytes) was incubated with 2 µl of each typing serum or each unknown serum for 30 min at room temperature. The wash step, described by [1], was included to remove excess antibody. The cells were then incubated for 1 h at room temperature with 4 µl of rabbit complement. Trypan blue dye was added and reactivity determined by dye exclusion. A cytotoxic reaction was considered positive if at least 20% of cells were killed.

Mixed Leucocyte Cultures. One-way mixed leucocyte cultures (MLC) were performed using modifications of techniques described by [4]. Heparinized venous blood was settled with plasmagel, and the leucocyte-rich plasma extruded and centrifuged. Erythrocytes were lysed with a mixture of Tris- and NH_4Cl. Cells were cultured in RPMI 1640 tissue culture medium, with streptomycin and penicillin, and with added 15% fetal calf serum. Stimulating cells were treated with mitomycin C (50µg per 1.5 $\times$ 10^6 cells) for 30 min at 37 °C and washed. Cell counts were adjusted for lymphocyte content. Responding lymphocytes and stimulating lymphocytes or tumor cells were mixed in a 1 : 1 ratio, 0.75 $\times$ 10^6 cells of each, or a total of 1.5 $\times$ 10^6 cells per ml, each culture being 1 ml, in 16 $\times$ 100 mm test tubes. Triplicate cultures were incubated in a humidified 5% CO_2 incubator at 37 °C. At about 100 h of incubation, 1.0 µCi of tritiated thymidine (specific activity 1.0 Ci/mM) was added. Cultures were harvested 16 h later and DNA precipitated on glass fiber filters with cold 5% trichloroacetic acid. Filters were dried with absolute ethanol, suspended in scintillation fluid and counted in a beta scintillation counter. Controls were done of all combinations of each family member and patient serving as responding or stimulating (mitomycin treated) cell source, and all cells were tested for ability to stimulate and to respond to an unrelated control, and for response to PHA. Controls of mitomycin-treated cells alone showed essentially no (less than 50 c.p.m.) thymidine incorporation. Standard error among triplicate cultures was in the range of ± 10 to 15%. As the MLC has a well-known day-to-day variation in absolute counts, due to technical variables, all tests and all appropriate controls on a given patient and his family were done simultaneously on a single day. Mean counts for triplicate cultures were calculated, and stimulation index (c.p.m. experimental lymphocyte mix divided by c.p.m. autologous lymphocyte mix) was determined in order to compare different patient families done on different days. A stimulation index of 2.0 or more was considered a significant response.

^{51}Chromium Release Cytotoxicity Test. Cytotoxicity testing, was done by cell-mediated ^{51}Cr release, essentially as described by [6]. Lymphocytes from heparinized venous blood were purified on a Ficoll-Hypaque gradient, washed in Hank's balanced salt solution with 6% heat-inactivated fetal calf serum, and suspended at a concentration of 1.0×10^7 cells per ml. in Minimal Eagle's Medium (MEM) with 12% fetal calf serum. Target cells were leukemic blasts similarly prepared, to a concentration of 1.5×10^7 cells per ml. To one ml of target cell suspension was added 250 μCi of ^{51}Cr (0.25 ml of $Na_2{}^{51}CrO_4$, specific activity 100—500 μCi/μg of sodium chromate) and the cells incubated for 45 min in a shaking water bath at 37 °C. Excess chromium was washed off, and target cells suspended in MEM with 12% fetal calf serum at a concentration of 2.0×10^6 cells per ml. Attacking cells (from family members or unrelated controls) and labelled target cells were set up in triplicate at a target: attacking cell ratio of 1 : 100 in a total volume of 1.05 ml in plastic Petri dishes. Cultures were incubated on a rocking platform at 37 °C in a humidified 5% CO_2 atmosphere for 4 h. After incubation, Petri dishes were emptied into test tubes, centrifuged, and released radioactivity counted in a gamma scintillation counter. The degree of cytotoxicity in the experimental cultures was expressed as a percentage of the total release of ^{51}Cr from labeled, freeze-thaw disrupted target cells. As a control for spontaneous leak, 1.0×10^5 labeled target cells were added to 1.0×10^7 unlabeled target cells and handled simultaneously with the experimental cultures. Spontaneous release of ^{51}Cr from the control tubes after 4 h was approximately 12—16% of release from freeze-thawed cells. Calculations for cytotoxicity were: Percent lysis = c.p.m. ^{51}Cr release from target cell lymphocyte mixture $\times$ 100, divided by c.p.m. ^{51}Cr release from freeze-thawed cells. The percent lysis of the experimental test was compared to the percent lysis of the control by the Student t-test. Significance was accepted at the 5% level, and usually corresponded to a 5% or greater release from the experimental over the control (spontaneous release, as above) cultures. In Table 3 results are expressed as number of family members whose lymphocytes caused ^{51}Cr release from labeled leukemic cells, over the number of such combinations tested.

Macrophage Migration Inhibition Test. Macrophage migration inhibition factor (MIF) tests were done by modifications of techniques described by [14, 16]. Lymphocytes were purified from heparinized venous blood by use of a Ficoll-Hypaque gradient. Leukemic blasts (stimulating cells) and lymphocytes (responding cells) from each family member were mixed in RPMI 1640 tissue culture medium, with 0.5% fetal calf serum, in a concentration of 2.5×10^6 cells per μl of each. Responding and stimulating cells were also cultured alone at a concentration of 5.0×10^6 cells per µl. Cultures were incubated in a humidified atmosphere of 37° in 5 % CO_2 for 72 h. Supernatants were harvested every 24 hr and pooled.

Supernatants from unmixed cultures were pooled together in the various test combinations as controls. After final harvesting, pooled supernatants were dialyzed against physiological saline and lyophilized. Lyophilized supernatants were reconstituted at ten times the original concentration in RPMI 1640 with 10% normal guinea-pig serum, and tested for inhibition of guinea-pig pertioneal exudate (mineral oil-induced) cells from capillary tubes in Sykes-Moore chambers. The area of migration was projected on paper and measured with a compensating planimeter. Experimental mixtures were supernatants from cultures where leukemic blasts and lymphocytes from family members were cultured together. Controls included supernatants mixed from independently cultured cells, cultures of tumor plus lymphocytes from unrelated controls, and positive controls of family members or unrelated controls whose lymphocytes were cultured with antigens to which they had shown a response in skin tests. The mean of the area of migfation of the test preparation was compared with the mean of the area of migration of the control (supernatants mixed from independently cultured cells) by the Student t test and significance accepted at the 5% level. In Table 3 positive results are shown as the number of family members showing significant macrophage migration inhibition when their lymphocytes were cultured with leukemic blasts, over the number of such cases tested.

Results

Skin Testing. The results of skin testing of 24 patients with acute leukemia and a control group of 20 unrelated normal volunteers are displayed in Table 1. The data clearly indicate that patients with acute leukemia are frequently unresponsive to the antigens tested, i.e. are "anergic". Those that are not totally anergic tend to show a smaller number of positive responses than normal controls, but in this non-anergic leukemic group the incidence of response to a given antigen tends to parallel

Table 1. Skin testing in acute leukemia [a]

	Number of persons positive						
	PPD	Mumps	SKSD	Candida	Tricho-phyton	Histo-plasmin	
Control (20)	1	19	20	10	2	1	
Akute Leukemia (24)	1	8	11	2	1	2	
	Number of persons in each reactivity score group [b]						
	0	**1**	**2**	**3**	**4**	**5**	**6**
Control (20)	0	1	8	9	1	1	0
Acute Leukemia (24)	10	5	7	2	0	0	0

[a] All patients negative to skin testing with autologous tumor.
[b] Number of persons responding to 0, 1, 2 etc. of the skin-test antigens.

that of the control group. In no instance was a delayed hypersensitivity response to intradermally injected autologous tumor cells found by our technique.

HL-A Typing and Mixed Leukocyte Cultures. Twenty-three of 75 siblings in the 30 families studied were found to have HL-A identical matches. Nine normal siblings were found to be HL-A identical to leukemic patients. In no case was there evidence, in the typing data, for deletion or addition of HL-A antigens on the leukemic blasts. Table 2 summarizes the results (obtained by means of the mixed leukocyte culture

Table 2. Mixed leukocyte culture. Responses of HL-A identical siblings to leukemic blasts (measured by tritiated thymidine incorporation)

	Number of tests	Mean stimulation index [a]	Standard error	p value
Sibling response to normal HL-A identical siblings	14	0.9	± 0.099	< 0.0005
Sibling response to HL-A identical leukemic blasts	9	2.5	± 0.300	

[a] Stimulation Index = c.p.m. experimental leukocyte mix. c.p.m. autologous leukocyte mix

(MLC) technique) of measuring the stimulation of siblings by HL-A identical normal sibling lymphocytes and by HL-A identical sibling leukemic blasts. Elsewhere we report the results of MLC testing in more detail [2]. Of 9 HL-A identical siblings tested for response to leukemic blasts, only one failed to show a stimulation index of 2.0 or greater. No responses were seen in mixed cultures of normal HL-A identical siblings. In one case of acute lymphoblastic leukemia, leukemic lymphoblasts stimulated an HL-A identical sibling's lymphocytes. Patient lymphocytes obtained during remission did not stimulate, but frozen, stored leukemic blasts continued to stimulate. Similar studies on further cases are pending.

^{51}Chromium Release Cytotoxicity and Macrophage Migration Inhibition Factor Tests. Table 3 summarizes the evidence for anti-tumor cellular immunity in family members, obtained by employing the ^{51}Cr and MIF tests. Positive cytotoxicity indicated by ^{51}Cr release from leukemic blasts was seen in 6 of 43 family members tested. Similarly, inhibition of macrophage migration by supernatants obtained from family members'

Table 3. Anti-tumor cellular immunity in family members

Fathers		Mothers		Brothers		Sisters	
MIF	^{51}Cr	MIF	^{51}Cr	MIF	^{51}Cr	MIF	^{51}Cr
0/2	0/3	0/1	1/3	4/15	2/17	2/16	3/20

No. tests with positive response/No. tests done.
MIF = macrophage migration inhibition factor test.
^{51}Cr = ^{51}Chromium release cytotoxicity test.

lymphocytes cultured with leukemic blasts was seen in 6 of 34 MIF tests. Positive responses in one mother and two sisters in the series may have been due to presensitization to HL-A antigens by virtue of multiple pregnancies. In none of the positive tests did serum obtained from the respective patients in relapse either reduce or block these positive responses, i.e. we did not find evidence for "blocking" activity in patient sera.

Cytotoxic Antibody. Sera from each patient and each family member were assayed for cytotoxicity to tumor cells of the patient and to lymphocytes of the other family members. Three cytotoxic sera were found: one (M.B.) from the father of a patient with acute lymphoblastic leukemia, one from a brother of another patient with ALL, and one from a brother of the patient with acute progranulocyticleukemia (APGL).

Table 4. Sera cytotoxic to acute lymphocytic leukemia [a]

	M. B. [c]	N. N. [c]	M. W. [c]
Acute lymphocytic leukemia	6/6	7/7	6/6
Acute lymphocytic leukemia remission	0/4	0/4	0/4
Acute myelocytic leukemia [b]	2/11	2/11	2/11
Acute progranulocyte leukemia	1/1	1/1	1/1
Acute monocytic leukemia	0/2	0/2	0/2
Leuko-lymphosarcoma	0/2	0/2	0/2
Normal lymphocytes	0/60	0/500	0/60

[a] All sera complement-dependent for cytotoxicity.

[b] Reactivity was $\pm$ in these 2 cases.

[c] Activity against ALL not removed by absorption with ALL remission lymphocytes, nor family member lymphocytes.

The latter two sera have not yet been characterized. The first serum (M.B.) and sera from two other unrelated normal individuals (N.N. and M.W.) appear to have cytotoxic specificity for acute lymphoblastic leukemic cells, as recently reported by [5].

These three sera have been tested against a number of freshly collected cells from other patients with different leukemias and against lymphocytes from normal donors. The results of this screening are shown in Table 4. The one unequivocally positive cytotoxic reaction to other than acute lymphoblastic leukemic cells was that to the single case of acute progranulocyte leukemia in our series. On the basis of our investigations (including absorption studies) with normal lymphocytes from unrelated and normal family donors, and with lymphocytes from acute lymphoblastic leukemia in remission, we have tentatively concluded that these sera are detecting antigens primarily associated with acute lymphoblastic leukemia [5].

Recently we have identified, but not yet fully characterized as to specificity, three additional sera cytotoxicity to ALL cells: one from a boy experiencing a 4-year clinical remission from ALL, another from his pediatrician, and another from a normal blood donor.

Discussion

The present findings of a marked degree of cutaneous anergy in patients in the florid stage of acute leukemia is consistent with the observations of others that patients with a variety of neoplasms may display cutaneous anergy when their disease is widespread and advanced. Future studies of cutaneous reactivity and *in vitro* studies of lymphocytes and sera of such patients done serially throughout their treatment courses and remission may provide further insight into the mechanisms and significance of these immune deficiencies. Preliminary work of [13], for instance, has indicated that a population of cells responsive in the MLC test may be separated from the peripheral blood of leukemic patients in which unseparated leukocytes showed little or no response. In addition, their data indicate that the lack of MLC response in unseparated leukocytes was not due to factors present in the leukemic sera.

In vitro humoral and cellular immunity to tumor cells in non-parous and non-transfused family members, and in other individuals, has been shown by others in a variety of solid tumors [11, 12]. In the present studies, about a quarter of the family members showed some form of humoral (cytotoxic antibody) or cellular (^{51}Cr release or MIF positivity) immunity to leukemic cells. The present data, as well as those reported by others, are compatible with and strongly suggestive of a viral etiology for these malignancies. Immunization by natural exposure to such putative oncogenic viruses could produce the type of results observed in family members.

In the present studies 8 of 9 HL-A identical siblings responded to leukemic blasts in MLC. The observation is in apparent contrast to the results reported by [10, 15] and but confirms the observations of [3]. Explanations for the discrepancy are not readily discernable. In the studies of Halterman and Leventhal the leukemic population was primarily pediatric, [15] studied identical twins. The significance of these differences in population is unknown.

The significance of positive reactivity in the MLC response is not readily apparent. At least three possibilities exist: 1) the leukemic blast cell surface expresses minor histocompatibility antigens and so stimulates in the MLC; 2) the leukemic blasts express blast or embryonic antigens not unique to leukemic cells; and 3) the leukemic cells possess a leukemia-specific tumor antigen. Our data do not at present allow a definitive choice from among these possibilities. However, the results of our studies with cytotoxic antibody, considered with observations of others, such as [8, 9, 10], that leukemic patients in remission can respond to autologous tumor cells in MLC, persuade us to favor the thrid possibility.

The discovery of cytotoxic antibody with apparent specificity for acute lymphoblastic leukemia cells needs further study and confirmation. The report [7], or recurrence of acute lymphoblastic leukemia in the donor cells after a marrow transplant, however, suggests to us that our preliminary serological studies are consistant with the notion of an infectious agent that may be associated with acute leukemia.

References

1. Amos, D. B., Bashir, H., Boyle, W., MacQueen, M., Tiilikainen, A.: A simple microcytotoxicity test. Transplantation **7**, 220 (1969).
2. Anderson, P. M., Santos, G. W., Bias, W. B., Mullins, G. M., Burke, P. J.: Response of HL-A identical siblings to leukemic blasts in mixed leucocyte culture (1972). (Manuscript in preparation.)
3. Bach, M. L., Bach, F. H., Joo, P.: Leukemia-associated antigens in the mixed leucocyte culture test. Science **166**, 1520 (1969).

4. BACH, M. L., BACH, F. H., WIDMER, M., ORANEN, H., WOLBERG, W. H.: Leucocyte reactivity *in vitro*. VII. The effect of polymorphonuclear leucocytes on lymphocyte response. Transplantation **12**, 283 (1971).
5 BIAS, W. B., SANTOS, G. W., BURKE, P. J., ANDERSON, P. N., KLEIN, D. L., MULLINS, G. M., HUMPHREY, R. L.: Human cytotoxic antibody to acute leukemia. Proc. Amer. Ass. Cancer Res. **13**, 73 (1972).
6. CANTY, T. J., WUNDERLICH, J. R., FLETCHER, F.: Qualitative and quantitative studies of cytotoxic immune cells. J. Immunol. **106**, 200 (1971).
7. FIALKOW, P. J., THOMAS, E. D., BRYANT, J. I., NEIMAN, P. E.: Leukemic transformation of engrafted human marrow cells *in vivo*. Lancet **1971 I**, 251.
8. FRIDMAN, W. H., KOURILSKY, F. M.: Stimulation of lymphocytes by autologous leukemic cells in acute leukemia. Nature **224**, 277 (1969).
9. GUTTERMAN, J. U., MCCREDIE, K. B., HERSH, E. M.: Lymphocyte blastogenic response to autologous leukemia cells and the demonstration of a serum inhibitory effect. Proc. Amer. Ass. Cancer Res. **13**, 80 (1972).
10. HALTERMAN, R. H., LEVENTHAL, B. G.: Mixed leukocyte cultures (MLC) reactivity to leukemia cells in patients, their twins, and HL-A identical siblings. Proc. Amer. Ass. Cancer Res. **13**, 6 (1972).
11. HELLSTRÖM, I., PIERCE, G. E., HELLSTRÖM, K. E.: Human tumor-specific antigens. Surgery **65**, 984 (1969).
12. MORTON, D. L., HOLMES, E. C., EILBER, F. R., WOOD, W. C.: Immunological aspects of neoplasia: A rational basis for immunotherapy. Ann. intern. Med. **74**, 487 (1971).
13. RAGAB, A. H., COWAN, D. H.: The response of cells from the peripheral blood of patients with acute leukemia to allogeneic cells. In: Proceedings of the fifth leukocyte culture conference (HARRIS, J. E., Eds.), p. 329. New York: Academic Press 1970.
14. ROCKLIN, R. E., DAVID, J. R.: Method for production of MIF by human blood lymphocytes. In: In vitro methods in cell mediated immunity (BLOOM, B. R., GLADE, P. R., Eds.), p. 281. New York: Academic Press 1971.
15. RUDOLPH, R. H., MICKELSON, E., THOMAS, E. D.: Mixed leukocyte reactivity and leukemia: Study of identical siblings. J. clin. Invest **49**, 2271 (1970).
16. THOR, D. E.: The capillary tube migration inhibition technique applied to human peripheral lymphocytes using the Guinea pig peritoneal exudate as the indicator cell population. In: In vitro methods in cell mediated immunity (BLOOM, B. R., GLADE, P. R., Eds.), p. 273. New York: Academic Press 1971.

Primary and Secondary Immune Responses in the Evaluation of Immunocompetence and Prognosis in Cancer Patients*

E. M. Hersh, E. J. Freireich, K. B. McCredie, J. U. Gutterman, G. P. Bodey Sr., J. P. Whitecar, G. Mavligit, and A. R. Cheema

Department of Developmental Therapeutics, The University of Texas, M. D. Anderson Hospital and Tumor Institute at Houston, Houston, Texas

Introduction

Tumor antigens and specific tumor immunity have been well-documented in several human malignant diseases [3]. There have also been several studies which have indicated that the degree or type of tumor immunity relates to the prognosis of the tumor-bearing patient [8]. Therefore if a patient's general immunocompetence is impaired, his tumor immunity is also likely to be impaired and his prognosis will be poor. Several studies have suggested that this is indeed true. Thus, several investigators [2, 7, 8, 11] have found that immunological evaluation of solid tumor and lymphoma patients prior to treatment could identify patients with a good prognosis on the basis of their immunocompetence.

Furthermore, the state of immunocompetence following therapy may be even more important than that prior to therapy in determining the patient's prognosis. We have shown in several studies [1, 5, 6], that recovery or overshoot of immunocompetence or both, after one or more courses of chemotherapy correlates with a good prognosis in both solid-tumor and acute leukemia patients.

The etiology of these relationships is unknown. An intrinsic lymphocyte defect [4], a defect in marcophage number or function [10] and the presence or absence of immunosuppresive serum factors [9] have all been advanced as possible etiologic factors. Irrespective of etiology, modern cancer management and progress in therapeutic research must be based on these factors.

We have summarized our past work in this field and attempted to synthesize it here. In addition we present new data on a study of immunocompetence and prognosis in a consecutive series of 51 patients with acute leukemia. A battery of primary and secondary immunological tests was used in this evaluation. Our data indicate

* Supported by: U. S. Public Health Service Contract PH 43 68 949 from the Collaborative Research Program, Transplantation Immunology Branch, National Institutes of Allergy and Infectious Diseases, National Institutes of Health and Grant CA 05831 and FR 05511 from the National Institutes of Health.

that competence and prognosis are indeed related in the cancer patient undergoing treatment, that immunocompetence relates to a good prognosis and that this must be determined with a battery of tests done both before and after therapy. Finally, on the basis of our own data plus data from the literature, we present a unifying hypothesis relating immunocompetence and immune responsiveness to the etiology and pathogenesis of malignant disease in man.

Materials and Methods

The present report comprises data from 4 separate studies. In the first study 91 patients with metastatic solid tumors were skin-tested with 5 established delayed-hypersensitivity antigens just before an early course in a chemotherapy program, and again just before the next course. Changes in established delayed-hypersensitivity skin-test reactivity were correlated with their subsequent prognosis.

In the second study, *in vitro* lymphocyte responses to phytohemagglutinin (PHA) and streptolysin O (SLO) of 40 patients with metastatic solid tumors were measured just before, one day after, and 9 days after a 5-day course of chemotherapy given early in a treatment program. Changes in *in vitro* lymphocyte reactivity were correlated with their subsequent prognosis.

In the third study *in vitro* lymphocyte responses, *in vivo* established delayed-hypersensitivity responses, and primary immune responses to keyhole limpet hemocyanin (KLH) were measured before and after an early course of chemotherapy in 25 patients with acute leukemia. Changes in and degrees of reactivity were correlated with subsequent prognosis.

In the final study a similar battery of tests was conducted in a consecutive series of 51 patients with acute leukemia. They were initially studied at monthly intervals and then followed approximately every 2 months for as long as possible. Degrees of and changes in reactivity were also correlated with prognosis.

In vitro lymphocyte responses were measured as previously described [6—8]. Peripheral blood was obtained by venipuncture, defibrinated by swirling with glass beads, the erythrocytes sedimented with dextran, and the resultant leukocyte-rich serum (1×10^6 lymphocytes per ml) used for the cultures. Cultures were stimulated with PHA, SLO and KLH, incubated for 5 days, and harvested and processed for liquid scintillation counting as previously described [6—8]. Results were recorded as net counts per minute per 10^6 lymphocytes (cpm) or as the stimulation index (cpm in the stimulated culture divided by the cpm in the control).

Established delayed-hypersensitivity skin-test antigens comprised the following: dermatophytin, dermatophytin-0, streptokinase-streptodornase (Varidase), *Candida*, and mumps. All antigens were injected intradermally in 0.1 ml aliquots. The resultant delayed hypersensitivity was measured at 24 and 48 h and the mean skin test diameter recorded. Only induration was measured.

Primary immunization with KLH was carried out as previously described. The immunizing and skin test doses were both 100 μg. The delayed hypersensitivity reaction to KLH was evaluated approximately two weeks after immunization, and in some studies serially thereafter. Lymphocyte cultures were set up with KLH as described above; the optimal stimulating dose being 100 μg per ml. Antibody titers to KLH were measured as previously described [6—8] by passive hemagglutination using chromic chloride-treated, KLH-coated red cells as the antigen.

Results

Table 1 shows the results of the first study in which established delayed-hypersensitivity skin-test reactions were measured before and after an early course of therapy in solid tumor patients. Patients whose negative pre-therapy skin tests converted to positive after chemotherapy, or from positive to more positive, showed tumor regression in the majority of instances. Patients whose pre-therapy skin tests were positive and after treatment either became negative or showed a significant

Table 1. Relationship between chemotherapy, delayed hypersensitivity and response to therapy in cancer patients

Skin test results		Course of Tumor		
		Progression	Regression	No change
Pre-therapy	*Post-therapy*			
Negative	Positive	0	11	1
Positive	Negative	19	0	1
Positive	>100% increase in diameter	0	10	17
Positive	>50% decrease in diameter	2	0	3
Positive	No change	1	4	6
Negative	Negative	15	1	0
	All improved	0	21	18
	All not improved	37	5	10

reduction in size generally had tumors which did not respond to treatment or which actually grew in size. Of patients with negative skin tests before and after treatment, 15 showed tumor progression while only one showed a tumor response. These differences were highly significant.

Table 2 shows data from the study in which *in vitro* lymphocyte blastogenic responses were used to evaluate immunocompetence of solid tumor patients, together with prognosis before and after therapy. It can be seen that in groups with both long and short survival or with both tumor regression and progression, respectively, chemotherapy suppressed the *in vitro* blastogenic responses asmeasured on day 6 (1 day after the end of therapy). However, the group with long survival and tumor regression showed not only recovery but actual rebound and overshoot of the *in vitro* blastogenic response. In contrast, in the group with short survival and tumor progression responses either remained suppressed or recovered only to the baseline after the end of chemotherapy. These groups were well balanced in terms of age, type of tumor, extent of metastatic disease, and type of chemotherapy. Therefore it seems reasonable to assume that relative sensitivity of the immune apparatus to chemotherapy must relate to prognosis.

Table 2. Relationship between chemotherapy, lymphocyte response and survival with metastatic cancer

Category	Lymphocyte response to mitogen						Tumor size after therapy		
Mitogen	PHA			SLO			Increase	Decrease	No change
Day tested	0	6	14	0	6	14			
Survival									
> 5 months	42[a]	31	76	2	1.1	7.5	0[b]	17	6
< 4 months	41	22	36	3.5	1.0	1.5	11	0	6

[a] CPM $\times 10^3$.
[b] No. of patients in category.

Table 3. Immunologic test results in patients responding and those not responding to remission induction therapy

Test	Effect of therapy on leukemia				Chi-square p value
	No major therapeutic response		Major therapeutic response		
	a[a]	b[b]	a[a]	b[b]	
Established delayed response:					
Before treatment	5	5	13	2	< 0.05
After treatment	2	6	14	1	< 0.005
PHA response:					
Before treatment	4	6	12	3	< 0.025
After treatment	4	6	13	2	< 0.005
SLO response:					
Before treatment	5	5	12	3	< 0.05
After treatment	3	7	12	3	< 0.005

[a] No. of patients exhibiting positive or normal immunological response.
[b] No. of patients exhibiting negative or subnormal response.

Tables 3, 4, and 5 show the relevant data from the study in which immunocompetence and prognosis were related in patients with acute leukemia. These patients included 16 receiving COAP[1], 5 receiving POMP, one receiving cytosine arabinoside and thioguanine simultaneously, 2 receiving cytosine arabinoside, thioguanine and cytosine arabinoside sequentially, and one receiving thioguanine alone. For immunological evaluation, patients were divided into those who did not show a major therapeutic response, and those who did (defined as complete or partial remission). These two groups were well balanced in terms of age, sex type of therapy and extent of leukemia. Only 3 patients had any prior therapy.

[1] COAP: Cyclophosphamide, Oncovin, arabinosyl cytosine, prednisone. POMP: Prednisone, Oncovin, methotrexate, purinethiol.

Table 4. Immunocompetence of treated patients with leukemia

Immunological test	Effect of therapy on leukemia	
	No major therapeutic response	Major therapeutic response
Established delayed response [a]:		
Before treatment	8.0	12.0
After treatment	0.0	13.0
Blastogenic response to PHA [b]:		
Before treatment	15,000	41,000
After treatment	9,000	42,000
Blastogenic response to SLO [c]:		
Before treatment	2,000	6,000
After treatment	0	14,000

[a] Diameter (mm). — [b] All values are medians. — [c] cpm/10^6 lymphocytes.

Table 5. Immune response to KLH

KLH response	Effect of therapy on leukemia		p value
	No major therapeutic response	Major therapeutic response	
Delayed hypersensitivity:			
No. positive/no. tested	3/8	9/15	< 0.025
Diameter in mm	0 (12) [a]	17/.0 (28)	
In vitro lymphocyte response (cpm)	0	5,000	< 0.05
Antibody (total/mercapto-ethanol-resistant):			
At 1 week	0.8/0	1.5/0.3	> 0.50
At 2 weeks	3.5/1.4	2.6/0.5	

[a] All values are medians; figures in parentheses indicate median of positive values only.

It can be seen in Tables 3 and 4 that both for established delayed-hypersensitivity responses and for the *in vitro* blastogenic responses to PHA and SLO, patients with a major therapeutic response were significantly more immunocompetent than those without. This was true both before and after treatment. In fact, immunocompetence in the group with no major therapeutic response declined dramatically after therapy while it was maintained or improved in the other group. This is also true for the primary cell-mediated immune response to KLH (Table 5). Thus only 3 of 8 in the "no major therapeutic response" group developed KLH delayed hypersensitivity, while 9 of 15 in the "major therapeutic response" group did so. In contrast, there was no difference in the antibody responses of the 2 groups. This suggested a selective relationship with cell-mediated immunity.

Table 6 shows the remission and prior therapy status of patients in the study reported here for the first time. 32 of 51 patients entered complete remission while 19 did not. 28 had received no prior therapy (defined as no more than one course of the current regimen) while 23 patients had had extensive prior therapy with other regimens, averaging 13 courses of treatment over 5—6 months. Of the 51 patients in this study, 14 were receiving DOAP[1], 13 COAP, 9 OAP, 7 a combination of cytosine arabinoside with either thioguanine or β-TGDR, 5 guanazole, 2 POMP, and 1 β-TGDR alone.

Table 6. Remission and prior therapy status of patients

Prior therapy status	Clinical status		
	Remission	No remission	Total
no	23	5	28
yes	9	14	23
total	32	19	51

Table 7. Association of clinical and immunological status of patients receiving therapy for acute leukemia

Immunological category and status on first evaluation	Status of leukemia after therapy [%]	
	Remission (32 patients)	No remission (19 patients)
PHA response, stimulation index (SI) < 20	9.3	21.0
SLO response, SI < 2	12.5	36.8
Varidase response, SI < 2	37.5	63.1
Dermatophytin skin test negative	40.6	78.9
Dermatophytin O skin test negative	21.8	68.4
Varidase skin test negative	28.1	73.6
Candida skin test negative	25.0	57.8
Mumps skin test negative	46.8	52.6
KLH skin test negative	34.4	41.1
All established delayed-hypersensitivity skin tests negative	12.5	42.1

The overall initial results of these studies are shown in Tables 7 and 8. It can be seen that the results of initial testing by *in vitro* lymphocyte culture with PHA and SLO, and of initial skin testing with a battery of 5 antigens, and the development of delayed hypersensitivity to KLH fully confirm the study outlined above. Thus, there was a striking difference in immunocompetence between the group which entered remission and the group which subsequently failed to enter remission, the latter group being significantly less immunocompetent.

Established delayed-hypersensitivity skin-test reactivity seems as good a parameter as any to demonstrate this difference. This is well illustrated in Table 9, in which

[1] DOAP: Daunomycin, Oncovin, arabinosyl cytosine, prednisone. OAP: Oncovin, arabinosyl cytosine prednisone. β-TGDR: β-thioguanine deoxyriboside.

Table 8. Immunological response of patients entering or failing to enter remission after therapy (CPM = counts per minute; SI = stimulation index; S.T. = skin test reaction; KLH = keyhole limpet hemocyanin)

Immunological stimulant	Measurement	Results of chemotherapy	
		Remission	No remission
PHA	CPM	60,500	52,000
	SI	110	53
SLO	CPM	11,700	2,300
	SI	8.5	2.0
Varidase	CPM	1,100	100
	SI	2.5	1.0
Dermatophytin	Diameter of S.T.	3	0
Dermatophytin O	Diameter of S.T.	8	0
Varidase	Diameter of S.T.	6	0
Candida	Diameter of S.T.	8	0
Mumps	Diameter of S.T.	3	0
KLH	Diameter of S.T.	7.5	5

Table 9. Relationship between established delayed hypersensitivity and the therapeutic response

Clinical status after therapy	Percent of patients with indicated number of positive skin tests		
	0—1	2—3	4—5
Remission (32 patients)	18.8	21.7	59.5
No remission (19 patients)	58.0	10.5	31.5

the percentage of patients with 0—1, 2—3, or 4—5 positive skin tests is tabulated. Approximately 60% of patients who entered complete remission had 4—5 positive skin tests, while approximately 60% of patients who failed to enter remission had 0—1 positive skin tests. These differences were highly significant.

Of great interest was a tendency to lower skin-test reactivity with continued chemotherapy. This occurred both in patients who failed to enter remission, and also in patients who achieved and remained in remission. This is shown in Table 10. The first skin test referred to was done at the onset of the study, the second skin test 1 month later, and the last at the very end of the study, an average of 12 months after the onset. This suggests that continued chemotherapy has a chronic immunosuppressive effect, even when given intermittently, and that this immunosuppression may indeed be the cause of subsequent relapses.

Since almost half of these patients had had prior therapy, it was also possible to investigate the effects of prior therapy on the immunological parameters and on the patient's prognosis. The data are shown in Tables 11, 12, and 13. Prior therapy indeed did have a suppressive effect on some of the initial immunological parameters.

Table 10. Changing pattern of immunological reactivity during the therapy of acute leukemia

Category	Remission Test period			No remission Test period		
	1st	2nd	last	1st	2nd	last
Number of patients evaluated	32	32	28	19	17	9
Number positive	28	26	15	11	12	4
Percent positive	87.5	81.4	53.5	58	70.5	44.5
Median diameter of positives (mm)	9	8.5	10	10	9	3.5
Number negative	4	6	13	8	5	5
Number negative to positive	—	1	3	—	5	2
Number positive of negative	—	3	12	-	3	4

Table 11. Relationship between prior therapy and initial immunological parameters in patients with leukemia

Immune category and status on first evaluation	No prior therapy	Prior therapy
PHA response, stimulation under 20,000 CPM (%)	10.7	8.7
SLO response stimulation under 2,000 CPM (%)	28.6	47.8
Varidase response, stimulation under 2,000 CPM (%)	57.2	69.6
KLH skin test negative (%)	32.2	38.1
All established delayed-hypersensitivity skin tests negative (%)	17.8	30.4

Table 12. Relationship between prior therapy status and initial delayed-hypersensitivity reactions

Clinical status after therapy	Percent of patients with indicated number of positive skin tests		
	0—1	2—3	4—5
No prior therapy (28 patients)	25	17.8	57.2
Prior therapy (23 patients)	43.5	21.8	34.7

This was particularly true for the responses to SLO and to established delayed-hypersensitivity skin-test antigens. However, as shown in Table 13, the remission status was still related to the immunological parameters. Thus in both categories, "prior therapy" and "no prior therapy", patients who entered remission tended to have significantly better immunocompetence than patients who did not enter remission.

Table 13. Interrelationship of prior therapy status, response to chemotherapy in terms of remission status and serial immunological parameters

Data categories			*In vitro* lymphocyte responses (CPM × 10^3)						Skin-test reactions (% pos.)			
Prior therapy status	Remission status	Number in category	PHA 1st test	PHA 2nd test	SLO 1st test	SLO 2nd test	VAR 1st test	VAR 2nd test	Battery 1st test	Battery 2nd test	Battery 3rd test	KLH
yes	no	14	69	62	2.0	4.7	0.05	1.3	64.3	75.0	42.8	66.7
yes	yes	9	62	71	15.9	22.0	0.30	0.9	77.8	77.8	71.4	55.6
none	no	5	51	76	2.9	2.2	0.0	0.8	40.0	60.0	0.0	60.0
none	yes	23	58	77	11.4	3.1	1.9	0.3	91.3	78.3	47.6	69.5

Discussion

These studies clearly indicate that immunocompetence is related to prognosis in patients with malignant disease. Patients with a good prognosis generally have better immunocompetence and immune responsiveness (measured by *in vitro* lymphocyte blastogenesis, established delayed hypersensitivity and primary immune response) than patients with a poor prognosis. As important, or perhaps more important than a pre-therapy evaluation of the immune response is an evaluation done after therapy. Some patients who are immunologically incompetent before therapy become immunocompetent after therapy; these have a good prognosis. Conversely, patients who are immunocompetent before therapy but who have prolonged and profound suppression of immune responsiveness after therapy have a poor prognosis. This is true, both for patients with acute leukemia and for those with a variety of solid tumors. In the last series of studies presented here duration and extent of prior therapy were also found to be related to the poor immune responsiveness and poor prognosis of some leukemia patients. However, even within the group of patients who had had extensive prior therapy, the immonocompetence relationship still held true (at least for some of the immunological parameters).

It is attractive to speculate that decreased immunocompetence of a general type is associated with decreased specific tumor immune responsiveness, that this permits immunogenic tumors to grow, and so results in a poor prognosis. However, alternative explanations are possible. First, decreased tumor immunity could be caused by the tumor: once the tumor came under control with chemotherapy these immunosuppressive factors would be dissipated and good immune responsiveness would result. Second, decreased immunity and progressive tumor growth could be unrelated to each other but both caused by the same factor (independently). If these factors were removed by effective chemotherapy, tumor regression and improved immune responsiveness would both result. Finally, decreased immune responsiveness is, at least in part, related to the extent of prior therapy. This is true for chemotherapy, radiotherapy, and surgery. Patients who have had extensive prior therapy for their malignancy tend to have fewer responses than previously untreated patients. Thus, we are not sure which is the cart and which is the horse in the relationship of poor immune responsiveness and poor prognosis.

Since most human tumors have been shown to have tumor-specific antigens and to induce tumor-specific immune responses, these considerations are very important. The observations outlined above can be combined into a unified hypothesis concerning the relationship between immunocompetence and prognosis in the etiology and pathogenesis of malignant disease. This hypothesis is outlined in Fig. 1. Malignant cells are constantly arising in the normal tissues of the body. The surveillance mechanism based on the recirculating thymus-dependent lymphocytes, normally eliminates these malignant foci when they number just a few cells. Transient episodes of immunological incompetence (such as those known to be associated with common viral infections) permit these foci to achieve a number of cells too great to be handled by the surveillance mechanism alone. The continued growth of the neoplastic focus is assured by the release of tumor antigens into the lymphatic drainage and the subsequent immunological paralysis of the draining lymph node. If curative surgery, radiotherapy, or chemotherapy is applied at this point and the tumor mass is reduced to a small number of cells, the specific immunosuppressive effects may be relieved and the few remaining tumor cells can be destroyed by the recovering specific anti-tumor immune response. If then another immunosuppressive event occurs and there are residual foci of tumor cells, they are released from immunological restraints and in-transit or disseminated metastases may appear. These have not only specific but also general immunosuppressive effects that lead to a breakdown in host defense and accelerated dissemination and growth of the tumor. Again, therapeutic intervention

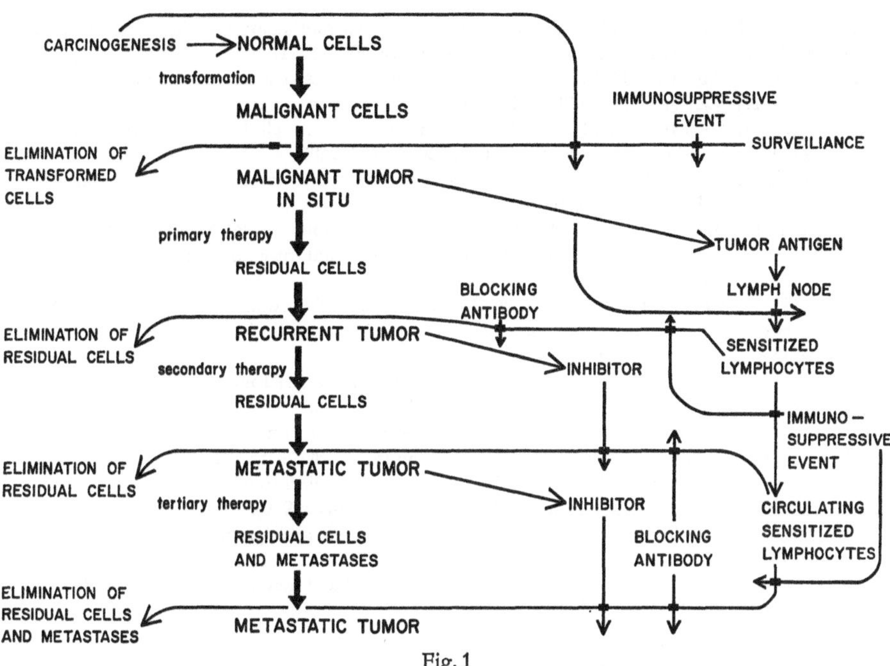

Fig. 1

may reduce the tumor burden sufficiently to allow the host defense mechanisms to recover. This would be particularly true for very responsive tumors such as neuroblastoma, choriocarcinoma, acute leukemia, malignant lymphoma, etc. It is at this point that attempts to augment specific tumor immunity or the general host defense mechanism through immunotherapy may tip the balance between failure or success of conventional therapy, and may result in cures of disseminated malignant disease.

On the basis of this hypothesis and the above observations, there are several things which are indicated for continuing immunological research in cancer therapy. *Firstly*, we must make serial studies of the immunocompetence of treated cancer patients to identify those who are immunologically incompetent. *Secondly*, we must attempt to identify the etiology of the immunological deficiency so that it can be attacked specifically. *Thirdly*, we must attempt to characterize and identify the immunosuppressive effects of the conventional therapies used to control cancer, such as radiotherapy, chemotherapy, and surgery. *Finally*, we must attempt to reverse the immunological deficiencies we detect by either specific or non-specific immunotherapy.

Acknowledgement

The authors wish to thank Mrs. Annette Matthews and Mrs. Donna Storms for their very capable technical assistance.

References

1. Cheema, A. R., Hersh, E. M.: Patient survival after chemotherapy and its relationship to in vitro lymphocyte blastogenesis. Cancer (Philad.) **28**, 851 (1971).
2. Eilber, F. R., Morton, D. L.: Impaired immunologic reactivity and recurrence following cancer surgery. Cancer (Philad.) **25**, 362 (1970).
3. Hellström, I., Hellström, K. E., Pierce, G. E., Yang, J. P. S.: Cellular and humoral immunity to different types of human neoplasms. Nature **220**, 1352 (1968).
4. Hersh, C. M., Oppenheim, J. J.: Impaired *in vitro* lymphocyte transformation in Hodgkin's disease. New Engl. J. Med. **273**, 1006 (1965).
5. Hersh, E. M., Whitecar, J. P., Jr., McCredie, K. B., Bodey, G. P., S., Freireich, E. J.: Chemotherapy, immunocompetence, immunosuppression and prognosis in acute leukemia. New Engl. J. Med. **285**, 1211 (1971).
6. Hersh, E. M., Curtis, J. E., Cheema, A. R.: Host defense failure in the etiology and pathogenesis of malignant disease. Proceedings of the M. D. Anderson Basic Science Symposium on Environmental Carcinogenesis (in press).
7. Krant, M. J., Manskopf, G., Brandrup, C. S., Madoff, A. A.: Immunologic alterations in bronchogenic cancer. Cancer (Philad.) **21**, 623 (1967).
8. Morton, D. L., Holmes, E. C., Eilber, F. R., Wood, W. C.: Immunological aspects of neoplasia: A rational basis for immunotherapy. Ann. intern. Med. **74**, 587 (1971).
9. Pisano, J. C., Di Luzio, N. R., Salky, N. K.: Absence of macrophage humoral recognition factor(s) in patients with carcinoma. J. Lab. clin. Med. **76**, 141 (1970).
10. Silk, M.: Effect of plasma from patients with carcinoma on *in vitro* lymphocyte transformation. Cancer (Philad.) **20**, 2088 (1967).
11. Sokal, J. E., Aungst, C. W.: Response to BCG vaccination and survival in advanced Hodgkin's disease. Cancer (Philad.) **24**, 128 (1969).

Delayed-Hypersensitivity Reactions in Patients with Cancer*

C. M. Pinsky, A. El Domeiri, A. S. Caron, W. H. Knapper, and H. F. Oettgen

Memorial Hospital for Cancer and Allied Diseases, Sloan-Kettering Institute for Cancer Research, Cornell University Medical College, New York

Introduction

A recent study of considerable interest has indicated that the ability to respond to the skin-sensitizer DNCB (2,4-dinitrochlorobenzene) signifies a favorable prognosis after cancer surgery whereas failure to respond heralds an unfavorable outcome [3]. This has also been our experience.

In addition, we have found that patients with cancer of the head and neck are often DNCB-negative in an early stage of their disease, while many patients with malignant melanoma or sarcoma are DNCB-positive when their disease is far advanced. Part of this work was reported previously [4].

Materials and Methods

Between November 1969 and February 1971, 234 patients with various types and stages of cancer and 17 patients with non-malignant disease were studied (Table 1). DNCB (Lot 81800) was purchased from K and K Laboratories, Inc., Plainview, N.Y. The skin tests were carried out according to the method previously described by others [2, 3]. The sensitizing dose of 2000 μg DNCB dissolved in 0.1 ml of acetone was applied to the inner aspect of the upper arm, inside a plastic ring 2 cm in diameter, and allowed to evaporate. Test doses of 100 μg and 25 or 50 μg were applied in the same way and at the same time to the ipsilateral forearm. The sites were covered by dressings for 48 h and kept dry. All sites were examined for erythema and induration at 2 weeks and, when possible, during the interval. In patients who showed no delayed-hypersensitivity reactions at the test sites at 48 h, erythema and induration beginning 9 to 10 days after sensitization were considered evidence of *de-novo* sensitivity. Patients who showed no reaction after 14—16 days were tested again with 100 μg and 25 or 50 μg of DNCB. These tests were considered positive if there was definite induration

* This investigation was supported in part by grants from the United States Public Health Service: CA 05110, CA 08748 and CA 05826, National Cancer Institute.

at least 10 mm in diameter after 48 h. (Equivocal reactions showing erythema but no induration were rarely encountered.)

174 patients were also tested for pre-existing delayed hypersensitivity to common antigens, including dermatophytin "0" (1 : 100, a Candida antigen)[1], mumps skin-test antigen[2], tuberculin (intermediate strength)[3], and streptokinase/streptodornase,

Table 1. Types of cancer studied

Histological diagnosis	Number of patients
Squamous cell carcinoma:	
Head and neck	25
Lung	19
Cervix	13
Adenocarcinoma:	
Colon and rectum	39
Breast	29
Endometrium	8
Ovary	5
Malignant melanoma	32
Sarcoma	23
Lymphoma	17
Hodgkin's disease	8
Miscellaneous	16
Total malignant	234
Benign disease	17

(SK = 4 units; SD = 1 unit)[4]. These antigens were injected intradermally in volumes of 0.1 ml. The tests were read at 24 or 48 h, and considered positive if the diameter of induration was more than 5 mm.

Results

Overall Results (Table 2)

In about one half of the patients at least one of the skin tests for pre-existing immunity to common antigens was positive. Previous studies indicate that 90—100% of normal individuals respond to at least one of a similar series of tests [1, 3] just as most normal individuals can be sensitized to DNCB by the method used in this study [2, 3].

Only 64% of our patients could be sensitized.

1 Hollister-Stier Laboratories, Yeadon, Pennsylvania.
2 Eli Lilly & Co., Indianapolis, Indiana.
3 Parke-Davis Co., Detroit, Michigan.
4 Lederle Laboratories, Pearl River, New York.

Table 2. Skin tests for delayed hypersensitivity in patients with cancer

Antigen	Number of patients tested	% positive
Dermatophytin 0	172	5
Mumps	172	20
Tuberculin	173	25
Streptokinase	172	26
Any of these	174	51
DNCB	234	64

Factors Influencing the Incidence of Positive DNCB Tests (Table 3)

Both extent of disease and performance status (as measured by severity of symptoms) affected the results of the DNCB test. Patients without metastases responded more often (83%) than those with regional metastases (67%) or with distant metastases (41%). As the severity of symptoms increased, the incidence of positive reactions decreased. Patients who were severely debilitated never developed sensitivity to DNCB.

Table 3. Correlation of the results of DNCB tests with the extent of disease or the performance status

	Number of patients tested	% positive
No metastases	76	83
Regional metastases	55	67
Distant metastases	80	41
No evidence of disease	18	67
Minimal symptoms	193	69
Moderate symptoms	34	44
Debilitating symptoms	7	0

Six patients with negative DNCB tests had no evidence of disease at the time of the test. Two had unusually long survival (11 and 19 years) after bilateral radical mastectomy for breast cancer where positive nodes were found in the upper axilla. Two were patients with acute leukemia in remission but on chemotherapy. The remaining two patients were debilitated from causes other than cancer (one from chronic progressive pulmonary disease and the other from intra-abdominal complications after radiotherapy for cancer of the cervix).

Results of DNCB Tests Classified According to the Type of Cancer (Table 4)

The incidence of positive reactions was much lower (42%) in patients with localized head and neck cancer (with or without regional metastases) than in patients

Table 4. Incidence of positive DNCB tests in patients with different types of cancer

	Localized		Generalized	
	Number of patients tested	% positive	Number of patients tested	% positive
Carcinoma of:				
Lung	10	100	10	80
Cervix	6	100	4	25
Breast	21	90	3	0
Colon and rectum	30	80	0	—
Head and neck	19	42	6	33
Sarcoma	5	100	15	73
Melanoma	11	91	19	74

with disseminated melanoma, sarcoma and lung cancer. In fact, several patients with melanoma or sarcoma had positive DNCB tests a few weeks before they died.

Correlation between Response to DNCB and Course of Disease after Surgery

73 patients were followed for at least 6 months after definitive surgery (i.e. after removal of all detectable tumor) (Table 5). Of 57 (78%) patients with positive DNCB skin tests only 3 (5%) had recurrence at that time. By contrast, 7 of 16 patients with a negative DNCB test had developed recurrent disease. According to contingency-table analysis, this indicates that a favorable short-term result was associated with a positive DNCB at a χ^2 of 12.5 ($p < 0.001$).

Table 5. Correlation of the result of DNCB tests at the time of definitive surgery with the incidence of recurrence at six months after surgery

	DNCB pos.	DNCB neg.	
No recurrence	54	9	63
Recurrence	3	7	10
	57	16	73

$\chi^2 = 12.5$, $p < 0.001$

Similarly, among patients followed for one year (Table 6), only 2 of 12 with positive DNCB tests but 5 of 7 with negative DNCB tests had recurrence. The numbers here are too small to perform χ^2 by contingency-table analysis, but a Fisher's Exact Test indicates that a favorable result was associated with a positive DNCB test ($p < 0.025$).

When the results of the skin tests for pre-existing immunity to common antigens were analyzed in a similar manner, the correlation was not close ($\chi^2 = 3.3$). This suggests that the ability to become immunized on initial exposure to an antigen is more important, as a measure of good prognosis in the patient with cancer, than the ability to respond to a previously encountered antigen.

Table 6. Correlation of the result of DNCB tests at the time of definitive surgery with the incidence of recurrence at twelve months after surgery

	DNCB pos.	DNCB neg.	
No recurrence	12	2	14
Recurrence	2	5	7
	14	7	21

Acknowledgement

The authors wish to thank DAVID SCHOTTENFELD for assistance in the statistical analysis.

References

1. AL-SARRAF, M., WONG, P., SARDESAI, S., VAITKEVICIUS, V. K.: Clinical immunologic responsiveness in malignant disease. I. Delayed hypersensitivity reaction and the effect of cytotoxic drugs. Cancer (Philad.) **26**, 262 (1970).
2. BROWN, R. S., HAYNES, H. A., FOLEY, T. H., GODWIN, H. S., BERARD, C. W., CARBONE, P. P.: Hodgkin's disease, immunologic, clinical, and histologic features of 50 untreated patients. Ann. Intern. Med. **67**, 291 (1967).
3. EILBER, F. R., MORTON, D. L.: Impaired immunologic reactivity and recurrence following cancer surgery. Cancer (Philad.) **25**, 362 (1970).
4. PINSKY, C. M., OETTGEN, H. F., EL DOMEIRI, A., OLD, L. J., BEATTIE, E. J., BURCHEANL, J. H.: Delayed hypersensitivity reactions in patients with cancer. Proc. Amer. Ass. Cancer Res. **12**, 100 (1971).

Nonspecific Immune Responses in Hematosarcomas and Acute Leukemias

M. Schneider, G. Mathé, L. Schwarzenberg, P. Pouillart, R. Weiner, J. L. Amiel, M. Hayat, C. Jasmin, and F. de Vassal

Unite Fred-Siguier de l'Hôpital Paul-Brousse
et Service d'Hématologie de l'Institut Gustave-Roussy, Villejuif, France

Non-specific immune responses in cancer patients have been explored in several studies of both cell-mediated and humoral immunity [1, 2, 3, 4, 5, 6]. Since 1968 we have been systematically studying non-specific immune responses in leukemia and hematosarcoma patients [7]. The results are presented below.

Patients and Methods

Immune studies were carried out in 550 patients (322 male and 228 female), aged from 3 to 78 years. These patients have been routinely given the following tests (Table 1): delayed cutaneous hypersensitivity to BCG, candidin and streptokinase; transformation of lymphocytes *in vitro* in the presence of phytohemagglutinin; counts of small and large lymphocytes, monocytes, and so-called immunoblasts in the peripheral blood; and measurement of the concentration of IgG, IgA and IgM immunoglobulins. These tests are neither very precise nor very sensitive, but they can be applied routinely to many patients.

Results

In *Hodgkin's disease* a constant change of cellular responses is seen in patients in the clinically apparent phase of the disease (Table 2). Cutaneous responses are frequently negative, and the rate of transformation of lymphocytes is low, as is the number of circulating small lymphocytes. In contrast, the relative number of circulating immunoblasts is increased. The immunoglobulins do not vary significantly. During remission, responses improve but never reach normal levels. If we consider the extent of the lesions (Table 3), we see that the cutaneous responses are more often positive in stages I and II than in stages III and IV. The transformation of lymphocytes and the relative number of small lymphocytes are also higher in these two stages. The abnormalities were even more pronounced in patients who died within 6 months of the investigation. If we classify patients according to the histological

Table 1. Routine tests of clinical immune response

Cellular responses								Humoral responses		
Positive responders to (%)			TL[a] PHA (%)	Circulating/mm³ (means)				Immunoglobulins mg/100 ml (means)		
				Lymphocytes		Mono-cytes	"Immuno-blasts"			
BCG	CD[b]	SK[c]		Small	Large			IgG	IgA	IgM

[a] TL PHA = mean of the percentage of transformed lymphocytes *in vitro* in the presence of phytohemagglutinin.
[b] CD = Candidin. — [c] SK = Streptokinase.

Table 2. Routine "immune investigation" of patients with Hodgkin's disease. I. Perceptible phases and "complete remissions"

	Number of patients	Cellular responses								Humoral responses		
		Positive responders to (%)			TL[a] PHA %	Circulating/mm³ (means)				Immunoglobulins mg/100 ml (means)		
						Lymphocytes		Mono-cytes	"Immuno-blasts"			
		BCG	CD[b]	SK[c]		small	large			IgG	IgA	IgM
Normal controls	22	88	65	50	73	1560	410	300	4.2	1180	175	80
Patients in perceptible phase of the disease	149	**33.1**	**31.2**	**20**	**37** ± 3[d]	**1030** ± 56	260	250	**18.4** ± 2.1	1276	227	75
Patients in remission	34	56.4	52.1	**26**	**44** ± 4	**1100** ± 110	270	170	11.3	1515	250	76

[a] TL PHA = mean of the percentage of transformed lymphocytes *in vitro* in the presence of phytohemagglutinin.
[b] CD = Candidin. — [c] SK = Streptokinase. — [d] Standard error of the means.

Table 3. Routine "immune investigation" of patients with Hodgkin's disease. II. Clinical Stages

	Number of patients	Cellular responses								Humoral responses		
		Positive responders to (%)			TL[a] PHA %	Circulating/mm^3 (means)				Immunoglobulins mg/100 ml (means)		
						Lymphocytes		Mono- cytes	"Immuno- blasts"			
		BCG	CD[b]	SK[c]		small	large			IgG	IgA	IgM
Normal controls	22	88	65	50	73	1560	410	300	4.2	1180	175	80
Patients in perceptible phase of the disease	149	33.1	31.2	20	37	1030	260	250	18.4	1276	227	75
Stages I and II	42	30.8	44	30	43	1390	250	330	18.2	1307	238	106
Stages III and IV	107	33	**18.4**	**10.5**	**32** ± 4[d]	**803** ± 52	250	220	18.9	1150	189	59
Patients who died in the 6 months following the investigation	49	32.8	**13.3**	**20**	**30** ± 3.2	**610** ± 49	270	300	13.8	1170	182	55

[a] TL PHA = mean of the percentage of transformed lymphocytes *in vitro* in the presence of phytohemagglutinin.
[b] CD = Candidin. — [c] SK = Streptokinase. — [d] Standard error of the means.

type of their disease (Table 4), we can see that the mixed cellularity and lymphocyte depletion types have the lowest incidence of cutaneous responses to BCG, candidin, and streptokinase.

Such changes in the cellular immune responses are not specific to Hodgkin's disease. We also find them in *reticulosarcoma* at stages III and IV (Table 5). There is a fall in the frequency of cutaneous responses, a decline in the ability of the lymphocytes to transform *in vitro*, a decrease in small lymphocytes, and a considerable increase in immunoblasts. In patients who died during the 6 months following the investigation the defect in delayed hypersensitivity is even more significant and the relative number of circulating lymphocytes even lower.

In *poorly differentiated lymphosarcoma* at stages III and IV, too, there are similar abnormalities of delayed hypersensitivity, transformation of lymphocytes, relative numbers of circulating small lymphocytes and circulating immunoblasts (Table 6).

In patients with *acute myeloid leukemia* (Table 7) in the perceptible phase of their disease, the transformation of lymphocytes approaches normal values. There is, in particular, a decrease in positive cutaneous responses as well as an increase in immunoblasts. Delayed hypersensitivity does not improve significantly during remission, with the exception of response to the BCG test.

In patients with *acute lymphoid leukemia* in the clinically apparent phase (Table 8) delayed cutaneous hypersensitivity is altered and the immunoblasts have increased. These abnormalities do not entirely disappear during remission. A slight decrease in IgG and IgA is also noted. It is in the first perceptible phase of the disease (Table 9) that the cutaneous responses to BCG and to candidin are most often negative. *In patients who relapse under immunotherapy, however, cutaneous responses are frequently positive. This suggests that the relapse is more likely to be due to immunoresistance than to a decrease in immune responses.* Patients who died during the month following the investigation showed the lowest relative number of positive responses to streptokinase, the highest relative number of circulating immunoblasts and the lowest level of IgG. If we analyse the results observed in patients in first remission according to their subsequent treatment (Table 10), we see that IgG first decreases slightly under chemotherapy which reduces complementary cells and then tends to become normal. The most interesting modifications, however, are seen in the incidence of positive delayed-hypersensitivity reactions, the level of transformation of lymphocytes, and the level of immunoblasts. As Fig. 1 shows, the cutaneous responses to BCG, candidin and streptokinase slowly improve when a complete remission has been obtained, and also during the course of complementary cell-reducing chemotherapy. The increase of positive responses is considerable after a month of immunotherapy and more moderate thereafter. The capacity of lymphocytes to transform *in vitro*, which increases with remission, has a great tendency to decrease under complementary cell-reducing chemotherapy and then to increase progressively in the course of immunotherapy. Immunoblasts decrease with remission, decrease even more under complementary cell-reducing chemotherapy, and then increase from the first month of immunotherapy.

In conclusion, this battery of tests permits us to confirm the frequent decline of cell-mediated immunity in leukemias and hematosarcomas. This alteration is frequently correlated with the severity of the disease, the stage of progression, and a

Table 4. Routine "immune investigation" of patients with Hodgkin's disease. III. Histological classification

Histological type	Number of patients	Cellular responses								Humoral responses		
		Positive responders to (%)			TL[a] PHA %	Circulating/mm³ (means)				Immunoglobulins mg/100 ml (means)		
						Lymphocytes		Mono-cytes	"Immuno-blasts"			
		BCG	CD[b]	SK[c]		small	large			IgG	IgA	IgM
Normal controls	22	88	65	50	73	1560	410	300	4.2	1180	175	80
Lymphocyte predominance	43	40.5	55.5	37.5	42	1100	250	100	16.5	1417	134	66
Nodular sclerosis	40	43.4	55.5	33.3	42	970	230	290	12.5	1445	256	87
Mixed cellularity	61	**29.9**	**33.3**	**21.7**	48	1280	310	220	14	1441	233	84
Lymphocyte depletion	21	**33.3**	**25**	**7**	38	910	290	230	11.8	1283	330	66

[a] TL PHA = mean of the percentage of transformed lymphocytes *in vitro* in the presence of phytohemagglutinin.
[b] CD = Candidin. — [c] SK = Streptokinase.

Table 5. Routine "immune investigation" of patients with reticulosarcoma, in perceptible phase of the disease. Clinical Stages III and IV

	Number of patients	Cellular responses								Humoral responses		
		Positive responders to (%)			TL[a] PHA %	Circulating/mm³ (means)				Immunoglobulins mg/100 ml (means)		
						Lymphocytes		Mono-cytes	"Immuno-blasts"			
		BCG	CD[b]	SK[c]		small	large			IgG	IgA	IgM
Normal controls	22	88	65	50	73	1560	410	300	4.2	1180	175	80
Reticulosarcoma well differentiated	12	**30.7**	**33.3**	**10**	**38** ± 5[d]	**990** ± 434	530 ± 220	450 ± 125	**51.4** ± 19.6	854 ± 86	206 ± 56	62 ± 5.88
Reticulosarcoma porly differentiated	60	**44**	**42**	**17.8**	**41** ± 2	**880** ± 98	220 ± 34	370 ± 48	**33.3** ± 2.01	1020 ± 57	238 ± 21	77 ± 5
Patients who died in the 6 months following the investigation	14	**24.2**	**21.4**	**0/14**	**41** ± 4	**608** ± 206	170 ± 110	290 ± 116	8.9 ± 1.5	1090 ± 116	259 ± 56	72 ± 9

[a] TL PHA = mean of the percentage of transformed lymphocytes *in vitro* in the presence of phytohemagglutinin.
[b] CD = Candidin. — [c] SK = Streptokinase. — [d] Standard error of the means.

Table 6. Routine "immune investigation" in patients with poorly differentiated lymphosarcoma in perceptible phase. Clinical Stages III und IV

	Number of patients	Cellular responses								Humoral responses		
		Positive responders to (%)			TL [a] PHA %	Circulating/mm³ (means)				Immunoglobulins mg/100 ml (means)		
						Lymphocytes		Mono-cytes	"Immuno-blasts"			
		BCG	CD [b]	SK [c]		small	large			IgG	IgA	IgM
Normal controls	22	88	65	50	73	1560	410	300	4.2	1180	175	80
Patients in perceptible phase of the disease	39	**36**	**23**	**16**	**50** ± 2.[d]	**807** ± 100	229 ± 46	305 ± 75	**17.7** ± 2.9	1012 ± 57	204 ± 24	78 ± 6.9

[a] TL PHA = mean of the percentage of transformed lymphocytes *in vitro* in the presence of phytohemagglutinin.
[b] CD = Candidin. — [c] SK = Streptokinase. — [d] Standard error of the means.

Table 7. Routine "immune investigation" of patients with acute myeloid leukemia

	Number of patients	Cellular responses								Humoral responses		
		Positive responders to (%)			TL[a] PHA %	Circulating/mm³ (means)				Immunoglobulins mg/100 ml (means)		
						Lymphocytes		Mono-cytes	"Immuno-blasts"			
		BCG	CD[b]	SK[c]		small	large			IgG	IgA	IgM
Normal controls	22	88	65	50	73	1560	410	300	4.2	1180	175	80
Patients in perceptible phase of the disease	52	**42.8**	**39**	**21.8**	58 ± 2.7[d]	2300 ± 396	750 ± 127	370 ± 7.9	**26.2** ± 5	1317 ± 89	277 ± 55	116 ± 9
Patients in Remission	13	62	**35**	**20**	67 ± 5.7	2750 ± 745	500 ± 190	290 ± 133.2	12.4 ± 2.9	1338 ± 125	287 ± 36	168 ± 56

[a] TL PHA = mean of the percentage of transformed lymphocytes *in vitro* in the presence of phytohemagglutinin.
[b] CD = Candidin. — [c] SK = Streptokinase. — [d] Standard error of the means.

Table 8. Routine "immune investigation" of patients with acute lymphoid leukemia. I. Perceptible phases and "complete remissions"

	Number of patients	Cellular responses								Humoral responses		
		positive responders to (%)			TL[a] PHA %	Circulating/mm³ (means)				Immunoglobulins mg/100 ml (means)		
						Lymphocytes		Mono-cytes	"Immuno-blasts"			
		BCG	CD[b]	SK[c]		small	large			IgG	IgA	IgM
Normal controls	22	88	65	50	73	1560	410	300	4.2	1180	175	80
Patients in perceptible phase of the disease	200	**39.5**	**24**	**14.2**	50	3382	717	339	**40.2** ± 6.6[d]	978	154	83
Patients in remission	301	60	**35**	**21**	59 ± 1.3	1650	290	270	**18.9** ± 2.4	882	135	80

[a] TL PHA = mean of the percentage of transformed lymphocytes *in vitro* in the presence of phytohemagglutinin.
[b] CD = Candidin. — [c] SK = Streptokinase. — [d] Standard error of the means.

Table 9. Routine "immune investigation" of patients with acute lymphoid leukemia. II. Perceptible phases

	Number of patients	Cellular responses								Humoral responses		
		Positive responders to (%)			TL[a] PHA %	Circulating/mm³ (means)				Immunoglobulins mg/100 ml (means)		
						Lymphocytes		Mono-cytes	"Immuno-blasts"			
		BCG	CD[b]	SK[c]		small	large			IgG	IgA	IgM
Normal controls	22	88	65	50	73	1560	410	300	4.2	1180	175	80
Patients in all perceptible phases of the disease	200	39.5	24	14.2	50	3382	717	339	40.2	978	154	83
Patients in first perceptible phase of the disease	57	**18.4**	**18.9**	16.6	49	6264	955	263	44	938	166	92
Patients in perceptible phase after immunotherapy	43	78.9	42.8	17.1	51	2961	1210	475	53	928	163	87
Patients who died in the month following the investigation	37	21.4	19.3	**6.4**	46	5777	1585	430	**61.8** ± 20[d]	820 ± 93	141	75

[a] TL PHA = mean of the percentage of transformed lymphocytes *in vitro* in the presence of phytohemagglutinin.
[b] CD = Candidin. — [c] SK = Streptokinase. — [d] Standard error of the means.

Table 10. Routine "immune investigation" of patients with acute lymphoid leukemia. III. Complementary cell reducing chemotherapy (CCRC) and immunotherapy in first complete remission

	Number of patients	Cellular responses								Humoral responses		
		Positive responders to (%)			TL[a] PHA %	Circulating/mm³ (means)				Immunoglobulins mg/100 ml (means)		
						Lymphocytes		Monocytes	"Immunoblasts"			
		BCG	CD[b]	SK[c]		small	large			IgG	IgA	IgM
Normal controls	22	88	65	50	73	1560	410	300	4.2	1180	175	80
Patients in first perceptible phase of the disease	57	**18.4**	**18.9**	16.6	49	6264	955	263	44	938	166	92
Patients in first remission at the beginning of CCRC	51	40.3	21.4	19.8	63 ± 2.9[d]	1992	263	225	**19.5** ± 5.4	**803** ± 31	125	83
Patients in first remission during CCRC	53	**44.4**	**25.9**	**16.6**	64 ± 3	1945	242	303	**14.3** ± 4	**754** ± 71	122	68
Patients in first remission at the end of CCRC	56	**53.7**	**28.5**	**17.5**	**56** ± 3.8	1324	137	219	**12.2** ± 2.4	**913** ± 78	139	90
Patients in first remission after one month of immunotherapy	28	**93.3**	**68.5**	**25**	**55** ± 3.9	1823	413	378	**22.3** ± 6.2	**991** ± 53	157	101
Patients in first remission after 6 months of immunotherapy	22	**100**	**66.6**	**46.6**	**64** ± 4.1	1743	301	295	**34.2** ± 15.6	**1061** ± 92	184	78

[a] TL PHA = mean of the percentage of transformed lymphocytes *in vitro* in the presence of phytohemagglutinin.
[b] CD = Candidin. — [c] SK = Streptokinase. — [d] Standard error of the means.

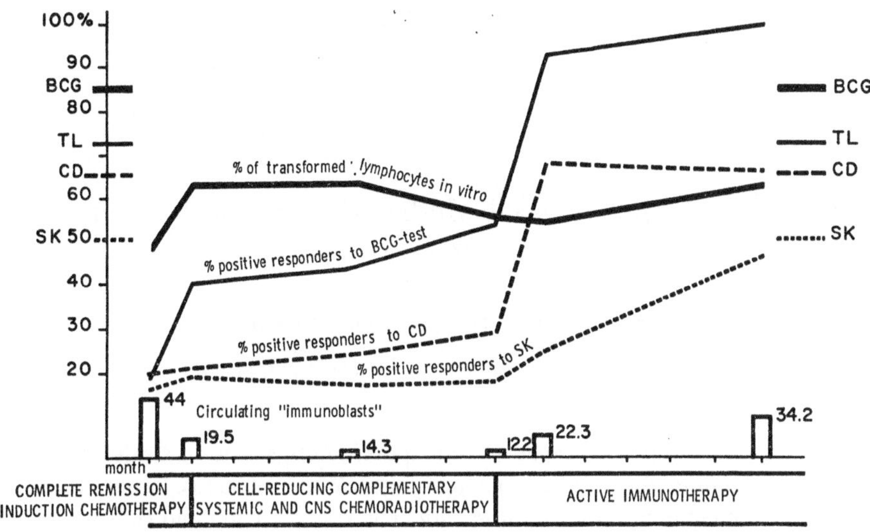

Fig. 1. Acute lymphoid leukemia: 54 patients. Kinetics of immune responses evaluated by a routine battery of tests

poor short-term prognosis. One notes as well that there is an improvement in the results of the tests while the patient is undergoing immunotherapy.

However, we must point out that these results have only statistical value, that they apply to a patient population, not to any single patient, and it is thus impossible to draw any therapeutic conclusions from this information. We need more precise and sensitive tests. At present this is one of the objectives of our group.

References

1. Aisenberg, A. C.: Studies on delayed hypersensitivity in Hodgkin's disease. J. clin. Invest. **41**, 1964 (1962).
2. Aisenberg, A. C.: Manifestations of immunologic unresponsiveness in Hodgkin's disease. Cancer Res. **26**, 1152 (1966).
3. Arends, T., Coonrad, C. V., Rundles, R. W.: Serum proteins in Hodgkin's disease and malignant lymphomas. Amer. J. Med. **16**, 833 (1954).
4. Barr, M., Hamilton-Fairley, G.: Circulating antibodies in reticuloses. Lancet **1961 I**, 1305.
5. Dubin, I. N.: Poverty of immunological mechanism in patients with Hodgkin's disease. Ann. intern. Med. **27**, 898 (1947).
6. Hersh, E. M., Oppenheim, J. J.: Impaired in vitro lymphocyte transformation in Hodgkin's disease. New Engl. J. Med. **273**, 1006 (1965).
7. Schneider, M., Schwarzenberg, L., Amiel, J. L., Hayat, M., Mascaro, G., Otmezguine, Y., Mathé, G.: Les réponses immunitaires au cours de la maladie de Hodgkin. Presse Med. **78**, 1969 (1970).

2. *Specific*

Kinetics of Specific Cell-Mediated Immune Response in Cancer-Bearing Hosts

G. BARSKI, J. K. YOUN, and D. LE FRANÇOIS

Institut Gustave-Roussy and C.N.R.S., Villejuif, France

Several recently published papers [1—4] report investigations on the development of cell-mediated immunity in mice carrying syngeneic transplantable tumors with the aid of the colony-inhibition (CI) test *in vitro*. The reactive lymphoid cells were collected by peritoneal washings performed in the same animals at different stages of tumor growth or treatment and associated in standard conditions with the tumor target cells maintained in permanent cultures *in vitro*, thus securing reproducible conditions of colony formation by these cells in parallel or successive experiments. Three different host-tumor systems were studied, comprising three malignant cell lines and their corresponding syngeneic host animals: a) a BALB/c cell line (T5) having an antigen induced by a low leukemogenic Rauscher virus variant, b) a C3H mammary tumor line (TM1) and c) a C57BL/6 methylcholanthrene-induced sarcoma line.

The general conclusion drawn from these investigations was that, in all three systems studied, cell-mediated immunity, expressed as specific cytotoxicity of peritoneal cells (PC) directed against the target tumor cells *in vitro*, appeared at the beginning of palpable tumor growth, then declined, and finally disappeared in mice bearing tumors exceeding an average diameter of 10 mm. This kind of immunological "eclipse" was very marked in animals with progressing tumors but could be reversed if the tumors were radically excised, in which case the specific immunological activity of the PC reappeared. This reappearance could be significantly accelerated if the animals were reinoculated a few days after surgery with their own frozen and irradiated tumor cells.

Experiments were undertaken to confirm that the "eclipse" phenomenon was immunologically specific. Two antigenically distinct malignant cell lines of BALB/c mouse origin were used: T5, as already described, and the T2BA line developed from a methylcholanthrene-induced sarcoma. Both were highly malignant and strongly antigenic; irradiated cells readily immunized mice against challenge with tumorigenic doses of the corresponding non-irradiated cells. No cross-resistance was observed in the mice immunized with the two different tumors. In these conditions mice sensitized to one tumor (e.g. T5) and supplying active PC that were cytotoxic towards T5 cells *in vitro* retained this activity while carrying a sizeable T2BA tumor. Consequently, immunological "eclipse" in tumor-beaiing animals was assumed to be specific rather than general.

Our observations on the loss of specific immunological activity in lymphoid cells from hosts with progressing tumors were in agreement with reported observations on chemically induced sarcomas in rats [5], on transplanted Rous sarcomas in rats [6], on Gross-type lymphomas in rats [7] and on metastatic nephroblastomas in human patients [8].

However, the HELLSTRÖMS and their group [9, 10] found that lymphoid cells from different sources (chiefly lymph nodes and blood), taken from hosts at different stages of tumor development or after their removal, rather uniformly inhibited the corresponding tumor target cells *in vitro*. More recently, the HELLSTRÖMS, SJÖGREN and their group have suggested [11] that sera from tumor-bearing animals contain blocking factors (antibodies, or antigen-antibody complexes) capable of binding to specific antigenic sites of the target tumor cells, and that this mechanism protects them against the specific cytotoxic activity of the sensitized lymphoid cells.

However, in our experiments the target tumor cells escaped the cytotoxic effect of the PC taken from tumor-bearing, "progressor" hosts, although these tumor cells supplied from *in vitro* cultures had not had any previous protective exposure to sera from these animals.

To explain this phenomenon, two possibilities may be envisaged.

1. If there is a peripheral mechanism acting at the level of the target cells, as suggested by HELLSTRÖM *et al.* [12], one has to suppose that the PC population is a mixture of two functional types of cells, including both "killer" and antibody-producing cells. The latter would produce blocking antibodies that would oppose or abolish the activity of the former. Certain observations of HALL and DAY [13] support this concept. This author, using the MMI (macrophage migration inhibition) test, has shown that PC from tumor-bearing "progressor" animals (immunologically inactive, as in our experiments) produce a "blocking factor" that is able to abolish the activity of PC from "regressor" animals. So far, we have not been able to verify that a factor is produced by the immunologically "eclipsed" PC *in vitro*.

2. Alternatively, the mechanism responsible for the immunological "eclipse" we observed in tumor-bearing animals might be ascribed to a centrally operating block of the sensitized lymphoid effector cells.

To check this possibility, we postulated that a "blocking factor" may be present in detectable quantities in the serum of immunologically "eclipsed" tumor-bearing mice. If this is so, it should be able to cancel out, at least to some extent, the specific cytotoxicity of immunologically active PC from immunized mice.

Experiments were designed [14] in which active PC, taken from BALB/c mice immunized against T5 cells, were associated with T5 cells plated as usual for the CI test. In parallel assays either the plated T5 cells or the PC were incubated prior to the association with pooled sera from BALB/c mice bearing T5 tumors exceeding 10 mm in diameter. The necessary precautions were taken to eliminate excess serum before the association. In a control series, sera from normal mice were subjected to the same conditions.

Three replications were carried out according to this protocol. In all three, sera from "eclipsed" tumor-bearing mice reduced the CI activity of sensitized PC by some 24% as compared with normal sera. This result was significant at the 0.05 to 0.001 level of p.

In one replication only, a significant reduction of cytotoxicity was also seen with serum from immunologically "eclipsed" mice acting on the target T5 cells.

Similar experiments with the TM1-C3HeB system showed significant abrogation of the CI activity of PC from immunized mice only when these cells were exposed to the sera of tumor-bearing mice. No statistically significant blocking of CI activity could be demonstrated when the target cells were incubated with the same sera in a similar way.

When the tumor-bearing mice were sublethally irradiated prior to the inoculation of the tumor cells, the abrogating activity of the "progressor" sera on the CI capacity of the PC did not increase but tended to decrease.

Taken as a whole, these data support the idea that progressive tumor growth is associated with the presence in the host's serum of a factor that blocks the specific "killer" activity of the sensitized lymphoid cells collected in the peritoneal cavity. Thus, the block may operate as a central mechanism directed against the effector lymphoid cells. This could explain the immunological "eclipse" we observed, the PC from tumor-bearing animals appearing to be already blocked when used in the CI tests.

The nature of the "blocking factor" is still not quite clear. Recently, Brawn [15] reported that the *in vitro* cytotoxic anti-target cell activity of lymphoid cells from mice sensitized against homologous histocompatibility antigens could be abolished by normal sera from the sensitizing mouse strain. He concluded that the "blocking factors" are circulating histocompatibility antigens that act on effector lymphoid cells, but not on the target cells.

On the other hand, Sjögren [16] have demonstrated that the blocking factor found in the sera of tumor-bearing animals and capable of abolishing the specific cytotoxic effect of sensitized lymphocytes in CI tests is in fact an antigen-antibody complex.

We found a certain ambivalence in the results of our experiments on sera from tumor-bearing "eclipsed" mice: they acted chiefly on the effector lymphoid cells, but also showed some activity against target tumor cells. This lends support to the above hypothesis.

Further experiments will certainly elucidate the nature of the "blocking factor" that opposes the "killer" activity of sensitized lymphoid cells. In due course it may be possible to regulate the impact of this factor on the mechanism of cell-mediated immunity.

References

1. Barski, G., Youn, J. K.: Evolution of cell-mediated immunity in mice bearing an antigenic tumor. Influence of tumor growth and surgical removal. J. nat. Cancer Inst. **43**, 111 (1969).
2. Le François, D., Youn, J. K., Belehradek, J., jr., Barski, G.: Evolution of cell-mediated immunity in mice bearing tumors produced by a mammary carcinoma cell line. Influence of tumor growth, surgical removal and treatment with irradiated tumor cells. J. nat. Cancer Inst. **46**, 981 (1971).
3. Belehradek, J., jr., Barski, G., Thonier, M.: Evolution of cell-mediated antitumor immunity in mice bearing a syngeneic chemically induced tumor. Influence of tumor growth, surgical removal and treatment with irradiated tumor cells. Int. J. Cancer **9**, 461 (1972).
4. Barski, G., Youn, J. K., Belehradek, J., jr., Le François, D.: Variations des mécanismes de défense immunologique spécifique de type cellulaire en fonction de la croissance tumorale Ann. Inst. Pasteur **122**, 633 (1972).

5. MIKULSKA, Z. B., SMITH, C., ALEXANDER, P.: Evidence for an immunological reaction of the host directed against its own actively growing primary tumor. J. nat. Cancer Inst. **36**, 29 (1966).
6. BELLONE, C. J., POLLARD, M.: A transient cytotoxic host response to the Rous sarcoma virus-induced transplantation antigen. Proc. Soc. exp. Biol. (N.Y.) **134**, 640 (1970).
7. OREN, M. E., HERBERMAN, R. B., CANTY, T. G.: Immune response to Gross-virus-induced lymphoma. II. Kinetics of the cellular immune response. J. nat. Cancer Inst. **46**, 621 (1971).
8. DIEHL, V., JEREB, B., STJERNSWÄRD, J., O'TOOLE, C., AHSTRÖM, L.: Cellular immunity to nephroblastoma. Inst. J. Cancer **7**, 277 (1971).
9. HELLSTRÖM, I., HELLSTRÖM, K. E., PIERCE, G. E.: In vitro studies of immune reactions against autochthonous and syngeneic mouse tumors induced by methylcholanthrene and plastic discs. Int. J. Cancer **3**, 467 (1968).
10. HELLSTRÖM, I., HELLSTRÖM, K. E., PIERCE, G. E.: Cellular and humoral immunity to different types of human neoplasms. Nature (Lond.) **220**, 1352 (1968).
11. HELLSTRÖM, I., SJÖGREN, H. O., WARNER, G., HELLSTRÖM, K. E.: Blocking of cell-mediated tumor immunity by sera from patients with growing neoplasms. Int. J. Cancer **7**, 226 (1971).
12. HELLSTRÖM, I., HELLSTRÖM, K. E., SJÖGREN, H. O.: Serum mediated inhibition of cellular immunity to methylcholanthrene-induced murine sarcomas. Cell. Immunol. **1**, 18 (1970).
13. HALLIDAY, W. J.: Macrophage migration inhibition with mouse tumor antigens: properties of serum and peritoneal cells during tumor growth and after tumor loss. Cell. Immunol. **3**, 113 (1972).
14. YOUN, J. K., LE FRANÇOIS, D., BARSKI, G.: *In vitro* studies on mechanism of the "eclipse" of cell-mediated immunity in mice bearing advanced tumors. J. nat. Cancer Inst. **50**, 921 (1973).
15. BRAWN, R. J.: *In vitro* desensitization of sensitized murine lymphocytes by a serum factor (soluble antigen?). Proc. nat. Acad. Sci. (Wash.) **68**, 1634 (1971).
16. SJÖGREN, H. O., HELLSTRÖM, I., BANSAL, S. C., HELLSTRÖM, K. E.: Suggestive evidence that the "blocking antibodies" of tumor-bearing individuals may be antigen-antibody complexes. Proc. nat. Acad. Sci. (Wash.) **68**, 1372 (1971).

Technical and Interpretative Problems with Immunofluorescence

M. G. Lewis

McGill University Cancer Research Unit, Montreal

Introduction

The publication of a paper entitled "Immunological properties of an antibody containing a fluorescent group" inaugurated use of the now rapidly expanding technique of immunofluorescence [1]. This was the first real approach to the use of a chemical attached to antibody as a tracer enabling the identification and localization of antigen [6]. Following this work, [12] localized adrenocorticotrophin in normal tissue, thus demonstrating the remarkable degree of specificity of the reagents used in the immunofluorescent technique. This set the scene for what is now a very widespread, complex subject, the localization of tissue antigens by a variety of sensitive antisera. One of the major obstacles to the widespread acceptance of this technique was the difficulty of obtaining suitable microscopes, since the main way of identifying the antibody/antigen complex linked to a fluorochrome was to excite the fluorochrome with UV or blue light [6]. The first commercial fluorescent microscopes were developed in 1955 and this problem has now been largely overcome, some form of immunofluorescent technique being applied in almost every laboratory throughout the world [6]. Its application to a variety of topics, including diagnostic bacteriology and the study of autoimmune disease, has established this method as one of the most important and sensitive available in biology and medicine.

The problem of nonspecific reactions and unwanted fluorescence was soon encountered, and between 1958 and 1961 the relationship between the fluorescent dye and the labeled globulin was shown to be of great importance; a more heavily loaded protein was shown to possess the greatest nonspecific activity [2, 3]. The use of column chromatography enabled fractions to be prepared with high antibody content and low nonspecific activity [2, 3]. In addition, the use of various types of tissue powder to absorb the antiserum and conjugate allowed the specific reaction to be more easily determined [9]. The applicability of the fluorescent antibody technique to tumor immunology was largely established [10, 13] in the late 1950's and early 1960's. The production of fluorescent labeled antibody against the surface components of Burkitt's lymphoma was probably one of the most important stages in this development. Since then a variety of tumors, both animal and human, have been studied. Despite the obvious value of immunofluorescence, there still remain problems of interpretation, standardization and nonspecificity of labeling [7] and

DIRECT FLUORESCENT METHOD

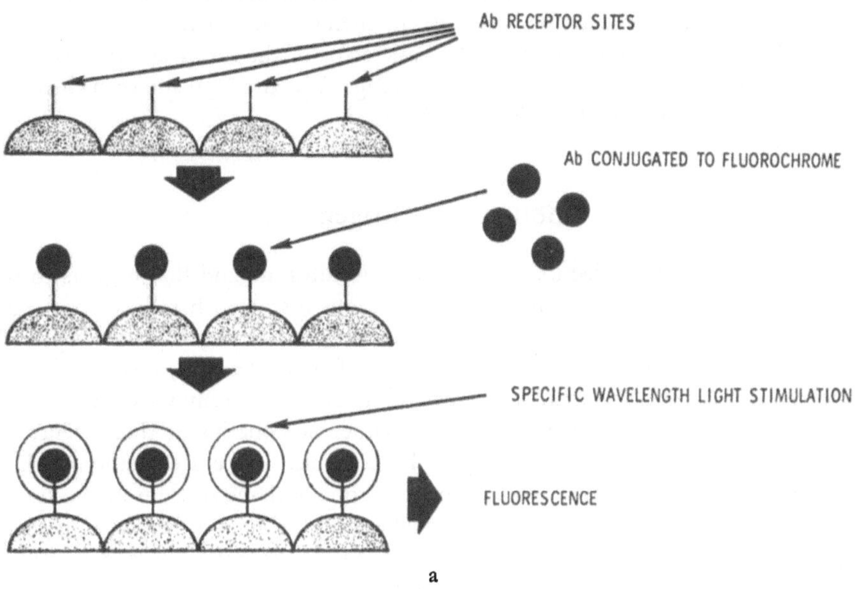

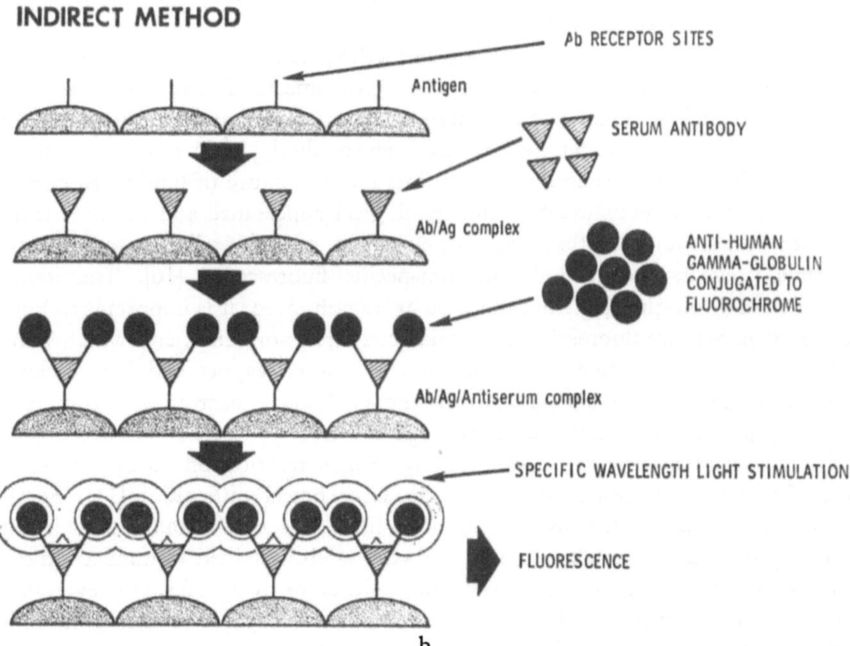

Fig. 1. a Diagrammatic summary of the direct immunofluorescence technique, b Indirect immunofluorescence technique

different research groups using this technique appear to obtain different results with the same type of tumor. The best way to investigate these seems to be to examine each stage in the immunofluorescent methods and determine where the greatest likelihood of variability lies. The basic steps of the direct and indirect immunofluorescent techniques are summarized in Figs. 1 (a) and 1 (b) and the principles underlying specific immune blocking are discussed.

Source of Antigen

The first stage is the selection of the antigenic substrate and the reagents to be used in the test. The substrate, under the conditions discussed here, is tumor cells or tumor material. Tissue sections of tumor give less clearcut results than dispersed cells, largely due to the difficulty of penetration of tissue sections, however thinly cut, by the antisera and the conjugate. Equally difficult is the removal of serum and conjugate during the washing procedure, and either one obtains no fluorescence at all, or all the sections fluoresce including the controls. There are methods available to make this a great deal easier, and the technique of tissue sections in the study of autoimmune and tissue antigens is now well established [6, 14]. However, certain types of tumor, including those of the skin, present considerable difficulties under these circumstances. To make a cell suspension or individual cell separation first and then apply the technique to the individual cells eliminates much of this problem and the picture becomes clearer. The method of preparing the cells is obviously an area of variability and the type of cell is yet another variable, since the cells can be used either in a fixed state or a living state.

Fixed Cells. One of the most widespread methods is to produce a cell suspension or an imprint of cells, as for preparing cytological smears. The cells then are fixed in either methanol or acetone and the fluorescent conjugate and the sera applied in much the same way as for cytological stains. The method [14] in which the cells are shap-frozen by placing the smears or imprints into a mixture of liquid nitrogen and isopentane, gives a very much better cytological appearance and to some extent a cleaner background, so that less proteinaceous material adheres to the glass and thus prevents background and nonspecific fluorescence [16]. The importance of clear cytological control cannot be overemphasized; it is important to know not only that cells are fluorescing but which cells are fluorescing, and whether they are the right ones. In some recent experiments, my colleagues and I have clearly identified brightly fluorescent plasma cells and occasional macrophages containing fluorescing particles of conjugate in some specimens.

Living Cells. The production of antibody-antigen reaction on the surface membrane of a living cell presents certain additional technical difficulties [11]. Firstly, it is desirable to have a cell suspension with a high degree of viability. This is relatively easy to obtain in animal tumors but very rarely obtained in human tumors; therefore, one has to accept a high proportion of dead or dying cells. However, dead cells take up other dyes in addition to fluorochrome so they can be distinguished by the use of other markers. In addition, the whole cell becomes fluorescent if it is dead or dying. Cells which have been stored in liquid nitrogen and protected by dimethylsulphoxide must be thoroughly washed, otherwise the fluorescent reaction is considerably reduced; sometimes a rather diffuse flare-like reaction occurs, presumably due to alterations produced in the cell membrane by DMSO [11]. Following removal from liquid nitrogen, a certain period of time, varying from tumor ot tumor, must be allowed for recovery after washing away the DMSO. The use of enzymes, such as trypsin, in the preparation of cell suspensions can also produce difficulties. In trials to compare the use of trypsin with mechanical means of producing cell suspensions of human tumors, we obtained some very variable results after trypsinization, sometimes again with a flare-like diffuse reaction over the entire cell surface; on other occasions we detected no surface antibody–antigen reaction even though the same cell suspension produced by mechanical means gave a positive result.

The Reagents Used in Immunofluorescent Technique

The main reagent, the conjugate (or fluorochrome–labeled antiglobulin), constitutes one of the greatest sources of variability in this technique. There are numerous ways of preparing antihuman globulin and several methods are available for conjugating it to a fluorochrome [6, 8, 14]. The most commonly used dye is fluorescein isothiocyanate, isomer I giving the most consistent results [2]. The protein–fluorescein ratio is very critical so that the ideal conjugate is one which contains high antibody activity and minimal or no free fluorescein. By means of extensive chromatography and careful chemical preparation it is now possible to produce a conjugate which contains minimal quantities of fluorescein, thus reducing the liability of the dye to diffuse or become nonconjugated. To be able to use such conjugates one needs to increase the sensitivity of the microscope, and this will be discussed later. The problem of standardization of fluorescent reagents and techniques has been discussed at great length [7, 14].

We have investigated a series of commercially available prepared conjugates against some known tumor cells and compared them with highly purified antiserum conjugated to a known degree of specificity. Many of the commercial conjugates contained not only free fluorochrome but also non-gamma proteins, including albumin and beta lipoproteins [11, 15]. This can produce quite a high degree of nonspecific reactivity.

The steps of the fluorescent techniques are summarized in Fig. 2. Let us go through this technique step by step, studying each stage and determining its weak points.

Staining Technique. The antigenic substrate is prepared as a section, smear or suspension, and to this is added the patient's or the control serum. After 20 min incubation, any unreacted serum is washed off and then the conjugate is applied for the same length of time as the sera. Following incubation, usually for twice the period applied to the serum, the unreacted conjugate is removed by washing and the preparation is viewed under the microscope. There are four stages at which error can easily be introduced.

a) Lack of *serum dilution* can produce nonspecific effects because both albumin and beta-lipoproteins can adhere to cell preparations, especially membranes of living cells. In some systems, i.e. autoimmune studies, there is low-titre positivity to a variety of tissues.

b) *Inadequate washing* can fail to remove all unreacted sera or conjugate, causing fluorescence in areas where no specific reaction has taken place.

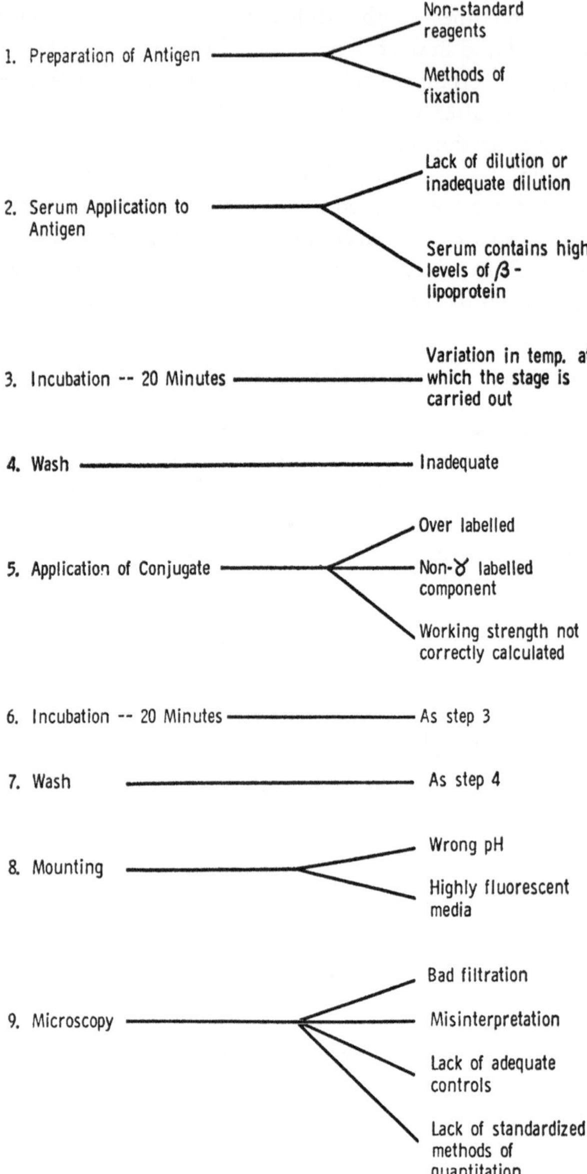

Fig. 2 Steps in indirect immunofluorescence including areas where technical errors may be introduced

c) The *conjugated antiserum* needs to be strictly *controlled* since the difference between positivity and negativity rests solely on the amount and location of the fluorescence observed. The use of wrong or mixed antibody, free fluorochrome, overlabeling and labeling of non-gamma components all adds to the possibility that the observed fluorescence is nonspecific.

d) *Microscopy and interpretation.* The final result is usually obtained by subjecting the preparation to fluorescent microscopy. There are many forms of fluorescence microscopes and numerous methods of light excitation and filtration. The procedure chosen should ideally excite the fluorochrome at its maximum absorbance peak and the filter system should correspond to this peak as closely as possible [17]. This enables the pure fluorescent emission to be observed without distortion. The usual procedure is to use transmitted light, corrected by the use of either primary and secondary filters or close-wavelength interference filters [19]. The selection of filter systems and light sources determines the sensitivity of the reaction and therefore certainly influences the interpretation.

It has been stated that the use of fluorochrome–labeled antisera increases the microscopical sensitivity about a thousandfold over standard staining techniques. It is not sufficient, therefore, merely to record positive or negative fluorescence; the pattern of fluorescence is also very important and, even more so, the cell type fluorescing.

Methods of Illumination

[17] introduced an epi-illumination system for the study of cell surface reactions or tissue sections where the light is focused on the surface of the material through the objective, which acts as a condenser; the emitted fluorescence is then reflected back along the same pathway. This prevents the loss of light that usually occurs in any transilluminated specimen, and therefore increases both the fluorescence emission and sensitivity.

One of the main problems in interpreting the results obtained with fluorescein-conjugated antisera and UV light is the need to distinguish between the apple-green positive fluorescence and the rather yellowish or bluish-green background, depending on the system used. However, by maneuvering various secondary filters or using interference filter systems, one can obtain a situation where the positive fluorescence is apple-green but the background is red [19]. Except for sufferers from red/green color blindness, who should not really be involved in this type of work, this presents much less difficulty for most people. This is particularly emphasized by a report indicating that only 50% of a group of observers were suitable for scanning immunofluorescence slides [20]. We have found this type of fluorescent microscopy very useful. The pattern of fluorescence is of great importance. A cell can be made to fluoresce very easily, either by coating it with albumin or with lipoprotein, or simply by not washing thoroughly enough after the application of the sera or antisera. Usually the type of fluorescence obtained under these circumstances is a rather bland, complete partial covering of the cell with no discrete localization [11, 15]. It is interesting that the same picture is produced immediately following trypsinization, but after a recovery period the cell membrane produces a discrete, localized, beaded appearance which cannot be washed away.

Specific Immune Blocking

The use of specific immune blocking is a very important way of distinguishing between specific and nonspecific reactions. The technique consists essentially of first applying the nonconjugated antiserum and then the conjugate; the effect is blocked only in cases where a specific reaction has occurred [6]. The other method, which we have recently demonstrated clearly in one particular human tumor, malignant melanoma, is the use of cross-absorption techniques. Positive sera can only be absorbed on the surface of their own tumor cells, absorption with other living tumor cell preparations yielding positive fluorescence against the autologous cells [11].

Controls

Controls are essential in all experimental or technical procedures. A positive control is often the most difficult to obtain in this type of work. Usually one has to be content with controlling the degree of positive reaction of the conjugate itself. This can be done by using any known positive cell plus serum preparation and then applying the conjugated antiserum or, as we usually do routinely, setting up a series of anti-nuclear factor preparations from the sera of patients with disseminated lupus erythematosis or rheumatoid arthritis and then applying the conjugate. When it is thought that sera which may contain autoantibodies against normal components that might complicate any of these procedures, some form of autoantibody scan is performed on each serum. This usually involved screening the serum against a battery of frozen organ sections.

Negative Controls

There is a variety of possible negative controls but they need to be standardized. Usually we use a serum from a patient known to be negative to a particular tumor. Of course, any test system should include one slide containing only phosphate buffered saline to which no serum has been added, as a check against contamination and nonspecificity of the conjugate itself. This is a very important control. The use of a pool of normal human serum as well as negative cancer-patient serum is recommended.

Measurements, or Quantitation of the Results

Quantitation presents one of the greatest difficulties in the fluorescent antibody technique. Until recently, one had to be content with some form of semi-quantitative measurement. This is usually expressed either as a fluorescent index, that is the proportion of the cells which specifically fluoresce, or one may set a particular fluorescent index as the base line and then measure the titer of the serum which gives this reaction. This is one of the areas of greatest variability in results, since different methods of quantitation in such a sensitive technique can result in quite dramatic differences. The establishment of a baseline is fundamental to all laboratory procedures since there are no tests that give absolute values in any biological system. It is this question of establishment of the baseline which has caused most discrepancies.

In a large series of patients with malignant melanoma we recently matched a variety of measurements of both fluorescent indices and titers against a fluorescent index of 0.30. It became very clear to us that at a serum dilution of 1 in 4 or above nonspecific reactions are reduced to a minimum; this was apparent in both the membrane technique and against the cytoplasm of snap-frozen melanoma cells. This is further evidence of the danger of using undiluted serum for these procedures. Although our study was semiquantitative, it was important in determining the degree of patient specificity in the membrane technique. Whereas the cytoplasmic reaction showed multiple cross-reactivity between positive melanoma sera cells at both low and high titers [16], in the membrane technique the majority of high-titer reactions were seen in the autologous situation and only the very low-titer reactions gave rise to some degree of cross-reactivity. This was confirmed by the cross-absorption technqiue described earlier. The importance of standardizing all procedures concerning interpretation and quantitation is obvious if one is seeking to obtain sera from large numbers of patients in order to establish the basic lines along which this work must proceed. This is, indeed, one of the objects which the melanoma group of the E.O.R.T.C. is at present pursuing, and already a series of workshops have been held in an attempt to establish such a standardized approach. At the moment the data are being collected and analysed and discrepancies investigated.

Finally, a word about more sophisticated methods of quantitation. The ideal situation, of course, would be to have some real quantitation in terms of the amount of fluorescent emission. There are now several prototype instruments enabling photometric measurements of fluorescence to be made [4, 5]. Many of them are so complicated to use that large groups of specimens are impractical. There are, however, microscopes now available, particularly those with the epi-illumination system which increases sensitivity, where a photometric measurement can be made by means of a photometer with a range of focus from whole groups of cells down to the membrane or nucleus of an individual cell [18]. We may thus look forward to the day when it will no longer be necessary to express, or see expressed, results of fluorescence in terms of fluorescent indices or titers, but in terms of absolute emission spectra. There is, however, one very great danger in this, i.e. that the photometer will measure cell fluorescence and not distinguish between specific and nonspecific fluorescence. Just as "all that glitters is not gold", "all that fluoresces is not specific nor significant". Therefore, the art of microscopy will not be superceded and the need for microscopical monitoring of what is fluorescing will remain. Nevertheless, despite its problems, this technique can be, and I think already has proven itself to be, one of the most useful available, not only in tumor immunology but in many aspects of biology and medicine.

Acknowledgements

I would like to express my thanks to Mr. T. M. Phillips for assistance with this presentation, and to the Medical Research Council of Canada and the National Cancer Institute of Canada for financial support.

References

1. Coons, A. H., Creech, H. J., Jones, R. N.: Immunological properties of an antibody containing a fluorescent group. Proc. Soc. exp. Biol. (N.Y.) **47**, 200 (1941).
2. Fothergill, J. E.: Fluorescent protein tracing (Nairn, R. C., Ed.), Ch. 2, p. 14. Edinburgh, London: Livingstone 1969.

3. Fothergill, J. E.: Fluorescent protein tracing (Nairn, R. C., Ed.), Ch. 2, p. 28. Edinburgh, London: Livingstone 1969.
4. Goldman, M.: Antigenic analysis of *Entamoeba histolytica* by means of fluorescent antibody. I. Instrumentation for microfluorimetry of stained amoebae. Exp. Parasit. **9**, 25 (1960).
5. Goldman, M.: An improved microfluorimeter for measuring brightness of fluorescent antibody reactions. J. Histochem. Cytochem. **15**, 38 (1967).
6. Goldman, M.: Fluorescent antibody methods. New York: Academic Press 1968.
7. Holborow, E. J.: Standardization in immunofluorescence. Oxford: Blackwell 1970.
8. Holborow, E. J., Johnson, G. D.: Immunofluorescence. In: Handbook of experimental immunology (Weir, D. M., Ed.), p. 571. Oxford: Blackwell 1967.
9. Johnson, G. C.: Simplified procedure for removing non-specific staining components from fluorescein-labelled conjugates. Nature (Lond.) **191**, 70 (1961).
10. Klein, G., Clifford, P., Klein, E., Stjernsward, J.: Search for tumour-specific reactions in Burkitt lymphoma patients by the membrane immunofluorescence reaction. Proc. nat. Acad. Sci. (Wash.) **55**, 1628 (1966).
11. Lewis, M. G., Phillips, T. M.: The specificity of surface membrane immunofluorescence in human malignant melanoma. Int. J. Cancer **10**, 105 (1972).
12. Marshall, J. M.: Localization of adrenocorticotrophic hormone by histochemical and immunochemical methods. J. exp. Med. **94**, 21 (1951).
13. Moller, G.: Demonstration of mouse isoantigens on the cellular level by the fluorescent antibody technique. J. exp. Med. **114**, 415 (1961).
14. Nairn, R. C.: Fluorescent protein tracing, 3rd Ed. Edinburgh, London: Livingstone 1969.
15. Phillips, T. M.: Immunofluorescent techniques in the study of malignant melanoma. Rev. Inst. Pasteur (Lyon) **4**, 59 (1971).
16. Phillips, T. M., Lewis, M. G.: A system of immunofluorescence in the study of tumour cells. Rev. Europ. Etud. clin. biol. **15**, 1016 (1970).
17. Ploem, J. S.: The use of a vertical illuminator with interchengeable dichroic mirrors for fluorescence microscopy with incident light. Z. wiss. Mikr. **68**, 129 (1967).
18. Ploem, J. S.: Standardization in immunofluorescence (Holborow, E. J., Ed.), Ch. 10, p. 63. Oxford: Blackwell 1970.
19. Rygaard, J., Olsen, W.: Interference filters for improved immunofluorescence microscopy. Acta path. microbiol. scand. **76**, 146 (1969).
20. Sander, G.: Standardization in immunofluorescence (Holborow, E. J., Ed.), Ch. 21, p. 155. Oxford: Blackwell 1970.

Patterns of Cellular Immunity in Malignant Melanoma*

D. A. Clark and L. Nathanson

Medical Oncology Service, Department of Medicine, New England Medical Center Hospital and Tufts University School of Medicine, Boston, Mass.

Introduction

Rejection of a growing solid tumor, such as malignant melanoma, appears to depend on an effective cell-mediated immune response. For example, the primary lesions of melanoma often contain areas of flattening and depigmentation overlying sites of dense lymphoid infiltration [26]; metastatic deposits regressing either spontaneously [16] or as a result of immunologic stimulation [45] show features of delayed hypersensitivity [4[. Cellular immunity can also be detected in patients who do not show these phenomena either by a positive delayed hypersensitivity skin test to tumor antigens [4], or by *in vitro* testing. Data from *in vitro* tests indicate that cell-mediated immunity is present [18, 21, 31] in cancer patients, even with advanced disease, but is antagonized by serum blocking factors [6, 21, 24] which allow the tumor to grow through the mechanism of immunological enhancement.

Three *in vitro* techniques have been used by us and by our collaborators to study the quantitative interrelationships of cell-mediated immunity and humoral blocking responses in melanoma. These include: 1. lymphocyte stimulation by soluble tumor-specific antigen; 2. inhibition of leukocyte migration induced by this antigen; 3. studies of lymphocytotoxicity and serum blocking factors by mixed lymphocyte-tumor cell culture. We must emphasize at the outset that such studies have a dual purpose: to define fundamental immunological mechanisms in the host's response to his tumor, and to predict clinical behaviour of the disease and to serve as a guidance system in applying chemo-immunotherapy. This report focuses on the latter goal.

Lymphocyte Transformation

Our lymphocyte stimulation studies [25] demonstrated both autochthonous and allogeneic responses to a soluble melanoma-associated antigen present in the cyst fluid of a necrotic tumor. This antigen did not stimulate normal control lymphocytes or lymphocytes from cancer patients with a different type of tumor. Dimethyl-

* Supported by Grants: T-550, American Cancer Society Ca 12924-01, National Cancer Institute (U.S.P.H.S.) DRG-1067, Damon Runyon Memorial Fund.

triazenoimidazole carboxamide (DTIC) therapy suppressed lymphocyte responsiveness to the antigen, and also reduced the levels of antigen circulating in the blood and present in the urine [32].

Inhibition of Leukocyte Migration

COCHRANE [10] studied our antigen and found migration inhibition in 10 of 16 disease-free melanoma patients, whereas only 1 of 6 with recurrent disease and 2 of 16 normal controls reacted. Purification of the antigen by Sephadex G100 gel chromatography yielded a low-molecular-weight (less than 60,000) preparation giving similar results. A deficiency in cell-mediated immunity was correlated with recurrent or metastatic disease; this deficiency was not apparent in the lymphocyte stimulation experiments, although the fact that the patients had good survival [25] perhaps signified a quantitatively greater immune response.

Mixed Lymphocyte-Tumor Culture

The *in vitro* studies of the HELLSTROMS [21, 23, 24] suggested that most tumors grow progressively in the face of cell-mediated immunity due to the presence of serum blocking factors (antibodies). We, therefore, set out to study blocking antibody levels and the effect of BCG and chemotherapy-induced tumor regression on both cell-mediated immunity and blocking antibody. The principal steps in our assay of cell-mediated immunity (microcytotoxicity assay) are shown in Fig. 1. Tumor cells were obtained by excision of metastatic nodules, mincing, and growth in monolayer in Ham's F-10, 20% fetal calf serum (Microbiologic Associates), with penicillin (50 u/ml) and streptomycin (50 μg/ml). After several subcultures, antibiotics were discontinued and bacterial and PPLO (pleuropneumonia-like organism)

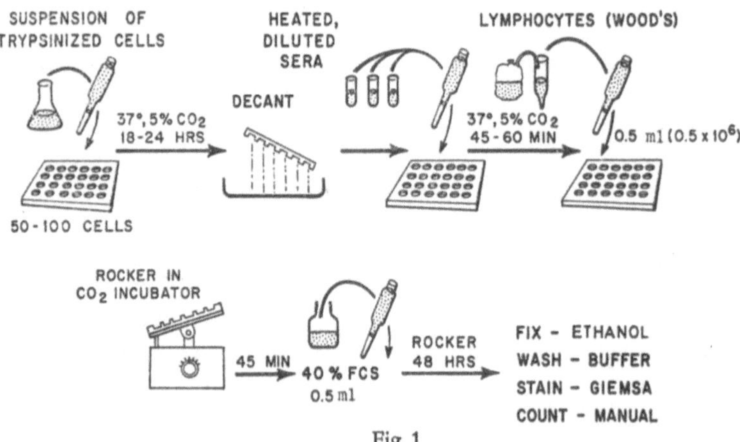

Fig. 1

cultures carried out. Cell lines LeCa and MeGo were kindly provided by Dr. M. ROMSDAHL. Whenever PPLO were found, intensive antibiotic therapy was applied to suppress them before the cells were used. The cell lines were identified as melanoma by their aneuploid karyotype, positive DOPA-oxidase staining, electron-microscopic demonstration of premelanosomes and, in one case, by growth of a typically pigmented tumor after heterotransplantation into an immunosuppressed neonatal Wistar-Furth rat [30]. Tumor cells were harvested from monolayer by trypsinization (0.25%—0.025%, Grand Island Biologicals), suspended in a medium with 20% heat-inactivated fetal calf serum, and seeded at a concentration of 50—100

Table 1. Definition of terms

Lymphocyte donor	Serum	
	Control	Patient
Tumor patient	A	C
Control	B	D

% CMI = ((B — A[a])/B) × 100%) — % kill on control target

% Blocking = ((C — A)/(B — A)) × 100%
C must be larger than A at $P < 0.05$

Arming = Negative blocking or C less than at $P < 0.05$ or D less than B at $P < 0.05$

[a] A must differ from B at $P < 0.05$.

cells in a volume of 0.2—0.5 ml per well in Linbro FB 16-24 TC Disposotrays. The following day, the medium was decanted, and 0.2—0.5 ml of a 1 : 6 dilution of serum added. Patient and control sera were heat-inactivated at 56° for 30 minutes, filtered through a 0.22 micron Millipore filter, and stored at —20°C until use. A 1 : 6 dilution was made in 0.01 M phosphate buffered saline, pH 6.8, or in Ham's F-10. After incubation for 45—60 minutes at 37° in 5% CO_2, the test sera were dumped out and 0.5×10^6 lymphocytes in 0.5 ml F-10 added. Lymphocytes were obtained by the Woods method [46] wherein the plasmagel-sedimented supernatant from lightly heparinized blood is defibrinated with a mixture of nylon powder and glass beads. After this treatment, the preparations contained 95—99% pure lymphocytes, were depleted of monocytes, fibrin, and platelets, and showed greater than 90% viability as determined by trypan blue exclusion. Occasionally, polymorphonuclear leukocytes were not completely removed. The lymphocytes were washed once in 20 ml Hanks solutions, resuspended in serum-free F-10, and added to replicate wells of the Disposotray. The trays were rocked for 45 min on a Bellco rocker in a CO_2 incubator and an additional 0.5 ml of 40% fetal calf serum in F-10 added. The rocking was continued for 48 h then the plates were washed with saline, fixed with ethanol, and stained with Wright's or Giemsa stain. Cell-mediated immunity was reflected in a reduced tumor cell count in wells exposed to immune as compared to control lymphocytes. Statistical analysis was carried out using Student's T-test for predesignated comparisons of two samples. Comparability was established by computing the ratio of the variances, and T-test results were confirmed by one-way analysis of variance and the Duncan range test [42].

A randomized arrangement of sera and lymphocyte seeding was adopted to obviate any bias due to nonspecific growth and plating effects. The specificity of the reactions for melanoma were confirmed by using control non-melanoma tumor cell lines, and testing lymphocytes from other types of cancer patients. Inhibition of lymphocytoxicity with mitomycin C [8, 9] excluded allogeneic inhibition and agglutination cytotoxicity as major mechanisms of target cell damage [29]. ABO and HLA typing was done, and ABO compatibility of tumor cell-line donor, test sera, and lymphocytes determined.

Results

A pilot study of 7 melanoma patients using 6-mm diameter Falcon wells and lymphocytes separated by a variety of methods [8, 9] failed to demonstrate cell-mediated immunity except in two controls. By the use of larger, 16-mm wells, a striking improvement in assay sensitivity was achieved (Table 2). Only in the larger wells was

Table 2. Comparison of well diameters

Lymphocytes	Target melanoma BR [c]					
	6 mm well diameter			16 mm well diameter		
	Control serum treated					
Progressor BR	125 ± 19.7	NS [a]		332 ± 26.8	NS [a]	
Regressor AP	154 ± 27.4	NS		181 ± 9.9	0.0025	
Control JC	132 ± 19.9	—		412 ± 50.0	—	
	Progressor serum treated					
Progressor BR	145 ± 15.6	NS [a]	NS [b]	572 ± 32.2	NS [a]	0.05 [b]
Regressor AP	150 ± 27.4	NS	NS	657 ± 28.5	0.01	0.001
Control JC	122 ± 4.1	—	NS	530 ± 32.2	—	NS

[a] P value testing null hypothesis that lymphocytes from melanoma patients are more cytotoxic than control lymphocytes. Student's t-test and analysis of variance with Duncan's range test.

[b] P value testing null hypothesis that progressor serum is no more effective than control serum in reducing the observed lymphocytotoxicity.

[c] All data given as mean ± 1 S.E.M.

significant cytotoxicity of regressor patient's lymphocytes detected. These were significantly more potent than progressor lymphocytes. Progressor serum blocked cytotoxicity and induced stimulation of cell growth in the presence of both progressor and regressor lymphocytes. Three additional experiments comparing the two well sizes confirmed the superiority of the large wells (Table 3). Only in one instance was cell-mediated immunity detected in the smaller wells, and in this case, a technical accident caused tilting of the plates and settling of the lymphocytes to one side. The precise reason for the superiority of the larger wells remains unclear; it could be due to inadequate mixing on the rocker in the smaller wells, the presence of red blood cells, or the scarcity of certain species of mononuclear leucocytes in our lymphocyte preparations.

Table 3. Comparison of well diameter

Lymphocytes	6 mm wells	16 mm wells
Melanoma T	39 ± 15	57 ± 6.7
Control JC	57 ± 10	105 ± 8.8
	NS	P < 0.05
Positive control LN	25 ± 5	146 ± 13
Control JC	15 ± 2	195 ± 11
	NS	P < 0.05
Tilt		
Melanoma D	194 ± 27	668 ± 40
Control JC	280 ± 34	798 ± 29
	P < 0.05	P < 0.01

Table 4. Human melanoma cell-mediated immunity: specificity controls

Lymphocyte donor	Target cells		
	Melanoma MG	Colon carcinoma	Parotid carcinoma
Melanoma SH	24 ± 3.7 [a]	322 ± 27.8	60 ± 4.0
Positive control N	23 ± 4.3 [a]	310 ± 20.0	63 ± 5.6
Control JC	36 ± 6.0	285 ± 24.3	60 ± 3.7
	Melanoma MG	Colon carcinoma	
Melanoma AP	448 ± 17.7 [a]	11 ± 1.1	
Control JC	513 ± 29.4	11 ± 1.0	
Colon CA B (Post 5-FU)	514 ± 29.5	14 ± 1.4	
	Melanoma LC	Carcinoma ovary	
Melanoma G	128 ± 7.9 [b]	78 ± 7.9 [a]	
Control AF	222 ± 14.3	98 ± 4.8	
	Melanoma ME	Melanoma LC	Carcinoma ovary
Melanoma F	80 ± 6.8 [a]	963 ± 22.3 [b]	135 ± 10.4
Control JC	99 ± 8.2	1330 ± 72.0	138 ± 18.8
	Melanoma LC	Carcinoma ovary	
Positive control N	146 ± 12.7 [a]	681 ± 66.6	
Control JC	195 ± 11.1	596 ± 51.7	

[a] $P \leqq 0.05$. — [b] $P \leqq 0.001$.

Demonstration of specificity entailed the use of tumor target cell lines other than melanoma (Table 4). Here lines derived from human colon, parotid and ovarian carcinoma were all unaffected by melanoma lymphocytes, while melanoma cells were uniformly killed to a significant extent. The only exception was one ovarian carcinoma cell line.

Where patients with different stages and activity of disease had been included in the same assay, we observed significantly higher levels of cell-mediated immunity in patients free of disease or with disease regressing after therapy. Following chemotherapy (5-day courses of DTIC), a 4-week rest period was allowed prior to performing the assay. To compare the levels of cell-mediated immunity (CMI) among all patients tested, the actual percentage of cytotoxicity was adjusted for variations in sensitivity between target cell lines and within a line from time to time by the use of a positive control as a standard. The control subject had a family history of melanoma, no evident disease, and had melanoma-specific immunity on repeat testing. The same negative control was used in the majority of assays. The median cytotoxicity values (Table 5) were higher in disease-free or regressing patients than in BCG

Table 5. Correlation of cell-mediated immunity with clinical status

	% cell-mediated cytotoxicity (corrected values)		
	No systemic treatment	BCG then DTIC therapy (chemotherapy)	
Disease-free or Regressing	Positive control = 40%		
	SH 36%	AP 59%	
	F 44%	TH 39%	
	Median = 40%	Median = 47%	
Progressing	JM 33%	ME 23%	BR 20%
	D 17/33%	KPL 23%	CY 0%
		LH 32%	ET 0%
		GR 35%	JB 0%
	Median = 24/33%	Median = 26% (zero values excluded)	

progressors and patients in whom chemotherapy had failed. The explanation for this may be the recently reported phenomenon of rebound hyperimmunity in chemotherapy responders and persistent immunosuppression in nonresponders [7, 19, 20]. The two untreated "progressor" patients showed higher levels of immunity, but one had progression only in the central nervous system, and the other was clinically free of disease 6 weeks after excision of positive axillary nodes and re-excision of a wound abcess containing tumor in its margins; on the basis of node metastases the likelihood of distant spread was considered high. The double value shown was the result of the technical mishap described earlier.

Blocking effects of sera are shown in Table 6.

All but two progressors showed blocking. The two without blocking were unusual, as noted above; if these are excluded from the table, the P value associating blocking with progression increases from 0.027 to 0.004 (Fisher's Exact Test). Patient sera produced several other striking effects. An example is shown in Table 7. The upper panel illustrates the typical cytotoxic effect of autochthonous immune lymphocytes compared with control cells. Patient serum produced blocking but, in the presence of control lymphocytes, significant tumor cell death was induced. That this effect was reproducible is shown in the lower set of data obtained with 6-mm diameter wells, and lymphocytes purified by glass absorption after gelatin sedimentation. Significant CMI was not detected in any of the melanoma patients compared to controls. The effect of ME serum, however, may be discerned as similar to that seen in the first experiment. There was slight blocking with ME lymphocytes, and an opposite effect with allogeneic melanoma and cancer control lymphocytes. The pooled statistics on the latter group show significant induction of cyto-

Table 6. Serum blocking factors

	Absent or negative	Positive
Disease-free or regressing	5	0
Progressing	2	5

(Patients without significant cell-mediated immunity excluded from table.)

Table 7. Serum "arming" factors

Lymphocyte donor	Melanoma ME pretreated with		
	Control serum	ME serum	P
Melanoma ME [a]	149 ± 9.8	264 ± 16.0	0.01
Control C	193 ± 10.6	140 ± 9.0	0.01
Melanoma ME [b]	27 ± 2.0	37 ± 3.5	NS
Melanoma KPL	51 ± 4.3	28 ± 5.0	NS
Melanoma M	28 ± 7.3	14 ± 4.7	NS
Colon carcinoma	34 ± 5.3	18 ± 2.9	NS
Breast carcinoma B [c]	7.8 ± 1.4	2.8 ± 0.75	NS
Pooled minus ME	30 ± 2.6	16 ± 1.9	0.01+

[a] Large wells.
[b] 6 mm wells.
[c] Significant contamination with polymorphonuclear leukocytes.

toxicity by serum. This effect we have termed "arming". Such phenomena include: 1. cytotoxicity induced with control lymphocytes by blocking serum; 2. augmentation of cytotoxicity of autochthonous lymphocytes or "negative blocking"; and 3. augmentation or negative blocking with allogeneic melanoma lymphocytes, a phenomenon similar to the deblocking reaction.

Arming of control lymphocytes was seen with four sera, all from progressors. Three patients (ME, KPL, LH) also showed blocking effect for autochthonous immune cells. One patient, (D), free of gross disease following axillary dissection, showed "negative blocking" of her own cytotoxic lymphocytes. Patient F, disease-free one year after local excision of a melanoma, showed autochthonous arming without arming of control lymphocytes. Regressor AP's serum was tested for deblocking, but alone at a 1 : 6 dilution increased the median cytotoxicity of progressor lymphocytes from 23% to 53%. When diluted further and added to progressor serum (which had no blocking activity), cytotoxicity increased significantly to 66%. There was no effect on control lymphocytes.

Discussion

There are *three* fundamental questions one must consider in evaluating the data from our assay. First, does the *in vitro* phenomenon represent an immunologic reaction? The evidence for this is apparent specificity shown in Table 4 and more rigorously demonstrated by the Hellstroms elsewhere [21]. Second, does the antigen against which the *in vitro* reaction is directed exist on tumor cells *in vivo*? There is are suggestions that the cross-reactive membrane antigen of melanoma cells is only expressed after a period of *in vivo* culture [13, 15, 28, 33]. This would imply that fluctuations in the levels of CMI *in vivo* could represent nonspecific or anamnestic changes in the host. The recent demonstration in animal-tumor models that blocking factors may be antigen–antibody complexes [2, 41] is the only evidence we know of apart from data on CEA (carcinoembryonic antigen) which indicates that the cross-reactive membrane antigen may persist in man even in advanced disease. Even though we have not been able to demonstrate it on the surface of freshly prepared tumor cells, immune reactions to it may possibly be useful. Nevertheless, uncertainty remains on this third question: "Is such an immune reaction detected *in vitro* beneficial to the tumor-bearing host, and if not, can it be made so?" We think it more appropriate to speak at present of *cell-mediated killing* (CMK) *in vitro*, rather than CMI. The inference that CMK represents a true state of immunity *in vivo* depends entirely on clinical correlations!

The correlation between the levels of CMK and disease behavior interests us greatly. We find a decreased level of measurable CMK in progressors, although the possible contribution of chemotherapy to this observation has been noted. Although the Hellströms originally denied significant correlations between CMK and tumor behavior [21, 23], recently after titrating their effector cell concentrations they admitted that the correlation does exist [22]. The MIF studies of Cochrane [10] and Spitler [43] also support our observation. Barski *et al.* [27] found markedly decreased immunity in peritoneal exidate cells as tumor size increased. O'Toole and Perlmann [34, 37], using Teresaki microplates, obtained similar data in human bladder carcinoma. de Vries did not find the decrease, but did not titrate his effector cell dose [15]. Others such as Currie [13] and Fossatti [18] have had less success with the microplates (Teresaki type): our experience suggests that larger wells improve the sensitivity of the assay. Using microplates, O'Toole and Perlmann [34, 35, 37] found that immunity waned in tumor-free patients, in contrast to the results obtained by the Hellströms [21] and ourselves, that reactions can be demonstrated in patients who have been tumor-free for several years. These discrepancies emphasize the difficulties inherent in *in vitro* assays; these arise both from technical factors and from the heterogeneity of the effector cell population being studied.

Technical factors include such variables as washing the plates at the end of the incubation period, growth state of the target cell, number of target cells plated, fetal calf serum, method of preparation of lymphocytes. The latter may be critical. So-called "pure" lymphocyte preparations contain small numbers of polymorphonuclear leukocytes, esterase-positive monocytes [47], hemopoietic progenitor cells (CFU-C for example), and may be enriched or depleted of certain subtypes of B and T cells. Some of these cell types may produce nonspecific toxicity in either control or tumor-patient test wells; others may be essential in amplifying a very weak T-cell response. Moreover, the purification may alter the inherent character of the effector T lymphocytes. Such cells may be made tolerant, or inactivated, by surface-bound antigen *in vivo,* both in normal hosts [5] where such antigen may prevent autoaggression, and in tumor-bearing animals [2, 41]. Washing the cells free of such antigen and increasing their agglutination to target cells, as seems to occur with Hypaque-Ficoll separation [8] may change the *in vitro* reaction of such cells completely. The addition of such cells to targets in the absence of serum may also be important. In the MIF system, a positive reaction to allogeneic membranes by lymphocytes of kidney transplant recipients or melanoma patients (using tumor membranes) can easily be demonstrated if the reaction takes place in serum-free medium. However, normal human AB serum abrogates the reaction except in those transplant recipients who have only recently converted to positive [17]. This serum effect does not occur when an antigen such as PPD is tested. A component of the *in vitro* killing may be due to "tolerant" T lymphocytes which would never act aggressively *in vivo.*

In addition to these variables, the observation that non-T cells may kill tumor targets [14, 38] may account for discrepant observations among investigators. Evidence that "killer cells" in man may be other than T cells is provided by the reduction in killing by some cell preparations after passage through an anti-immunoglobulin coated column [37]. Denham has reported a dual effector population [14]. The arming phenomenon, in contrast to direct lymphocyto-toxicity appears to be mitomycin resistant [8, 9, 29]. By rigorously investigating which cell is producing the *in vitro* killing, we hope to understand which *in vitro* reactions indicate whether the tumor will regress in the patient.

Blocking reactions seem to correlate with tumor progression [24], but exceptions occur. In one patient followed serially, blocking was absent after a 5-day course of DTIC therapy. Several months later, striking blocking was seen, but two months before death, blocking was again absent. On each occasion, however, the tumor progressed during periods of blocking, but did not regress in the face of measurable CMI and no blocking. A similar phenomenon has been reported by Byrne *et al.* [6] and more recently by Cummings *et al.* [12]. In part the explanation may lie in the observations of Baldwin [2], who noted that tumor-specific antibody blocks colony inhibition by killer lymphocytes as antigen is added; and then blocking diminishes to zero as the antigen concentration increases still further. Antigen may block *in vivo* [5, 37, 41] and may lower the level of cytotoxic lymphocytes by sequestration in the reticulo-endothelial system [1, 40], sometimes with the assistance of antibody [44]. If effector cells are washed free of this "tolerogen", they may not be reblocked on exposure to serum *in vitro.* We would be less misled about the true state of circulating cell-mediated immunity *in vivo* if unmodified (i.e. not extensively washed) effector cells, albeit ineffective killers, were used. Serum antibodies have fallen into disrepute as a result of the association of immunologic enhancement *in vivo* with blocking *in vitro*. Antibodies may prevent metastasis [28, 39] and stop tumor growth [3, 36], while enhancing antibodies may render macrophages cytotoxic *in vitro* [11]. It is clear by now that before meaningful correlations can be put to clinical use, we must critically analyze the assays. To obtain cause-effect correlation, we must study these parameters in tumor model systems which closely mirror the human disease.

Conclusions

1. Cell-mediated immunity and serum blocking may be monitored *in vitro* using cell lines.

2. Failure of systemic therapy is associated with reduced levels of cell-mediated immunity and the presence of serum blocking factors at some time in the course of the patient's illness.

3. Tumors progress in the face of cell-mediated immunity and the absence of blocking for reasons which are not yet clear.

4. Serum effects, particularly the induction of cytotoxicity are far more striking than the effects of immune lymphocytes alone. It would be premature to define humoral reaction and B cells as harmful to the tumor-bearing host.

5. Tumor patient X's serum cannot be reliably tested for blocking with allogeneic immune lymphocytes from patient Y and tumor from patient X, Y, or Z because an "arming" reaction may obscure a blocking effect which is actually occurring in X.

References

1. Alexander, P., Hall, J. G.: The role of immunoblasts in host resistance and immunotherapy of primary sarcomata. Advanc. Cancer Res. **13**, 1 (1970).
2. Baldwin, R. W., Price, M. R., Robins, R. A.: Blocking of lymphocyte mediated cytotoxicity for rat hepatoma cells by tumor-specific antigen-antibody complexes. Nature New Biol. **238**, 185 (1972).
3. Bansal, S. C., Sjogren, H. O.: Counteraction of the blocking of cell-mediated tumor immunity by inoculation of unblocking sera and splenectomy: Immunotherapeutic effects in primary polyoma tumor in rats. Int. J. Cancer **9**, 490 (1972).
4. Bluming, A. A., Vogel, C. L., Ziegler, J. L., Kiryabwire, J. W. M.: Delayed cutaneous sensitivity reactions to extracts of autologous malignant melanoma: A second look. J. nat. Cancer Inst. **48**, 17 (1972).
5. Brawn, R. J.: *In vitro* desensitization of sensitized murine lymphocytes by a serum factor (soluble antigen?). Proc. nat. Acad. Sci. (Wash.) **68**, 1634 (1971).
6. Byrne, M. J., Heppner, G., Stolbach, L., Cummings, F. J., McDonough, E., Calabresi, P.: Correlation of tumor specific immunity with extent of disease in malignant melanoma. Proc. Amer. Ass. Cancer Res. **13**, 46 (1972).
7. Cheema, A. R., Hersh, E. M.: Patient survival after chemotherapy and its relationship to *in vitro* lymphocyte blastogenesis. Cancer (Philad.) **28**, 851 (1971).
8. Clark, D. A., Nathanson, L.: Cellular immunity in malignant melanoma. Proc. Int. Cancer Conference and VIIIth Int. Pigment Cell Meeting pp. 350-359. Basel: Karger 1973.
9. Clark, D. A., Nathanson, L.: Cellular immunity (CMI) in malignant melanoma. Proc. Amer. Ass. Cancer Res. **13**, 79 (1972).
10. Cochrane, A. J., Jehn, U., Cothoskar, B.: Cell mediated immunity to malignant melanoma. Lancet **1972 I**, 1340.

11. CRUSE, J. M., WHITTEN, H. D., LEWIS, G. K., WATSON, E. S.: Facilitation of macrophage-mediated destruction of allogeneic fibrosarcoma cells by tumor-enhancing IgG 2 *in vitro*. Transplant. Proc. **5**, 961 (1973).
12. CUMMINGS, F. J., HEPPNER, G. H., BYRNE, M., STOLBACH, L., CALABRESI, P.: Effects of chemotherapy on cell-mediated immunity and serum blocking factors in malignant melanoma. Proc. Amer. Ass. Cancer Res. **14**, 122 (1973).
13. CURRIE, G. A., LEJEUNE, F., HAMILTON, FAIRLEY G.: Immunization with irradiated tumor cells and specific lymphocyte cytotoxicity in malignant melanoma. Brit. med. J. **1971 I**, 305.
14. DENHAM, S., GRANT, C. K., J. G. ALEXANDER, P.: The occurance of two types of cytotoxic lymphoid cells in mice immunized with allogeneic tumor cells. Transplantation **9**, 366 (1970).
15. DE VRIES, J. E., RUMKLE, P., BERNHEIM, J. L.: Cytotoxic lymphocytes in melanoma patients. Int. J. Cancer **9**, 567 (1972).
16. EVERSON, T. C., COLE, W. H.: In: The spontaneous regression of cancer. Philadelphia: Saunders 1966.
17. FALK, R. E., MANN, P. L., COWAN, D., LANGER, B.: A study of cell-mediated immunity in human neoplasia. Ann. roy. Coll. Phys. Surg. Canad. **42**, 33 (1973).
18. FOSSATI, G., COLNAGHI, M. I., DELLA PORTA, G., CASCINELLI, N., VERONESI, U.: Cellular and humoral immunity against human malignant melanoma. Int. J. Cancer **8**, 344 (1971).
19. HALTERMAN, R. H., LEVENTHAL, B. G.: Enhanced immune response to leukemia. Lancet **1971 II**, 704.
20. HARRIS, J., BAGAI, R., STEWART, T.: Immunocompentence and response to antitumor treatment. New Engl. J. Med. **286**, 494 (1972).
21. HELLSTROM, I., HELLSTROM, K. E., SJOGREN, H. O., WARNER, G. A.: Demonstration of cell-mediated immunity to human neoplasms of various histologic types. Int. J. Cancer **7**, 1 (1971).
22. HELLSTROM, I., HELLSTROM, K. E.: Some recent studies on cellular immunity to human melannomas. Fed. Prod. **32**, 156 (1973).
23. HELLSTROM, I., HELLSTROM, K. E., SJOGREN, H. O.: Serum mediated inhibition of cellular immunity to methylcholanthrene-induced sarcomas. Cell. Immunol. **1**, 18 (1970).
24. HELLSTROM, I., SJOGREN, H. O., WARNER, G. A., HELLSTROM, K. E.: Blocking of cell-mediated tumor immunity by sera from patients with growing neoplasms. Int. J. Cancer **7**, 226 (1971).
25. JEHN, U., NATHANSON, L., SCHWARTZ, R. S.: *In vitro* lymphocyte stimulation by a soluble antigen from malignant melanoma. New Engl. J. Med. **283**, 329 (1970).
26. LLOYD, O. C.: Regression of malignant melanoma as a manifestation of a cellular immune response. Proc. roy. Soc. Med. **62**, 543 (1969).
27. LEFRANCOIS, D., YOUN, J. K., BLECHRADEK, J., BARSKI, G.: Evolution of cell-mediated immunity in mice bearing tumors produced by a mammary carcinoma cell line: Influence of tumor growth, surgical removal, and treatment with irradiated tumor cells. J. nat. Cancer Inst. **46**, 981 (1971).
28. LEWIS, M. G., IKONOPISOV, R. C., NAIRN, R. C., PHILLIPS, T. M., HAMILTON FAIRLEY, G. H., BODENHAM, D. C., ALEXANDER, P.: Tumor specific antibodies in human malignant melanoma and their relationship to extent of disease. Brit. med. J. **1969 III**, 547.
29. MOLLER, G., LUNDGREN, G.: Aggressive lymphocytes and sensitive target cells: Two pathways for cytotoxicity. In: Cellular recognition (SMITH, R. T., GOOD, R. A., Eds.). New York: Appleton-Century-Crofts 1969.
30. MUKHERJI, B., FLOWERS, A., NATHANSON, L., CLARK, D. A.: Heterotransplantation study of human melanoma. Cancer Research **34**, 43 (1974).
31. NAGEL, G. A., ST.-ARNEAULT, G., HOLLAND, J. F., KIRKPATRICK, D., KIRKPATRICK, K. R.: Cell-mediated immunity against malignant melanoma in monozygous twins. Cancer Res. **30**, 1828 (1970).
32. NATHANSON, L., JEHN, U., SCHWARTZ, R. S.: Disappearance of a tumor-associated antigen in malignant melanoma after imidazole carboxamide therapy. Cancer (Philad.) **27**, 411 (1971).
33. OETTGEN, H. F., BEAN, M. A., KLEIN, G.: Workshop in human tumor immunology. Cancer Res. **32**, 2845 (1972).
34. O'TOOLE, C. O., PERLMANN, P., UNSGAARD, B., MOBERGER, G., EDSMYR, F.: Cellular immunity in human urinary bladder carcinoma. I. Correlation to clinical stage and radiotherapy Int. J. Cancer **10**, 77 (1972)

35. O'TOOLE, C. O., PERLMANN, P., UNSGAARD, B., MOBERGER, G., EDSMYR, F.: Cellular immunity to human urinary bladder carcinoma. II. Effect of surgery and pre-operative irradiation. Int. J. Cancer **10**, 92 (1972).
36. PEARSON, G. R., REDMAN, L. W., BASS, L. R.: Protective effect of immune sera against transplantable moloney virus-induced sarcoma and lymphoma. Cancer Res. **33**, 171 (1973).
37. PERLMANN, P., O'TOOLE, C. O.: Cellular and humoral mechanisms of tumor destruction. In: Proc. Immunol. Carcinogenesis Conference, May 1972. Nat. Cancer Inst. Monograph 35 (in press).
38. PERLMANN, P., HOLM, G.: Cytotoxic effect of lymphoid cell *in vitro*. Adv. Immunol. **11**, 117 (1969).
39. PROCTOR, J. W., RUDENSTAN, C. M., ALEXANDER, P.: A factor preventing the development of lung metastases in rats with sarcomas. Nature (Lond.) **242**, 29 (1973).
40. SCHLOSSMAN, S. F., LEVIN, J. A., ROCKLIN, R. E., DAVID, J. R.: The compartmentalization of antigen-reactive lymphocytes in desensitized guinea pigs. J. exp. Med. **134**, 741 (1971).
41. SJOGREN, H. O., HELLSTROM, I., BANSAL, S. C., WARNER, G. A., HELLSTROM, K. E.: Elution of blocking factors from human tumors, capable of abrogating tumor cell destruction by specifically immune lymphocytes. Int. J. Cancer **9**, 274 (1972).
42. SNEDECOR, G. W., COCHRANE, W. G.: In: Statistical methods. Ames, Iowa: Iowa State University Press 1971.
43. SPITLER, L. E.: Transfer factor therapy of malignant melanoma. Clin. Res. **21**, 654 (1973).
44. STUTMAN, O.: Lymphocyte sequestration: Its possible role in tumor immunity. Transplant. Proc. **5**, 969 (1973).
45. TAYLOR, G., ODILI, J. L. I.: Histologic evidence of tumor regression after active immunotherapy in human malignant disease. Brit. med. J. **1972 II**, 183.
46. WOODS, A. H.: A closed system for large scale lymphocyte purification. Blood **35**, 39 (1970).
47. YAM, L. T., LI, C. Y., CROSBY, W. H.: Cytochemical identification of monocytes and granulocytes. Amer. J. clin. Path. **55**, 283 (1971).

Lymphocyte-Defined Histocompatibility Differences as a Model for Tumor Antigens*

M. B. WIDMER, MIRIAM SEGALL [1], F. H. BACH, and MARILYN L. BACH [2]

Laboratory of Genetics, University of Wisconsin, Madison, Wisconsin

Reactivity of lymphocytes in mixed leukocyte culture (MLC) [2, 8] for the most part reflects disparity for the major histocompatibility complex (MHC). The MHC contains loci which control the serologically defined antigens (H-2 of mouse or HL-A of man). However, evidence in the mouse points to the existence of other MHC differences which cannot be detected serologically, but which can lead to MLC activation, and in some cases to graft rejection. This evidence has been extensively reviewed in previous publications [4, 5] and will only be summarized here; the possible relationship of these findings to the detection and definition of tumor antigens will be discussed.

We use the following abbreviations and terms. The general term MHC refers to the chromosomal segment where the major histocompatibility loci are located. These loci are of two types: SD (serologically defined) loci controlling the serologically detectable antigens (H-2K and H-2D in the mouse, Four and LA in man); and LD (lymphocyte-defined) loci, the products of which are very difficult to detect serologically using standard methods of immunization and testing, but which can be detected by *in vitro* lymphocyte responses.

Mouse strains that have been studied have been maintained in our laboratory from pedigreed breeding pairs kindly supplied by Dr. G. SNELL, Bar Harbor Laboratories, Bar Harbor, Maine, or been obtained from Drs. J. KLEIN, D. SHREFFLER, and J. STIMPFLING whom we thank for their collaboration. Most of the strains used in these studies are either coisogenic (genetically identical except for differences due to a single mutation in the MHC, or congenic) genetically identical except for the MHC. The genotypes of the different strains are given (Table 1) to indicate which H-2 allele is present for the two SD loci (H-2K and H-2D) and for the immune response (Ir-1) locus [15]. Also included are the alleles of the Ss locus (Ss^h determining a high level of the Ss serum protein, Ss^l a 20-fold lower amount) and the Slp locus (which may be the same as the Ss locus) [16]. The Slp antigen is present only in males and then only when the Slp^a allele is present; this antigen is not detected when

* Supported by NIH grants AI 08439 and GM 15422, ONR grant N 00014-67-A-0128-0003, and National Foundation March of Dimes grant CRBS 246.

[1] NIH trainee from NIGMS (Grant No. GM 00398).

[2] MLB is a recipient of the Faculty Research Award of the American Cancer Society.

the Slp° allele is present. The mice can differ for any one or more of these 4 loci and for other, as yet undefined loci within each region.

The method for culturing is similar to that used for human cultures [12]. A brief description of the method follows. Mouse spleen cells are cultured in RPMI 1640 (Gibco, Grand Island, New York) supplemented with penicillin (100 units/ml), streptomycin 100 μg/ml) and heat-treated (56° for 30 min) human plasma obtained from a frozen pool (5 ml/100 ml) [6]. Responding cells and mitomycin C-treated stimulating cells [3] are cultured in 0.2 ml volumes in Linbro microtiter plates (IS-FB-96-TC) at concentrations of 10^6 stimulating and responding cells per well. After 72 h of incubation in a humidified 5% CO^2, 95% air atmosphere, 2 μCi tritiated

Table 1. MHC regions of various mouse strains

		H-2K	Ir-1	Ss-Slp	H-2D
a)		H-2K	Ir-1	Ss-Slp	H-2D
b)	H-2a/b	$H\text{-}2K^k$	$Ir\text{-}1^k$	$Ss\text{-}Slp^d$	$H\text{-}2D^d$
	heterozygote	$H\text{-}2K^b$	$Ir\text{-}1^b$	$Ss\text{-}Slp^b$	$H\text{-}2D^b$
	B 10.A(1R)	$H\text{-}2K^k$	$Ir\text{-}1^k$	$Ss\text{-}Slp^d$	$H\text{-}2D^b$
	B 10.A(2R)	$H\text{-}2K^k$	$Ir\text{-}1^k$	$Ss\text{-}Slp^d$	$H\text{-}2D^b$
	B 10.A(4R)	$H\text{-}2K^k$	$Ir\text{-}1^k$	$Ss\text{-}Slp^b$	$H\text{-}2D^b$
c)	AQR	$H\text{-}2K^q$	$Ir\text{-}1^k$	$Ss\text{-}Slp^d$	$H\text{-}2D^d$
	B 10.T(6R)	$H\text{-}2K^q$	$Ir\text{-}1^q$	$Ss\text{-}Slp^d$	$H\text{-}2D^d$
	B 10.A	$H\text{-}2K^k$	$Ir\text{-}1^k$	$Ss\text{-}Slp^d$	$H\text{-}2D^d$

Superscripts in this table refer to the MHC chromosomes from which a given region is derived. There is evidence which suggests that more than one Ir locus may be present in the Ir-1 region. It has recently been reported that B10.A(2R) and B10.A(4R) mice differ in their Ir loci (R. LIEBERMAN, Fed. Proc. 31, 777, 1972). The B10.T(6R) strain was derived from a B10.A/B10.G heterozygote. AQR was derived from T-138 (H-2^q) which has an SD locus indistinguishable from B10.G.

thymidine (sp. act. 1.9 Ci/mmole; Schwartz Bioresearch, Orangeburg, New York) is added to the cultures. 16 h later, cultures are precipitated onto glass-fiber filters [13] and assayed for uptake of ^{3}H-TdR by liquid scintillation spectrophotometry.

We have recently obtained evidence for the existence of LD differences in the MHC which are not detectable serologically with the usual methods of immunization and testing but which cause stimulation in MLC. BAILEY *et al.* have discovered a spontaneous mutation in the MHC of C57BL/6 mice [7]. Except for this mutation, the mutant mice (H(z1)) are genetically identical to C57BL/6 mice, including serological identity for H-2K and H-2D; however, there is reciprocal skin graft rejection. The position of the mutation within the MHC is not further defined except that it is to the left of Ss-Slp (Table 1a). Despite extensive immunization schedules, BAILEY *et al.* were unable to produce agglutinating or cytotoxic antisera against the "difference" [7]. There is stimulation in both directions in 4 separate MLC tests; a representative experiment is shown in Table 2a. In each case there is a significantly higher incorporation of tritiated thymidine in the allogeneic mixtures than in the control isogeneic ones. There is thus reciprocal MLC stimulation as there is reciprocal skin-graft rejection.

Table 2. Mixed lymphocyte culture results in various mouse strain combinations

Responding cells	Stimulating cells		
	C 57 B L/6	H(z1)	B 10.D2
C 57 B L/6	(5567 ± 516)[a]	23756 ± 1191 $p < 0.001$[b]	66305 ± 7512 $p < 0.001$
H(z 1)	15545 ± 2496 $p < 0.001$	(5453 ± 494)	103279 ± 3567 $p < 0.001$
B 10.D2	139685 ± 5501 $p < 0.001$	84931 ± 7211 $p < 0.001$	(3569 ± 650)

Responding cells	Stimulating cells			
	B 10.A (1 R)	B 10.A (2 R)	B 10.A (4 R)	B 10.D2
B 10.A (1 R)	(5500 ± 1100)	5058 ± 1517 $p > 0.5$	5081 ± 1410 $p > 0.5$	27691 ± 3080 $p < 0.001$
B 10.A (2 R)	5590 ± 1045 $p > 0.2$	(5644 ± 1816)	5947 ± 1316 $p > 0.5$	25462 ± 1457 $p < 0.001$
B 10.A (4 R)	5976 ± 1412 $p < 0.001$	5472 ± 201 $p < 0.001$	(1926 ± 304)	22952 ± 2487 $p < 0.001$
B 10.D 2	49868 ± 8010 $p < 0.001$	41911 ± 11244 $p < 0.001$	23918 ± 5667 $p < 0.001$	(3898 ± 472)

Responding cells	Stimulating cells		
	AQR	B 10.T (6 R)	B 10.A
AQR	(3567 ± 1190)	32087 ± 1900 $p < 0.001$	7869 ± 439 $0.01 < p < 0.025$
B 10.T (6 R)	44181 ± 2071 $p < 0.001$	(3440 ± 1409)	52402 ± 4292 $p < 0.001$
B 10.A	8425 ± 722 $0.01 < p < 0.2$	25823 ± 1583 $p < 0.001$	(6856 ± 1416)

[a] Counts per minute ± standard deviation.

[b] p value for t-test on log transformed data comparing each allogeneic mixture with the appropriate isogeneic control (given in parentheses).

Several strain combinations with SD loci identity have been tested. One set of 3 strains, B10.A(1R), B10.A(2R) and B10.A(4R), is of special interest since these strains were derived from different crossovers from the same F_1 genotype. The genotypes of the H-2^a/H-2^b F_1 heterozygote and the three resultant recombinant chromosomes are given in Table 1b. 1R and 2R are identical for the available markers, although the recombinational events may well have taken place at different positions. Both 1R and 2R cells reproducibly and significantly stimulate cells of the 4R strain; however, there is very weak or no response of 1R and 2R cells to 4R stimulating cells (Table 2b). Since this unidirectional response is an unusual finding, we have tested the cells of these strains at multiple concentrations of stimulating and responding cells assayed on several days to maximize response; an occasional weak but significant response of 1R or 2R to 4R stimulating cells was seen, but for the most part there has been no stimulation in these mixtures. The Slp antigen does not appear to be responsible for these results, as stimulation occurs in mixtures of female cells where the Slp antigen is not expressed [4, 5]. It is known that there are loci in the MHC which affect susceptibility to viral infections; perhaps the 1R and 2R cells carry viral antigens which are recognized by the 4R cells.

The other strain combination of great interest is AQR, B10.T(6R) and B10.A, the MHC genotypes of which are given in Table 1c. AQR and B10.T(6R) mice differ for Ir-1 [14] and Slp (Klein, unpublished) are identical for H-2K and H-2D, yet their cells stimulate in MLC. One representative MLC experiment of the 4 we have done is shown in Table 2c.

There are two possible interpretations for the reciprocal stimulation in the AQR-6R combination: a) there may be a gene or genes between H-2K and H-2D the product of which can lead to stimulation of the responding cells in MLC; b) since AQR and 6R mice have different minor histocompatibility loci as well as different MHC, differences in minor histocompatibility loci may cause the MLC stimulation. Arguing against the second possibility is the negative or weak MLC response between AQR and B10.A cells as compared to the much stronger response between AQR and 6R, even though B10.A and 6R are congenic resistant and therefore carry the same alleles at minor loci. Whereas one might still argue that there is an interaction between the MHC and the minor loci in the AQR-6R mixtures, such a hypothesis requires further assumptions and thus seems less likely. The Slp antigen would seem an unlikely cause for the MLC stimulation since reciprocal one-way MLC tests are positive and the Slp antigen incompatibility exists in only one direction. Extensive studies have tended to rule out a role for the Slp antigen in homograft reactions [16].

The suggestion by Amos and Bach [1] that there may be an LD locus linked to the SD loci in man has received support from similar studies [17], the more informative family studies of Yunis and Amos [18], and other extensive studies [10]. Our present studies in the mouse provide direct evidence for the existence of genetic differences in the MHC which lead to MLC activation and which cannot be defined serologically by means of the usual methods for immunization and testing. In some cases the LD loci of the MHC are genetically separable from the SD loci.

The nature of these LD loci is presently unknown. In some combinations which are described here, and in other combinations which we have studied, the LD locus (loci) maps genetically with the Ir-1 locus [4]. Our studies of a number of mouse strains suggest that the greatest responses in MLC are frequently associated with Ir region differences [5] whereas Ir region identity is at least sometimes associated with very weak or absent stimulation in MLC. It may be, in fact, that although no cytotoxic or agglutinating antibody is produced against the LD product, a blocking antibody is synthesized [9].

The LD loci discussed above have been mapped within the MHC. There is evidence for LD loci segregating independently of the MHC, differences for which also result in MLC stimulation [11]. The existence of such loci is obviously of importance in the consideration of tumor-specefic antigens which may provoke the formation of blocking antibody but which are difficult to detect serologically by agglutination or cytotoxicity determinations.

A major problem in certain forms of tumors has been the apparent paradox that, while transplantation antigens are evidenced by *in vivo* studies, there is inability to produce satisfactory agglutinating or cytotoxic antibodies against the presumed transplantation antigen. The work we have presented in this paper concerning the lymphocyte-defined differences of the MHC in mice, which likewise have not so far been defined with the usual methods of immunization and serological testing but which can lead to MLC activation and in some cases graft rejection, may provide a model for the tumor system. The importance of obtaining a molecular, cellular and (hopefully) serological (blocking antibody) definition of the phenotypic products of the LD loci is obvious. It should be possible to extrapolate the results of such studies to questions of tumor immunity.

References

1. Amos, D. B., Bach, F. H.: Phenotypic expressions of the major histocompatibility locus in man (HL-A): leukocyte antigens and mixed leukocyte culture reactivity. J. exp. Med. **128**, 623 (1968).
2. Bach, F H., Hirschhorn, K.: Lymphocyte interaction: a potential *in vitro* histocompatibility test. Science **143**, 813 (1964).
3. Bach, F. H., Voynow, N. K.: One-way stimulation in mixed leukocyte culture. Science **153**, 545 (1966).
4. Bach, F. H., Widmer, M. B., Segall, M., Bach, M. L., Klein, J.: Genetic and immunological complexity of major histocompatibility regions. Science **176**, 1024 (1972a)
5. Bach, F. H., Widmer, M. B., Bach, M. L., Klein, J.: Serologically defined and lymphocyte-defined components of the major histocompatibility complex in the mouse. J. exp. Med. **136**, 1430 (1972b).
6. Bach, M. L., Solliday, S., Stambuk, M.: Detection of disparity in the mixed leukocyte culture test: a more rapid assay. In: Histocompatibility Testing 1970 (Terasaki, P. I., Ed.), p. 643. Copenhagen: Munksgaard 1970.
7. Bailey, D. W., Snell, G. D., Cheery, M.: Complementation and serological analysis of an H-2 mutant. In: Proc. Symp. Immunogenetics of the H-2 System, p. 165. Basel: Karger 1971.
8. Bain, B., Vas, M. R., Lowenstein, L.: The development of large immature mononuclear cells in mixed leukocyte cultures. Blood **23**, 108 (1964).
9. Ceppellini, R.: Old and new facts and speculations about transplantation antigens of man. In: Progress in Immunology (Amos, E. B., Ed.), p. 973. New York, London: Academic Press 1971.
10. Eijsvoogel, V. P., Koning, L., Groot-Kooy, L., Huismans, L., van Rood, J. J., *et al.*: Mixed lymphocyte culture and HL-A Transplant Proc **4**, 199 (1972)
11 Festenstein, H , Abbasi, K , Sachs, J A , Oliver, R T : Serologically undetectable immune responses in transplantation Transplant Proc **4**, 219 (1972)
12 Hartzman, R H, Segall, M , Bach, M L , Bach, F H : Histocompatibility matching VI Miniaturization of the mixed leukocyte culture test: a preliminary report. Transplant. **11**, 268 (1971).
13. Hartzman, R. H., Bach, M. L., Bach, F. H., Thurman, G. B., Sell, K. W.: Precipitation of radioactively labeled samples: a semi-automatic multiple-sample processor. Cell. Immunol. **4**, 182 (1972).
14. Klein, J., Klein, D., Shreffler, D. C.: H-2 types of stocks T(2; 9)138Ca, T(9; 13)190Ca and an H-2 recombinant. Transplant. **10**, 309 (1970).
15. McDevitt, H. O., Benacerraf, B.: Histocompatibility-linked immune response genes. Science **175**, 273 (1972).
16. Passmore, H. C., Shreffler, D. C.: A sex-linked serum protein variant in the mouse: inheritance and association with the H-2 region. Biochem. Genet. **4**, 351 (1970).
17. Plate, J. M., Ward, F. E., Amos, D. B.: The mixed leukocyte culture response between HL-A identical siblings. In: Histocompatibility Testing 1970 (Terasaki, P. I., Ed.), p. 531. Kopenhagen: Munksgaard 1970.
18. Yunis, E. J., Amos, D. B.: Three closely linked genetic systems relevant to transplantation. Proc. nat. Acad. Sci. (Wash.) **68**, 3031 (1971).

Cell-Mediated Immunity to Human Solid Tumors: *in vitro* Detection by Lymphocyte Blastogenic Responses to Cell-Associated and Solubilized Tumor Antigens*

G. M. Mavligit, J. U. Gutterman, Ch. M. McBride, and E. M. Hersh

Section of Immunology Department of Developmental Therapeutics and Department of Surgery, The University of Texas, M. D. Anderson Hospital and Tumor Institute at Houston, Houston, Texas

Introduction

Studies during the past 7 years have demonstrated tumor-specific antigens in most human solid tumors [15, 27, 28]. In general, more importance was attached to cell-mediated immunity than to humoral immunity in the host's immune defense against solid tumors, since transplantation experiments have shown that effective tumor immunity is based on lymphocytic mechanisms similar to those of homograft rejection [26].

In vitro lymphocyte blastogenic responses to tumor cells were first studied by Stjernsward [35, 36, 41] using techniques similar to those of the mixed leukocyte reaction [2]. A positive blastogenic response to autochthonous tumor cells could be interpreted as a primary cellular recognition of non-self, tumor cell-surface antigens. On the other hand, sensitization to these antigens should occur *in vivo* and subsequent blastogenic response of circulating memory cells to tumor cells *in vitro* could reflect established tumor immunity. Two pieces of information tend to support the latter view. Firstly, soluble tumor antigens obtained from a cystic melanoma induced blastogenic responses in autologous lymphocytes and lymphocytes from other patients with melanoma but not in lymphocytes from normal subjects [20]. Secondly the intensity of lymphocyte blastogenic responses to leukemia cells can be enhanced temporarily by active immunization with irradiated leukemia cells [29].

In this report we present our experience with the lymphocyte blastogenesis assay for tumor immunity. We confirm previous reports that freshly obtained tumor cells from a variety of solid tumors can stimulate blastogenic responses among autologous lymphocytes from the majority of patients. For the most effective study of tumor immunity with this system, viable tumor cells are superior to non-viable cells, and irradiated tumor cells are superior to mitomycin C-treated tumor cells. The degree of blastogenic response is related to the stage of disease and a vigorous response

* Supported by Grant ACS CI 22 from the American Cancer Society and Grants CA 05831 and FR 05511 from the National Institutes of Health, Bethesda, Maryland.

indicates a good prognosis. Serum effects were complex and patient's sera had both suppressive and enhancing effects on the blastogenic response to tumor cells. Finally, we present preliminary evidence that human tumor-associated antigen can be separated by salt extraction and effectively used to detect cell-mediated tumor immunity.

Materials and Methods

Patients

This study included 42 patients aged 18 to 81 years. 12 had melanoma, 8 carcinoma of the colon, 6 sarcoma, 4 lymphoma, 3 squamous cell carcinoma of the lung, 2 gastric carcinoma, 2 carcinoma of the ovary, 2 basal cell carcinoma, and the remaining 3 had carcinoma of the breast, hypernephroma and carcinoma of unknown origin, respectively. 15 patients were studied prior to any form of treatment, 17 patients had previous surgery, 8 had received chemotherapy (but not within 4 weeks prior to study), 7 patients had received radiotherapy (but not within 3 months prior to study). Patients differed in stage of disease. Localized disease was defined as primary tumor, either without spread, or with spread but not beyond the reionalg lymph nodes. Widespread disase was defined as spread beyond the regional lymph nodes.

Tumor Cells and Tumor Antigens

Single tumor-cell suspensions were prepared mechanically from fresh tumor biopsies by teasing, scraping, and sieving through a 60-mesh screen into Medium 199 (Gibco Laboratories, Grand Island, New York) containing 1 unit of penicillin and 1 μg of streptomycin per ml. Cells were washed once, counted, and their viability determined by exclusion of trypan blue [9].

Samples for bacteriological cultures were taken frequently. Unseparated (viable from nonviable) tumor cells were either irradiated with 4000 rad or remained untreated before use as lymphocyte stimulants.

For separation of viable from nonviable tumor cells, a solution of specific density made up of Ficoll (Pharmacia Fine Chemicals, Uppsala, Sweden) and Hypaque (Winthrop Laboratories, New York, New York) was prepared as follows. 24 parts of 9% Ficoll and 10 parts of 33.9% Hypaque were thoroughly mixed to give a solution of density 1.080 g/ml. This solution was sterilized by autoclaving. Approximately 10^8 tumor cells in 2 ml of Medium 199 were carefully layered on top of 10 ml of the specific-density solution in a 25×150 mm screw-cap centrifuge tube and centrifuged at 1,500 g for 15 min. The cells in the fraction floating between the Medium 199 and the Hypaque-Ficoll solution, and the cells in the pellet at the bottom of the tube were removed separately, washed twice in minimal essential medium (MEM, Gibco Laboratories) and each fraction was separated into three parts: in the first, tumor cells were treated with mitomycin C (Bristol Laboratories, Syracuse, New York) as previously described, [41]): In the second, they were irradiated with 4,000 rad, and in the third they remained untreated.

For extraction of tumor antigens, a single cell suspension was prepared as described above. Red blood cells were lysed by tris-buffered ammonium chloride for

15 min [5], and 5×10^9 tumor cells were mixed with 50 ml of 3 M KCl made up in phosphate-buffered saline at pH 7.2 [25]. After equilibration on a rocker at 4°C for 16 h, the contents of the tube were centrifuged at 40,000 g for 60 min at 0°C. The slightly viscous supernatant was dialyzed against 20 vol. of deionized water for 1 h, followed by dialysis against 20 vol. of phosphate-buffered saline for 24 h, with a change of solution every 8 h. The dialyzed extract was centrifuged at 40,000 g for 30 min at 0°C and the supernatant concentrated by pervaporation. The concentrate was mixed with an equal volume of 4 M ammonium sulphate and the precipitate centrifuged at 40,000 g for 30 min at 0°C. The supernatant was discarded and the precipitate redissolved in 5 ml of phosphate-buffered saline, pH 7.2. It was finally dialyzed against phosphate-buffered saline for 4 h. The protein concentration was estimated by measuring optical density at a wavelength of 280 mm (O.D. 280). The final preparation was sterilized by passage through a 0.45 μ Millipore filter (Millipore Corporation, Bedford, Massachusetts) and stored at 4°C with frequent checks for bacterial contamination.

In selected cases, uninvolved organs were obtained from cancer patients. These normal organs included an adrenal gland from a patient with carcinoma of the breast, an ovary from another patient with carcinoma of the breast, a kidney from a patient with transitional carcinoma of the ureter, and a testis from a patient with carcinoma of the prostate. In all cases the gross pathological examination and the histological sections failed to reveal evidence of tumor involvement. Single-cell suspensions were prepared as described for tumor cells. Cells were either irradiated or remained untreated before use as lymphocyte stimulants.

Lymphocyte Cultures

For preparation of lymphocytes, venous blood was drawn on the day of surgical removal of tumor but before sedation, anesthesia, or surgery. It was defibrinated by swirling with glass beads for 10 min, and the red blood cells were sedimented with dextran [18]. The leukocyte-rich serum was collected, and the WBC and differential counts determined. For each experiment, venous blood was also drawn from a normal, healthy subject and lymphocytes similarly prepared. Lymphocytes of both patients' and normal subjects were centrifuged at 140 g for 10 min at room temperature (International Centrifuge, Model UV). Serum was removed and heat-inactivated at 56° for 30 min. The lymphocytes were washed with MEM.

Four groups of lymphocyte cultures were set up in 16×125 mm screw-cap centrifuge tubes. Each tube contained 10^6 lymphocytes, 2 ml of MEM and 1 ml of heat-inactivated serum. Cancer patients' lymphocytes were cultured in both autologous and allogeneic sera (groups 1 and 2) and normal subjects' lymphocytes were likewise cultured in their own serum and in serum from a cancer patient (groups 3 and 4).

In addition to unstimulated control cultures, each of the 4 groups described above was stimulated with phytohemagglutinin M (PHA, Difco Laboratories, Detroit, Michigan), allogeneic leukocytes (MLC) irradiated with 4,000 rad (usually exchanged between the cancer patient and the normal subject studied on the same day), and with autologous irradiated leukocytes.

Stimulation of lymphocyte cultures with tumor material was conducted in three ways: 1. with unseparated tumor cells; in this case, 10^4—2×10^6 irradiated or untreated tumor cells in half-log dose intervals were used. 2. With separated tumor cells; in this case, 5×10^4—1×10^6 viable and nonviable tumor cells untreated and treated separately with irradiation mitomycin-C, were used, again in half-log dose intervals. 3. With extracted tumor antigens over a dose range of 20 to 1,000 μg per ml of culture. Tumor cells in the above preparations were always cultured simultaneously in identical doses and after identical treatments but without lymphocytes.

In the selected cases where normal tissue from a cancer patient was available, 10^6 autologous lymphocytes were stimulated with 10^4—1×10^6 normal tissue cells. Simultaneously, normal tissue cells were also cultured in identical doses but without lymphocytes.

All cultures were incubated at 37° in an atmosphere of 5% CO_2 in air. Cultures containing tumor cells or normal tissue cells were incubated for 7 days and 2 μCi of ^{3}H-thymidine (specific activity 1.9 μCi per millimole, Schwarz-Mann, Orangeburg, New York) were added to each culture 3 h before harvesting as previously described [18]. Cultures stimulated with extracted tumor antigen were incubated under identical conditions for 3—5 days and 1 μCi of the isotope was added to each of the cultures, 8 h before harvesting. Blastogenesis was taken as incorporation of ^{3}H-thymidine in the acid insoluble fraction, measured by liquid scintillation counting, and expressed as counts per minute per 10^6 lymphocytes (c.p.m.). The true blastogenic response to tumor was defined as c.p.m. of cultures containing lymphocytes with tumor cells, minus c.p.m. of cultures containing tumor cells alone. The stimulation index was defined as the true blastogenic response divided by the c.p.m. of cultures containing unstimulated lymphocytes. A stimulation index of 3.0 or over was considered significant for reasons which will be discussed below.

Significant serum inhibition of the blastogenic response was defined as drop of 50% or more in the stimulation index in one serum compared to the other. Significant facilitation of blastogenesis was defined as arise of 100% or more in the stimulation index in one serum compared to the other. Statistical analysis of the data was performed with the Wilcoxon signed rank test [34].

Results

Blastogenic responses to autologous leukocytes were not significantly different from those of unstimulated control cultures. Lymphocyte blastogenic responses to optimal doses of normal autologous tissue cells in the selected cases studied never exceeded a stimulation index of 3.0. Positive or significant lymphocyte blastogenic responses to an optimal dose of autochthonous tumor cells were therefore defined as a stimulation index of 3.0 or over, as observed in 19 of 29 patients studied with unseparated tumor cells (Table 1). The median stimulation index among these responders was 13.6 and corresponded to a median true balstogenic response of 3,405 c.p.m. In contrast, lymphocytes from 24 of 27 normal subjects responded to optimal doses of these allogeneic tumor cells with a stimulation index equal to or greater than 3.0. The median stimulation index among these responders was 20.1 and corresponded to a median true blastogenic response of 9,475 c.p.m. The difference in blastogenic response to tumor as between patients and normal subjects was statistically significant at the 5% level and probably represented the response of the latter to histoincompatible MLC antigens.

The blastogenic response to tumor cells was dose-related (Table 2). A median stimulation index greater than 3.0 was observed among cancer-patient lymphocytes when 10^5 or more tumor cells were used for stimulation. A maximum stimulation index of 6.5 among cancer-patient lymphocytes was obtained with 10^6 tumor cells. This was equivalent to a tumor cell-lymphocyte ratio of 1 : 1. An excess of tumor

Table 1. Lymphocyte blastogenic responses to optimal doses of unseparated tumor cells

Responder cells	Stimulation index $\geqq 3.0$ Observed/studied	Median stimulation index among responders	Median c.p.m. among responders
Cancer patient lymphocytes	19/29 (65.5%)	13.6	3405
Normal donor lymphocytes	24/27 (88.8%)	20.1	9475

Table 2. Lymphocyte blastogenic responses (stimulation indices) to graded doses of unseparated tumor cells

	Tumor cell dose used for stimulation				
	10^4	10^5	5×10^5	10^6	2×10^6
Responses of cancer patients	2.0	3.6	4.0	6.5	4.4
Response of normal subjects	2.2	3.4	12.1	11.5	11.5

cells with a tumor cell-lymphocyte ratio of 2 : 1 not only failed to augment stimulation, but slightly inhibited it. Stimulation of normal-subject lymphocytes to an index above 3.0 was also achieved with the use of 10^5 or more tumor cells, and reached its maximum (12.1) when 5×10^5 tumor cells were used. This was equivalent to a tumor cell-lymphocyte ratio of 1 : 2. Increasing the tumor cell-lymphocyte ratio to 1 : 1 or 2 : 1 did not augment the blastogenic response. Although the dose-response relationship is similar in patients and normal subjects, the latter show considerably stronger responses to each tumor-cell dose above the critical level of 10^5 tumor cells per culture.

The relationship between the stage of disease and the blastogenic response to optimal doses of autochthonous tumor cells and to PHA is shown in Table 3. The median stimulation index of the 16 patients with localized disease was 13.2, in the 13 patients with widespread disease it was only 4.9 (statistically significant at the 6% level). In contrast, no such relationship was observed after stimulation of lymphocytes with PHA. The median stimulation index in the 16 patients with localized disease was 207, whereas in the 13 patients with widespread disease it was 266.

Table 3. Blastogenic responses (stimulation indices) of cancer-patient lymphocytes to tumor cells and to PHA. Relation to stage of disease

	Tumor cells		PHA	
	Localized disease	Widespread disease	Localized disease	Widespread disease
No.	16	13	16	13
Mean	20.0	8.0	231.0	300.0
S.D.	20.3	9.6	177.8	223.5
Median	13.2	4.9	207.5	266.4
Range	1.3—62.5	0—34.5	0.7—805.1	0.8—710.7
P	0.06		0.3	

The effect of heat-inactivated serum from cancer patients on the lymphocyte blastogenic response to optimal doses of tumor cells is shown in Table 4. The response was significantly inhibited by autologous serum in 7, and significantly enhanced in 9 of the 28 patients so studied. In only a small fraction of patients whose lymphocyte blastogenic responses were inhibited or facilitated by autologous serum was the effect tumor-specific. In most patients, the simultaneous responses of the same lymphocytes to PHA and to allogeneic leukocytes were changed by serum in the same direction as the response to the tumor cells. The reverse phenomenon of nonspecific inhibitory or facilitatory effects of serum on the blastogenic responses to PHA and to allogeneic leukocytes in the absence of an effect on the response to tumor was also observed in a number of patients. Similarly, the blastogenic responses of normal subjects to tumor cells were significantly inhibited by sera from the respective tumor-bearing hosts in 9, and facilitated in 6 of 27 subjects so studied. Again, the effect was tumor-specific only in a fraction of the normal subjects whose lymphocyte blastogenic responses were inhibited or facilitated by sera from tumor-bearing hosts. There was no correlation between any serum effect and the stage of disease, or between the effects on the responses of normal subjects compared to patients.

Table 4. Effect of cancer-patient sera on the blastogenic responses of autologous and normal donor lymphocytes to optimal doses of tumor cells, to PHA, and to allogeneic leukocytes (MLC)

Responder cells	Stimulation with tumor cells		Stimulation with PHA		Stimulation in MLC	
	Inhibition	Enhancement	Inhibition	Enhancement	Inhibition	Enhancement
	No. observed/no. studied					
Cancer patient lymphocytes	7/28	9/28	7/28	9/28	9/28	10/28
Normal donor lymphocytes	9/27	6/27	9/26	5/26	7/22	9/22

Separation of viable from non-viable tumor cells by means of specific density solution centrifugation (Table 5), increased the viable cell population from a median of 16% (range 2% to 57%) before separation, to a median of 77% (range 65% to 97%) in the floating fraction after separation ($p < 0.001$). The pellet consisted almost exclusively of non-viable cells with a median purity of 98.5%.

Table 5. Separation of viable from nonviable tumor cells on Ficoll-hypague specific-density solution. Results of 10 experiments

	% Viable tumor cells			Viable tumor cells recovered in floating fraction	
	Before separation	Floating fraction	Pellet	Absolute number (× 10^6)	% Initial total cell count
Mean	21.6	79.9	7.6	6.9	12.4
Median	16	77	1.5	4.6	6.5
Range	2—57	65—97	1—30	0.2—21	0.5—47
S.D.	18.3	12.8	10.0	6.9	14.9

Table 6. Incidence of stimulation index ≧ 3.0 in patient lymphocytes and median blastogenic responses to optimal doses of autochthonous viable and nonviable tumor cells, irradiated (XRT), treated with mitomycin C (Mito-C) or untreated

Tumor cells	True blastogenic response CPM/10^6 lymphocytes	Stimulation index	No. positive with stimulation index ≧ 3.0/no. tested (% positive)
Viable, XRT	4608	6.8	9/11 (82)
Viable	4068	4.5	8/11 (73)
Non-viable	4004	5.1	7/11 (64)
Non-viable, XRT	1780	4.7	7/11 (64)
Viable, Mito-C	1411	2.0	3/10 (30)
Non-viable, Mito-C	1359	1.7	3/10 (30)

Treatment of viable and non-viable tumor cells with irradiation or mitomycin C compared with no treatment in 11 patients so studied, resulted in populations of tumor cells which induced (at their optimal doses) the blastogenic responses shown in Table 6.

The median blastogenic response to irradiated viable tumor cells was 4,608 c.p.m. and exceeded the response to untreated viable tumor cells (4,068 c.p.m.) and to viable tumor cells treated with mitomycin C (1,411 c.p.m.). The median response to untreated non-viable tumor cells was 4,004 c.p.m. while the responses to non-viable tumor cells treated with irradiation or mitomycin C were 1,780 c.p.m. and 1,359 c.p.m., respectively. Thus, the efficiencies of the various tumor cell preparations in the induction of blastogenesis (in descending order) were: irradiate-viable, viable, non-viable, irradiated non-viable, and mitomycin C-treated viable and non-viable tumor cells.

Table 7. Blastogenic responses (CPM) of patient and normal donor lymphocytes to autochthonous, KCl-solubilized tumor antigens and other stimulants. Numbers in parentheses indicate stimulation index

	Patient 1 (Colon cancer)		Normal donor 1		Patient 2 (ovarian cancer)	Normal donor 2
Stimulants	Autologous serum	Normal serum	Autologous serum	Patient 1 serum	Autologous serum	Autologous serum
Unstimulated	112	111	209	247	197	1,463
PHA	40,468 (361)	48,522 (437)	149,856 (717)	176,990 (716)	43,878 (222)	78,982 (54)
10^6 allogeneic leukocytes	4,570 (41)	5,420 (49)	8,493 (40)	12,172 (49)	16,734 (85)	16,552 (11)
Tumor antigens μg/ml						
10	—	—	—	—	954 (4.8)	2,320 (1.6)
20	—	—	326 (1.5)	154 (0.6)	—	—
40	—	—	162 (0.8)	380 (1.5)	—	—
50	—	—	—		696 (3.5)	1,444 (0.9)
60	3,174 (28)	6,034 (54)	—	—	—	—
80	—	—	228 (1.1)	228 (0.9)	—	—
100	4,960 (44)	14,034 (126)	—	—	1,810 (9.2)	1,872 (1.3)
170	—	—	317 (1.5)	668 (2.7)	—	—
250	—	—	—	—	1,278 (6.5)	2,640 (1.8)
330	—	—	299 (1.4)	232 (0.9)	—	—
500	—	—	—	—	1,058 (5.4)	1,908 (1.3)
600	162 (1.4)	170 (1.5)	—	—	—	—
1000	46 (0.4)	332 (3.0)	—	—	—	—

The stimulation indices showed good correlation with the true blastogenic responses. Thus, stimulation with irradiated viable tumor cells resulted in an index of 6.8, while stimulation with viable and non-viable tumor cells treated with mitomycin C resulted in indices of 2.0 and 1.7, respectively. The incidence of stimulation indices equal to or greater than 3.0 is also shown in Table 6. An incidence of 82% was observed with irradiated viable tumor cells, and only 30% with either viable or non-viable tumor cells treated with mitomycin C.

Statistical analysis of the data showed that viable tumor cells, irradiated or untreated, were significantly superior to mitomycin C-treated viable and non-viable tumor cells. Although irradiated viable tumor cells were also superior to irradiated and untreated non-viable tumor cells, the difference was not significant at the 5% level. In addition, non-viable tumor cells, irradiated or untreated, were significantly superior to mitomycin C-treated non-viable tumor cells.

The blastogenic responses of the lymphocytes of two patients to extracted autochthonous tumor antigen were studied and compared with the responses of the lymphocytes of two normal healthy subjects. Maximal blastogenic response to tumor antigen was observed among the lymphocytes of the patients (Table 7) when a dose of 100 μg/ml was used. The blastogenic response was partially inhibited by one patient's serum. Higher doses of antigen resulted in inhibition of the blastogenic response. Blastogenic response to tumor antigens was not detected among the normal donor lymphocytes, despite an adequate response to PHA, to the patient's lymphocytes (MLC) and in the absence of serum inhibitory effect. Parenthetically, it is noteworthy that both antigen extracts induced positive skin reactions in the respective patients. These were proved by biopsy to be delayed hypersensitivity reactions.

Discussion

The results of this study indicate that lymphocyte blastogenic responses to optimal doses and preparations of autochthonous tumor cells can be detected in most patients with solid tumors. To rule out the possibility that the response to tumor cells may really be to non-specific tissue mitogens or tissue-specific antigens [32], rather than to tumor-specific antigens, we studied the patient's lymphocyte responses to cells from normal autochthonous tissues. A slight degree of blastogenesis, which did not exceed a stimulation index of 3.0 was observed. In consequence, we chose this value as a cut-off point to distinguish positive from negative blastogenic responses to tumor cells.

The relation of the blastogenic response to tumor cell dose, is pertinent to the role of cell density in lymphocyte cultures in general [18]. Maximum responses are obtained at a critical tumor cell-lymphocyte ratio, and once this ratio is exceeded, responses decline. The decline in blastogenic response with increase in tumor cell dose may be due to crowding and unfavorable culture conditions with nutritional deprivation of the responding lymphocytes, and, possibly, physical interference of an excess of tumor cells with uptake of the isotope.

The association between the intensity of the blastogenic response to tumor cells and the stage of disease, is a phenomenon of major clinical interest. In general, it has been suggested that immunological deficiency tends to parallel the extent of malignant disease [12]. Following tumor surgery, impaired immunologic reactivity in the presence of little or no detectable disease is associated with increased incidence of tumor recurrence and poor prognosis [7]. Recovery of general immunocompetence and the associated "rebound and overshoot" in lymphocyte function have been recognized as favorable prognostic signs in patients with solid tumors and leukemia who are receiving chemotherapy [6, 19].

The present study suggests that *in vitro* cell-mediated tumor immunity correlates quantitatively with the extent of disease: as the disease progresses, tumor immunity tends to decline. In contrast, the median response to PHA did not appear to be affected by the extent of disease in this group of patients. This dichotomy suggests a decrease in tumor antigenicity, a decrease in tumor recognition capacity by the lymphocytes or specific antigen or antibody-mediated suppression of tumor immunity in progressively growing tumors. Correlation between cell-mediated tumor immunity and stage of disease was also studied using cutaneous delayed-hypersensitivity reactions [28, 10, 11].

Localized solid tumors or remission in leukemia were associated with positive delayed-hypersensitivity reactions to tumor cell extracts. Also, the degree of blastogenic response of lymphocytes to autologous leukemic blast cells was correlated with the clinical status of leukemia patients [13]. A higher stimulation index was associated with an increased incidence of remission and a decreased incidence of relapse. In contrast, the Hellströms found no difference in anti-tumor immunity (microcytotoxicity assay) between patients who became symptom-free following a curative procedure, and patients with progressively growing tumors [16]. However, the presence of serum blocking factors did correlate with advanced disease. Also, their test system used cultured tumor-cell lines in which antigens may be grossly altered [4].

The complexity of serum effects deserves a critical comment. Our results differ from those of other investigators who found only blocking serum effects in patients with progressively growing tumors. In contrast to previously described *in vitro* assays for serum effects [17, 40], we use fresh rather than cultured tumor cells, and we incubate both tumor cells and lymphocytes together in the presence of serum for 7 days, rather than tumor cells alone for a few hours. Our system may be closer to *in vivo* conditions. Our results suggest that serum from cancer patients can exert both inhibitory and facilitory effects on lymphocyte blastogenic response to tumor cells. The mechanisms by which serum factors exert their effects are poorly understood. Elution studies in animal tumor models have revealed that tumor cells may be coated by antibodies [30] or by antigen-antibody complexes [33] which correlated with the presence of inhibitory factors in the serum from the tumor-bearing host. Also, such eluates could suppress antitumor immunity *in vivo* [38]. Facilitatory serum factors were detected in patients who became symptom-free after a curative manipulation [16]. These "unblocking" sera abrogated the *in vitro* inhibitory effect of serum from patients with progressively growing tumors. In the rat polyoma system, serum "unblocking" effect *in vitro* may correlate with its antitumor activity *in vivo* [3].

In the current study, no correlation was observed between the presence of any serum factors and the extent of disease, and in most cases serum factors were nonspecific, as reflected in the simultaneous effects on responses to PHA and allogeneic leukocytes (MLC).

The demonstration that tumor cells can induce blastogenic response among autologous lymphocytes *in vitro* supports the concept that tumor cells do contain non-self antigens on their surfaces.

It seems likely that these antigens are weak, since they induce mild blastogenic responses compared to other antigens and mitogens. However, one cannot rule out the possibility that various factors may interfere with the process of recognition and that this leads to a failure to evoke a more intense response.

Weak responses may have also been the result of a failure to select the ideal tumor cell preparation for the stimulation of blastogenesis. Our results emphasize the superiority of viable compared to non-viable tumor cells and the superiority of irradiated compared to mitomycin C-treated cells. The superiority of viable tumor cells deserves further comment. In some experimental systems, viable tumor cells are superior for immunotherapy [22]. In our system, viable tumor cells may be superior because they furnish a better source of tumor-associated antigen than non-viable cells. Cells in the process of disintegration may have lost a great deal of the surface antigen and certainly will not be able to synthesize new antigen. Further treatment of such fragile cells with irradiation or mitomycin C may remove more antigen or further reduce their ability to synthesize new antigen. Conversely, good cell viability and continued surface antigen production may be a requirement for vigorous stimulator cell activity both in the MLC and in the tumor cell stimulation of blastogenesis.

The mechanism by which mitomycin C reduces the blastogenic activity of both viable and non-viable tumor cells is unknown. The only well characterized activity of mitomycin C is to induce structural change in DNA and completely inhibit its synthesis [37]. In one-way mixed lymphocyte reaction, mitomycin C-treated lymphocytes appear to be satisfactory stimulator cells [2]. However F_1 hybrid lymphocytes which are unreactive to parental strains of cells in animal systems and yet are stimulatory in the MLC, their treatment with mitomycin C resulted in a markedly reduced stimulator cell reactivity [42]. In tumor cells, it might be postulated that some changes in membrane properties caused by this drug may lead to the diminished antigenicity. Leakage of mitomycin C from treated tumor cells with subsequent suppressing effect on the responding lymphocytes is also possible, despite the extensive washing to which they were subjected.

Irradiation may also be a cause of the reduction of cell surface antigens, especially the weak ones, and thus reduce MLC [24]. Studies of the one-way mixed lymphocyte reaction demonstrated satisfactory stimulation by lymphocytes irradiated with 4,000 rad. However, doses of 6,000 rad or more, always resulted in diminished stimulatory activity [21]. Ultra-violet irradiation of lymphocytes was also associate with their inability to stimulate allogeneic lymphocytes [23]. A comparative study of irradiation and mitomycin C pretreatment of stimulator cells for the one-way mixed lymphocyte reaction, resulted in two conflicting reports. One claims the superiority for irradiated stimulator cells [8] and the other found no significant difference [1]. In our system using tumor cells, irradiated tumor cells were superior to mitomycin C-treated tumor cells.

The question of whether a positive blastogenic response to tumor cells does merely represent a primary tumor recognition *in vitro*, or evidence of cellular immunity and memory cells in the peripheral blood is not settled yet. The current study furnishes a preliminary evidence to support the latter hypothesis. KCl-solubilized tumor antigen can stimulate autologous lymphocytes, but does not stimulate normal subjects' lymphocytes. Similar phenomenon was observed in patients with leukemia [14]. It is proposed that soluble antigen, in contrast to its cell-associated counterpart, can only stimulate blastogenesis among pre-sensitized lymphocytes. Hence, autologous lymphocytes responded *in vitro* to the soluble antigen because they were pre-sensitized to the tumor *in vivo*, while allogeneic lymphocytes failed to respond *in vitro*, because they were not pre-sensitized to either tumor-associated, or to HL-A antigens which were probably also present in the solubilized extract [31]. We consider this phenomenon strongly suggests that the blastogenic response of autologous lymphocytes to tumor cells is indeed a manifestation of cell-mediated immunity.

References

1. Bach, F. H., Bach, M. L.: Comparison of mitomycin-C and X-irradiation as blocking agents in one-way mixed leukocyte cultures. Nature New Biol. **235**, 243 (1972).
2. Bach, F. H., Voynow, N. K.: One-way stimulation in leukocyte cultures. Science **153**, 545 (1966).
3. Bansal, S. C., Sjogren, H. O.: "Unblocking" serum activity *in vitro* in the polyoma system may correlate with anti-tumor effects of antiserum *in vivo*. Nature New Biol. **233**, 76 (1971).
4. Birnbaum, G., Siskind, G. W., Weksler, M. E.: Autologous and allogeneic stimulation of peripheral human leukocytes. Cell Immunol. **3**, 44 (1972).
5. Boyle, W.: An extension of the Cr-release assay for the estimation of mouse cytotoxins. Transplantation **6**, 761 (1968).
6. Cheema, A. R., Hersh, E. M.: Patient survival after chemotherapy and its relationship to *in vitro* lymphocyte blastogenesis. Cancer (Philad.) **28**, 851 (1971).
7. Eilber, F. R., Morton, D. L.: Impaired immunologic reactivity and recurrence following cancer surgery. Cancer (Philad.) **25**, 362 (1970).
8. Elves, M. W.: Comparison of mitomycin-C and X-rays for the production of one-way stimulation in mixed leukocyte cultures. Nature **223**, 90 (1969).
9. Evans, H. M., Schulemann, W.: The action of vital stains belonging to the benzidine group. Science **39**, 443 (1914).
10. Fass, L., Herberman, R. B., Ziegler, J.: Delayed cutaneous hypersensitivity reaction to autologous extracts of Burkitt-lymphoma cells. New Engl. J. Med. **282**, 776 (1971).
11. Fass, L., Herberman, R. B., Ziegler, J. L., *et al.*: Cutaneous hypersensitivity reactions to autologous extracts of malignant melanoma cells. Lancet **1970 I**, 116.
12. Gross, L.: Immunological defect in aged population and its relationship to cancer. Cancer (Philad.) **18**, 201 (1965).
13. Gutterman, J. U., Hersh, E. M., McCredie, K. B., *et al.*: Lymphocyte blastogenesis to human leukemia cells and their relationship to serum factors, immunocompetence, and prognosis. Cancer Res. **32**, 2524 (1972).
14. Gutterman, J. U., Mavligit, G. M., Hersh, E. M., *et al.*: Antigen solubilized from human leukemia: Lymphocyte stimulation. Science **177**, 1114 (1972).
15. Hellström, I., Hellström, K. E., Sjogren, H. O., *et al.*: Demonstration of cell-mediated immunity to human neoplasms of various histological types. Int. J. Cancer **7**, 1 (1971).
16. Hellström, I., Hellström, K. E., Sjogren, H. O., *et al.*: Serum factors in tumor-free patients cancelling the blocking of cell-mediated tumor immunity. Int. J. Cancer **8**, 185 (1971).
17. Hellström, I., Sjogren, H. O., Warner, G., *et al.*: Blocking of cell-mediated tumor immunity by sera from patients with growing neoplasms. Int. J. Cancer **7**, 226 (1971).
18. Hersh, E. M., Harris, J. E., Rogers, E. A.: Influence of cell density on response of leukocytes and column-purified lymphocytes to mitogenic agents. J. reticuloendoth. Soc. **7**, 567 (1970).
19. Hersh, E. M., Whitecar, J. P., McCredie, K. B., *et al.*: Chemotherapy immunocompetence, immunosuppression and prognosis in acute leukemia. New Engl. J. Med. **285**, 1211 (1971).
20. Jehn, U. W., Nathanson, L., Schwartz, R. S., *et al.*: *In vitro* lymphocyte stimulation by a soluble antigen from malignant melanoma. New Engl. J. Med. **283**, 329 (1970).

21. KASAKURA, S., LOWENSTEIN, L.: The factors affecting the strength of "one-way" stimulation with irradiated leukocytes in mixed leukocyte cultures. J. Immunol. **101**, 12 (1971).
22. KRONMAN, B. S., WEPSIC, H. T., CHURCHILL, W. H. jr., *et al.*: Immunotherapy of cancer: An experimental model in syngeneic guinea pigs. Science **168**, 257 (1970).
23. LINDAHL-KIESSLING, K., SAFWENBERG, J.: Inability of UV-irradiated lymphocytes to stimulate allogeneic cells in mixed lymphocyte culture. Int. Arch. Allergy **41**, 670 (1971).
24. MCKHANN, C. F.: The effect of X-ray on the antigenicity of donor cells in transplantation immunity. J. Immunol. **92**, 811 (1964).
25. MELTZER, M. S., LEONARD, E. J., RAPP, H. J., *et al.*: Tumor-specific antigen solubilized by hypertonic potassium chloride. J. nat. Cancer Inst. **47**, 704 (1971).
26. MITCHISON, N. A.: Studies on the immunological response to foreign tumor transplants in the mouse. I. The role of the lymph node cells in conferring immunity by adoptive transfer. J. exp. Med. **102**, 157 (1955).
27. MORTON, D. L., MALMGREN, R. A., HOLMES, E. C., *et al.*: Demonstration of antibodies against human malignant melanoma by immunofluorescence. Surgery **64**, 233 (1968).
28. OREN, M. E., HERBERMAN, R. B.: Delayed cutaneous hypersensitivity reactions to membrane extracts of human tumor cells. Clin. exp. Immunol. **9**, 45 (1971).
29. POWLES, R. L., BALCHIN, L. A., FAIRLEY, G. H., *et al.*: Recognition of leukemia cells as foreign before and after autoimmunization. Brit. med. J. **1971 I**, 486.
30. RAN, M., WITZ, I. P.: Tumor-associated immunoglobulins. The elution of IgG_2 from mouse tumors. Int. J. Cancer **6**, 361 (1970).
31. REISFELD, R. A., PELLEGRINO, M. A., KAHAN, B. D.: Salt extraction of soluble HL-A antigens. Science **172**, 1134 (1971).
32. SHEFFIELD, J. B., EMMELOT, P.: Studies on plasma membranes. XVI. Tissue specific antigens in the liver cell surface. Exp. Cell Res. **71**, 97 (1971).
33. SJOGREN, H. O., HELLSTRÖM, I., BANSAL, S. C., *et al.*: Suggestive evidence that the "Blocking Antibodies" of tumor-bearing individuals may be antigen-antibody complexes. Proc. nat. Acad. Sci. (Wash.) **68**, 1372 (1971).
34. SNEDECOR, G. W., COCHRAN, W. G.: Statistical methods. Ames Iowa: The Iowa State University Press 1969.
35. STJERNSWARD, J., ALMGARD, L. E., VON SCHREEB, T., *et al.*: Tumor-distinctive cellular immunity to renal carcinoma. Clin. exp. Immunol. **6**, 963 (1970).
36. STJERNSWARD, J., CLIFFORD, P., SINGH, S., *et al.*: Indications of cellular immunological reactions against autochthonous tumor in cancer patients studied *in vitro*. E. Afr. med. J. **45**, 484 (1968).
37. SZYBALSKI, W., IYER, V. N.: Crosslinking of DNA by enzymatically or chemically activated mitomycins and porfiromycins, bifunctionally "Alkylating" antibodies. Fed. Proc. **23**, 946 (1964).
38. TAM, M. R., WEISER, R. S.: Passive transfer of immunological enhancement by low pH eluates of sarcoma I (sal) cells. Fed. Proc. (abstracts) **31**, 785 (1972).
39. VANKY, F., STJERNSWARD, J.: Tumor-distinctive cellular immunity to human sarcoma and carcinoma. Israel J. med. Sci. **7**, 211 (1971).
40. VANKY, F , STJERNSWARD, J., KLEIN, G., *et al.*: Serum-mediated inhibition of lymphocyte-stimulation by autochthonous human tumors. J. nat. Cancer Inst. **47**, 95 (1971).
41. VANKY, F., STJERNSWARD, J., NILSONNE, U.: Cellular immunity to human sarcoma. J. nat. Cancer Inst. **46**, 1145 (1971).
42. WILSON, D. B.: Quantitative studies on the mixed lymphocyte interaction in rats. I. Conditions and parameters of response. J. exp. Med. **126**, 625 (1967).

Cell-Mediated and Humoral Immune Response to Acute Leukemia Cells and Soluble Leukemia Antigen-Relationship to Immunocompetence and Prognosis*

J. U. Gutterman, E. M. Hersh, G. Mavligit, E. J. Freireich, R. D. Rossen, W. T. Butler, K. B. McCredie, G. P. Bodey, Sr., and V. Rodriguez

Section of Immunology Department of Developmental Therapeutics,
The University of Texas M. D. Anderson Hospital and Tumor Institute at Houston
Department of Microbiology, Baylor College of Medicine, Houston, Texas

Introduction

During the past several years there has been increasing evidence that tumor-associated antigens are present in a variety of human neoplasms [25]. In studying the immunological response to human leukemia, Yoshida found that the sera of 71% of patients with acute leukemia gave a positive immune adherence reaction with autologous leukemia cells [46]. In contrast, Dore *et al.* found by similar methods that only 22% of 140 patients with acute leukemia had antibody to autologous leukemia cells [7]. Cell-mediated immunity was studied by Oren and Herberman who reported that the majority patients with acute leukemia had positive delayed hypersensitivity skin tests to membrane preparation of their own leukemia cells [34]. Cellular reactivity to acute leukemia cells *in vitro* has also been demonstrated by the mixed leukocyte culture technique (MLC) and lymphocyte cytotoxicity [9, 14, 28, 36, 44].

An observation which may be relevant to the apparent failure of this tumor immunity to control clinical cancer is that the serum factors in solid tumor patients may interfere with *in vitro* cell-mediated immunity [11]. The Hellströms *et al.* have described a factor (presumably anti-tumor antibody) in the serum of patients with solid tumors which may block lymphocyte-mediated cytotoxicity to tumor cells [17].

There have been few studies designed to determine the role of serum factors in tumor immunity in patients with acute leukemia. Therefore, the current study was designed to determine the presence and possible interrelationship of humoral and cell-associated tumor immunity in acute leukemia. The interrelationship between general immunocompetence and specific tumor responsiveness was also studied. Evidence for both humoral and cell-mediated tumor immunity was found [15]. The

* Supported by Grant ACS CI 22 from the American Cancer Society and Grants CA 05831, FR 05511 and CA 11520 from the National Institutes of Health and Department of Health, Education, and Welfare, U.S. Public Health, Bethesda, Maryland.

presence of a vigorous lymphocyte blastogenic response to leukemia cells, its inhibition or facilitation by autologous serum, and the presence of immunoglobulin bound to leukemia cells were found to indicate good prognosis.

Recently, the technique for salt extraction of soluble HLA antigens [38] has been applied to the extraction of tumor-associated antigens in animal tumors [32]. We have used similar techniques for extraction of soluble antigens from human leukemia cells. These soluble preparations have been assayed in lymphocyte cultures from both autologous leukemia patients and allogeneic normal donors. In addition to demonstrating the feasibility of salt extraction of antigens from human leukemic cells, the current data strongly suggests that *in vitro* lymphocyte responsiveness represents specific tumor immunity.

Materials and Methods

Membrane immunofluorescence with anti-immunoglobulin antisera, blastogenic response, and skin-test reactivity to autologous leukemia cells were studied in 35 adult acute leukemic patients. In addition, 6 of these patients and one chronic myelogenous leukemia (CML) patient in "blast crisis" were tested for lymphocyte blastogenesis and skin-test reactivity to soluble antigen.

Leukemic blast cells were collected from the peripheral blood of untreated patients on admission to the hospital. The cells were collected with the IBM or the Aminco blood cell separators, which have previously been used to obtain lymphocytes [10]. The red blood cells were removed by exposure of the collected cells (in their original critic acid-dextrose suspending medium) to 5 volumes of tris-buffered ammonium chloride [3]. After centrifugation and washing, the leukemia cells were resuspended in RPMI 1640 with 20% fetal calf serum. This suspension was mixed with a 10% v/v of DMSO and 1 µl aliquots frozen at 1° per min to —120 °C in sterile glass ampules at a leukocyte concentration of 5×10^7 per ampule. The ampules were stored at —310 °C in liquid nitrogen. On the day fo study the ampules were thawed rapidly at 37 °C, washed 3 times in Spinner modified Eagle's minimal essential medium (MEM) (Hyland Laboratories, Los Angeles, California) and resuspended in MEM at room temperature. The cells were counted in hemocytometer chamber and viability determined by trypan blue dye exclusion [8].

Extraction of Tumor Antigen

The leukemia cells were collected as described above and the red blood cells were lysed by tris-buffered ammonium chloride for 15 min. Depending on the availability of cells, 3×10^8—3×10^{10} leukemia cells were used for antigen extraction. The method described by [32] was used with slight modifications. 10 ml of 3 m KCL in potassium phosphate-buffered saline at pH 7.2 were added to every 3×10^8 cells in 25×200 mm screw-cap glass tubes. This was equilibrated at 40 °C for 16—24 h and the contents were then centrifuged at 100,000 g and 40 °C for 60 min. This supernatant was dialyzed against 20 volumes of potassium phosphate-buffered saline for 24 h with a change of solution every 8 h. The dialyzed extract was centrifuged at 4 °C at 40,000 g for 15 min. The supernatant was then concentrated by ultrafiltration at 4 °C, and the concentrate was mixed with an equal volume of 3.8 molar ammonium sulfate for 1 h at 4 °C to precipitate the protein. This mixture was centrifuged at 40,000 g and 4 °C for 15 min. The precipitate was re-dissolved in 5 ml of phosphate-buffered saline pH 7.2 and was dialized against this buffer for 4 h. The protein concentration was estimated by measurement of optical density (O.D.) at a wave length of 280 nm (O.D. 280). The final preparation was sterilized by filtration through a 0.45 micron millipore filter (Millipore Corporation, Bedford, Massachusetts) and was stored at 4 °C.

For the lymphocyte culture and other lymphocyte studies, peripheral blood lymphocytes were collected, washed and cultured as previously described [18]. Cultures contained 1×10^6 washed lymphocytes, 1 ml of serum (either autologous or allogeneic), 2 ml of MEM and various stimulants including leukemia cells, phytohemagglutinin (PHA-M; Difco Laboratories, Detroit, Michigan), streptolysin O (SLO; Difco) and allogeneic normal leukocytes. The stimulator leukemia cells were added in doses varying from 10^4 to 10^6 in half-log increments. Both unirradiated and irradiated cells were studied (4,000 or 12,000 rad). Extracted tumor antigen was added in a dose range 10—1000 μg/ml of culture. Appropriate controls consisting of unstimulated lymphocytes, unirradiated leukemia cells cultured alone and irradiated leukemia cells cultured with irradiated lymphocytes were set up. Cultures were incubated at 37 °C in an atmosphere at 5% in air for 3—5 days (PHA, SLO), 5 days (tumor antigen) or for 7 days (MLC and tumor cells). Harvesting was accomplished as previously described [18] by adding 2 μc of ^{3}H-thymidine with a specific activity 1.9 Ci per mM for 3 h and measuring the acid-insoluble radioactivity by liquid scintillation counting (Schwarz Bioresearch, Orangeburg, New York).

Lymphocyte blastogenesis was measured as the net counts per minute (CPM) of tritiated thymidine incorporation per 1×10^6 cultured lymphocytes with the incorporation of the appropriate controls subtracted from that of the stimulated cultures (CPM). A 100% increase or 50% decrease in thymidine incorporation compared to the appropriate control indicated significant stimulation or inhibition at the 95% level of confidence [19] and a 300% increase or 75% decrease was significant at the 99% level of confidence. The stimulation index (S.I.) was defined as the CPM of a stimulated culture divided by the CPM of the appropriate unstimulated lymphocyte culture.

Membrane immunofluorescence using highly class specfic animal anti-human IgG, IgA or IgM purified by absorption to and elution from insoluble immunoabsorbant antigens [37] was performed according to the method of [33]. Leukemia cells were thawed rapidly, washed three times with MEM, and then incubated at room temperature for 60 min with patient's serum, serum from a normal donor with the blood type AB Rh positive, or McCoy's medium (modfied) with 30% fetal calf serum. These incubated cells were washed three times in phosphate-buffered saline PBS-McCoy's before being exposed to the fluorescein-conjugated antisera specific to human IgG, IgA, or IgM heavy chains as previously described [40]. Leukemia cells were resuspended in the appropriate fluorescein-conjugated antiserum and incubated for 30 min at 22 °C. After three washings in PBS-McCoy's, the cells were mounted in a solution of PBS and glycerin on glass slides and read immediately or fixed with glutaraldehyde and read within 7 days. A positive reaction was recorded when 20% or more of the cells showed surface membrane fluorescence with an antibody reagent against a single immunoglobulin class (100 cell count).

Skin Testing: 0.1 ml of live autologous leukemia cells in doses from 10^4 to 10^6 in half-long intervals was injected intradermally. Delayed hypersensitivity was evaluated with soluble tumor antigen by injecting 0.1 ml of the extracted antigen intradermally. No more than 0.33 mg of protein per 0.1 ml was injected. The ability of patients to react to skin tests was also evaluated by a battery of established skin testing antigens including dermatophytin, dermatophytin O, and Candida antigen or Monilia mixture (all from Hollister-Stier Labs, Downers Grove, Illinois and all given in 0.1 ml of a 1/20 dilution of the stock), streptokinase-streptodornase (Varidase; Lederle Laboratories, Pearl River, New York; 0.1 ml, 50 μ), and mumps antigen (Lyovac-Mumpsvax; Merck, Sharpe and Dohme, West Point, Pennsylvania: 0.1 ml of a 1/20 dilution of stock solution). The average diameter of right angle measurements in mm of induration was recorded at 24 and 48 hours.

35 patients with acute leukemia were studied. 25 had acute myelogenous leukemia (AML) and 10 had acute lymphoblastic leukemia (ALL). Their median age was 28 years (range 15—71). There were 21 males and 14 females. The various therapeutic regimens are listed in Table 1. All chemotherapeutic regimens consisted of 5 days of chemotherapy, with intervals without therapy of at least 9 days. The patients were studied as soon as their peripheral blood was free of leukemic cells, just prior to a

Table 1. Chemotherapy regimens

No. of patients treated	Regimen code	Drug (letter code)	Period during course when drug administered (days)	Average dose/day (Mg/M^2)	Schedule[b] (interval in days)
13	DOAP	Daunomycin (D)	1	60.0	14
		Vincristine (O)	1	2.0[a]	
		Ara-C (A)	1—5	100.0	
		Prednisone (P)	1—5	200.0[a]	
9	COAP	Cyclophosphamide (C)	1—5	100.0	14
		Vincristine (O)	1	2.0[a]	
		Ara-C (A)	1—5	100.0	
		Prednisone (P)	1—5	200.0[a]	
8	OAP	Vincristine (O)	1	2.0[a]	14
		Ara-C (A)	1—5	200.0	
		Prednisone (P)	1—5	200.0[a]	
2	Guanazole	Guanazole	1—5	25[c]	14
2	A-T	Ara-C (A)	1—5	100.0	14
		Thioguanine (T)	2—4	130.0	
1	POMP	6-Mercaptopurine (P)	1—5	500.0	14
		Vincristine (O)	1	2.0[a]	
		Methotrexate (M)	1—5	7.5	
		Prednisone (P)	1—5	200.0[a]	

[a] Total dose/patient/day.

[b] From day 1 of 1 course to day 1 of next course.

[c] Gm/M^2.

course of chemotherapy, and at least 5 days after the completion of the previous course. The patients were studied prior to the second or third course of therapy for induction of remission and again during remission maintenance therapy. 27 of the 35 patients had not been treated with chemotherapy previously while 8 had relapsed from previous chemotherapeutic regimens. The criteria for remission have been described previously [27].

Results

19 of 24 patients with AML and 6 of 11 with ALL had a positive blastogenic response (S.I. > 2) to autologous leukemia cells in autologous or allogeneic serum, or in both sera. Correlation between the degree of blastogenic response to leukemia cells and the clinical response is shown in Table 2. 17 of 20 (85%) patients with an

Table 2. Correlation between degree of blastogenic response to leukemia cells and clinical response

		S.I. < 3[a]	S.I. > 3	S.I. > 5	S.I. > 10
No. remission / No. tested	AML	5/8	13/16	12/13	8/8
	ALL	4/7	4/4	3/3	1/1
	Total	9/15 (60%)	17/20 (85%)	15/16 (94%)	9/9 (100%)
No. relapsed / No. remission	AML	3/5	2/13	2/12	0/8
	ALL	4/4	2/4	1/3	0/1
	Total	7/9 (78%)	4/17 (24%)	3/15 (20%)	0/9 (0%)
Median duration[b] of remission (weeks)		19	20 +	20 +	21 +

[a] Maximum stimulation index in either autologous or allogeneic serum.
[b] Difference between S.I. < 3, S.I. > 3, $P = 0.02$ (Wilcoxon).
Difference between S.I. < 3, S.I. > 10, $P = 0.002$ (Wilcoxon).

S.I. greater than 3 achieved remission. In contrast, only 60% of patients with an S.I. less than 3 achieved a clinical remission. All 9 patients with an S.I. greater than 10 had a clinical remission. Most patients with high S.I. had AML. The remission duration also correlated with the relapse rate. Thus, 78% of patients with an S.I. less than 3 who achieved remission relapsed subsequently. The median duration of remission was only 19 weeks. In contrast, only 24% of patients with an S.I. greater than 3 have relapsed, and none of the patients with an S.I. greater than 10 have relapsed. Their median duration of remission is greater than 21 weeks. 6 of the 8 ALL patients achieving remission have relapsed in contrast to onyl 5 of the 18 with AML.

The positive blastogenic response of 9 of the 24 positive patients was partially or completely abrogated when the cultures contained the patient's own serum instead of allogenic serum (Table 3). 8 of these patients had AML.

34 of the 35 patients had studies of direct membrane immunofluorescence with leukemia cells and the results are shown on Table 3. The cells of 8 of 24 patients

with AML, but 0 of 10 patients with ALL demonstrated immunofluorescence with anti-IgG antisera when the cells were incubated either in McCoy's medium or the patient's own sera, or both. The fluorescence staining appeared as large, non-uniform clumps on the surface of the leukemia cells.

The correlation between the blastogenic response, its serum inhibition, and the presence of membrane immunofluorescence is also shown in Table 3. 7 of the 9 patients with inhibition of blastogenesis by their own serum showed positive immunofluorescence with anti-IgG antisera. In contrast, only one of the 15 patients with a positive blastogenic response who did not have a serum inhibitory effect had a positive immunofluorescence. Finally, cells from patients who did not have a blastogenic response to leukemia cells failed to show this immunofluorescence reaction.

Table 3. Correlation between membrane immunofluorescence blastogenic response and serum inhibitory effect

Blastogenic response	Serum inhibition	Membrane immunofluorescence in types of leukemia			
		AML		ALL	
(S.I. > 2)		Yes	No	Yes	No
Yes	Yes	7[a]	1	0	1
Yes	No	1	10	0	4
No	No	0	5	0	5
Totals		8	16	0	10

[a] Difference between immunofluorescence in group with serum inhibition and other 2 groups without inhibition highly significant (Chi-square P value < 0.005).

The laboratory and clinical data on the 10 patients with the serum inhibitory effect or positive membrane immunofluorescence, or both, are shown in Table 4. 6 of the patients were males and 4 were females. All except patient 9 had AML. 6 of the 7 patients with positive blastogenesis, serum inhibition, and positive immunofluorescence experienced a complete clinical remission after chemotherapy. 4 of these patients have been studied serially, and the inhibitory effect has been constant in 3.

The percentage of fluorescence cells did not increase after the cells were incubated in the patient's own sera compared to incubation with McCoy's media (except for patient number 7). 50% of cells of 2 patients (number 6 and 10) also reacted with anti-IgM and IgA antisera.

6 of the 9 patients with inhibitory effect had complete abrogation of the blastogenic response when the leukemia cells were incubated in autologous serum and it was greater than 80% in the other 3 (numbers 3, 4 and 8). In contrast, only 4 of these 9 patients showed significant inhibition of the response to PHA by autologous serum and in 2 it was less than 70%. Thus, the inhibition of blastogenic response to leukemia cells was greater than 80% in 9 of 9, but that of PHA response was greater than 80% in only 2 of 9.

The response of normal allogeneic donor leukocytes to the leukemia cells of the 10 patients (serum inhibition or positive immunofluorescence, or both) is shown in Table 4. Cultures containing allogeneic lymphocytes were incubated in both the

Table 4. Patients with serum inhibitory effect and positive immunofluorescence

Test of clinical or immunological response	Parameter of evaluation	Source of serum	Patient number									
			1	2	3	4	5	6	7	8	9	10
Immuno- fluorescence	% Positive (IgG)	None	20	40	50	50	25	50	5	<5	<5	50
		AB +	20	ND [c]	ND	48	19	ND	23	<5	<5	50
		Autologous	20	40	50	50	15	50	20	<5	<5	50
Blastogenic response of patient lymphocytes	Tumor cells CPM [a]	Autologous	0.0	0.0	18.7	0.7	0.0	0.0	0.0	6.5	0.0	5.1
		Allogeneic	120.0	4.6	23.3	5.1	1.7	1.2	1.1	19.5	0.8	2.6
	Tumor cells S.I. [b]	Autologous	0.5	0.5	27	2.4	0.0	0.9	0.8	5.3	0.7	5.9
		Allogeneic	1250	27	517	14.8	3.1	2.5	5.4	38.0	2.4	3.2
	PHA CPM	Autologous	63.0	48.4	53.6	31.0	57.8	40.2	107.0	50.4	5.6	29.8
		Allogeneic	ND	55.1	64.4	58.5	107.0	41.7	ND	95.6	10.7	35.0
	PHA S.I.	Autologous	789	19.8	56.1	103	380	38.8	548	34.5	7.5	35.3
		Allogeneic	ND	23.2	771.0	164	200	107.0	ND	383.0	22.2	43.6
Therapeutic response	Complete remission		Yes	Yes	Yes	Yes	Yes	Yes	No	Yes	No	Yes
Blastogenic response allogeneic normal lymphocytes	Tumor cells CPM	Patient	0.0	4.2	28.8	0.0	16.1	40.5	ND	ND	13.1	24.8
		Normal	38.1	41.7	57.7	3.7	26.3	33.6	7.9	58.3	20.2	11.6
	Tumor cells S.I.	Patient	0.9	5.7	9.7	0.1	47	41	ND	ND	4	24
		Normal	376	47.3	18.5	2.4	77	18	15.2	58.0	5.6	32

[a] CPM: counts per minute, per 10^6 lymphocytes $\times 10^3$. — [b] SI: Stimulation index. — [c] ND: Not determined.

patient's serum and the donor (allogeneic) serum. In three instances, the response of donor allogeneic lymphocytes was significantly inhibited by the patient's serum as compared to the donor serum. Thus, in at least three instances, inhibitory serum was able to block both autologous and allogeneic lymphocyte responsiveness to leukemia cells.

The sera of 5 of the 25 patients with positive blastogeneic responses showed a facilitory effect on the blastogeneic response to autologous leukemia cells. There was a significant increase in the tumor response of the patients' lymphocytes cultured in

Table 5. Blastogenic response to autologous leukemia cells — Serum facilitory effect

Patient	Dx	CPM × 10^3		Stimulation index		Clinical response
		Auto.	Allo.	Auto.	Allo.	
1.	AML	3.6	1.08	5.7	1.9	R
2.	AML	9.5	0.09	59.7	1.0	R
3.	AML	4.5	0	80.9	0.9	R
4.	AML	1.82	0	12.9	1.0	R
5.	ALL	3.3	0.08	10.0	1.4	R
Median		3.6	0.08	12.9	0	

autologous serum compared to allogeneic serum. 4 of the 5 had AML and all experienced clinical remission. 3 also had a significant facilitation of the response to PHA in autologous serum. 2 of these and an additional patient also had an increase response to SLO in autologous serum. Thus, 4 or 5 had an increase response to either PHA or SLO in autologous serum, and therefore the facilitatory effect was non-specific.

The correlation between general immunocompetence as measured by the response to PHA and SLO in lymphocyte response to autologous leukemia cells is shown in Table 6. The overall median response to PHA in CPM was somewhat lower in the

Table 6. Correlation between blastogenic response to leukemia cells, PHA and SLO

Blastogenic response to leukemia cells	Stimulation-index	< 3	> 3	> 5	> 10
Blastogenic response to PHA	Net CPM × 10^3	62.0 [a] (11.0—114.0)	84.0 (13—148)	69.0 (13—145)	55.0 (13—145)
	S.I. [b]	139 (4.7—500)	322 (13—1116)	250 (13—1116)	464 (13—1116)
Blastogenic response to SLO	Net CPM × 10^3	2.3 (0—46.0)	13.2 (0—98)	13.5 (0—98)	17.7 (0—98)
	S.I. [c]	3.6 (0—162)	17.5 (1.5—843)	14.7 (1.5—843)	16.0 (1.5—843)

[a] All values are medians with ranges in parenthesis. Values represent maximum response in autologous or allogeneic serum.

[b] Difference in PHA response between S.I. < 3 and S.I. > 3 groups P = 0.05.

[c] Difference in SLO response between S.I. < 3 and S.I. > 3 groups P = 0.013.

group with the S.I. less than 3 than the group with an S.I. greater than 3. The S.I. of the former group was clearly lower than the latter. The response to SLO in these groups of patients was more interesting. Those with a stimulation index to autologous leukemia cells greater than 3 had a strikingly superior response to SLO than those with a response less than 3. A similar pattern was noted for the S.I. to SLO. Despite this difference only one of 15 patients with an S.I. to autologous leukemia cells less than 3 had a subnormal response to PHA (CPM less than 20,000) [21].

Table 7. Serial blastogenic response to leukemia cells in patients experiencing remission

Change in blastogenic response		Change in clinical status	
		Remission → remission	Remission → relapse
Initial study	Follow-up study		
Positive [a] →	positive	9	1
Negative →	positive	1	0
Positive →	negative	0	2
Negative →	negative	1	5

[a] Positive = stimulation index ≧ 2.
Negative = stimulation index ≦ 2.

Table 8. Blastogenic response to leukemia cells

	Net CPM × 10^3		Stimulation index		P value
	AML	ALL	AML	ALL	
Patient Lymphocytes	4.6 [a] (0—120.0)	0.449 (0—3.35)	5.4 (0.9—1250)	2.6 (0.7—12.1)	0.06
Normal Lymphocytes	34.9 (0.937—104.0)	11.1 (2.6—76.2)	35.9 (1.6—579.0)	17.7 (2.9—113)	0.35

[a] All values are medians with ranges in parenthesis.

However, 7 of 15 patients with an S.I. less than 3 had a subnormal response to SLO (CPM less than 2,000) [24], compared to 5 of 20 with an S.I. greater than 3. Thus, the proportion of patients considered immunoincompetent was only slightly greater in the group with a poor response to autologous leukemia cells. The overall response by AML and ALL patients to PHA was comparable (median net CPM 60×10^3 and 67×10^3 respectively). Patients with AML has a somewhat more vigorous response to SLO than those with ALL (8.5×10^3 compared to 3.7×10^3 CPM respectively).

19 patients achieving a clinical remission had repeat studies during the remission maintenance phase of their treatment. These results are shown in Table 7. 10 of 11 (91%) of the patients who had a positive blastogenic response during remission have

continued in remission. In contrast, 7 of the 8 patients who had a negative response to leukemia cells during remission have relapsed. 2 of these patients were positive initially. 5 of 6 of the patients whose negative (S.I. < 2) blastogenic responses persisted have relapsed.

The overall blastogenic responses to leukemia cells by patients' lymphocytes and allogeneic normal lymphocytes cultured concurrently are shown in Table 8. The median response of AML patients to their own leukemia cells was considerably

Table 9. Blastogenic response to autologous leukemia cells (LC) and soluble leukemia cell antigen. Maximum response in autologous or allogeneic serum

Cell and antigen number	Net CPM × 10^3		Stimulation index		Effect of therapy
	LC	Antigen	LC	Antigen	
1	1.7	2.4	3.1	5.4	R
2	5.9	21.8	10.8	39.6	R
3	9.2	1.0	30.5	4.4	R
4	19.5	1.6	38.0	6.4	R
5	0	0.62	0.9	1.1	R
6	0.72	0.56	3.6	2.8	F
7	0	0.64	0.8	3.1	F

Table 10. Blastogenic response of normal human lymphocytes to allogeneic leukemia cells (LC) and soluble leukemia cell antigen

Cell and antigen number	Net CPM × 10^3		Stimulation index	
	LC	Antigen	LC	Antigen
1	26.0	0.53	75.4	2.7
2	30.0	0.08	60.0	1.2
3	18.0	0	12.5	0.1
4	65.0	0	65.0	0.7
5	25.0	0	52.0	0.7
6	0.17	0.18	1.6	1.6
7	34.0	0.10	66.0	1.2

greater than the response of ALL patients to their own cells. Similarly, normal subject lymphocytes responded to a significantly greater degree to AML cells than to ALL cells.

Table 9 summarizes the patient's lymphocyte blastogenic responses to soluble antigen and autologous leukemia cells. 5 of the patients had AML, one had ALL and one had blast crisis of CML. 4 of the 5 patients with AML and the patient with ALL had significant blastogenic response to autologous leukemia cells. All 5 of these patients as well as the patient with blast crisis had significant blastogenic responses to soluble antigen. The response to soluble antigen was greater than the response to cells in patients 2 and 7. In contrast, the response to intact leukemia cells was greater in patients 3 and 4. 4 of the 5 patients achieving remission responded to antigen with an S.I. greater than 4. In contrast, the 2 patients who failed to achieve a bone marrow remission had S.I. less than 4.

The blastogenic response of normal allogeneic donor lymphocytes to leukemia cells and soluble antigen is shown in Table 10. 6 of the 7 leukemic cell preparations elicted a vigorous blastogenic response *in vitro*. In contrast, only one of the soluble antigen preparations (number 1) induced a significant response, and this was quite weak.

Although dose response relationships were noted in these studies, good stimulation was noted when doses were as low as 10—100 μg/ml. Because of the limited availability of the antigen, doses higher than 1000 μg/ml of culture were not used in the study. In at least 2 patients, the maximum stimulating dose of antigen may not have been used since th edose response curve was still rising at 1000 μg/ml.

None of the 34 patients have demonstrated positive delayed hypersensitivity reactions to intact leukemia cells with doses as high as 10^6 per 0.1 ml. 2 of the 7 patients skin tested with antigen have reacted with a positive skin test (patients 1 and 3). The positive delayed hypersensitivity skin reaction was confirmed by punch biopsies. 4 of the 5 patients who did not demonstrate delayed hypersensitivity to the soluble antigen, however, were anergic to the battery of 5 established skin test antigens at the time of testing.

Discussion

To acquire a more complete understanding of the patients immune responses to autologous tumor, it is important to consider both the cell-associated and humoral aspects of tumor immunity. The series of studies in acute leukemia reported here were designed to determined the interrelationship between lymphocyte blastogenic responses to leukemia cells, serum effects on these responses, and in the pressence or absence of immunoglobulin on the leukemia cells. In addition to the knowledge gained, this type of combined approach should form a background for the design of rational immunotherapy programs in acute leukemia and in other malignancies.

Previous work from this laboratory has demonstrated that immunocompetence is associated with a favorable prognosis in patients with acute leukemia [19]. The present study has identified several new features which may be of relevance to the prognosis of these patients. In addition to confirming previous observations that the lymphocytes of the majority of patients with acute leukemia show a blastogenic responce to their own leukemia cells [9], we have identified a strong correlation between the intensity of lymphocyte responsiveness to autologous leukemia cells early in therapy, and the likelihood of subsequent remission. Even more significant, the duration of remission is longer in patients with vigorous responses to their leukemia cells. Some previous studies have failed to demonstrate this correlation [28]. However, Oren and Herberman found a correlation between the positive response to skin tests with autologous leukemia membrances and clinical remissions in ALL patients [34].

It is interesting to speculate that the strong immune response to leukemia cells may augment the chemotherapeutic effects and play a role in the remission induction process. Similar speculations have been offered as an explanation for the dramatic responses seen with chemotherapy in patients with Burkitt's lymphoma [6] and choriocarcinoma [25].

This study has also shown the importance of serial studies of tumor immunity in patients with leukemia. The persistence of a positive blastogenic response in remission or a change from nagetive to positive was associated with a good prognosis. In contrast, patients who repeatedly had negative blastogenic response to their leukemia cells during remission or who have gone from positive to negative, relapsed early. Therefore, these techniques should be used to evaluate patients on long term chemotherapy and be used to guide future immunotherapy trials in acute leukemia.

Earlier studies of humoral responses to human leukemia cells have only rarely detected immunoglobulin on the cell surfaces. They current demonstration that positive membrane immunofluorescence occurred as frequently when the cells were incubated in McCoy's media or the patients' own sera suggests that immunoglobulin is already coated on the cells. Whether the cells themselves are producing the IgG immunoglobulin (as Burkitt lymphoma cells produce IgM [24]) or the cells are being coated from the outside as described for the IgG on some Buıkitt cells [26] cannot be determined by these studies.

The idea that the positive fluorescence represents bound immunoglobulin in our group of patients is substantiated by the morphological appearance of the immunoglobulin on the tumor cells. Immunoglobulin receptors on cells of B origin show either a fine uniform ring pattern of fluorescence or cap formation [35]. In contrast, the immunoglobulin in the leukemia cells in this study appears as none uniform, larger clumps of staining, and this is characteristic of bound immunoglobulin.

Evidence for bound immunoglobulin was found only by patients with AML. Thus, patients with ALL either do not make such antibody or perhaps their leukemia cells are not very immunogenic. The greater autologous blastogenic response to AML cells compared to ALL cells also suggests this possibility. The fact that ALL cells do not appear to produce surface immunoglobulin as do tumor cells from other lymphoid tumors such as chronic lymphocytic leukemia [12] and malignant lymphoma [23] suggest that these cells may be of thymic origin, may not have differentiated sufficiently to produce immunoglobulin or may not be of lymphoid origin.

It has been recognized previously that patients with cancer may have factors in their serum which inhibits cell-associated responses to various mitogens and tumor cells [11]. The HELLSTRÖMS *et al.* have demonstrated a tumor specific blocking or enhancing antibody in the serum as many patients with progressively growing solid tumors [17]. [30] and [43] have demonstrated serum inhibition of blastogenic reactivity to tumor cells in patients with solid tumors. Initial studies by the HELLSTRÖMS suggested that the blocking factor was a 7S immunoglobulin. Recently, [42] have suggested that the blocking factor may be a tumor antigen-antibody complex. Although our present study showed a strong correlation between the presence of immunoglobulin on leukemia cells and the blocking of the blastogenic response, it does not clarify whether antibody, antigen-antibody complexes, or perhaps other factors may be involved with the inhibitory phenomenon.

In the present study the presence of immunoglobulin on leukemia cells and the presence of an inhibitory effect on the blastogenic response was correlated with a good prognosis. 6 of the 7 such patients achieved a clinical remission. 5 of these patients remained in remission from 3 to 12 months later. The serum inhibitory effect has been consistent throughout the clinical course in 3/4 patients tested serially.

The demonstration of a serum facilitatory effect in 5 patients with acute leukemia demonstrates that the effect of serum factors on *in vitro* cell-associated immunity is complex and requires careful investigation in individual patients with all types of maligancies. The pathogenesis of this effect is unclear but it appears to be associated with a relatively good prognosis. None of these patients had demonstrable immunoglobulin on their leukemia-cell surfaces. There may be circulating antigen or antigen antibody complexes in autologous serum which evoke an additive blastogenic effect *in vitro*. We should also take into account the previous report by [1], that lymphocyte response to PHA is lower when incubated in allogeneic serum than in autologous serum. Therefore, rather than autologous facilitation we may be seeing inhibition by allogeneic serum. At any rate, the evaluation of serum factors in all studies of cell-mediated immunity is of great importance in attempting to understand the immune response to human tumors.

The lymphocyte responses to PHA and SLO *in vitro* do not always parallel the patient's response to autologous leukemia cells, although as a group patients not responding to their own leukemia cells tended to have a lower response to PHA than patients with a positive blastogenic response to leukemia cells. Only 1 patient in the former group could be considered immunoincompetent on the basis of response to PHA. However, several patients unresponsive to leukemia cells have poor responses to the antigen SLO. Since macrophages are required for *in vitro* lymphocyte responsiveness to antigens [20], one could speculate that perhaps impaired processing of antigen by macrophages may be one of the reasons for lack of tumor cell responsiveness in some patients. However, several patients with vigorous responses to leukemia cells also had poor SLO responsiveness. Hence, the evaluation of general immunocompetence does not invariably parallel the response to autologous leukemia cells.

Another factor which may be important in the tumor responsiveness of patients is the antigenicity of leukemia cells. Our data strongly suggest that patients with AML have a more intense immune response to their own tumor cells compared to patients with ALL. As a group, there was no difference between AML and ALL patients in their response to PHA and only a slight difference in response to SLO. The evidence that AML may be associated with a more intense immune response is further substantiated by the superior response to AML cells of allogeneic normal lymphocytes compared to ALL cells. It is possible that there may be antigen deletion of some ALL cells. This has been suspected in a patient with malignant lymphoma [41] and some animal leukemias [4]. Alternatively, there may be antigen masking by sialic acid residues [47].

Our data indicate that antigen extracted from human leukemia cells by 3 m KCL can be used to stimulate autologous lymphocytes in lymphocyte cultures. The results correspond quite well with the lymphocyte response to autologous leukemia cells.

Except for one report to the contrary [45], most workers have reported that soluble histocompatibility antigens can stimulate lymphocyte blastogenesis only after prior sensitization [22, 29]. Only one of the normal donors in the current study responded to the allogeneic soluble antigen preparations, and even that response was very weak, while 6 of the 7 leukemia patients responded to their autologous antigen. Thus, the data strongly supports the idea that this lymphocyte stimulation indicates prior sensitization to the antigen and represents specific tumor immunity [1–]. A similar observation has recently been made in a patient with colon carcinoma [3–]. It was suggested that peripheral blood and lymphocytes can undergo primary *in vitro* blastogenic responses to foreign antigens only if the latter are cell-associated. If they are solubilized, a response will occur if the subject is immune. Whether presensitization is required to respond to cell-associated leukemia antigen is unclear [2, 16, 39].

Thus, the study has demonstrated the usefulness of soluble antigen in the study of tumor immunity in patients with leukemia. Hopefully, the use of soluble antigen will identify subjects previously sensitized with leukemia-associated antigens and may be helpful in the search for common antigens in leukemia cells. In addition, as the preliminary observations with skin testing has suggested, such antigen preparations should be useful in the other assays of cell-mediated immunity such as migration inhibition and delayed hypersensitivity.

References

1. AL-SARRAF, M., SARDESSI, S., VAITKEVICIUS, V. K.: Effect of syngeneic and allogeneic plasma on lymphocytes from cancer patients with non-neoplastic diseases, and normal subjects. Cancer (Philad.) **27**, 1426 (1971).
2. BACK, M. L., BACH, F. H., JOO, P.: Leukemia-associated antigens in the mixed leukocyte culture test. Science **166**, 1520 (1969).
3. BOYLE, W.: An extension of the ^{51}Cr release assay for the estimation of mouse cytotoxins. Transplantation **6**, 761 (1968).
4. BOYSE, A. B., OLD, L. J., STOCKERT, E., SHIGENO, N.: Genetic origin of tumor antigens. Cancer Res. **28**, 1280 (1968).
5. BURCHENAL, J. H.: Features suggesting curability in leukemia and lymphoma. In: Leukemia-lymphoma year book, pp. 93—104. New York: Medical Publishers 1970.
6. BURCHENAL, J. H.: Geographic chemotherapy — Burkitt's tumor as a stalking horse for leukemia. Presidential Adress. Cancer Res. **26**, 2393 (1966).
7. DORÉ, J. F., MORHOLEY, L., AJURIA, E., DORE, M., PAINTRAND, M., DE THE, G., MATHÈ, G.: Seriological evidence for immune reaction to leukemia in man. (Abstract volume), pp. 276. XIII. International Congress of Hematology 1970.
8. EVANS, H. M., SCHULEMANN, W.: The action of vital stains belonging to the benzidine group. Science **39**, 443 (1914).
9. FRIDMAN, W. H., KOURILSKY, F. M.: Stimulation of lymphocytes by autologous leukemic cells in acute leukemia. Nature **224**, 277 (1969).
10. FREIREICH, E. J., CURTIS, J. E., HERSH, E. M.: Use of the blood cell separator to collect lymphocytes: Characteristics of the collection and effects on the donor. In: White cell transfunsions (MATHÉ, F., Ed.), pp. 259. Paris: Centre National de la Recherche Scientifique 1970.
11. GATTI, R. A., GARRIOCH, D. H., GOOD, R. A.: In: Proceedings of Fifth Leukocyte Culture Conference (HARRIS, J., Ed.), p. 339. New York: Academic Press 1970.
12. GREY, H. M., RABELLINO, E., PIROFSKY, B.: Immunoglobulins on the surface of lymphocytes. IV. Distribution of hypogammaglobulinemia, cellular immune deficiency, and chronic lymphatic leukemia. J. clin. Invest. **50**, 2368 (1971).
13. GUTTERMAN, J. U., G. MAVLIGIT, MCCREDIE, K. B., BODYE, G. P., FREIREICH, E. J., HERSH, E. M.: Antigen solubilized from human leukemia: Lymphocyte stimulation. Science **177**, 1114 (1972).
14. GUTTERMAN, J. U., HERSH, W. M., MCCREDIE, K. B., BODEY, G., RODRIQUEZ, V., FREIREICH, E. J.: Lymphocyte blastogenesis to human leukemia cells and their relationship to serum factors, immunocompetence, and prognosis. Cancer Res. **32**, 2524 (1972).

15. Gutterman, J. U., Rossen, R. D., Butler, W. T., McCredie, K. B., Godey, G. P., Freireich, E. J., Hersh, E. M.: Immunoglobulin on tumor cells and tumor-induced lymphocyte blastogenesis in human acute leukemia. New Engl. J. Med. **288**, 169 (1973).
16. Halterman, R. H., Leventhal, B. G.: Mixed leukocyte cultures (MLC) reactivity to leukemia cells in patients, their twins, and HL-A identical siblings. Proc. Amer. Ass. Cancer Res. **13**, 6 (1972).
17. Hellström, K. E., Hellström, I.: Immunological enhancement as studied by cell culture techniques. Ann. Rev. Microbiol. **24**, 373 (1970).
18. Hersh, E. M.: Blastogenic responses of human lymphocytes to xenogeneic cell *in vitro*. Transplantation **12**, 287 (1971).
19. Hersh, E. M., Brown, B.: Inhibition of the immune response by glutamine antagonist-effects of azotomycin on lymphocyte blastogenesis. Cancer Res. **31**, 834 (1971).
20. Hersh, E. M., Harris, J. E.: Macrophage-lymphocyte interaction in the antigen-induced blastogenic response of human peripheral blood leukocytes. J. Immunol. **100**, 1184 (1968).
21. Hersh, E. M., Whitecar, J. P., McCredie, K. B., Bodey, G. P., Freireich, E. J.: Chemotherapy, immunocompetence, immunosuppression and prognosis in acute leukemia. New Engl. J. Med. **285**, 1211 (1971).
22. Kahan, B. D., Reisfield, R. A., Epstein, L. B., Southworth, J. G.: In: Histocompatibility testing (Curtoni, E. S., Martiuz, P. L., Tose, R. M., Eds.)
23. Klein, E., Clifford, P., Klein, G., Hamberger, C. A.: Further studies on the membrane immunofluorescence reaction of Burkitt lymphoma cells. Int. J. Cancer **2**, 27 (1967).
24. Klein, E., Klein, G., Nadkarni, J. J., Nadkarni, J. S., Wigzell, H., Clifford, P.: Surface IgM-kappa specificity on a Burkitt lymphoma cell *in vivo* and in derived culture lines. Cancer Res. **28**, 1300 (1968).
25. Klein, G.: Experimental studies in tumor immunology. Fed. Proc. **28**, 1739 (1969).
26. Klein, G.: Immunological studies on human tumor. Israel J. med. Sci. **7**, 111 (1971).
27. Leikin, S. L., Brubaker, C., Hartmann, J. R., Murphy, M., Wolff, J., Perrin, E.: Varying prednisone dosage in remission induction of previously untreated childhood leukemia. Cancer (Philad.) **21**, 346 (1968).
28. Leventhal, B. G., Halterman, R. H., Rosenberg, E. B., Herberman, R. B.: Immune reactivity of leukemia patients to autologous blast cells. Cancer Res. **32**, 1820 (1972).
29. Leventhal, B. G., Mann, D. L., Rogentine, G. N., jr.: Sensitization to water soluble HL-A antigens. Transplant. Proc. **3**, 243 (1971).
30. Mavligit, G., Gutterman, J.U., McBride, C. M., Hersh, E. M.: Multifaceted evaluation of human tumor immunity using a salt extracted colon carcinoma antigen. Proc. Soc. exp. Biol. Med. (N.Y.) **140**, 1240 (1972).
31. Mavligit, G. M., Hersh, E. M., McBride, C. M.: Influence of tumor irradiation and specific serum factors (s) on lymphocyte blastogenic response to solid tumors. Proc. Amer. Ass. Cancer Res. **13**, 67 (1972).
32. Meltzer, M. S., Leonard, E. J., Rapp, H. J., Borsos, T.: Tumor-specific antigen solubilized by hypertonic potassium chloride. J. nat. Cancer Inst. **47**, 703 (1971).
33. Möller, G.: Demonstration of mouse isoantigens at the cellular level by the fluorescent antibody technique. J. exp. Med. **114**, 415 (1961).
34. Oren, M. E., Herberman, R. B.: Delayed cutaneous hypersensitivity reactions to membrane extracts of human tumor cells. Clin. exp. Immunol. **9**, 45 (1971).
35. Papamichail, M., Brown, J. C., Holoborow, E. J.: Immunoglobulins on the surface of human lymphocytes. Lancet **1971 I**, 840.
36. Powles, R. L., Balchin, L. A., Fairley, G. H., Alexander, P.: Recognition of leukemic cells as foreign before and after autoimmunization. Brit. med. J. **1971 I**, 486.
37. Reisberg, M. A., Rossen, R. D., Butler, W. T.: A method for preparing specific fluorescein-conjugated antibody reagents using bentonite immunoadsorbents. J. Immunol. **105**, 1151 (1970).
38. Reisfeld, R. A., Pellegrino, M. A., Kahan, B. D.: Salt-extraction of soluble HLA-A antigens. Science **172**, 1134 (1971).
39. Rudolph, R. H., Mickelson, E., Thomas, E. D.: Mixed leukocyte reactivity and leukemia: Study of identical siblings. J. clin. Invest. **49**, 2275 (1970).
40. Rossen, R. D., Butler, W. T., Reisberg, M. A., Brooks, D. K., Leachmen, R. D., Milam, J. D., Mittal, K. K., Montgomery, J. R., Nora, J. J., Rochelle, D. G.: Immunofluorescent

localization of human immunoglobulin in tissues from cardiac allograft recipients. J. Immunol. **106**, 171 (1971).
41. Seigler, H. F., Kremer, W. B., Metzgar, R. S., Ward, F. E., Huang, A. T., Amos, D. B.: HL-A antigenic loss in malignant transformation. J. nat. Cancer Inst. **46**, 577 (1971).
42. Sjogren, H. O., Hellström, I., Bansal, S. C., Hellström, K. E.: Suggestive evidence that the "blocking antibodies" of tumor-bearing individuals may be antigen-antibody complexes. Proc. nat. Acad. Sci. (Wash.) **68**, 1372 (1971).
43. Vanky, F., Stjernsward, J., Klein, G., Nilsenne, U.: Serum-mediated inhibition of lymphocyte stimulation by autochthonous human tumors. J. nat. Cancer Inst. **47**, 95 (1971).
44. Viza, D. C., Bernard-Degani, O., Bernard, C., Harris, R.: Leukemia antigens. Lancet **1969 II**, 493.
45. Viza, D. C., Degani, O., Dausset, J., Davies, D. A. L.: Lymphocyte stimulation by soluble human HL-A transplantation antigens. Nature **219**, 704 (1968).
46. Yoshida, T. O., Imai, K.: Auto-antibody to human leukemic cell membrane as detected by immune adherence. Europ. J. clin. biol. Res. **15**, 61 (1970).
47. Watkins, E. Jr., Ogata, Y., Anderson, L. L., Watkins, E. III., Waters, M. F.: Activation of host lymphocytes cultured with cancer cells treated with neuraminidase. Nature New Biol. **231**, 83 (1971).

Lymphocyte Cytotoxicity in Human Acute Leukemia*

B. G. LEVENTHAL [1], R. H. HALTERMAN [1], E. B. ROSENBERG [2], J. L. McCOY [3], and R. B. HERBERMAN [2]

[1] Leukemia Service and [2] Laboratory of Cell Biology, National Cancer Institute and [3] Bionetics Research Laboratories, Bethesda, Maryland

Introduction

There are several mechanisms of lymphocyte-mediated target cell killing which can be assayed *in vitro*. Lymphocytes which have been sensitized either *in vivo* or *in vitro* to transplantation antigens can kill target cells directly. These activated cells are thought to be thymus-derived (T) killer cells. Non-sensitized lymphocytes with immunoglobulin receptor sites (B lymphocytes) can attach to and kill specific antibody coated target cells. This mechanism has been called lymphocyte-dependent antibody-induced cytotoxicity. Lymphocytes which are sensitive to antigen can also indirectly kill target cells coated with the same antigen [18]. These same mechanisms have also been shown to result in tumor cell destruction *in vitro*, although presumably only the direct and antibody-mediated mechanisms could be assumed to be active against tumor cells *in vivo*.

Most of these observations have been made with *in vitro* methods which use solid tumor cells or allogeneic tissue culture cell lines as targets and they generally utilize the capacity of these cells to stick to glass or plastic surfaces as they grow. The degree of cell killing is assessed by direct cell counts after varying periods of incubation with attacker lymphocytes [9, 20]. In all studies the incubation period is short (usually less than 2 days) to avoid *in vitro* sensitization.

Acute leukemia cells remain in suspension in culture and will not adhere to culture flasks. The method used in this study was an adaptation by CANTY and WUNDERLICH [3] of a method originally described by BRUNNER [2] using ^{51}Cr-labeled target cells. This assay has been useful in measuring tumor-specific cellular immunity to a virus-induced lymphoma in inbred rats [17]. Reactivity of patients' remission cells to autologous and allogeneic blast cells was seen.

Methods

All patients had either acute lymphatic leukemia (ALL) or acute myelogeneous leukemia (AML) as diagnosed by bone marrow morphology at the National Cancer

* Supported in part by U.S.P.H.S. contracts, NIH-NCI 69-2160 and NIH-NCI 72-3227. We thank G. JOHNSON, D. SIWARSKI, F. DONNELLY and G. FISCHETTI for their excellent technical assistance.

Institute. Normal individuals were usually laboratory workers or blood bank donors.

Acute leukemia blast cells were obtained from patients by leukopheresis and stored in liquid nitrogen with 10% DMSO (dimethylsulfoxide) as preservative. After the patients had been treated, normal peripheral blood lymphocytes were obtained and used as attacking cells for the lymphocyte cytotoxicity assay (LCA). Target leukemia cells were labeled with ^{51}Cr. The attacker to target-cell ratio was 60:1. The incubation period was 4 h with constant agitation, after which the supernatants were collected and the amount of ^{51}Cr released was counted and expressed as the percentage of total ^{51}Cr which could be released from the cells by rapid freeze-thawing repeated three times. Cultures were set up in quadruplicate and statistical differences between experimental and control cultures analyzed for significance with Student's t test. A test was considered positive if the p value was less than 0.05. Details of the method have been previously reported [19].

A standard cell line against which the majority of normal individuals do show cytotoxic activity was used as a positive control target in many experiments. This lymphoblast line (F-265) was originally started with cells from a normal individual and has been maintained in long-term culture [15].

Mixed leukocyte cultures (MLC) using autologous mitomycin-treated leukemia cells as stimulators [12] and skin tests with autologous blast membrane preparations [16] were performed by methods previously described.

Results

None of the leukemia patients showed cytotoxic reactivity against target cells from normal individuals but 8/20 ALL and 6/19 AML patients showed reactivity against autologous blast cells (Table 1).

Table 1. Lymphocyte cytotoxicity reactions against autochthonous target cells
Positive tests/total number of tests (%)

Attacking lymphocytes	Target cells	
	Blasts	Normal
ALL	8/20 (40)	0/22 (0)
AML	6/19 (32)	0/10 (0)
Normal		0/30 (0)

This reactivity was not correlated with clinical state since 11/31 studies of patients in remission and 3/9 patients in relapse gave positive results.

When response of cells to allogeneic targets were studied, there was a high degree of cross-reactivity. Leukemia patients with ALL reacted to both ALL and AML blast cells and leukemia patients with AML reacted to both AML and ALL blast cells from other individuals, but the patients did not react to normal leukocytes nor to remission leukemia cells. In contrast there was a high degree of reactivity of the normal individuals' cells against both relapse and remission cells from leukemia patients but not against the cells from the other normal individuals (Table 2).

Two other tests of cellular reactivity were also used; delayed hypersensitivity skin testing with membrane extracts from autologous leukemia cells, and mixed leukocyte cultures using autologous mitomycin-treated leukemia cells as stimulating cells. There was no apparent correlation between different tests run at approximately the same time in 20 patients. Skin test and LCA results were the same 6 times and different 6 times. Skin test and MLC results were the same 7 times and different 9 times. The MLC and LCA were the same 6 times and different 6 times [12].

Table 2. Lymphocyte cytotoxicity reactions against allogeneic target cells
Positive tests/total number of tests (%)

Target cell	Attacking lymphocytes		
	Normal	ALL patients	AML patients
Normal lymphocytes	5/220 (2.3)	0/20 (0)	0/15 (0)
ALL blasts	55/117 (47)	9/23 (39)	4/15 (27)
ALL remission lymphocytes	15/79 (19)	0/5 (0)	0/2 (0)
AML blasts	40/95 (42)	6/14 (43)	6/25 (24)
AML remission lymphocytes	13/47 (28)	0	0/5 (5)

Recently it has been demonstrated that intermittent chemotherapy can lead to an increase in the degree of *in vitro* reactivity to standard antigens [4], in MLC [8] and to autologous leukemia cells [5]. In two patients in whom the MLC and LCA tests were performed simultaneously at varying intervals after 5 days of high dose combination chemotherapy there was no significant change in cytotoxic activity against autologous blast cells despite a marked increase in MLC reactivity at about 15 days after therapy [10].

Discussion

Patients with acute leukemia do have cell-mediated immune reactions to autologous leukemia cells [12]. In the skin test, patients react to membranes prepared from autologous and allogeneic leukemia cells but not to those from normal allogeneic leukocytes [17]. In the MLC, HL-A identical siblings do not react to blast cell preparations which are stimulatory to the patient [6]. Thus the specificity of these two immune cellular reactions appears to be established.

In studies using human tissue culture cell membrane fractions to immunize rabbits, cytotoxic antisera have been produced which are active against both AML and ALL relapse cells, but not to cells from these same patients in remission [7], nor to normal white blood cells [14]. These antisera were also cytotoxic to all cultured human lymphoblast lines tested, but were unreactive to non-human cell lines [13].

In the present studies, lymphocytes from the leukemia patients were seen to be cytotoxic to autologous and allogeneic blast cells and to cultured human lymphoblasts but not to remission leukemia cells or normal cells.

All of this data taken together may be best interpreted as showing that a human antigen is expressed on the surface of the "transformed" acute leukemia blast cell and on human tissue culture cell lines which is not present on normal leukocytes. The patient has been sensitized and is therefore reactive to this antigen because he has leukemia: the antigen is not recognizable when the patient is in remission.

In the cytotoxicity assay the high degree of reactivity of normals against both the relapse and remission leukemia cells is difficult to explain, particularly since it differs from the pattern shown by the patients who, although the numbers are small, react to relapse but not to remission cells. Several possible explanations for this data come to mind. It may be that leukemic patients are less responsive than normal to the smaller quantity of antigen which still persists on the surface of the leukemic patients' blood cells even when the patient is in remission. Alternatively the antigen recognized on the remission cells by the normal controls may be different from the blast antigen. This possibility of two distinct antigens is supported by the pattern of reactivity of many of the normal controls: some had reactivity against one cell type but not the other. A third possibility is that the leukemic patients' cells are coated with antibody and the normals are showing a lymphocyte-dependent cytotoxic reaction. However, when this type of lymphocyte-dependent cytotoxic reactivity was directly determined in the sera of 40 patients with acute leukemia, no consistent activity was found [11].

A high degree of cross-reactivity using solid tumor target cells with normal individuals and individuals with cancer different from those of the target cell line is now being reported by workers using the microcytotoxicity method [21]. In the earlier studies with these methods there was a greater specificity but less overall cytotoxicity at low attacker to target cell ratios than at high ratios [20]. The most likely explanation for this high degree of cross-reactivity seems to be a loss of specificity in the assay as the sensitivity has increased.

The lack of correlation of the LCA with other assays of cellular immunity is puzzling but best explained if one assumes that the tests are measuring different aspects of the immune response.

The failure of the cytotoxic reaction to show an "overshoot" after chemotherapy as is seen in the MLC is disappointing since a reaction during which an immune cell clearly kills its malignant target would seem the most useful type of reaction to attempt to induce during chemoimmunotherapy. However, the four-drug combination employed in these two patients may not have been appropriate for demonstrating such an effect. Animal experiments have already shown that at least two types of cells can be responsible for direct *in vitro* cytotoxicity. One type arises 6—12 days after immunization and is resistant to irradiation and drugs which inhibit DNA synthesis. The other, arising later, at about 21 days, is radiation-sensitive and killed by agents affecting DNA [21]. Although it may not be valid to generalize these results to human tumor systems, it is clear that further studies may show a relationship between chemotherapy and the lymphocyte responsible for cytotoxicity.

References

1. BLOOM, B. R.: In vitro approaches to the mechanism of cell mediated immune reactions. Advanc. Immunology **13**, 101 (1971).
2. BRUNNER, K. T., MANUEL, J., RUDOLF, H., CHAPIUS, B.: Studies of allograft immunity in mice. I. Induction, development and in vitro assay of cellular immunity. Immunology **18**, 501 (1970).

3. CANTY, T. G., WUNDERLICH, J. R.: Quantitative *in vitro* assay of cytotoxic cellular immunity. J. Nat. Cancer Inst. **45**, 761 (1970).
4. CHEEMA, A. R., HERSH, E. M.: Patient survival after chemotherapy and its relationship to *in vitro* blastogenesis. Cancer (Philad.) **28**, 851 (1971).
5. HALTERMAN, R. H., LEVENTHAL, B. G.: Enhanced immune response to leukemia. Lancet **1971 II**, 704.
6. HALTERMAN, R. H., LEVENTHAL, B. G.: Mixed leukocyte cultures (MLC) reactivity of leukemia cells in patients, their twins and HL-A identical siblings. Proc. Amer. Ass. Cancer Res. **13**, 6 (1972).
7. HALTERMAN, R. H., LEVENTHAL, B. G., MANN, D. L.: An acute leukemia antigen: Its correlation with clinical status. New Engl. J. Med. **287**, 1272 (1972).
8. HARRIS, J. E., STEWART, T. H. M.: Recovery of mixed lymphocyte reactivity (MLR) following cancer chemotherapy. In: Proceedings of the Sixth leukocyte Culture Conference (SCHWARZ, M. R., Ed.), p. 555. New York: Academic Press 1972.
9. HELLSTRÖM, I., HELLSTRÖM, K. E.: Colony inhibition and cytotoxic assays. In: *in vitro* methods of cell mediated immunity (BLOOM, B. R., GLADE, P. R., Eds.), p. 409. New York: Academic Press 1971.
10. HERBERMAN, R. B., ROSENBERG, E. B., HALTERMAN, R. H., MCCOY, J. L., LEVENTHAL, B. G.: Cellular immune reactions to human leukemia. Nat. Cancer Inst. Monogr. **35**, 259 (1972).
11. LEPOURHIET, A., HALTERMAN, R. H., MANN, D. L.: Detection and isolation of a blocking factor (circulating antigen?). In Acute leukemia sera. In: Proc. IVth Intern. Congress of the Transplantation Society 1972.
12. LEVENTHAL, B. G., HALTERMAN, R. H., ROSENBERG, E. B., HERBERMAN, R. B.: Immune reactivity of leukemia patients to autologous blast cells. Cancer Res. **32**, 1820 (1972).
13. MANN, D. L. HALTERMAN, R., LEVENTHAL, B. G.: Crossreactive antigens on human cells infected with Rauscher leukemia virus and on human acute leukemia cells. Proc. Nat. Acad. Sci. USA, 70, 495, 1973.
14. MANN, D. L., ROGENTINE, G. N., HALTERMAN, R. H., LEVENTHAL, B. G.: Detection of an antigen associated with acute leukemia. Science **174**, 1136 (1971).
15. MCCOY, J. L., HERBERMAN, R. B., ROSENBERG, E. B., DONNELLY, F. C., LEVINE, P. H., ALFORD, C.: 51 Chromium-release assay for cell-mediated cytotoxicity of human leukemia and lymphoid tissue-culture cells, Nat. Canc. Inst. Monograph **37**, 59 (1973).
16. OREN, M. E., HERBERMAN, R. B.: Delayed cutaneous hypersensitivity reactions to membrane extracts of human tumor cells. Clin. exp. Immunol. **9**, 45 (1971).
17. OREN, M. E., HERBERMAN, R. B., CANTY, T. G.: Immune response to gross virus induced lymphoma: II. Kinetics of cellular immune response. J. nat. Cancer Inst. **46**, 621 (1971).
18. PERLMANN, P., HOLM, G.: Cytotoxic effects of lymphoid cells *in vitro*. Advanc. Immunology **11**, 117 (1969).
19. ROSENBERG, E. B., HERBERMAN, R. B., LEVINE, P. H., HALTERMAN, R. H., MCCOY, J. L., WUNDERLICH, J. R.: Lymphocyte cytotoxicity reactions to leukemia antigens. Int. J. Cancer **9**, 648 (1972).
20. TAKASUGI, M., KLEIN, E.: A microassay for cell mediated immunity. Transplantation **9**, 219 (1970).
21. TAKASUGI, M., MICKEY, M. R., TERASAKI, P.: Specificities in cell mediated reactions: relationships to cancer types Proc. Amer. Assoc. Canc. Res. **15**, 115 (1974).

Lymphocyte-Mediated Cytotoxicity and Tumor Immunity

J.-C. Cerottini

Department of Immunology, Swiss Institute for Experimental Cancer Research, Lausanne

In vitro assay systems based on destruction of tumor cells by blood lymphocytes are being used in studies of the immune response of cancer patients to tumor-associated antigens (TAA). In the last few years, lymphocyte-mediated cytotoxicity (LMC) has been demonstrated in a variety of human tumor systems. This suggests not only that TAA are present on the surface of human cancer cells but also that cancer patients have an immune response to the TAA of their own tumor. Because of the clinical importance of these observations, it is necessary to make a critical assessment of the relevance of the *in vitro* reactions to protective immunity in the cancer patient. We briefly review here the various methods used to detect LMC, with special reference to some of the technical problems associated with these *in vitro* assay systems. We then discuss the possible mechanisms for LMC in human tumor systems in the light of the results obtained in various experimental model systems and analyze the value of such *in vitro* tests for longitudinal studies of cancer patients.

Assay Systems

Two main procedures are presently employed. The first, developed by [12], is generally termed microcytotoxicity assay. It consists of plating 100—500 tumor cells into individual wells of microtitration plates. After attachment of the tumor cells, lymphocyte-enriched cell populations are added, usually at a lymphocyte–target ratio of 100 : 1 or more. The plates are incubated for 48—72 h; the wells are then washed out and the remaining target cells fixed, stained and counted. Cytotoxicity is usually expressed as the percentage reduction in the number of surviving target cells as against the controls. However, the number of tumor cells reamaining at the end of the incubation period is influenced by several factors, including spontaneous cell death, proliferation rate, detachment, and direct lysis. Therefore, it is of prime importance to use appropriate controls, i.e. tumor cells incubated with or without lymphocytes from several normal donors, in order to rule out as far as possible any nonspecific influence on tumor cell proliferation or survival, or both, and any *in vitro* sensitization to irrelevant antigens, such as histocompatibility antigens, during the long incubation time required. The latter possibility should be seriously considered, as cytotoxic lymphocytes are known to appear during a unidirectional mixed lymphocyte culture. In addition, a dose-response analysis using different lymphocyte–tumor cell ratios is necessary before the significance of any reduction in the number of tumor cells can be assessed.

An alternative to this visual method is the test proposed by [7], where the target cells are labeled with ^{3}H-thymidine. The amount of radioactivity remaining in the wells at the end of the incubation period is then taken as a measure of the number of tumor cells surviving. However, the interpretation of the data is complicated by the fact that the isotope can be reutilized after release from lysed cells. Recently, ^{125}I-iododeoxyuridine (^{125}IUdR) has been used to label target cells [3]. After incorporation of this compound into DNA, there is no spontaneous release and very little reutilization. However, its toxicity to culture cells has to be carefully evaluated in each system. Since proliferation of tumor cells appears to be inhibited after incorporation of ^{125}IUdR, isotope release depends mainly on cell lysis. [11] have suggested that, in addition to the use of prelabeled target cells, cytostasis (or growth inhibition) of tumor cells might be measured by pulse labeling with ^{125}IUdR at the end of the incubation period.

The second method measures direct lysis of tumor cells labeled with ^{51}Cr (sodium chromate). After incubation of target cells and lymphocytes for a few hours, the cell mixtures are spun down and ^{51}Cr release in the supernatant fluid is measured [1]. With the specific activity of ^{51}Cr presently available, a minimum of $5—10 \times 10^{3}$ labeled tumor cells per tube is required in order to obtain a measurable reaction, so that more lymphocytes are needed to achieve appropriate lymphocyte–target cell ratios than in the microplate assay. This disadvantage, however, is offset by the reduction in the number of controls required, since *in vitro* sensitization and various feeder effects of lymphocytes can be excluded in short-term incubations. One difficulty often encountered with the ^{51}Cr assay is that the spontaneous release of the isotope label can vary from one source of tumor cells to another, so that ^{51}Cr cannot be used in long-term assays. Quantitation of lymphocyte-mediated cytotoxicity is more precise than the microplate assay, especially when a dose-response analysis is performed. Thus the ^{51}Cr assay appears to be of greater value for studying factors such as the "blocking" or "unblocking" activity of patient serum.

With both assay systems the main problem is the appropriate choice of target cells. Freshly explanted cells kept in culture for a few passages or established cell lines are used as the source of tumor cells. It should be realized that antigenic expression at the cell surface can vary during cultivation; moreover, changes may occur in lytic susceptibility according to proliferation rate or cell cycle. The choice of normal target cells is particularly difficult, since in most instances normal cells of the same histological type as the tumor cells are not available and cannot be cultured. Use of cultured skin fibroblasts as the source of normal cells is highly questionable because of the various factors involved in susceptibility to lysis.

Mechanisms of LMC

Recent studies, based on various experimental model systems and extensively reviewed by [2], have suggested two mechanisms for lymphocyte-mediated cytotoxicity: 1) sensitized thymus-derived (T) lymphocytes specifically destroy target cells carrying the sensitizing antigen(s); 2) normal thymus-independent lymphocytes interact with target cells coated with small amounts of IgG antibody. In neither case is addition of complement required; target-cell lysis depends on close contact between target cells and lymphocytes and there is no detectable release of nonspecific cytotoxic factors in the supernatant. The experimental data indicate that the two mechanisms could be distinguished by selective removal prior to the cytotoxicity assay of either thymus-derived cells or lymphoid cells with affinity for antigen-antibody complexes. In human systems the feasibility of these studies depends on the availability of methods allowing separation of lymphocyte subpopulations. Preliminary results suggest that such methods will soon be available [13]. Identification of the lymphocytes responsible for *in vitro* cytotoxicity would be very useful. Not only would it allow us to clarify the mechanisms of LMC, it would also increase the sensitivity of the assay systems because lymphocyte populations enriched in cytotoxic lymphocytes could be obtained by physicochemical or immunological methods.

Recent studies suggest that the different assay methods for measuring LMC do not necessarily detect the same mechanism of cell destruction. For example, [6], using a colony-inhibition technique, found that cytotoxic lymphoid cells were present in mice with Moloney sarcoma virus (MSV)-induced tumor either at the time of tumor growth or after spontaneous regression. [9] reported a sharp fall in cytotoxic lymphocytes, as measured by the ^{51}Cr assay method, in mice with progressive MSV tumors. Analysis of the nature of the effector cells gave conflicting results, since only T cells were involved in the ^{51}Cr assay, whereas both T and non-T cells contributed to the effects measured by the microplate assay [8, 10]. Further experiments are needed to establish the validity of these findings in different tumor systems.

Relevance of *in-vitro* LMC to Protective Immunity in Cancer Patients

It is generally assumed that LMC is the *in vitro* correlate of the cell-mediated immunity involved in tumor rejection. Evidence for this assumption, however, is far from complete, even in experimental tumor systems. Very few studies have been undertaken to establish a quantitative correlation between *in vitro* LMC and tumor-cell destruction *in vivo*. Recent work in this laboratory has confirmed such a correlation in an allogeneic tumor system involving thymus-derived cytotoxic lymphocytes [5]. In this particular situation, a pure population of sensitized thymus-derived cells having high cytotoxic activity *in vitro* was able to protect an immunologically incompetent host against allogeneic tumor cells. Similar studies in syngeneic tumor systems are in progress in order to analyze the relative importance *in vivo* of the two LMC mechanisms described above, and to assess the possible role of non-lymphoid cells such as activated macrophages [4] in tumor-cell destruction.

It is difficult to draw any firm conclusion from LMC studies concerning protective immunity in cancer patients. It is thus not too surprising that no correlation between LMC and the clinical stage of the disease has been noticed in some studies. These observations do not mean that LMC is not potentially useful. They simply indicate that the clinical interpretation of a positive LMC is still difficult because of the technical problems associated with the assay systems, the complexity of the phenomenon of *in vitro* cytotoxicity, and the lack of information concerning the precise mechanisms underlying tumor immunity. Careful studies in cancer patients should be combined with extensive animal experimentation to elucidate the problems mentioned and to assess the true value of LMC in the diagnosis, prognosis and therapy of human cancer.

References

1. Brunner, K. T., Mauel, J., Cerottini, J.-C., Chapuis, B.: Quantitative assay of the lytic action of immune lymphoid cells on ^{51}Cr-labeled allogeneic target cells *in vitro*. Inhibition by isoantibody and by drugs. Immunology **14**, 181 (1968).
2. Cerottini, J.-C., Brunner, K. T.: Cell-mediated cytotoxicity, allograft rejection and tumor immunity. Advanc. Immunol. **18**, 67 (1974).
3. Cohen, A. M., Burdick, J. F., Ketcham, A. S.: Cell-mediated cytotoxicity: An assay using ^{125}I-iododeoxyuridine-labeled target cells. J. Immunol. **107**, 895 (1971).
4. Evans, R., Alexander, P.: Mechanism of immunologically specific killing of tumor cells by macrophages. Nature (Lond.) **236**, 168 (1972).
5. Freedman, L. R., Cerottini, J.-C., Brunner, K. T.: *In vivo* studies of the role of cytotoxic T cells in tumor allograft immunity. J. Immunol. **109**, 1371 (1972).
6. Hellström, I., Hellström, K. E.: Studies on cellular immunity and its serum-mediated inhibition in Moloney virus-induced mouse sarcomas. Int. J. Cancer **4**, 587 (1969).
7. Jagarlamoody, S. M., Aust, J. C., Tew, R. H., McKhann, C. F.: *In vitro* detection of cytotoxic cellular immunity against tumor-specific antigens by a radioisotopic technique. Proc. nat. Acad. Sci. (Wash.) **68**, 1346 (1971).
8. Lamon, E. W., Wigzell, H., Klein, E., Andersson, B., Skurzak, H. M.: The lymphocyte response to primary Moloney sarcoma cirus tumors in Balb/c mice: Definition of the active subpopulations at different times after infection. J. exp. Med. **137**, 1472 (1973).
9. Leclerc, J.-C., Gomard, E., Lecy, J.-P.: Cell-mediated reaction against tumors induced by oncornaviruses. I. Kinetic and specificity of the immune response in murine sarcoma virus (MSV)-induced tumors and transplanted lymphomas. Int. J. Cancer **10**, 589 (1972).
10. Leclerc, J.-C., Gomard, E., Plata, F., Levy, J.-P.: Cell-mediated immune reaction against tumors induced by oncornaviruses. II. Nature of the effector cells in tumor cell cytolysis. Int. J. Cancer **11**, 426 (1973).
11. Seeger, R. C., Owen, J. J. T.: Measurement of tumor immunity *in vitro* with ^{125}I-iododeoxyuridine labeled target cells. Transplantation **15**, 404 (1973).
12. Takasugi, M., Klein, E.: A microassay for cell-mediated immunity. Transplantation **9**, 219 (1970).
13. Wigzell, H., Golstein, P., Svedmyr, E. A. J., Jondahl, M.: Impact of fractionation procedures on lymphocyte activities *in vitro* and *in vivo*. Separation of cells with high concentrations of surface immunoglobulin. Transplantation Proc. **4**, 311 (1972).

Cell-Mediated Immunity in Allogeneic and Tumor-Systems: Nature of the Cells Involved in Killing Target Cells

J. C. Leclerc, J. P. Levy, E. Gomard, F. Plata, F. M. Kourilsky

Institut de Recherches sur les Maladies du Sang — Hôpital Saint Louis, Paris

The method of [2] for studying lymphocyte-mediated tumor cytotoxicity in the Moloney Sarcoma virus (MSV) tumor system has revealed several discrepancies in the results obtained in the same isologous tumor system by the colony-inhibition test (CIT) [5, 6] or by the microcytotoxicity assay (MA) [7, 14]. The discrepancies concern the kinetics of cytotoxic lymphoid cell populations, the action of progressor and regressor sera [6, 8, 10, 13, 14] and the nature of the effector cells.

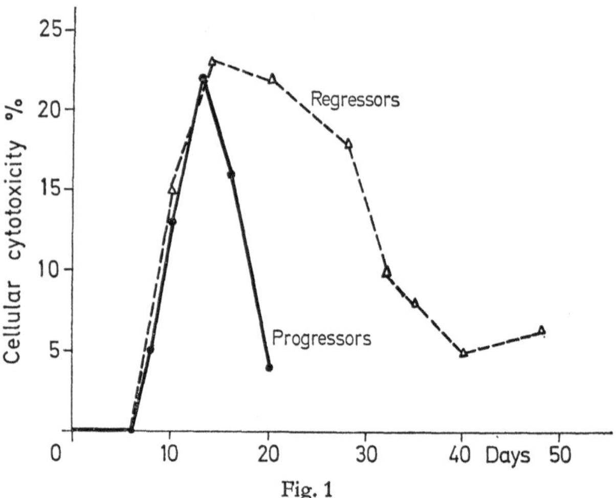

Fig. 1

Fig. 1 shows the kinetics of the cytotoxic activity of spleen cells from BALB/c mice following MSV inoculation. All tests were made by the chromium-release test (CRT) in isologous conditions with a ratio of 100 spleen cells to one tumor target cell, as previously described [8, 9, 10]. The cytotoxic activity is first detected at days 7—8 and rises sharply to a peak at days 13—15. In adult mice ("regressors") the tumor is rejected when cytotoxic activity is around its maximum; thereafter this activity declines slowly to become barely detectable after day 40. In younger mice injected with MSV ("progressors") cytotoxic activity declines much more rapidly after the peak and the tumor continuous to grow. Such a difference in the course of the immune response in regressors and progressors has not been reported in CIT or MA studies. In addition, some long-lasting cytostatic activity of the lymphoid cells seems to be detectable by MA in regressor mice [6, 14].

Table 1. The cytotoxic activity of anti-MSV spleen cells against GiL4 lymphoma cells in CRT. All sera have been tested from 1/2 to 1/20 dilution with the same results

Lymphoid cells from	Sera	% chromium release	Blocking
BALB/c anti-MSV	No	32	/
BALB/c anti-MSV	Normal sera 1/5	31	No
BALB/c anti-MSV	Progressors sera 1/5	33	No
BALB/c anti-MSV	Regressors sera 1/5	32	No
BALB/c anti-MSV	Hyperimmune sera 1/5	32	No

Table 1 shows some representative results of attempts to block the cytotoxic cellular reactions by incubating sera from isologous pregressor mice with target cells or with lymphoid cells. It appears that they failed to block the immune reactions in CRT. These observations do not agree with those obtained by CIT [6] or MA [14] which showed that progressor sera are blocking, probably by interaction with receptors of the lymphoid cells [13] (Fig. 2b).

In CRT the nature of blocking phenomena is probably different (Fig. 2c). In an allogeneic system (Table 2) hyperimmune anti-H-2 sera which are not able to block the reaction after preincubation with the lymphoid cells become clearly effective

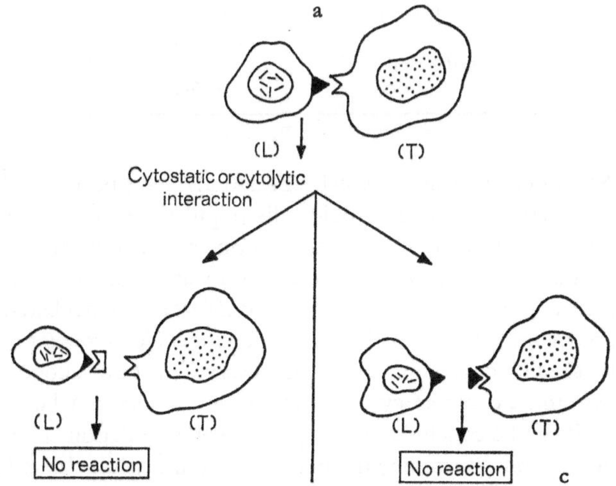

Fig. 2. a Effective interaction between lymphoid cells (L) and target cells (T), b Blocking as detected in CIT and MA (inhibition of lymphoid cells by antigen or antigen-antibody complexes?), c Blocking as detected in CRT (inhibition of target cells by antibodies)

when preincubated with the target cells. Hyperimmune anti-H-2 serae ffectively block cytolysis of the target cells (as indicated in CRT) only at low dilution. This probably explains why regressor and even hyperimmune anti-MSV sera, which are always weak antisera, have failed to block the reaction in our experiments (Table 1).

B cells and possibly macrophages may play a role in CIT [12], in MA [7], and in cytostasis induced by lymphocytes (FESTENSTEIN, personal communication). In CRT, it was shown that T cells are exclusively involved, at least in allogeneic systems [3, 4]. It is therefore important to determine whether T cells or non-T cells are involved

Table 2. Blockade cytotoxic activity of anti-H-2 spleen cells in an allogeneic system

Cells	Dilution of BALB/c anti-C 57 B 1/6 serum	% chromium release	Blocking %
BALB/c anti-C 57 B 1/6 spleen cells and GiL 4 (C 57 B 1/6) lymphoma cells: ration 25/1	1/10	0	100
	1/20	9	75
	1/50	13	60
	1/100	21	30
	1/200	30	0
	1/500	31	0
	Normal serum 1/10 1/500	30—32	

Table 3. Effect of anti-θ antisera on cytotoxic lymphoid cells in CRT (% inhibition of cytotoxicity)

		6 hours	12 hours	24 hours
Allogeneic system (anti H-2) BALB/c anti-C 57 B 1/6	Normal serum + C′	0	0	0
	Anti θ' + C′	100	100	100
Syngeneic system BALB/c anti-MSV	Normal serum + C′	No activity at that time	0	0
	Anti θ serum + C′	No activity at that time	100	100

in syngeneic MSV-tumor systems for which CIT and MA have been well documented: a difference in the nature of the cytotoxic cells populations could explain the discrepancies in kinetics and blocking. Several experiments have been designed to test this hypothesis. First the action of anti-θ antiserum was tested. Table 3 summarizes the results of typical experiments where spleen cells were preincubated with anti-θ serum and complement. As previously shown in allogeneic systems [3], a complete inhibition of the specific chromium release is observed in both allogeneic and syngeneic tumor systems. So far as cytolysis by an anti-θ sera can be considered as acting on T cells, it can be concluded that a pure T-cell population is involved in the anti-MSV tumor reaction detected by the Brunner method, while the action of non-T cells in MA has been shown by others [7]. Similar results in CRT have been found from day 5 to day 50 after MSV inoculation [11]. Recent experiments have shown that pure T-cell populations obtained by fractionation by the method of [15] are fully active in CRT, while they are slightly active in MA [7] (GOMARD, personal communication).

[12] have shown in the MSV-tumor system that normal lymphocytes can be specially cytotoxic in the presence of progressor sera against MSV tumor cells. [1] have shown that a specific property of B cells (but not of T cells) is to acquire immune activity when incubated with specific antibodies or antigen-antibody complexes. Therefore we tried to determine whether non-immune spleen cells could acquire cytotoxic activity detectable in CRT. Non-immune cells incubated with specific anti H-2 antibodies or with sera of MSV progressors at various dilutions were used in CRT. These cells do not become cytotoxic except in rare instances where a weak activity was detected after incubation for 24 h in CRT.

Therefore it is clear that, of the tests which detect cell-mediated immune reactions in syngeneic tumor systems, MA and CIT on the one hand and CRT on the other do not express the same phenomena.

It can be concluded that in the MSV-tumor system, T cells alone are involved in CRT. Conversely, it has been shown with purified lymphoid cell populations that B cells are predominantly active in MA [7], (GOMARD, personal communication).

The role of these different cells *in vivo* remains to be determined; meanwhile a comparison of several *in vitro* methods appears necessary to explore the phenomenon of *in vivo* tumor rejection further.

References

1. BASTEN, A., MILLER, J. F. A. P., SPRENT, J., PYE, J.: A receptor for antibody on B lymphocytes. I. Method of detection and functional significance. J. exp. Med. **135**, 610 (1972).
2. BRUNNER, K. T., MAUEL, J., CEROTTINI, J. C., CHAPUIS, B.: Quantitative assay of the lytic action of immune lymphoid cells on ^{51}Cr labeled allogeneic target cells in vitro; inhibition by iso-antibody and by drugs. Immunology **14**, 181 (1968).
3. CEROTTINI, J. C., NORDIN, A. A., BRUNNER, K. T.: Specific in vitro cytotoxicity of thymus derived lymphocytes sensitized to alloantigens. Nature (Lond.) **228**, 1308 (1970).
4. GOLSTEIN, P., SVEDMYR, E. J., WIGZELL, H.: Cells mediating specific in vitro cytotoxicity. I. Detection of receptor bearing lymphocytes. J. exp. Med. **134**, 1385 (1971).
5. HELLSTRÖM, I., HELLSTRÖM, K. E.: Studies on cellular immunity and its serum mediated inhibition in Moloney-virus induced mouse sarcoma. Int. J. Cancer **4**, 587 (1969).
6. HELLSTRÖM, I., HELLSTRÖM, K. E.: Colony inhibition studies on blocking and non-blocking serum effects on cellular immunity to Moloney Sarcoma. Int. J. Cancer **5**, 195 (1970).
7. LAMON, E. W., SKURZAK, H. M., KLEIN, E., WIGZELL, H.: In vitro cytotoxicity by a non thymus-processed lymphocyte population with specificity for a virally determined cell-surface antigen. J. exp. Med. **136**, 1072 (1972).
8. LECLERC, J. C., GOMARD, E., LEVY, J. P.: Cell-mediated reaction against tumors induced by oncornaviruses. I. Kinetic and specificity of the immune response in murine sarcoma virus (MSV) induced tumors and transplanted lymphomas. Int. J. Cancer **10**, 589 (1972).
9. LECLERC, J. C., GOMARD, E., PAVIE, J., LEVY, J. P.: Evolution de l'activité cytotoxique des lymphocytes immuns en réponse à une greffe de cellules leucémiques chez la souris. C.R. Acad. Sci. (Paris) **274**, 1233 (1972).
10. LEVY, L. P., LECLERC, J. C., GOMARD, E., PAVIE, J., KOURILSKY, F. M.: Decrease of cytotoxic immune lymphoid cells following regression of virus induced sarcoma in mice. The Vth International Symposium on Comparative Leukemia Research. Unifying Concepts of leukemia. Bibl. Haemat. **39**, 689 (1973).
11. PLATA, F., GOMARD, E., LECLERC, J. C., LEVY, J. P.: Further evidence for the involvement of thymus-processed lymphocytes in syngeneic tumor cell cytolysis. J. Immunol. **111**, 667 (1973).

12. Pollack, S., Heppner, G., Brawn, R. J., Nelson, K.: Specific killing of tumor cells in vitro in the presence of normal lymphoid cells and sera from hosts immune to the tumor antigens. Int. J. Cancer **9**, 316 (1972).
13. Sjogren, H. O., Hellström, I., Bansal, S. C., Hellström, K. E.: Suggestive evidence that the blocking antibodies of tumor-bearing individuals may be antigen-antibody complexes. Proc. nat. Acad. Sci. (Wash.) **68**, 1372 (1971).
14. Skurzak, H. M., Klein, E., Yoshida, T. O., Lamon, E. W.: Synergestic and antagonistic effect of different antibody concentrations on in vitro lymphocyte cytotoxicity in the Moloney Sarcoma Virus system. J. exp. Med. **135**, 997 (1972).
15. Wigzell, H., Sundqvist, K. G., Yoshida, T. O.: Separation of cells according to surface antigens by the use of antibody coated-columns. Fractionation of cells carrying immunoglobulins and blood group antigen. Scand. J. Immunol. **1**, 75 (1972).

Inhibition of Leukocyte Migration in Man

H. G. Remold

Robert B. Brigham Hospital, Harvard Medical School, Boston, Mass.

For the study of the role of delayed hypersensitivity in a variety of human diseases reliable *in vitro* assays are of major importance. There are a number of assays which measure the results of lymphocyte activation such as cytotoxicity, proliferation and inhibition of leukocyte migration. We will confine ourselves here to the migration inhibition assays.

In order to determine how *in vitro* assays of delayed hypersensitivity correlate with delayed hypersensitivity in man, it is useful to review the correlation of migration inhibition with delayed hypersensitivity in animals. It is now well known that inhibition of migration of peritoneal exudate (PE) cells from guinea pigs correlates with cellular immunity skin reactions and not with antibody production [3], and studies with split tolerance [1] and DNP-carrier protein antigens [4] have further defined this relationship. It is more difficult to correlate migration inhibition with cellular immunity in man.

There are two different types of migration inhibition assays applicable to man. The indirect assay [6, 9] has the advantage that it measures the activity of migration inhibiting factor (MIF) produced by sensitized lymphocytes. In this assay, human blood lymphocytes are stimulated with antigen in tissue culture. The cell-free supernatants are added to guinea-pig peritoneal cells in capillary tubes and the cells are inhibited from migrating out of the capillaries when the donors or the lymphocytes have delayed hypersensitivity to the antigen used. Furthermore, patients who acquire delayed hypersensitivity following treatment with transfer factor are able to inhibit migration of guinea pig macrophages in the presence of specific antigen. However, the indirect assay is not very sensitive and requires at least 50 ml of blood.

The same principle is applied in a new microassay, the agarose drop method, which might be useful in studies of delayed hypersensitivity in man [5]. Here PE cells are mixed with agarose and applied as 2 μl droplets to wells filled with tissue culture medium to be tested for activity; as before, the migration of the cells out of the droplets is measured. This method requires minute amounts of cells and is simpler than the capillary migration inhibition method once the problem of quantification of this assay has been satisfactorily solved.

The direct assay is based on the inhibition of migration of human blood leukocytes out of capillary tubes in the presence of specific antigen [7, 8]. This method is fast and requires only a small amount of blood from the patient but has the disadvantage of lack of sensitivity and occasional irreproducibility when soluble antigens are used. There has been some question about the role of polymorphonuclear leukocyte in this test system. Recently, Rocklin has shown [10] that leukocyte migration inhibition is mediated by a separate factor, leucocyte inhibitory factor (LIF) of molecular weight 69,000 daltons, which inhibits the migration of polymorphonuclear leukocytes but has no effect on guinea pig macrophages or human monocytes. Thus, LIF is separable from MIF, which has a MW 25,000 and inhibits the migration of guinea pig macrophages or human monocytes, but has no effect on polymorphonuclear leukocytes.

A modification of the direct assay is Clausen's agarose plate method [2]. Buffy-coat cells are placed in wells in agarose plates with or without preincubation with antigen. After incubation the migration of the cells between the agarose and the plastic dish is measured. This rapid method has the same disadvantages as the direct assay; the mode of inhibition is poorly understood. These assays can be used to assess cellular immunity to many antigens and in consequence they are being used in a wide variety of human diseases.

References

1. Borel, Y., David, J. R.: *In vitro* studies of the suppression of delayed hypersensitivity by the induction of a partial tolerance. J. exp. Med. **131**, 602 (1970).
2. Clausen, J. E.: Tuberculin-induced migration inhibition of human peripheral leucocytes in agarose medium. Acta allerg. (Kbh.) **26**, 56 (1971).
3. David, J. R., Al-Askari, S., Lawrence, H. S., Thomas, L.: Delayed hypersensitivity *in vitro*. I. The specificity of cell migration by antigen. J. Immunol. **93**, 264 (1964).
4. David, J. R., Schlossman, S. F.: Immunochemical studies on the specificity of cellular hypersensitivity: the *in vitro* inhibition of peritoneal exudate cell migration by chemically defined antigens. J. exp. Med. **128**, 1451 (1968).
5. Harrington, J. T., Stastny, P.: Macrophage migration from an agarose droplet: a new MIF assay. Fed. Proc. **31**, 780 Abs. (1972).
6. Rocklin, R. E., Meyers, O. L., David, J. R.: An *in vitro* assay for cellular hypersensitivity in man. J. Immunol. **104**, 95 (1970).
7. Rosenberg, S. A., David, J. R.: Inhibition of leukocyte migration: an evaluation of this *in vitro* assay of delayed hypersensitivity in man to a soluble antigen. J. Immunol. **105**, 1447 (1970).
8. Søborg, M., Bendixen, G.: Human lymphocyte migration as a parameter of hypersensitivity. Acta med. scand. **181**, 247 (1967).
9. Thor, D., Jureziz, R. E., Veach, S. R., Miller, E., Dray, S.: Cell migration inhibition factor released by antigen from human peripheral lymphocytes. Nature **219**, 5155 (1968).
10. Rocklin, R. E.: Products of activated lymphocytes: leukocyte inhibitory factor (LIF) distinct from migration inhibitory factor (MIF). J. Immunol. **112**, 1461 (1974).

Effect of Autologous Serum on *in vitro* Inhibition of Leukocyte Migration by Autochthonous Tumor Extracts from Human Patients*

F. Lacour, J. Lacour, A. Spira, and S. Bayet

Institut Gustave-Roussy, Villejuif

Introduction

An earlier study on cell-mediated immunity based on an *in vitro* leukocyte migration test (LMT) has been made on patients with a variety of operable carcinomas [5]. In the LMT blood leukocytes migrate from a capillary tube into the surrounding medium: the migration is inhibited when antigen to which the leukocyte donor displays cellular hypersensitivity is added to the medium [4, 6]. A significant inhibition of leukocyte migration was observed in the presence of autologous tumor

Table 1. Effects of autologous tumor extracts from different patients on leukocyte migration *in vitro*

Histological type	No. of patients whose tumor extracts inhibited leukocyte migration/ Total number of patients
Hodgkin's disease and lymphomas	10/17
Malignant bone and soft-tissue tumors	10/15
Breast carcinomas	8/13
Malignant melanomas	2/4
Miscellaneous malignant tumors	3/8

extract in 33 out of 57 patients studied. These results indicate a previous sensitization of the lymphocytes to some tumor antigens in 58% of the patients. These patients were placed in 5 groups according to the histological type of the tumors. No significant difference in the results from LMT was observed among the 5 groups (Table 1). Further, no correlation was observed between the LMT results and the clinical status of the disease. However, in this study there were only a few patients in each group, and to obtain additional information a second study was undertaken on 2 groups of patients: Group I with operable breast carcinoma and Group II with

* This work was supported by C.N.R.S. and by the Annie Dalsace Grant.

malignant melanoma. In the present study we tested the effect of tumor extracts, serum and tumor extracts in conjunction with serum on the migration of autologous leukocytes.

Methods

Methods for the preparation of leukocyte suspension, tumor extracts and the test for leukocyte migration were as described previously [5].

Medium M199 was used for the LMT tests and the following test substances were used in the 4 series of tests.

1. T : 10% horse serum plus tumor extracts (100 μg/ml protein).
2. S : 10% patients serum.
3. T + S : 10% patients serum plus tumor extracts.
4. Control : 10% horse serum.

The 4 tests were performed at the same time, each in quadruplicate. Tumor cells, serum and leukocytes were obtained from the same patients. The migration index of autologous lymphocytes is given by the formula:

$$MI = \frac{\text{Mean of migration of experimental test}}{\text{Mean of migration of control}}$$

Values between 0.80 and 1.20 are considered normal whereas those below 0.80 reflect an inhibition of migration.

Studies of leukocyte migration were carried out with blood obtained during the first post-operative week.

Results

In confirmation of our previous results, inhibition of leukocyte migration was found in the same proportion in presence of autologous tumor extracts (Table 2).

Table 2. Effects of autologous tumor extracts from different patients on leukocyte migration *in vitro*

Histological type	No. of patients whose tumor extracts inhibited leukocyte migration/ Total number of patients
Breast carcinomas	22/48
Malignant melanomas	11/19

These results are not significantly different from those of ANDERSEN *et al.* [1], who also observed positive results in the LMT in the presence of autologous tumor extracts in 8 out of 22 carcinoma-bearing patients.

The effect on leukocyte migration of tumor extract, serum alone and serum in conjunction with tumor extract could be tested at the same time in the samples from

34 of 44 breast carcinoma cases. The purpose of this study was to investigate whether sera from patients with breast carcinoma could abolish the inhibitory effect of autologous tumor extracts on leukocyte migration. The serum of patients with breast carcinoma did not abolish the inhibition of leukocyte migration and no "blocking" factor like those described by HELLSTRÖM *et al.* [3] in cytotoxic system (using lymphocytes and live tumor cells) could be noted.

Moreover, in the present case a synergistic effect of the serum on inhibition of leukocyte migration was evident. Thus, the mean migration index in the test with tumor extract in the presence of serum (0.71 ± 0.9) was significantly ($p < 0.01$) lower than in the corresponding test with the autologous tumor extract alone (0.88 ± 0.8). In 5 patients this synergistic effect of serum was particularly manifest (Table 3).

Table 3. Effect of tumor extract (T), serum (S) and tumor extract in presence of serum (TS) on the migration of autologous leukocytes

Case	Nodes	Histological grading [2]	Migration index of leukocytes		
			T	S	T + S
1	—	I	0.98 ± 0.13	1.1 ± 0.17	0.47 ± 0.07
2	—	I	$0.59 \pm 0\ 08$	0.85 ± 0.15	0.20 ± 0.04
3	+	II	0.68 ± 0.11	0.81 ± 0.15	0.38 ± 0.07
4	+	I	0.71 ± 0.10	0.69 ± 0.10	0.31 ± 0.06
5	+	I	0.99 ± 0.13	0.57 ± 0.10	0.19 ± 0.03

Table 4. Relationship between the grade of anaplasia of mammary carcinoma and the synergistic serum factor (SSF) on inhibition of leukocyte migration by autologous tumor extract

Grade of anaplasia [2]	SS factor pos.	SS factor neg.	% of cases with SSF
Grade I	4	1	80
Grades II and III	1	28	3.4

It is interesting to note that this effect was observable in Case 1 where neither tumor extract nor serum given separately were inhibitory. Thus a synergistic serum factor (SS factor) which inhibits leukocyte migration may exist in some patients with breast carcinoma. We have found that decomplemented and fresh sera have the same effect, so the SS factor is not the complement-dependent.

We investigated the relationship between the presence of SS factor in the serum and histological or clinical status of the tumor. A reverse correlation appears to exist between presence of SS factor and degree of malignancy. Thus, on the basis of BLOOM *et al.* [2] grading system (performed on 34 cases) the SS factor was observed only in tumors of a low degree of malignancy.

The difference between the presence of SS factor in 80% of tumors with grade I anaplasia and in only 3% of grades II and III tumors is obviously significant (Table 4). The prognostic significance of the presence of SS factor is of practical and theoretical importance.

In contrast to the sera from patients with breast carcinoma, those from patients with malignant melanomas did not show any synergistic effect on the inhibition of leukocyte migration by tumor extract.

Discussion and Conclusion

The important aspects of our study are the autologous nature of the lymphocytes, the tumor extracts, and the serum.

The migration index of leukocyte is much lower in presence of tumor extracts plus serum than in the presence of tumor extract alone in the case of patients with breast carcinoma. The synergistic effect which was observed in 14% of cases could be correlated with the best histological prognostic factors.

Immunoglobulin may be involved in this type of synergistic action but we cannot exclude other factors, e.g. hormones. Further studies are needed to characterize this synergistic serum factor and to understand its mechanism of action.

The results of our study may indicate that interactions of lymphocytes, tumor extract and serum are in some way a reflection of the host defense of a particular patient to his own tumor.

References

1. Andersen, V., Bjerrum, O., Bendixen, G., Schiodt, T., Dissing, I.: Effect of autologous mammary tumour extracts on human leukocyte migration *in vitro*. Int. J. Cancer **5**, 357 (1970).
2. Bloom, H. J. G., Richardson, W. W.: Histologic grading and prognosis in breast cancer. A study of 1409 cases of which 359 have been followed for 15 years. Brit. J. Cancer **11**, 359 (1957).
3. Hellström, I., Hellström, K. E., Evans, C. A., Heppner, G. H., Pierce, G. E., Yang, J. P. S.: Serum mediated protection of neoplastic cells from inhibition of lymphocytes immune to their tumor specific antigens. Proc. nat. Acad. Sci. (Wash.) **62**, 326 (1969).
4. Rosenberg, A. S., David, J. R.: Inhibition of leukocyte migration: an evaluation of this *in vitro* assay of delayed hypersensitivity in man to a soluble antigen. J. Immunol. **105**, 1447 (1970).
5. Segal, A., Weiler, O., Genin, J., Lacour, J., Lacour, F.: *In vitro* study of cellular immunity against autochthonous human cancer. Int. J. Cancer **9**, 417 (1972).
6. Søborg, M., Bendixen, G.: Human lymphocyte migration as a parameter of hypersensitivity. Acta med. scand. **181**, 247 (1967).

Serum Inhibitory Factors in Acute Leukemia

C. B. FREEMAN, J. S. WALKER, D. DAVIES, H. COCKING, and R. HARRIS

Department of Medical Genetics, St. Mary's Hospital,
Hathersage Road, Manchester

Introduction

The *in vitro* response of lymphocytes to phytohemagglutinin (PHA) has been used by many workers to assess possible disturbances in cell-mediated immunity in acute leukemia.

We have found that washed lymphocytes from patients with acute leukemia may react normally *in vitro* although inhibitory factors may be present in autologous serum. These factors play an unknown part in leukemogenesis and in the *in vivo* immune response.

Patients and Method

Venous blood samples obtained from patients with acute myeloblastic leukemia (AML) and acute lymphoblastic leukemia (ALL) were used for the study of lymphocyte reactivity to PHA. In many cases samples were obtained before and during various treatment protocols.

DNA synthesis in response to PHA (Difco PHA-P control) was measured in 3-day cultures by determining the uptake of ^{125}I-5-iodo-2'-deoxyuridine (^{125}IUDR); [12]. The rates of ^{125}IUDR uptake were expressed as dpm/hr/0.5×10^6 lymphocytes present in cultures at zero time.

Sera were stored at —20 °C for up to 3 months and frozen and thawed only once before use. Sera were used only in AB0-compatible systems.

Results

Inhibition of Normal Lymphocyte Response by Leukemic Sera

The effect of normal and leukemic serum on the rate of PHA-stimulated DNA synthesis was measured in cultures of washed lymphocytes obtained from healthy donors. In a typical experiment (Fig. 1) serum from patients with untreated acute leukemia (ALL and AML) inhibited the PHA response as compared with normal autologous serum. However, inhibition was observed only at PHA concentrations of less than 15 µg/ml culture. At concentrations about 15 µg/ml culture the rates of DNA synthesis in the presence of normal and leukemic serum were usually similar.

A PHA concentration was selected (7.0 µg/ml) which allowed maximum discrimination between the leukemic and normal serum. The rates of DNA synthesis in cultures of normal lymphocytes in allogeneic normal human serum or acute leu-

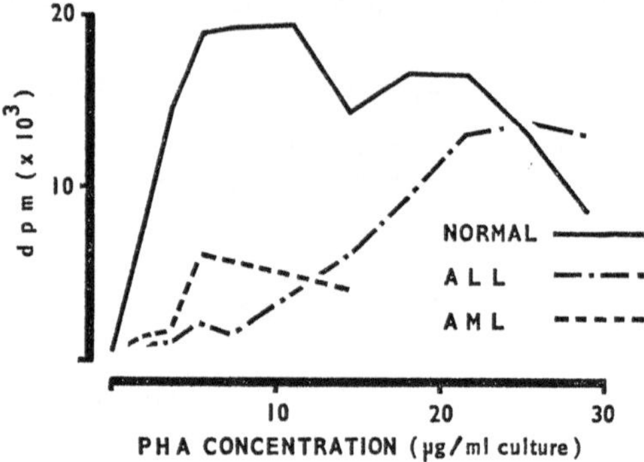

Fig. 1. Inhibitory effect of leukemic serum on ^{125}IUDR uptake by PHA-stimulated lymphocytes from *normal* donor. Normal autologous serum ———; serum from untreated ALL —·—·—; serum from untreated AML -------

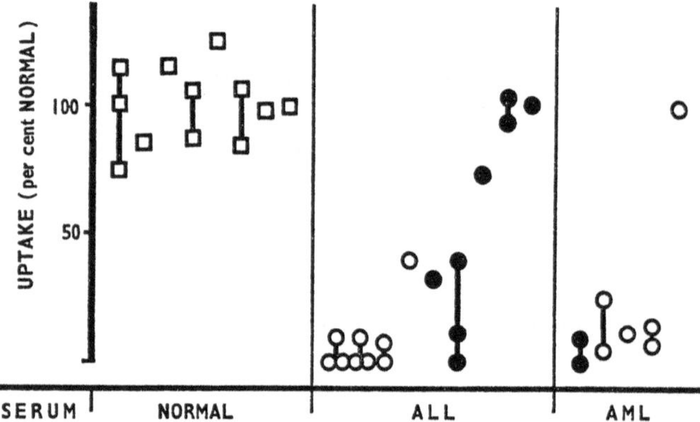

Fig. 2. Inhibitory effect of leukemic serum on ^{125}IUDR uptake by PHA-stimulated lymphocytes from normal donors at the maximum discriminatory dose of 7 µg/ml. □ Normal serum; ○ serum from untreated acute leukemia; ● serum from leukemia patients receiving chemotherapy

kemic serum were expressed as a percentage of the rate of DNA synthesis in autologous normal serum after subtraction of control values without PHA (Fig. 2). The range of response in allogeneic normal serum was 75—125% (mean 102%) compared with autologous serum. Quite marked inhibition was encountered in many of the leukemic sera and 7 out of 8 sera from untreated patients were inhibitory.

Further studies on a wider range of sera from patients with AML (Table 1) confirmed that leukemic serum was frequently but not always inhibitory. This was most commonly observed in serum obtained before chemotherapy.

Table 1. Inhibitory effect of serum from AML patients on ^{125}IUDR uptake by PHA-stimulated lymphocytes from normal donors at the maximum discriminatory dose of 7 μg/ml (Numbers in brackets denote number of patients)

Serum source	Number of sera % of PHA response (7.0 μg/ml culture) in autologous serum				
	0—25	25—75	75—125	125	Total
Pre-treatment patients	3 (3)	5 (5)	10 (10)	0 (0)	18
Patients receiving chemotherapy	5 (4)	15 (7)	84 (13)	1 (1)	105

Except in the case of a single AML patient following immunization with allogeneic blast cells there was no evidence that the inhibition observed was due to cytotoxic HL-A antibodies. Firstly, antibodies were not detected in a two-stage modification of the microcytotoxicity test [7]. Secondly, leukemic sera found to inhibit the PHA response of normal lymphocytes also inhibited autologous lymphocytes, although these lymphocytes from leukemics had a normal PHA response when cultured in normal allogeneic serum. Thirdly, 4 sera tested after heat inactivation at 56 °C for 30 min retained their ability to inhibit the PHA response.

One patient, A. R., showed marked inhibition before starting treatment. At this stage cytotoxic HL-A antibodies were not detected. The inhibitory effect rapidly disappeared after the start of induction chemotherapy and the PHA response remained within the normal range as she went into remission and during the cytoreductive phase of chemotherapy. The inhibitory effect that A. R.'s serum developed

Table 2. Development of cytotoxic HL-A antibodies in the serum of AML patient A. R. during immunotherapy: inhibition of the PHA response of normal lymphocytes

	Normal lymphocyte donor				
	B. P.		J. F.		patient's [a] PHA response
	PHA [a] response	serum [b] cyto-toxicity	PHA [a] response	serum [b] cyto-toxicity	
Pre-Immunotherapy					
1. 11. 71	NT	—	NT	—	
20. 12. 71	NT	—	NT	—	
Post-Immunotherapy					
3. 3. 72	106	—	4	(+)	
10. 3. 72	62	—	1	+	
24. 3. 72	NT	—	2	++	
31. 3. 72	NT	—	2	++	
21. 4. 72	78	—	2	++	120

[a] PHA response = % of lymphocyte response (7.0 μg PHA/ml culture) in normal autologous serum.

[b] Cytotoxic test score — = 0—10% kill; ± = 10—20% kill; (+) = 20—40% kill; + = 40—80% kill; ++ = 80—100% kill.

during immunotherapy is probably related to HL-A antibodies. Although A.R.'s serum reacted negatively in the lymphocytotoxic test initially, within 6 weeks antibodies reacting with HL-A 10, 12 ,13 and W10 lymphocytes developed. In the PHA stimulation system inhibition of J.F.'s response was noted, whereas only minimal depression of response of B.P.'s lymphocytes occurred (Table 2). J.F.'s lymphocytes typed as HL-A 3, 12 and W18 and B.P.'s as HL-A 2, 9.2 and W15*.

PHA Response of Washed Lymphocytes from Leukemic Patients

Our results show that potentially inhibitory autologous serum must be removed if the PHA response of lymphocytes from leukemic patients is to be studied. Consequently, lymphocytes were washed and cultured in TC 199 medium containing serum obtained from a panel of healthy donors whose serum was known from repeated testing not to be inhibitory.

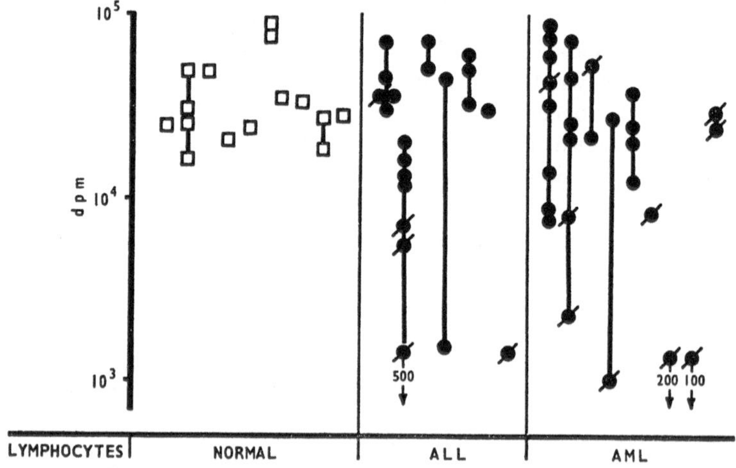

Fig. 3. Response ($\log_{10}$) of lymphocytes from leukemia patients and normal donors incubated with the maximum discriminatory dose of PHA (7 µg/ml). □ Normal lymphocytes; ● lymphocyte suspensions from leukemia patients; ● lymphocyte suspensions with many primitive cells

Fig. 3 shows the response ($\log_{10}$) of lymphocytes from leukemic patients and normal donors incubated with the maximum discriminating dose of PHA (7.0 µg/ml). 35 of 48 cultures of lymphocytes from 12 patients had PHA responses within the normal range (1.6—8.5 $\times$ 10^4 dpm/hr/0.5 $\times$ 10^6 lymphocytes), or only slightly less than normal (1.2—1.5 $\times$ 10^4 dpm/hr/0.5 $\times$ 10^6 lymphocytes). 13 cultures from 9 leukemic patients showed a reduction of the PHA response (less than 10^4 dpm/hr/0.5 $\times$ 10^6 lymphocytes). However, of these, 10 initially contained lymphoblasts, myeloblasts or other primitive cells.

A poor response of the patient's lymphocytes to PHA usually (but not invariably) occurred when numerous blast cells were present in the culture medium (Fig. 4); with blast counts under 5,000/cm^3 the PHA response was almost invariably normal. Marked depression of the PHA response usually occurred with blast counts over 5,000/cm^3.

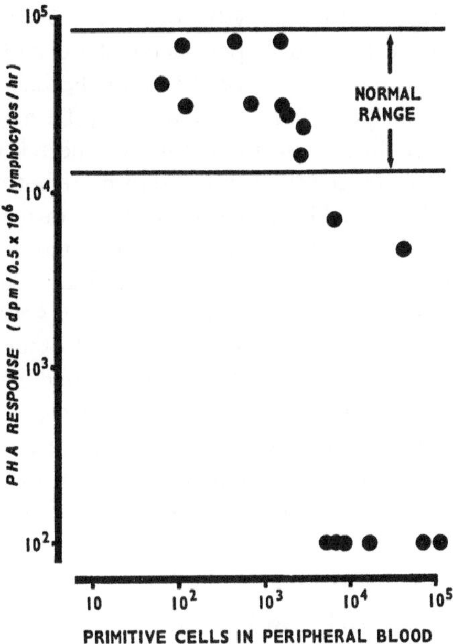

Fig. 4. Relationship between the absolute blast count of the peripheral blood and the response ($\log_{10}$) of lymphocytes from leukemia patients incubated with the maximum discriminatory dose of PHA (7 µg/ml)

Discussion

Most workers believe that the *in vitro* lymphocyte response to PHA is normal in untreated patients with acute leukemic and, although depressed by chemotherapy, probably recovers rapidly when treatment is stopped, especially in patients who have a good prognosis [1, 2, 3, 4, 8, 10]. However, the dose of PHA used in many studies is much in excess of that which gives the most sensitive discrimination between normal and abnormal responses [5, 11].

The response of lymphocytes from normals or leukemics to low (7.0 µg/ml) doses of PHA is often greatly reduced in the presence of serum obtained from patients with untreated AML or ALL. Inhibition is much less frequently observed following chemotherapy. We attribute these findings to the presence of inhibitory factors in the serum of leukemics.

In only one case was there evidence that inhibition resulted from the presence of complement-dependent cytotoxic HL-A antibodies, and in this patient (A.R.) HL-A antibodies probably developed as a result of immunization with allogeneic myeloblastic cells. Inhibition of the PHA response noted in this patient before any treatment was given was shown not to be due to the presence of HL-A antibodies.

A normal response to the 7.0 µg dose of PHA can usually be observed when lymphocytes from leukemic patients are resuspended in normal allogeneic serum. This is not always the case, however, and some leukemic cell preparations remain poorly responsive to a low PHA dose. Such results are usually, but not invariably, encountered when investigating the reactivity of lymphocytes from untreated patients who have many primitive cells in their peripheral blood and consequently in the cultures. Culture conditions, e.g. pH, may be altered by the inclusion of large numbers of blast cells. Alternatively, poor PHA response may be a result of inclusion of proportionately few T lymphocytes in the culture or the release by leukemic blast cells of inhibitors similar to those found in the serum, or both.

Serum inhibitors of the lymphocyte response occur in many different diseases, and not only in malignant disease [6, 9, 11]. They are often, as reported here, characterized by loss of inhibition at high PHA concentrations. One may only speculate as to the role of these inhibitors in *in vivo* immune responses generally and in leukemic in particular. Perhaps they interfere with the function of otherwise normal lymphocytes and thus provide a mechanism by which the leukemic blast cell can escape the host's immune reaction. If this is ultimately shown to be so, we may have to modify our approaches to immunotherapy. Not only should we attempt to increase the immune response but we should also attempt to remove or oppose the action of factors that may inhibit or block various parts of the host's immune response.

Acknowledgements

We are grateful to our hematologist colleagues for their co-operation and to Miss G. MARRIOTT and Mrs. E. QUINN for their invaluable assistance in obtaining blood samples. Mr. and Mrs. J. WENTZEL provided able technical assistance. We are also grateful to Mrs. S. BROOKS for secretarial assistance. This research is supported by the Leukemia Research Fund, the Medical Research Council and the Board of Governors, United Manchester Hospitals.

References

1. ASTALDI, G., MASSIMO, L., AIRO, R., MORI, P. G.: P.H.A. and lymphocytes from A.L.L. Lancet **1966 I**, 1265.
2. BARDARE, M., ACCORSI, A., APOLLONIO, T., CAREDDU, P.: Blastigenesis linfocitaria *in vitro* da PHA in babbini affettida leucemia acuta. Minerva pediat. **21**, 1019 (1969).
3. BORELLA, L., WEBSTER, R. G.: The immunosuppressive effects of long term combination chemotherapy in children with acute leukemia in remission. Cancer Res. **31**, 420 (1971).
4. DUPUY, J. M., KOURILSKY, F. M., FRADELIZZI, D., FEINGOLD, N., JACQUILLAT, C., BERNARD, J., DAUSSET, J.: Depression of immunologic reactivity of patients with acute leukemia. Cancer (Philad.) **27**, 323 (1971).
5. FITZGERALD, M. G.: The establishment of a normal human population dose response curve for lymphocytes cultured with PHA (Phytohemagglutinin). Clin. exp. Immunol. **8**, 421 (1971).
6. GATTI, R. A.: Serum inhibitors of lymphocyte responses. Lancet **1971 I**, 1351.
7. HARRIS, R., WENTZEL, J., COCKING, H., DODSWORTH, H., UKAEJIOFO, E. O.: Errors in allograft donor typing: A modified microcytotoxic test. In: Histocompatibility testing, p. 604. Kopenhagen: Munksgaard 1970.
8. HERSH, E. M., WHITECAR, J. P., Jr., MCCREDIE, K. B., BODEY, G. P., Sr., FREIREICH, E. J.: Chemotherapy, immunocompetence, immunosuppression and prognosis in acute leukemia. New Engl. J. Med. **285**, 1211 (1971).

9. Hsu, C. C. S., Leevy, C. M.: Inhibition of PHA stimulated lymphocyte transformation by plasma from patients with advanced alcoholic cirrhosis. Clin. exp. Immunol. **8**, 749 (1971).
10. Jones, L. H., Hardisty, R. M., Wells, D. G., Kay, H. E. M.: Lymphocyte transformation in patients with acute lymphoblastic leukemia. Brit. med. J. **1971 II**, 329.
11. Oppenheim, J. J., Blaese, R. M., Waldmann, T. A.: Defective lymphocyte transformation and delayed hypersensitivity in Wiskott-Aldrich syndrome. J. Immunol. **104**, 853 (1970).
12. Walker, J. S., Davis, D., Cocking, H., Freeman, C. B., Harris, R.: Immunological studies in acute myeloid leukemia: PHA responsiveness und serum inhibitory factors. Brit. J. Cancer **27**, 203 (1973).

Delayed Hypersensitivity Response toward Autochthonous Tumor Extracts

R. B. Herberman

Cellular and Tumor Immunology Section, Laboratory of Cell Biology, National Cancer Institute, Bethesda

In the past few years, there has been increasing evidence for cell-mediated immunological reactions against antigens associated with human neoplasms. Most studies have been performed with *in vitro* assays. It has also been possible to measure cellular immunity *in vivo* by skin testing for delayed hypersensitivity reactions. This *in vivo* test might be a closer reflection of the state of immunity in tumor patients than an *in vitro* assay. [9, 12] prepared crude extracts of carcinomas and skin-tested

Appendix 1. Preparation of membrane extracts

1. Prepare single cell suspension in 0.14 m NaCl.
2. Freeze at — 70° and thaw.
3. Extraction[1] with 0.14 m NaCl.
4. Extraction[1] with 0.07 m NaCl.
5. Extraction[1] with 0.035 m NaCl.
6. Membrane pellet obtained from pooled supernatant fluids by centrifugation at 105,000 g for one hour.
7. Suspension of membranes in 0.14 m NaCl.
8. Adjustment of concentration with 0.14 m NaCl, as determined by protein concentration.

[1] Extraction consisted of suspension in saline, incubation at 4 °C for 10 min and centrifugation at 500 g for 10 min.

the autologous patients. Positive reactions were seen in about 25% of the patients. The reactivity of the patients did not correlate well with their clinical state. The specificity of the reactions was not well characterized. Some control extracts produced positive skin reactions. In addition, bacterial contamination of some of the reactions could have contributed to the reactions [12].

Our group has also observed delayed skin reactions to extracts of a variety of human tumors. Most of the skin tests have been performed with membrane extracts of tumor cells and of normal tissues [11]. A summary of the extraction procedure is given in Appendix 1. At the same time that patients were tested intradermally with 0.1 ml of the membrane preparations, they were also tested with a battery of standard recall antigens[1] to determine whether general cellular reactivity was intact. At least one of these antigens produced positive reactions in all normal volunteers tested. Only nonanergic patients were found to have positive reactions to tumor extracts. A positive reaction was defined as 5 mm or more of induration at 48 h after inoculation. Biopsies of positive reactions showed histological reactions consistent with a delayed-hypersensitivity reaction, i.e. lymphocytes and histiocytes clustered around small blood vessels in the upper dermis.

Membrane extracts of autologous tumor cells have produced positive skin reactions in patients with acute leukemia [6, 11]. In patients with acute lymphocytic leukemia, positive reactions were seen in most of those in remission, whereas there was only one positive reaction during relapse (Table 1). A similar pattern was found

Table 1. Skin tests of acute leukemia patients with membrane extracts of autochthonous cells

Test material[a]	Tests positive/total number of tests	
	Remission	Relapse
Acute lymphocytic leukemia		
leukemia cells	18/23	1/16
remission cells	0/14	0/5
Acute myelogenous leukemia		
leukemia cells	18/20	7/19
remission cells	0/5	0/4

[a] All tests performed with 0.1 ml membrane extracts at a protein concentration of 1 mg/ml.

in patients with acute myelogenous leukemia, although the incidence of reactivity in relapse was higher. No positive reactions have been elicited by extracts of remission cells tested at the same protein concentration (1 mg/ml). For 15 of 18 patients on whom serial skin tests with tumor extracts were performed, results of skin tests correlated well with clinical state: tests were positive in remission and became negative in relapse. When the patients went back into remission, the skin tests became positive again. These changes in reactivity to the membrane extracts could not be accounted for by a generalized change in skin reactivity. Tests with the battery of recall antigens were not affected by the changes in clinical condition; the same tests were positive during remission and relapse.

In collaboration with L. Fass, A. Bluming and J. Ziegler, a series of patients with Burkitt's tumor were tested with extracts of autologous tumor and of normal lymphocytes [2, 4]. As with the acute leukemia patients, reactivity to tumor extracts correlated with the clinical state of the patients. Before treatment, with tumor present, only 1 of 16 patients gave positive reactions; in remission, about half of the patients gave positive reactions (Table 2). The incidence of relapse or mortality was the same in patients with positive and negative skin tests. However, patients with positive

[1] Dermatophyton "O" (1:100; Hollister-Stier), SKSD (Varidase; Lederle), mumps (Eli Lilly) and Dermatophyton (1:30; Hollister-Stier).

reactions remained in remission significantly longer than those with negative reactions. 7 patients with positive reactions subsequently relapsed and 10 had negative reactions. Upon re-induction of remission, positive reactions were again seen.

In studies with A. HOLLINSHEAD and T. C. ALFORD, we have detected tumor-associated antigens in patients with intestinal cancer [5, 7, 8]. It proved possible to solubilize the specific skin-reactive antigen from the tumor membranes by low-frequency sonication. Table 3 shows a representative test in which the membrane

Table 2. Skin tests in patients with Burkitt's tumor. Correlation with clinical course of disease

	Skin test in remission	
	Positive	Negative
Total number of patients	15	15
Patients with subsequent relapse	7	9
Mortality [a]	3	5
Remission duration [b]	25	6

[a] Number of patients. — [b] Median in weeks.

Table 3. Skin tests of a rectal cancer patient with autologous extracts and with fetal intestinal extracts

Materials	Protein concentration (μg/0.1 ml)	Delayed skin reaction	CEA [a]
Rectal cancer			
membranes	230	+	+
soluble fraction III	184	+	+
Normal rectum			
membranes	296	—	—
soluble fraction III	270	—	—
Fetal intestine			
membranes	186	+	ND [b]
soluble fraction III	270	+	—

[a] As detected by GOLD in radioimmunoassay. — [b] Not done.

extract and a Sephadex G-200 fraction of the solubilized tumor extract gave positive reactions. No reactions were seen with comparable extracts from normal tissues, nor with other Sephadex fractions of the tumor sonicate. Extracts of fetal intestine and liver have also given positive reactions. The Sephadex fractions containing the skin-reactive antigen usually contained the carcinoembryonic antigen (CEA) of Gold, as detected by inhibition in the radioimmunoassay [13]. However, on further fractionation of the antigens by acrylamide gel electrophoresis, CEA was clearly separated from the skin reactive antigen. Therefore, the skin-reactive antigen in intestinal cancer appears to be a carcinoembryonic antigen which is different from the CEA of Gold.

We have also performed skin tests in patients with malignant melanoma (HOLLINSHEAD *et al*, personal comm.). As shown in Table 4, membrane extracts and two different Sephadex G-200 fractions of the soluble sonicate of tumor have given positive reactions, as also have some comparable fractions of normal skin. A similar observation of reactivity of melanoma patients to antigens in normal skin has been made by [3]. 6 of 9 patients giving positive reactions to tumor extracts also reacted positively to the skin extracts. It is, therefore, likely that at least some of the observed reactivity of melanoma patients was directed against tissue-specific antigens, which are probably present in normal skin and absent on lymphocytes. These findings emphasize the importance of using control tissues as close in type to the tumor as possible in order to distinguish between tumor-associated and tissue-associated antigens. Despite the apparent lack of tumor specificity, there has been some correlation between reactivity to one of the melanoma fractions and clinical stage of disease (Table 5). The E antigen gave a high incidence of reactivity in localized disease, but was negative in patients with disseminated tumor.

Table 4. Delayed hypersensitivity reactions in melanoma patients

Antigen	Number of positive tests/total number of tests		
	Autologous	Allogeneic	Total
Melanoma			
Membranes	1/10	2/10	3/20
Sonicates	0/3	0/1	0/4
Sephadex fraction E	6/7	11/17	17/24
Sephadex fraction C	2/4	9/11	11/15
Normal skin			
Membranes	1/3	0/5	1/8
Sephadex fraction E		1/8	1/8
Sephadex fraction C		1/8	1/8

Table 5. Delayed skin reactions in melanoma patients. Correlation with stage of disease

Antigen (Sephadex fraction of melanoma sonicate)	Number positive tests/total number of tests			
	Stage [a] I	Stage II	Stage IV	Stage IV advanced
E (MW ~ 38,000)	7/7	10/13	0/2	0/2
C (MW ~ 10,000)	4/4	4/4	3/3	0/4

[a] Stage I: tumor confined to primary site; II: involvement of regional lymph nodes; III: regional lymph nodes plus other lymph nodes involved; IV: disseminated disease.

Studies in breast cancer also point toward a tissue-specific in addition to a tumor-specific antigen [1]. With membrane extracts (Table 6), tumor-associated reactivity was observed. With one exception, only breast tumor membranes produced positive reactions. However, soluble fractions, obtained from the membranes by sonication and separation on Sephadex G-200, produced a different pattern of reactions (Table 7). Patients with breast cancer reacted to soluble fractions from breast tumor, normal breast from the tumor patient, and to normal breast tissue from patients with benign disease. Patients with benign breast disease also had positive reactions to the normal breast extracts, but patients with other benign diseases did not.

Table 6. Delayed hypersensitivity skin reactions to breast membrane extracts

Type of patient	Membrane extracts (number of positive tests/number of patients tested)		
	Ca breast	N-Ca breast [a]	N-N breast [b]
Breast cancer			
Autologous	3/9	0/4	
Allogeneic	3/4	0/4	1/5
Other cancer	0/4	0/3	0/2
Benign disease			
Breast			0/3
Other			0/2

[a] Normal breast tissue from mastectomy specimen of cancer patient.
[b] Normal breast tissue from patients with benign breast disease.

Table 7. Delayed hypersensitivity reactions to soluble fractions from breast membranes

Type of patient	Soluble fractions [a] (number of positive tests/number of patients tested)		
	Ca breast	N-Ca breast	N-N breast
Breast cancer			
Autologous	5/6	3/5	
Allogeneic	4/4	3/4	4/5
Other cancer	2/4	1/4	1/4
Benign disease			
Breast			3/4
Other			0/3

[a] Membrane extracts sonicated and soluble proteins separated on Sephadex G-200. Reactive fraction contained proteins in 42—56,000 molecular weight range.

Discussion

Skin testing for delayed hypersensitivity is a useful method for studying cellular immune responses to human tumor-associated antigens. In patients with acute leukemia and with Burkitt's tumor, skin testing has detected reactivity to antigens which appear to be tumor-specific. With malignant melanoma and carcinoma of the breast, antigens not related to the tumors have also been demonstrated. The antigens associated with these diseases need to be separated further to determine whether tumor-specific as well as tissue-specific antigens are present.

In addition to the skin tests with autochthonous tumor extracts, tests with allogeneic preparations have also given some positive reactions. It is often assumed in tumor immunology that reactions to common antigens suggest a viral etiology for the tumor. Although this is one major explanation for reactivity to allogeneic antigens, the present work illustrates that two other causes exist. Carcinoembryonic antigens can be found in a variety of tumors, presumably due to derepression in the tumor of host genetic information. In intestinal cancer, such antigens can elicit cell-mediated immune responses. Tissue- or organ-specific antigens can also account for common antigenicity in tumors. This rather neglected category which may actually account for many observed reactions.

Since skin testing is an alternative to the various *in vitro* assays for cellular immunity, it is worthwhile to consider the relative advantages and disadvantages of this method. The following could be cited as advantages of the *in vivo* assay:

1. It is a relatively simple technique, which does not require specialized equipment or extensive training of personnel.

2. It allows use of tumor tissues taken directly from the patient, obviating the need for tissue culture, which also makes it much easier to perform controls with appropriate normal tissues. In contrast, it has been difficult or impossible in most cases to have tissue cultures of normal cells of the same morphologic type as the tumor available for *in vitro* testing.

3. The skin tests may be a closer reflection of the *in vivo* immune state. When skin tests and two *in vitro* assays were used to study patients with acute leukemia, only the skin tests correlated well with the clinical state of the patients [10].

The possible disadvantages of the skin test assay are:

1. Precise measurement of reactivity is difficult: tests are arbitrarily defined as positive when there is 5 mm or greater of induration at 48 h, yet some reactions have a peak earlier or later than 48 h. Tests with various concentrations of the same material do not give a clear dose-response curve. One of the problems here is that the depth of induration cannot be measured in addition to the diameter.

2. Skin tests require a fair amount of time and cooperation from the patients, both for inoculation and for readings.

3. The test procedure could produce sensitization to the antigens. However, in the skin tests with tumor extracts, we have not seen any clear evidence for this.

Further studies, particularly comparative studies with other assays of cellular immunity, will be needed before the role of skin testing can be defined more clearly.

References

1. Alford, C., Hollinshead, A. C., Herberman, R. B.: Delayed cutaneous hypersensitivity reactions to extracts of malignant and normal human breast cells. Ann. Surg. **18**, 20 (1973).
2. Bluming, A. Z., Ziegler, J. L., Fass, L., Herberman, R. B.: Delayed cutaneous sensitivity reactions to autologous Burkitt lymphoma protein extracts: Results of a prospective two and a half year study. Clin. exp. Immunol. **9**, 713 (1971).
3. Bluming, A. Z., Vogel, C. L., Ziegler, J. L., Kiryabwire, J. W. M.: Delayed cutaneous sensitivity reactions to extracts of autologous malignant melanoma: A second look. J. nat. Cancer Inst. **48**, 17 (1972).

4. FASS, L., HERBERMAN, R. B., ZIEGLER, J. L.: Delayed cutaneous hypersensitivity reactions to autologous extracts of Burkitt-lymphoma cells. New Engl. J. Med. **282**, 776 (1970).
5. HERBERMAN, R. B., HOLLINSHEAD, A., ALFORD, T. C.: Skin reactive soluble antigens from intestinal cancer cell membranes and from fetal cell membranes. In: Proc. First confer. and workshop on embryonic and fetal antigens in cancer, p. 331. Oak Ridge: Oak Ridge National Laboratory 1972.
6. HERBERMAN, R. B., ROSENBERG, E. B., HALTERMAN, R. H., MCCOY, J. L., LEVENTHAL, B. G.: Cellular immune reactions to human leukemia. Nat. Cancer Inst. Monogr. **35**, 259 (1973).
7. HOLLINSHEAD, A., GLEW, D., BUNNAG, B., GOLD, P., HERBERMAN, R.: Skin-reactive soluble antigen from intestinal cancer-cell membranes and relationship to carcinoembryonic antigens. Lancet **1970 I**, 1191.
8. HOLLINSHEAD, A. C., MCWRIGHT, C. G., ALFORD, T. C., GLEW, D. H., GOLD, P., HERBERMAN, R. B.: Separation of skin-reactive intestinal cancer antigen from the carcinoembryonic antigen of Gold. Science **177**, 887 (1972).
9. HUGHES, L. E., LYTTON, B.: Antigenic properties of human tumors: Delayed cutaneous hypersensitivity reactions. Brit. med. J. **1964 I**, 209.
10. LEVENTHAL, B. G., HALTERMAN, R. H., ROSENBERG, E. B., HERBERMAN, R. B.: Immune reactivity of leukemia patients to autologous blast cells. Cancer Res. **32**, 1820 (1972).
11. OREN, M. E., HERBERMAN, R. B.: Delayed cutaneous hypersensitivity reactions to membrane extracts of human tumour cells. Clin. exp. Immunol. **9**, 45 (1971).
12. STEWART, T. H. M.: The presence of delayed hypersensitivity reactions in patients toward cellular extracts of their malignant tumors. 1. The role of tissue antigen, nonspecific reactions of nuclear material, and bacterial antigen as a cause for this phenomenon. Cancer (Philad.) **23**, 1368 (1969).
13. THOMSON, D., KRUPEY, J., FREEDMAN, S., GOLD, P.: The radioimmunoassay of circulating carcinoembryonic antigen of the human digestive system. Proc. nat. Acad. Sci. (Wash.) **64**, 161 (1969).

Second Part

Stimulation of Immunity and Cancer Immunotherapy

1. Experimental

Experimental Screening for "Systemic Adjuvants of Immunity" Applicable in Cancer Immunotherapy

G. Mathé, M. Kamel, M. Dezfulian, O. Halle-Pannenko, and C. Bourut

Institut de Cancérologie et d'Immunogénétique, Hôpital Paul-Brousse, Villejuif

Introduction

The term "adjuvant" was introduced in immunology to designate an agent wich, when injected *locally* in a mixture with an antigen, was able to increase the immune (humoral) response to the antigen. Freund's adjuvant [12] has been the most widely used. The stimulatory effect of such "adjuvants" on proliferation and phagocytic ativity of macrophages, as well as some undefined action on the physicochemical presentation of the antigenic sites of the immunizing substances have been the conventionally accepted hypotheses for their mechanisms of action [9, 12].

It was observed that some agents, especially BCG, when administered *systemically* and *before* the inoculation of microorganisms [7] or tumors (allogeneic or isogeneic) known to carry tumor-associated antigens [1, 3, 13, 29, 34] were able to *prevent* the development of the infection or the growth of the tumor. Stimulation of the phagocytic capacity of the host was the generally accepted explanation for this effect [42].

The fact that chemotherapy is not able to eradicate most tumors even when cytostatic drugs are given in large, toxic doses [28] is partially explained by obedience of the tumor to first-order kinetics [37, 38, 39]. Moreover, many patients with localized tumors relapse after apparently complete surgical resection or radiotherapeutic destruction, indicating that these two classic weapons often leave residual diesease. There are thus pressing reasons to search for new types of treatment, able to kill the "last cancer cell".

The fact that the semi-allogeneic tumor, placental choriocarcinoma, induces intense immune reactions [25], first directed our attention to *active immunotherapy* [20, 29, 30]. Foley had described tumor-associated antigens (TAA) 19 years earlier [10].

Active immunotherapy (AI) is defined as the stimulation of the patient's own immune reactions *after* the establishment of the tumor. It can be *specific*, as when derícted against TAA, or *nonspecific*, producing a general stimulation of the host's immune reactions by "systemic adjuvants of immunity". We have given this name to the agents that have this effect, even when not mixed with the antigen or administered simultaneously [21].

Our first experiments with AI in murine models showed that AI can eradicate leukemia under certain conditions [20, 29]. It is effective only if the number of tumor cells does not exceed 10^5, and usually only with the combination of specific stimulation by (irradiated) tumor cells plus an adjuvant (the most efficient adjuvant being BCG). BCG given alone after the establishment of the tumor is rarely effective.

This is the *systemic* immunotherapy approach, the object of which is to eradicate the residual disease left after a previous treatment. Obviously, it differs from the *local* immunotherapy approach, which consists of injecting BCG into a perceptible tumor, as used recently by [8, 46].

The first clinical trials on residual disease in acute lymphoid leukemia [23] and subsequent trials [31] have shown that the concept of systemic active immunotherapy is applicable to human tumors. AI was shown to be capable of maintaining more than one third of acute lymphoid leukemia patients in complete remission for 4—6 years; after the number of tumor cells in these cases had been reduced by chemoradiotherapy. Powles *et al.* [35] have obtained similar results with AI in acute myeloid leukemia. These authors showed that the combination of irradiated tumor cells and BCG prolongs remission for longer than maintenance chemotherapy.

The difficulty of administering BCG, the variability of clinical results obtained with different BCG preparations, and the modality of administration [4, 32] have revealed a need for systemic adjuvants that can be administered, more easily and with a more scientific, especially quantitative, method.

The aim of this paper is to report the results of a study with a battery of screening tests set up a) to explore the validity of the information yielded on adjuvants, such as BCG, already used in experimental and/or clinical trials [26]; b) to learn more about the adjuvant effect of other agents which have been reported to exert a comparable effect, e.g. extracts from mycobacteria like the methanol-extract residue (MER) [44, 45], the insoluble component of the BCG membrane (Hiu I) [16] or the watersoluble component of the BCG membrane Hiu II) [15]. Other agents tested include microorganisms such as *Corynebacterium parvum* (CP), three preparations of *Corynebacterium granulosum* (CG) [36] and finally two synthetic compounds, polyinosinic-polycytidylic acid (poly IC) [5, 27] and polyadenylic-polyuridylic acid (poly AU) [5].

Methods and Materials

Methods

The tests included in the battery were chosen mainly because of the conclusions we drew from our "operational" results [20, 29]. The systemic immunity adjuvants we have studied are rarely effective when given alone as immunotherapy, but do work immunoprophylactically. Therefore, immunoprophylaxis of selected murine tumors was studied. Administration of the potential adjuvant before the inoculation of tumor cells is also necessary, in order to distinguish between the immunostimulating effect we are looking for and a possible cytostatic effect. If an agent produces an effect, when administered before the tumor, there will be little chance that it is due to a cytostatic effect; however, it will be quite consistent, in view of our previous experiments, with an immunostimulating action [29].

We chose 3 tumors for the immunoprophylaxis tests: a) L 1210 leukemia, has been the experimental model for our "operational" preclinical research; b) Lewis lung tumor, a solid tumor which gives lung metastases and is very sensitive to immunological enhancement; and c) ICIG CI_1 solid tumor, a tumor recently induced with dimethylbenzanthracene in our Institute. This tumor has been transferred by grafts only a few times and seems to be as sensitive to immunological enhancement as Lewis tumor. Enhancement [18], whether blocking [14, 33, 43] or exerting a central effect on the immune machinery [2], has to be considered as a possible side-effect of active immunotherapy trials [41].

Tests of activity in the three tumor systems were preceded by screening for immunological activity in two non-tumor systems. After preliminary experiments [26, 27] we chose the following: a) the hemolytic plaque-forming cell test [17] because it is simple and inexpensive and enabled us to study the dose factor, the time factor, and the effect of the route of administration ;b) the graft-versus-host reaction (GVHR) (in which the potential adjuvant is administered to donors) because it is a reaction which involves only T lymphocytes [40], while the Jerne test involves both T and B lymphocytes [6]. The second test enabled us to detect possible immuno-inhibition as well as immunostimulation in response to cell-surface antigens.

This battery of tests was designed to answer the questions: Is a given agent an immuno-adjuvant or an immuno-inhibitor, or both, depending on time and route of administration? Does it influence a pure T-lymphocyte reaction? Does it induce a growth-retarding effect or a growth-enhancing effect, or both, depending on various factors, such as route of administration and variety of tumor?

For all tests, the same animals (DBA/2 × C 57 BL/6) F_1 pathogen-free mice, 3 months of age were used. These are the most readily available F_1 animals in France, and the three tumors are semi-allogeneic for them.

A summary of the methods used for the different tests is given in Table 1.

For the *hemolytic plaque-forming tests* (HPFT), 192 mice were used for each potential adjuvant. They were randomized into 32 experimental groups, each comprising 6 animals. These 32 groups were randomized in 4 series which were submitted to the test on different days. The agents were injected by 4 routes, i.v., i.p., s.c., and i.d. once, on day — 14 or — 5 or — 2½ before the day of the administration of the sheep red blood cells (SRBC), or on day 0 (the same as the antigens), or day + 1, + 2, or + 3 after the SRBC. The plaques were counted on day + 4 after i.p. injection of SRBC. For the statistical analysis of the results, the Student-Fisher test was used.

For the *graft-versus-host* reaction, 40 mice were used for each potential adjuvant. They were randomized into 5 experimental groups. The (DBA/2 × C 57 BL/6) F_1 recipients were irradiated with 500 rads (225 kV, 12 mA, 0.2 Ci, D 50 cm). They were injected i.v. with 10^7 bone marrow and 2.5 × 10^7 lymph node cells of C57BL/6 mice, which were normal for the control group and which had been treated either i.v., i.p., s.c., or i.d. with one of the potential adjuvants at the doses indicated in Table 2. This treatment was administered to the donors 60 h before sacrifice for all the potential adjuvants except BCG, where it was injected 14 days before. This difference in the administration time of the potential adjuvant as between BCG and the others was based on previous experiments [26] and the results obtained with the hemolytic plaque-forming tests. The mortality of the recipients was studied and

Table 1. Tests and methods employed

Techniques	Day 0	Injection of the adjuvant		Results
		Before[a]	After[a]	
Hemolytic plaque-forming cell test (Jerne)	10^9 Sheep red blood cells i.p.	Days —14, or —5, or — 2.5	Days 0, or +1, or + 2, or +3	PFC at day + 4
GVH	10^7 Bone marrow and 2.5×10^7 lymph node C 57 Bl/6 cells to (C 57 Bl/6 × DBA/2) F_1	Day —14 (BCG) Day —2.5 (others)	— —	Mortality
L 1210	10^3 Leukemic cells i.v.	Day —14 (BCG) Day —2.5 (others)	— —	Mortality
Lewis T	2×10^6 Tumor cells s.c.	Day —14 (BCG) Day —2.5 (others)	— —	 Mortality
ICIG Ci_1	2×10^6 Tumor cells s.c.	Day —14 (BCG) Day —2.5 (others)	— —	Mortality

[a] The administration of the antigen (Jerne test), the transfer of the lymphocytes (GVH) or the inoculation of the tumors.

Table 2. Immunity systemic adjuvant-candidates submitted to the screening tests

Agents	Obtained from	Composition	Doses per mouse[a]
BCG	Institut Pasteur	Suspension of living bacteria	1 mg
MER	ICIG (Weiss's method)	BCG without lipid fraction extracted in methanol and acetone	1 mg
Hiu I	ICIG	Component of the BCG membrane (non-soluble)	1 mg
Hiu II	ICIG	Component of the BCG membrane (soluble)	0.5 mg
C. parvum	Institut Pasteur	Suspension of dead bacteria	400 γ
C. granulosum A	Institut Pasteur	Killed bacilli	400 γ
C. granulosum B	Institut Pasteur	Membranes treated by phenol in the cold	100 γ
C. granulosum C	Institut Pasteur	Membranes prepared by mechanic action	100 γ
Poly IC	CHOAY	Polyinosinic acid-Polycytidylic acid	300 γ
Poly AU	CHOAY	Polyadenylic acid-Polyuridilic acid	150 γ

[a] Determined by preliminary studies.

compared with that of controls. This is a test we established in 1960 [22] and it has been used in many experiments since then. It is, in our experience, the most reproducible test for studying GVHR. For the statistical analysis of the results we used the Wilcoxon test.

For the *immunoprophylaxis of L 1210 leukemia, Lewis tumor, and ICIG CI_1*, 40 mice were used for each tumor and each potential adjuvant. They were randomized into 5 experimental groups. The numbers and the routes of administration of the tumor cells are mentioned in Table 1, and the adjuvants to be tested had all been injected on day — 2½ before the tumor cells, except BCG which was injected on day — 14, as explained above. The same 4 routes of administration were used. The mortality of the animals was recorded and a cumulative mortality curve established. The different experimental groups were compared with controls. The Student-Fisher test was used to evaluate statistically L 1210 leukemia (where all animals die within a few days of each other) and the non-parametric Wilcoxon test was used for the other 2 tumors (where mortality is more spread out).

It must be noted that, because of the large number of groups we had to study, we had to randomize not only the animals, but also the different experimental protocols. Each experiment included controls, so that the curves for the controls are multiple and may differ slightly from one experiment to another.

To express the results the following index has been calculated:

for the HPFT (JERNE)

$$I = \frac{\text{mean number of PFC/spleen of the tested mice}}{\text{mean number of PFC/spleen of the controls}}$$

for GVHR and tumors

$$I = \frac{\text{median of survival of experimental animals}}{\text{median of survival of the controls}}$$

In each group that produced a significant result the same experiment was repeated to increase the probability that a given positive result was due to the material studied, and not appreciably influenced by the animals or the laboratory environment. The final significance of the result (given as S +) has been calculated from the results of both experiments.

All these assays were not done in the same experiment, and although they were randomly distributed, the degree of immunomodification found in each group of animals may not correlate perfectly with the statistical significance of the result. The immunomodification indicates the pharmacological effect in the experiments and the statistical significance indicates the variability within each group.

Materials

The potential adjuvants submitted to the battery of tests, their source, composition, and the dosage we used for each of them are listed in Table 2. These doses were determined from our own preliminary experiments for BCG, poly IC, and poly AU [26, 27] by HIU for Hiu I and II [15, 16, 36] for *C. parvum* and *C. granulosum* preparations.

Pasteur Institute BCG comprises 7×10^6 viable units per mg. It is a fresh non-lyophilized preparation less than 7 days old.

We prepared according to the procedure of [44, 45], and prepared Hiu I and Hiu II according to HIU [15, 16]. Hiu II is a soluble extract obtained by electrolysis. *C. parvum* and *C. granulosum* preparation methods have been published by [36]. Poly IC is prepared by the Choay Laboratory (for method, see [26, 27]). Polyadenylic acid and polyuridylic acid are synthesized enzymatically from the corresponding ribonucleoside diphosphates in the presence of a polynucleotide phosphatase extracted from *Azotobacter vinelandii*. For purification, the synthesized polymers are treated several times with phenol. Short-chain oligonucleotides and nucleolytic enzymes are removed by exhaustive dialysis and fraction on Biogel P 10. The concentration of each polymer is estimated chemically (by phosphorus determination) and physically (from UV absorption spectra). The chain length corresponding to the molecular weight is estimated from the sedimentation coefficient of each polymer. Poly AU is prepared under the conditions of pH, ionic strength, and temperature described by [11, 19]. The molecular association is controlled by varying the transition temperature.

Results

The Hemolytic Plaque-Forming Cell (HPFC) Test (Jerne)

We used this test to determine the effect of the time and the route of administration for each potential adjuvant at a dose which previous experiments had indicated to be the most efficient. Two different results have been obtained compared to controls: an increase or a decrease of the HPFC.

Table 3 shows that BCG induces a significant increase in number of PFC when administered i.v. and at day — 14 before the antigen.

MER exerts two kinds of action, an immunostimulative action when administered i.d. at day + 1 after the antigen, and an immunodepressive action when given s.c. at days — 14 and — 2½ (Table 4).

Table 3. Hemolytic plaque-forming cell test (JERNE) effect of Pasteur institute BCG (1 mg/mouse) on PFC/spleen

Days	Routes							
	i.v.		i.p.		i.d.		s.c.	
— 14	I[b] = 2.8 ↗	S[c] at 2%	I = 0.75	NS[c]	I = 0.75	NS	I = 0.75	NS
— 5	I = 1.1	NS	I = 0.75	NS	I = 0.75	NS	I = 1.1	NS
— 2.5	I = 1.1	NS	I = 0.8	NS	I = 0.75	NS	I = 1.1	NS
0	I = 1.1	NS	I = 0.75	NS	I = 1.1	NS	I = 1	NS
+ 1	I = 1.1	NS	I = 1	NS	I = 1.1	NS	I = 1	NS
+ 2	I = 1.1	NS	I = 0.8	NS	I = 1.1	NS	I = 0.75	NS
+ 3	I = 1	NS	I = 1	NS	I = 1.1	NS	I = 1	NS

[a] — = Before, + = after the injection of sheep red cells.

[b] $I = \frac{\text{Mean number of PFC/spleen of the tested mice}}{\text{Mean number of PFC/spleen of controls}}$.

[c] Statistics: Student-Fisher test. S = Significant. NS = Not significant.

Table 4. Hemolytic plaque-forming cell test (JERNE) effect of MER (1 mg/mouse) on PFC/spleen

Days[a]	Routes			
	i.v.	i.p.	i.d.	s.c.
— 14	I[b] = 1.1 NS[c]	I = 1.1 NS	I = 0.75 NS	I = 0.5 ↘ S[c] at 5%
— 5	I = 1.1 NS	I = 1.1 NS	I = 1.1 NS	I = 0.8 NS
— 2.5	I = 1.1 NS	I = 1.1 NS	I = 1.1 NS	I = 0.3 ↘ S at 1%
0	I = 0.75 NS	I = 0.75 NS	I = 1.1 NS	I = 0.75 NS
+ 1	I = 1.1 NS	I = 0.75 NS	I = 2.4 ↗ S at 2%	I = 0.75 NS
+ 2	I = 0.75 NS	I = 1.1 NS	I = 0.75 NS	I = 0.8 NS
+ 3	I = 0.75 NS	I = 1.1 NS	I = 1.1 NS	I = 1.07 NS

a — = Before, + = after the injection of sheep red cells.

b $I = \frac{\text{Mean number of PFC/spleen of the tested mice}}{\text{Mean number of PFC/spleen of controls}}$.

c Statistics: Student-Fisher test. S = Significant. NS = Not significant.

Table 5. Hemolytic plaque-forming cell test (JERNE) effect of Hiu I (insoluble) (1 mg/mouse) on PFC/spleen

Days[a]	Routes			
	i.v.	i.p.	i.d.	s.c.
— 14	I[b] = 0.75 NS[c]	I = 0.75 NS	I = 1.1 NS	I = 0.9 NS
— 5	I = 0.75 NS	I = 0.75 NS	I = 1.1 NS	I = 0.9 NS
— 2.5	I = 0.5 ↘ S[c] at 5%	I = 0.75 NS	I = 0.75 NS	I = 1.1 NS
0	I = 0.75 NS	I = 0.9 NS	I = 1.08 NS	I = 0.9 NS
+ 1	I = 0.9 NS	I = 0.75 NS	I = 1.1 NS	I = 1.1 NS
+ 2	I = 1 NS	I = 0.75 NS	I = 1.10 NS	I = 0.75 NS
+ 3	I = 0.75 NS	I = 0.9 NS	I = 0.75 NS	I = 0.9 NS

a — = Before, + = after the injection of sheep red cells.

b $I = \frac{\text{Mean number of PFC/spleen of the tested mice}}{\text{Mean number of PFC/spleen of controls}}$.

c Statistics: Student-Fisher test. S = Significant. NS = Not significant.

Hiu induces only immunodepression and is optimally administered i.v. at day — 2½ before the antigen (Table 5).

Hiu II, the water-soluble factor extracted from mycobacteria, induced only immunostimulation and did so when injected i.v. at day — 2½ and i.p. at day + 1, + 2, and + 3 (Table 6).

C. parvum (CP) induced only immunostimulation when given i.v. at days — 14, 0, + 2, and + 3, when given i.p. at days — 5 and — 2½, and when given s.c. at day + 1 (Table 7).

Table 6. Hemolytic plaque-forming cell test (Jerne) effect of Hiu II (soluble) (0.5 mg/mouse) on PFC/spleen

Days[a]	Routes							
	i.v.		i.p.		i.v.		s.c.	
— 14	I[b] = 0.75	NS[c]	I = 1.1	NS	I = 0.75	NS	I = 0.75	NS
— 5	I = 0.75	NS	I = 1.1	NS	I = 0.75	NS	I = 0.75	NS
— 2.5	I = 1.6 ↗	S[c] at 5%	I = 1.1	NS	I = 0.75	NS	I = 0.8	NS
0	I = 0.75	NS	I = 1.1	NS	I = 0.75	NS	I = 0.75	NS
+ 1	I = 0.9	NS	I = 2 ↗	S at 5%	I = 0.75	NS	I = 0.9	NS
+ 2	I = 0.75	NS	I = 2.4 ↗	S at 2%	I = 0.75	NS	I = 1	NS
+ 3	I = 0.75	NS	I = 2.4 ↗	S at 5%	I = 0.75	NS	I = 0.75	NS

[a] — = Before, + = after the injection of sheep red cells.

[b] $I = \frac{\text{Mean number of PFC/spleen of the tested mice}}{\text{Mean number of PFC/spleen of controls}}$.

[c] Statistics: Student-Fisher test. S = Significant. NS = Not significant.

Table 7. Hemolytic plaque-forming cell test (Jerne) effect of C. parvum (400 γ/mouse) on PFC/spleen

Days[a]	Routes							
	i.v.		i.p.		i.d.		s.c.	
— 14	I[b] = 1.5 ↗	S[c] at 1%	I = 1.1	NS[c]	I = 0.75	NS	I = 0.75	NS
— 5	I = 1.1	NS	I = 1.2 ↗	S at 5%	I = 0.75	NS	I = 1.1	NS
— 2.5	I = 1.1	NS	I = 1.3 ↗	S at 1%	I = 0.8	NS	I = 1.1	NS
0	I = 1.6 ↗	S at 2%	I = 1.1	NS	I = 1.1	NS	I = 0.75	NS
+ 1	I = 1.1	NS	I = 1.1	NS	I = 1.1	NS	I = 1.8 ↗	S at 2%
+ 2	I = 2 ↗	S at 1%	I = 1.1	NS	I = 1.1	NS	I = 1.1	NS
+ 3	I = 1.8 ↗	S at 2%	I = 1.1	NS	I = 1.02	NS	I = 1.1	NS

[a] — = Before, + = after the injection of sheep red cells.

[b] $I = \frac{\text{Mean number of PFC/spleen of the tested mice}}{\text{Mean number of PFC/spleen of controls}}$.

[c] Statistics: Student-Fisher test. S = Significant. NS = Not significant.

C. granulosum A (killed bacillus) induced only immunostimulation when given i.v. at day — 14, when given i.p. at days — 5 and — 2½, and when given s.c. at day — 14 and day 0 (Table 8).

Table 8. Hemolytic plaque-forming cell test (JERNE) effect of C. granulosum A (400 γ/mouse) on PFC/spleen

Days[a]	Routes							
	i.v.		i.p.		i.d.		s.c.	
— 14	I[b] = 1.7 ↗	S[c] at 1%	I = 1.01	NS[c]	I = 1.1	NS	I = 1.19 ↗	S at 5%
— 5	I = 1.1	NS	I = 1.2 ↗	S at 5%	I = 1.1	NS	I = 0.54	NS
— 2.5	I = 1.1	NS	I = 1.2 ↗	S at 2%	I = 1.1	NS	I = 1	NS
0	I = 0.75	NS	I = 1.01	NS	I = 1.1	NS	I = 1.32 ↗	S at 5%
+ 1	I = 0.8	NS	I = 0.85	NS	I = 1.09	NS	I = 1	NS
+ 2	I = 1	NS	I = 1.1	NS	I = 0.9	NS	I = 1	NS
+ 3	I = 1.1	NS	I = 0.75	NS	I = 0.75	NS	I = 1.1	NS

[a] — = Before, + = after the injection of sheep red cells.

[b] $I = \frac{\text{Mean number of PFC/spleen of the tested mice}}{\text{Mean number of PFC/spleen of controls}}$.

[c] Statistics: Student-Fisher test. S = Significant. NS = Not significant.

Table 9. Hemolytic plaque-forming cell test (JERNE) effect of C. granulosum B (100 γ/mouse) on PFC/spleen

Days[c]	Routes							
	i.v.		i.p.		i.d.		s.c.	
— 14	I[b] = 1.75 ↗	S[c] at 5%	I = 1.1	NS[c]	I = 0.75	NS	I = 1.1	NS
— 5	I = 0.75	NS	I = 1.5 ↗	S at 5%	I = 0.75	NS	I = 1.1	NS
— 2.5	I = 0.90	NS	I = 1.5 ↗	S at 5%	I = 0.8	NS	I = 1.1	NS
0	I = 0.75	NS	I = 1.7 ↗	S at 1%	I = 1.1	NS	I = 3 ↗	S at 2%
+ 1	I = 1.2	NS	I = 1.1	NS	I = 1.1	NS	I = 1.1	NS
+ 2	I = 1.75 ↗	S at 1%	I = 1.1	NS	I = 1.1	NS	I = 3 ↗	S at 5%
+ 3	I = 1.1	NS	I = 1.5 ↗	S at 5%	I = 1.1	NS	I = 3.8 ↗	S at 2%

[a] — = Before, + = after the injection of sheep red cells.

[b] $I = \frac{\text{Mean number of PFC/spleen of the tested mice}}{\text{Mean number of PFC/spleen of controls}}$.

[c] Statistics: Student-Fisher test. S = Significant. NS = Not significant.

C. granulosum B (membranes treated by phenol in the cold) is immunostimulating only when given i.v. at days — 14 and + 2, when given i.p. at days — 5, — 2½, 0 and + 3, and when given s.c. at days 0, + 2, and + 3 (Table 9).

C. granulosum C (membranes prepared by mechanical action) is only immunostimulant and exerts its effect only when given i.v. at day — 5 (Table 10).

Table 10. Hemolytic plaque-forming cell test (JERNE) effect of C. granulosum C (100 γ/mouse) on PFC/spleen

Days[a]	Routes			
	i.v.	i.p.	i.d.	s.c.
— 14	I[b] = 1.06 NS[c]	I = 0.75 NS	I = 0.80 NS	I = 0.82 NS
— 5	I = 2.01 ↗ S[c] at 1‰	I = 0.87 NS	I = 0.93 NS	I = 0.81 NS
— 2.5	I = 1.10 NS	I = 1.10 NS	I = 0.80 NS	I = 1.10 NS
0	I = 0.75 NS	I = 0.75 NS	I = 0.82 NS	I = 1.10 NS
+ 1	I = 0.80 NS	I = 1.06 NS	I = 1.01 NS	I = 1.10 NS
+ 2	I = 0.83 NS	I = 0.75 NS	I = 0.94 NS	I = 1.10 NS
+ 3	I = 1.03 NS	I = 0.90 NS	I = 0.76 NS	I = 1.10 NS

[a] — = Before, + = after the injection of sheep red cells.

[b] $I = \frac{\text{Mean number of PFC/spleen of the tested mice}}{\text{Mean number of PFC/spleen of controls}}$.

[c] Statistics: Student-Fisher test. S = Significant. NS = Not significant.

Table 11. Hemolytic plaque-forming cell test (JERNE) effect of poly I poly C (300 γ/mouse) on PFC/spleen

Days[a]	Routes			
	i.v.	i.p.	i.d.	s.c.
— 14	I[b] = 0.75 NS[c]	I = 1.8 ↗ S[c] at 1%	I = 1.1 NS	I = 1.1 NS
— 5	I = 0.75 NS	I = 0.77 NS	I = 0.75 NS	I = 1.1 NS
— 2.5	I = 0.73 ↗ S at 1%	I = 1.1 NS	I = 1.1 NS	I = 1.1 NS
0	I = 1 NS	I = 1.8 ↗ S at 5%	I = 0.75 NS	I = 1 NS
+ 1	I = 0.75 NS	I = 1.1 NS	I = 1.1 NS	I = 1.1 NS
+ 2	I = 0.75 NS	I = 1.1 NS	I = 1.1 NS	I = 1.8 ↗ S at 1%
+ 3	I = 0.75 NS	I = 0.75 NS	I = 1.1 NS	I = 1.1 NS

[a] — = Before, + = after the injection of sheep red cells.

[b] $I = \frac{\text{Mean number of PFC/spleen of the tested mice}}{\text{Mean number of PFC/spleen of controls}}$.

[c] Statistics: Student-Fisher test. S = Significant. NS = Not significant.

Poly IC exerts both kinds of actions, being immunostimulating when given i.p. at days — 14 and 0, and s.c. at day + 2 and immunosuppressive when given i.v. at days — 2½ (Table 11).

Poly AU is only immunostimulating and exerts its effect only when given i.v. at days + 1 or + 2 and i.p. at day + 3 (Table 12).

The GVHR test also reveals two kinds of results. *Mortality may be either unaffected or accelerated* in the case of BCG injected i.v., CGA injected i.v., and CGB injected

Table 12. Hemolytic plaque-forming cell test (JERNE) effect of poly A poly U (150 γ/mouse) on PFC/spleen

Days[a]	Routes							
	i.v.		i.p.		i.d.		s.c.	
— 14	I[b] = 1.1	NS[c]	I = 0.86	NS	I = 0.75	NS	I = 1.1	NS
— 5	I = 1.1	NS	I = 1.1	NS	I = 1.1	NS	I = 1.1	NS
— 2.5	I = 0.86	NS	I = 1.1	NS	I = 0.8	NS	I = 0.93	NS
0	I = 1.1	NS	I = 1.1	NS	I = 1.1	NS	I = 1.1	NS
+ 1	I = 2.2 ↗	S[c] at 1%	I = 0.77	NS	I = 0.75	NS	I = 1.1	NS
+ 2	I = 2.1 ↗	S at 2%	I = 1.1	NS	I = 0.8	NS	I = 1.1	NS
+ 3	I = 1.1	NS	I = 1.7 ↗	S at 5%	I = 0.87	NS	I = 1.1	NS

[a] — = Before, + = after the injection of sheep red cells.

[b] $I = \frac{\text{Mean number of PFC/spleen of the tested mice}}{\text{Mean number of PFC/spleen of controls}}$.

[c] Statistics: Student-Fisher test. S = Significant. NS = Not significant.

Table 13. Effect of "SIA"[a] (injected to the donor at day — 2.5)[d] on GVH lethality summary of the results

"SIA"	Routes							
	i.v.		i.p.		i.d.		s.c.	
Pasteur Inst. BCG	I[b] = 0.21 ↗	S[c] 2%	I = 1.20	NS	I = 1	NS	I = 1.30	NS
MER	I = 1.93 ↘	S 2%	I = 0.85	NS	I = 1.07	NS	I = 0.85	NS
Hiu I	I = 1.43 ↘	S 3%	I = 1.15	NS	I = 1	NS	I = 0.85	NS
Hiu II	I = 1	NS	I = 1.30	NS	I = 1.21	NS	I = 1.21	NS
CP	I = 0.85	NS	I = 1.30	NS	I = 1.28	NS	I = 1.30	NS
CG. A	I = 0.80 ↗	S 4%	I = 1.20	NS	I = 1.30	NS	I = 1.20	NS
CG. B	I = 1.35 ↘	S 2%	I = 1	NS	I = 1.20	NS	I = 0.07 ↗	S 2%
CG. C	I = 1	NS	I = 1.80 ↘	S 1%	I = 1.15	NS	I = 1	NS
Poly IC	I = 1.28	NS	I = 0.85	NS	I = 1.30	NS	I = 1.14	NS
Poly AU	I = 0.90	NS	I = 0.90	NS	I = 1.27	NS	I = 0.90	NS

[a] "SIA" = Systemic Immunity Adjuvant.

[b] $I = \frac{\text{Median of survival of experimental animals}}{\text{Median of the controls}}$.

[c] Statistics: Non-parametric test of Wilcoxon. S = Significant, NS = Not Significant.

[d] Except for BCG which is injected at day — 14.

Table 14. Effect of "SIA"[a] (injected at day — 2.5)[d] for immunoprophylaxis of L 1210 leukemia summary of the results

"SIA"	Routes							
	i.v.		i.p.		i.d.		s.c.	
Pasteur Inst. BCG	I[b] = 1.6 ↗	S[c] 5%	I = 1	NS	I = 1	NS	I = 1	NS
MER	I = 1	NS	I = 1.09	NS	I = 1	NS	I = 1.5 ↗	S 5%
Hiu I	I = 1	NS	I = 1	NS	I = 1	NS	I = 1	NS
Hiu II	I = 1	NS	I = 1	NS	I = 1	NS	I = 1	NS
CP	I = 1.15 ↗	S 1‰	I = 1	NS	I = 1	NS	I = 1	NS
CG. A	I = 1.2 ↗	S 1‰	I = 1.4 ↗	S 5%	I = 1	NS	I = 1.15 ↗	S 2%
CG. B	I = 1.09	NS	I = 1.10	NS	I = 1	NS	I = 1	NS
CG. C	I = 1.2 ↗	S 1%	I = 1.2 ↗	S 5%	I = 1	NS	I = 1	NS
Poly IC	I = 1.5 ↗	S 5%	I = 1	NS	I = 1	NS	I = 1	NS
Poly AU	I = 1	NS	I = 1	NS	I = 1	NS	I = 1	NS

[a] "SIA" = Systemic Immunity Adjuvant.

[b] $$I = \frac{\text{Median of survival of experimental animals}}{\text{Median of the controls}}.$$

[c] Statistics: Student test. S = Significant. NS = Not significant.

[d] Except for BCG which is injected at day — 14.

Table 15. Effect of "SIA"[a] (injected at day — 2.5)[d] for immunoprophylaxis of Lewis tumor summary of the results

"SIA"	Routes							
	i.v.		i.p.		i.d.		s.c.	
Pasteur Inst. BCG	I[b] = 2.6 ↗	S[c] 1%	I = 1	NS	I = 1	NS	I = 0.8 ↘	S 2%
MER	I = 1.2 ↗	S 4%	I = 1.1	NS	I = 1	NS	I = 1	NS
Hiu I	I = 1	NS	I = 1	NS	I = 1	NS	I = 1	NS
Hiu II	I = 1	NS	I = 1	NS	I = 1.10	NS	I = 1.08	NS
CP	I = 1.2 ↗	S 2%	I = 1	NS	I = 0.9	NS	I = 0.9	NS
CG. A	I = 1.2 ↗	S 2%	I = 1.1	NS	I = 1	NS	I = 1.1	NS
CG. B	I = 1.2 ↗	S 1%	I = 1.1	NS	I = 0.9	NS	I = 1.1	NS
CG. C	I = 1.1	NS	I = 1	NS	I = 1	NS	I = 1.8 ↗	S 2%
Poly IC	I = 1	NS	I = 1	NS	I = 1.1	NS	I = 1.1	NS
Poly AU	I = 1.1	NS	I = 0.9	NS	I = 1.1	NS	I = 1.1	NS

[a] "SIA" = Systemic Immunity Adjuvant.

[b] $$I = \frac{\text{Median of survival of experimental animals}}{\text{Median of the controls}}.$$

[c] Statistics: Non parametric test of Wilcoxon. S = Significant. NS = Not significant.

[d] Except for BCG which is injected at day — 14.

s.c., or it may be *delayed*, which is the case for MER injected i.v., Hiu i.v., CBG i.v., and CGC i.p. (Table 13).

L 1210 leukemia mortality is either *unaffected or delayed*, as is the case with BCG i.v., MER s.c., CP i.v., CGA i.v., i.p. and s.c., CGC i.v. and i.p., and poly IC i.v. (Table 14).

Lewis solid tumor mortality is either *unaffected, delayed, or enhanced*. It is delayed with BCG i.v., MER i.v., CP i.v., CGA i.v., CGB i.v., and CGC s.c. It is enhanced with BCG s.c. (Table 15).

ICIG CI_1 solid tumor mortality is similarly either not affected, *delayed*, or *enhanced* (Table 16). It is delayed by BCG i.v. and enhanced by MER i.d. and Hiu i.p.

Table 16. Effect of "SIA"[a] (injected at day — 2.5)[d] for immunoprophylaxis of ICIG Cil
Summary of the results

"SIA"	Routes							
	i.v.		i.p.		i.d.		s.c.	
Pasteur Inst. BCG	I[b] = 1.19	↗ S at 1%	I = 1.14	NS	I = 1.1	NS	I = 1	NS
MER	I = 0.97	NS	I = 0.75	NS	I = 0.65	↘ S[c] 2%	I = 0.84	NS
Hiu I	I = 1.1	NS	I = 0.70	↘ S 3%	I = 0.94	NS	I = 1	NS
Hiu II	I = 1	NS	I = 1	NS	I = 1	NS	I = 1	NS
CP	I = 1	NS	I = 1.07	NS	I = 0.77	NS	I = 0.95	NS
CG. A	I = 1.09	NS	I = 1.01	NS	I = 0.75	NS	I = 0.91	NS
CG. B	I = 1.06	NS	I = 0.83	NS	I = 0.81	NS	I = 1	NS
CG. C	I = 1	NS	I = 0.92	NS	I = 0.81	NS	I = 0.90	NS
Poly IC	I = 1.07	NS	I = 0.74	NS	I = 1.05	NS	I = 0.80	NS
Poly AU	I = 1	NS	I = 1	NS	I = 1	NS	I = 1	NS

[c] "SIA" = Systemic Immunity Adjuvants.

[b] $I = \frac{\text{Median of survival of experimental animals}}{\text{Median of the controls}}$.

[c] Statistics: Non-parametric Wilcoxon test. S = Significant. NS = Not significant.

[d] Except for BCG which is injected at day — 14.

Discussion

All these adjuvants and several others (see [21]) had been studied before and results had been published indicating one of the kinds of action we describe in this paper. No single systematic study has been conducted with several agents and several tests, taking into account several parameters such as time and route of administration. It is also possible that some agents have been designated adjuvants on the basis of the immunostimulating action they exerted in a given experiment. On the other hand, when they produced an opposite effect in other experiments conducted by the same or other researchers, this result was not published, either because it was not what the researchers were looking for, or because their paper was not accepted, for it has long been considered that an "adjuvant" could only be immunostimulating.

The screening work reported here definitely confirms that some agents have immunostimulant activity. This is true of reactions that require the cooperation of

T and B lymphocytes (Jerne test) [6] and of reactions that involve only T lymphocytes (GVHR) [40]. They delay mortality in tumor-carrying animals when the agent is administered before the neoplastic cells, thus eliminating any cytostatic action. This effect is at present attributable to immunoprophylaxis, a mechanism that is substantiated by many experiments [1, 3, 13, 29].

This work, however, demonstrates that the results are not unidirectional nor always beneficial as far as tumor immunoprophylaxis is concerned. This is not surprising; many experiments have shown that immune stimulation may enhance tumor growth [18, 41]. This could be explained by the fact that the agents may stimulate humoral immunity more than they do cell-mediated immunity. It has been reported that antibodies may be blocking factors, protecting tumor cells against cell-mediated immunity [14]. One possible explanation for the enhancing effect on tumor growth we have sometimes observed may be that some agents stimulate the production of "blocking" antibodies. Experiments are presently being conducted by explore this possibility. We do know, however, that enhancement of tumor growth has never been obtained with L 1210 leukemia and has been observed only with the two solid tumors. It is well known that it is easy to enhance solid tumors but most difficult to enhance leukemias [21].

Another explanation of possible enhancement of mortality may be inhibition of cell-mediated immunity. We have shown that the agents we call systemic immunity adjuvants can depress immune reactions requiring T- and B-cell cooperation (Jerne test) or those based only on T cells (GVHR). Therefore, such agents should be considered more as *immunomodulators* than immunostimulators. However, inhibition of cell-mediated immunity has never been observed with L 1210 leukemia.

Although we studied several factors thought to be capable of modifying the effect of immunomodification, results were inconclusive. Some preliminary conclusions may be proposed as working hypotheses for later studies of factors that influence immune responses, especially their effect on tumor growth.

Some agents are better candidates than others for tumor prevention (and treatment) because they induce, for a given modality of administration, immune stimulation in a T-B cooperation test, and immune stimulation of a T-lymphocyte reaction, and delay mortality for the two solid tumors and one leukemia studied. The best agent we have found so far is BCG. This agent illustrates the importance of the *route of administration*. While it delays mortality of Lewis tumor when administered i.v., it enhances it when given s.c. This does not mean that the s.c. route always results in enhancement; MER and CGA given s.c. delayed mortality of L 1210 leukemia, while CGC delayed mortality of Lewis tumor. Therefore, no general rule can be made concerning route of administration. Its effect is variable, at least with these agents.

The time factor appeared to be important for the result of the Jerne test. It was generally considered that SIA could work only if administered before the antigen. Our experimental research on active immunotherapy has suggested that this concept is not correct [20, 29], and the present work has definitely confirmed this view. With the Jerne test, several agents (MER, Hiu II, CP, CGB, poly IC, poly AU) were able to increase the number of HPFT, even when administered *after* the SRBC.

Another important factor to be considered is the physicochemical state of the agent. Important differences are observed in the effects of different preparations of

C. granulosum and of different extracts of mycobacteria. With mycobacteria, one has to emphasize that the water-soluble Hiu II compound shows stimulant activity in the HPFT test (which needs T and B lymphocyte cooperation) under many conditions. It has never, however, affected phenomena which depend exclusively on T cells, such as GVHR or tumor inhibition. Perhaps the water-solubility of the compound depresses such action.

Such factors may play an important role in SIA pharmacokinetics and, if not considered, may cause test results to be misinterpreted. Hence, the necessity for a battery of screening tests taking several factors into account. The number of tests in the present battery is limited, and some responses may be influenced by ecological factors (such as the microbiological environment, even though our mice and animal rooms are pathogen-free). Nevertheless, it can be proposed as a screening system to detect systemic immunity adjuvants useful in cancer immunoprophylaxis, and hence in immunotherapy. This is well illustrated by the diversity of the results given by the various tests for the ten different potential adjuvants. The enhancement induced by some agents must make us careful about their use in the treatment of solid tumors. Demonstration of tumor enhancement induced by the same agent that is stimulatory in the HPFT dramatically emphasizes the need for caution in the use of these agents in the treatment of solid tumor masses.

The data given by this screening system have to be completed by three more studies of the agents which it shows to be systemic immunity adjuvants:

a) Screening of SIA in humans; we have set up a battery of tests for the study of T lymphocytes including the delayed-hypersensitivity reaction to DNFB, picryl chloride, tuberculin, candidin and mumps antigen, as well as *in vitro* transformation by PHA and PPD, and the MLC, the study of IgG, IgA, IgM and the rheumatoid factor from B lymphocytes, and the transformation by pokeweed for the study of T and B lymphocytes.

b) A systematic study in animals to define, for each therapeutic situation in the clinic, the place and the modality of administration of the SIA. Our previous research [20, 29] had shown that BCG alone was not effective in the therapy of established leukemia and that active immunization should comprise BCG plus tumor cells. A MRC trial on ALL conducted with BCG alone gave a negative result [32] while [35] studied the effect of BCG and leukemia cells on acute myeloid leukemia and found a positive result which confirmed our work on ALL.

c) Finally, since these preclinical experiments could benefit from a better knowledge of the mechanism of action of the different SIA and the parameters which influence their action, we are presently conducting an experiment to compare the effects of fresh Pasteur Institute BCG injected i.v. and s.c. in a series of tests set up to indicate their effect on T and B lymphocytes, the killer and the helper cells respectively, and on macrophages at different anatomical sites such as lymph nodes, spleen, and bone marrow. Bone marrow may indeed be most important for eradicating "the last tumor cell" in leukemia by active immunotherapy.

Acknowledgements

We are grateful to the Pasteur Institute for supplying us with BCG and to the Choay Laboratory for their preparations of poly IC and poly AU.

References

1. Amiel, J. L.: Immunothérapie active non spécifique par le BCG de la leucémie E♂ G2 chez des receveurs isogéniques. Rev. franç. Étud. clin. biol. **12**, 912 (1967).
2. Amos, D. B., Cohen, J., Klein, W. J., jr.: Mechanisms of immunologic enhancement. Transplant. Proc. **2**, 68 (1970).
3. Biozzi, G., Stiffel, C., Halpern, B. N., Mouton, D.: Effet de l'inoculation du bacille Calmette-Guérin sur le développement de la tumeur ascitique d'Ehrlich chez la souris. C.R. Soc. Biol. (Paris) **153**, 987 (1959).
4. Bluming, A. Z., Vogel, C. L., Ziegler, J. L., Mody, N., Kamya, G.: Immunological effects of BCG in patients with malignant melanoma. A comparison of two modes of administration. Ann. intern. Med. **76**, 405 (1972).
5. Braun, W.: New approaches to immunology as potential adjuncts to chemotherapy. In: Progress in Antimicrobial and Anticancer Chemotherapy. Tokyo: University Tokyo Press 1970.
6. Claman, H. N., Chaperon, A. E., Triplett, R. F.: Thymus marrow cell combination. Synergism in antibody production. Proc. Soc. exp. Biol. (N.Y.) **122**, 1167 (1966).
7. Dubos, R. J., Schaedler, R. W.: Effects of cellular constituents of mycobacteria on the resistance of mice to heterologous infections, I. Protective effect. J. exp. Med. **106**, 703 (1957).
8. Eilber, F. R., Morton, D. L.: Immunologic response to human sarcomas: relation of antitumor antibody to the clinical course. In: Progress in Immunology: First Int. Congress of Immunology (Amos, D. B., Ed.), Vol. I, p. 951. New York: Academic Press 1971.
9. Finger, H.: Das freundsche Adjuvants: Wesen und Bedeutung. Arb. Paul-Ehrlich-Inst. **60**, 1 (1964).
10. Foley, E. J.: Antigenic properties of methylcholanthrene-induced tumors in mice of the strain of origin. Cancer Res. **13**, 835 (1953).
11. Fresco, J. R., Duty, P.: Polynucleotides. I. Molecular properties and configurations of polyriboadenylic acid in solution. J. Amer. chem. Soc. **79**, 3928 (1957).
12. Freund, J.: The mode of action of immunological adjuvants. Advanc. Tuberculosis Res. **7**, 130 (1956).
13. Harveit, F.: Evidence of induced immunity to Ehrlich's ascites carcinoma brought about through the combination of Freund's adjuvant with living tumor. Brit. J. Cancer **16**, 323 (1962).
14. Hellström, J., Hellström, K. E., Sjogren, H. O.: Serum mediated inhibition of cellular immunity to methylcholanthrene induced murine sarcoma. Cell. Immunol. **1**, 18 (1970).
15. Hiu, I. J.: Water-soluble and lipid-free fraction from BCG with adjuvant and antitumor activity. Nature New Biology **238**, 241 (1972).
16. Hiu, I. J., Amiel, J. L., Nikdjar, K.: Immunochemical study of mycobacterial firmly bound lipids. Europ. J. clin. biol. Res. **15**, 887 (1970).
17. Jerne, N. K., Nordin, A. A., Henry, C. C.: The agar plaque technique for recognizing antibody producing cells. In: Cell Bound Antibodies, Vol. I, p. 109. Philadelphia: Wistar Institute 1963.
18. Kaliss, N.: Immunological enhancement of tumor homografts in mice. Cancer Res. **18**, 992 (1958).
19. Leng, M., Felsenfeld, G.: A study of polyadenylic acid at neutral pH. J. molec. Biol. **15**, 455 (1966).
20. Mathé, G.: Immunothérapie active de la leucémie L 1210 appliquée après la greffe tumorale. Rev. franç. Étud. clin. biol. **13**, 881 (1968).
21. Mathé, G.: Active immunotherapy. Advanc. Cancer Res. **14**, 1 (1971).
22. Mathé, G., Amiel, J. L.: Aspects histologiques des lésions induites dans les organes hématopoiétiques par l'injection à des hybrides F_1 irradiés de cellules ganglionnaires d'une des lignées parentales. Rev. franç. Étud. clin. biol. **5**, 20 (1960).
23. Mathé, G., Amiel, J. L., Schwarzenberg, L., Schneider, M., Cattan, A., Schlumberger, J. R., Hayat, M., de Vassal, F.: Active immunotherapy for acute lymphoid leukaemia. Lancet **I**, 697 (1969).
24. Mathé, G., Amiel, J. L., Schwarzenberg, L., Schneider, M., Hayat, M., de Vassal, F., Jasmin, C., Rosenfeld, C., Sakouhi, M., Choay, J.: Remission induction with poly IC in patients with acute lymphoblastic leukaemia. Europ. J. clin. biol. Res. **15**, 671 (1970).

25. Mathé, G., Dausset, J., Hervet, E., Amiel, J. L., Colombani, J., Brule, G.: Immunological studies in patients with placental choriocarcinoma. J. nat. Cancer Inst. **33**, 193 (1964).
26. Mathé, G., Hayat, M., Amiel, J. L., Hiu, I. J.: Systemic immunity adjuvants and their use in cancer treatment. Proc. Amer. Ass. Cancer Res. **12**, 32 (abstr. 128) (1971a).
27. Mathé, G., Hayat, M., Sakouhi, M., Choay, J.: L'action immuno-adjuvante du poly IC chez la souris et son application au traitement de la leucémie L 1210. C.R. Acad. Sci. (Paris) **272**, 170 (1971b).
28. Mathé, G., Kenis, Y.: La chimiothérapie des cancers (leucémies, hématosarcomes et tumeurs solides), 3rd ed. Paris: l'Expansion Scientifique Françcaise, in press 1974.
29. Mathé, G., Pouillart, P., Lapeyraque, F.: Active immunotherapy of L 1210 leukaemia applied after the graft of tumour cells. Brit. J. Cancer **23**, 814 (1969b).
30. Mathé, G., Pouillart, P., Lapeyraque, F.: Active immunotherapy of mouse RC 19 and E♀ K1 leukaemias applied after the intravenous transplantation of the tumour cells. Experientia (Basel) **27**, 446 (1971c).
31. Mathé, G., Pouillart, P., Schwarzenberg, L., Amiel, J. L., Schneider, M., Hayat, M., de Vassal, F., Jasmin, C., Rosenfeld, C., Weiner, R., Rappaport, H.: Attempts at immunotherapy of 100 acute lymphoid leukemia patients. Some factors influencing results. Nat. Cancer Inst. Monogr. **35**, 316 (1973).
32. *Medical Research Council*: Treatment of acute lymphoblastic leukaemia. Comparison of immuntherapy (BCG), intermittent methotrexate and no therapy after a five month intensive cytotoxic regimen (concord trial). Brit. med. J. **IV**, 189 (**1971**).
33. Möller, G.: Prolonged survival of allogenic (homologous) normal tissues in antiserum treated recipients. Transplantation **2**, 281 (1964).
34. Old, L. J., Clarke, D. A., Benacerraf, S.: Effect of bacillus Calmette-Guérin infection of transplanted tumors in the mouse. Nature (Lond.) **18**, 291 (1959).
35. Powles, R., Kay, H. E. M., McElwain, T. J., Alexander, P., Crowther, D., Hamilton-Fairley, G., Pike, M.: Immunotherapy of acute myeloblastic leukemia in man. This volume.
36. Raynaud, M., Kouznetzova, B., Bizzini, B., Chermann, J. C.: Etude de l'effet immunostimulant de diverses espèces de corynebactéries anaérobies et de leur fractions. Ann. Inst. Pasteur **122**, 695 (1972).
37. Skipper, H. E., Schabel, F. M., Wilcox, W. S.: Experimental evaluation of potential anticancer agents. XIII. On the criteria and kinetics associated with "curability" of experimental leukemia. Cancer Chemother. Abstr. **35**, 1 (1964).
38. Skipper, H. E., Schnabel, F. M., Wilcox, W. S.: Further study of certain basic concepts underlying chemotherapy of leukemia. Cancer Chemother. Abstr. **45**, 5 (1965).
39. Skipper, H. E., Schnabel, F. M., Wilcox, W. S.: XXI. Scheduling of arabinosylcytosine to take advantage of its S-phase specificity against leukaemic cells. Cancer Chemother. Abstr. **51**, 125 (1967).
40. Stutman, O., Good, R. A.: Absence of synergism between thymus and bone marrow in graft-versus-host reaction. Proc. Soc. exp. Biol. (N.Y.) **130**, 848 (1969).
41. Thompson, R. B., Alberola, V., Mathé, G.: Evaluation of surgery, chemotherapy and immunotherapy on Lewis lung tumor. Europ. J. clin. biol. Res. **17**, 900 (1972).
42. Unanue, E. R., Askonas, B. A., Allison, A. C.: A role of macrophasges in the stimulation of immune responses by adjuvants. J. Immunol. **103**, 71 (1969).
43. Voisin, G. A., Kinsky, R. G., Maillard, J.: Réactivité immunitaire et anticorps facilitants chez des animaux tolérants aux homogreffes. Ann. Inst. Pasteur **115**, 855 (1968).
44. Weiss, D. W., Bonhag, R. S., Parks, J. A.: Studies on the heterologous immunogenecity of a methanol-insoluble fraction of attenuated tubercule bacilli (BCG). I. Antimicrobial protection. J. exp. Med. **119**, 53 (1964).
45. Weiss, D. W., Bonhag, R. S., Leslie, P.: Studies on the heterologous immunogenecity of a methanol-insoluble fraction of attenuated tubercle bacilli (BCG). II. Protection against tumors isografts. J. exp. Med. **124**, 1039 (1966).
46. Zbar, B., Bernstein, I. D., Rapp, H. J.: Suppression of tumor growth at the site of infection with living bacillus Calmette-Guérin. J. nat. Cancer Inst. **46**, 831 (1971).

Experimental Screening of Systemic Adjuvants Extracted from Mycobacteria

L. Chedid and A. Lamensans

C.N.R.S. and Pasteur Institute, Paris

It has long been recognized that certain microorganisms or bacterial extracts increase the host's resistance to a variety of unrelated bacterial or viral infections and also stimulate immunity against tumors [4, 14, 16, 21, 24, 31, 18]. It seems reasonable to assume that evolutionary pressure has preserved feedback mechanisms in the host-parasite relationship, such as stimulation of the host by certain substances of the infective agent, e.g. the lipopolysaccharide of gram-negative bacteria [9]. However, when compared to endotoxins, which also enhance nonspecific immunity very strongly [8, 24] mycobacteria appear to possess 2 major advantages: 1. they can trigger cell-mediated immunity [1], which probably plays the major role in resistance, particularly to tumors; 2. some of the varied biological activities of mycobacteria can be related to different components which can be separated by chemical fractionation.

The purpose of this paper is to stress that biological evaluation should determine not only that a given sample has retained a required activity, but also that it has no undesirable properties.

In the field of tumor immunity, mycobacteria have been used either as adjuvants or as stimulants of nonspecific immunity [20, 31, 18]. As a functional definition of these two different approaches, one can say that an immuno-adjuvant increases the immune response to a given antigen when administered simultaneously. In contrast, a nonspecific immunostimulant must not be administered at the same site or at the same time as the tumor cells (it is usually more active if injected several days before), and its response is unrelated to a specific antigen. Whether the nonspecificity resides only in the first step (stimulation) or whether these substances induce nonspecific responses in the second phase is debatable [30]. In any case our aim is to show that preparations can be obtained which have retained their capacity to stimulate immunity although they no longer exert the "toxic" effects observed after administration of whole mycobacterial cells.

Results comparable to those observed with Mycobacteria have been reported by authors who administered either *Corynebacteria* [12] or *Hemophilus pertussis* [11, 29, 30, 18]. However, there are conflicting opinions on the latter. Both organisms

---

[1] It must be remembered that historically, cell-mediated immunity was discovered and recognized during investigation of tuberculosis.

can sensitize mice to histamine and to passive anaphylaxis [2, 23], whereas such an effect is not observed with BCG [26] or with various mycobacterial preparations (CHEDID, L., LAMENSANS, A., PARANT, M., unpublished results). Nevertheless every new active mycobacterial preparation should be tested to determine that it does not sensitize to histamine. Although BCG does not sensitize to histamine, it shares with *H. pertussis* and *C. parvum* the capacity to render mice very susceptible to endotoxins and to induce granuloma formation. Furthermore, mycobacteria elicit tuberculin sensitivity and, when administered in FCA, induce auto-immune diseases.

Hyper-reactivity of BCG-treated mice to endotoxins was first observed and studied by SUTER who showed that this phenomenon was unrelated to delayed hypersensitivity and that it was mediated by a component of the cell wall (cord factor) [25, 27].

Many situations of immunological imbalance produce hyper-reactivity to endotoxins, and it has been postulated that the "wasting" syndrome is the consequence of endotoxemia [6, 15]. Because of our permanent exposure to endotoxins of intestinal origin, this hyper-reactivity may be a major cause of pathophysiological disturbances and therefore a very real hazard in the present period of immunological engineering [7]. In contrast to previous observations [28], it has been shown that the active component of mycobacteria in Freund's complete adjuvant is a water-soluble oligomer of the cell wall containing few, if any, fatty acids [1]. Analogous water-soluble fractions have been described more recently [13, 19].

Unlike most adjuvants, including Freund's incomplete adjuvant (FIA), Freund's complete adjuvant (FCA) not only increases humoral antibodies but can also induce delayed hypersensitivity and autoimmune diseases [3].

We have previously reported that a cell-wall component WSA (Water-Soluble Adjuvant), which is capable of increasing the level of precipitins and of inducing delayed hypersensitivity towards a given antigen, nevertheless does not induce allergic polyarthritis [10]. Such results prove that arthrogenicity is not strictly related to an auto-immune disease and also that this response should no longer be used as a test of adjuvant activity. All these effects were demonstrated by using WSA with FIA. Other results [5, 17, 22] have confirmed that in certain systems WSA can increase the immune response in the absence of mineral oil (FUKUI, G. M., BERGER, F. M., pers. comm.). Care was taken to evaluate the toxicity of the preparation. It was clearly established that WSA did not sensitize to histamine nor induce and liver hypertrophy, hyper-reactivity to endotoxins or tuberculin sensitivity [10]. WSA therefore seems to be a good candidate for investigation of adjuvant activity directed against tumors. However, we were unable to demonstrate any nonspecific stimulation by injection of WSA before inoculating the tumor cells, in contrast to the protection conferred by phenol-killed BCG or whole bacterial cells injected under the same conditions. However, such an effect can also be obtained with delipidated whole cells, or even with delipidated and enzyme-treated cell walls. All results included in the following tables were obtained with products prepared for us by LEDERER *et al.* As can be seen from Table 1, the preparations do not induce hyper-reactivity to endotoxin.

Table 1 represents the cumulative results of several experiments done under the same conditions. 14 days before being challenged with endotoxin, mice were injected with various dosages (dry weight) of mycobacterial preparations. Three strains were used as phenol-killed whole cells: BCG, *Mycobacterium smegmatis* and *M. kansasii.* The other preparations consisted either of cells delipidated by acetone alone (a) or by four solvents, acetone, alcohol-ether and chloroform (a, ae, c), or of purified cell walls (c.w.) obtained by delipidating crude cell walls and treating them with trypsin and chymotrypsin. Some purified cell walls were further treated by pronase (c.w.pr.).

Table 1. Hyper-reactivity to endotoxins of mice pretreated with BCG or other mycobacterial immunostimulants (a, ae, c = acetone, alcohol plus ether, and chloroform; c.w. = cell walls; c.w.pr. = cell walls digested by pronase)

Mycobacteria [a]	Dose [b] (μg)	LD_{50} of ET (μg) in mice pretreated with mycobacteria suspended in			
		Saline		Oil	
Controls		230	(62) [c]	> 50	(21)
BCG	100	< 1.5	(59)	—	
	300	< 1.4	(938)	—	
	1000	1.5	(32)	—	
BCG (a)	300	26	(59)	9	(87)
BCG (a, ae, c)	300	> 50	(24)	—	
M. smegmatis	300	41.4	(92)	< 2	(72)
M. smegmatis (a)	300	> 39	(118)	—	
M. kansasii	1000	2.9	(26)	—	
M. kansasii (a)	300	> 135	(87)	—	
	1000	6	(31)	—	
M. kansasii (a, ae, c)	100	> 300	(27)	180	(46)
	300	290	(80)	—	
M. kansasii (c.w.)	100	> 300	(27)	240	(58)
	300	140	(160)	—	
	1000	< 50	(7)	—	
M. kansasii (c.w.pr.)	100	> 50	(21)	> 50	(21)
	300	> 50	(21)	—	

[a] All mycobacterial immunostimulants (prepared by A. ADAM, R. CIORBARU, E. LEDERER, J. F. PETIT and J. WIETZEWBIN-FALSZPAN) were injected i.v. 14 days before endotoxin challenge by the same route.

[b] Dry weight.

[c] ( ) Total number of mice.

In certain cases, the preparations were injected i.v. in a water-oil emulsion instead of saline. The details of all the following experiments will be published elsewhere (CHEDID, L., LAMENSANS, A., PARANT, M., unpublished results).

As Table 1 shows 100 μg of BCG is sufficient to sensitize mice to endotoxins, the LD_{50} falling to 1.5 μg against 230 μg for the untreated controls. In contrast, whole cells which have been delipidated by acetone (or better, by the four solvents) do not increase the susceptibility of mice even if injected with oil. It was also shown that, contrary to SUTER's results (by injecting crude cell walls), purified enzyme-treated cell walls do not sensitize to endotoxins, whether injected with saline or with mineral oil. Care was taken to ensure that these various preparations do not sensitize to histamine as do *H. pertussis* or *C. parvum* preparations.

Table 2. Ehrlich ascites carcinoma. Comparison between BCG and various mycobacterial immunostimulants (a, ae, c = acetone, alcohol plus ether, and chloroform; c.w. = cell walls; c.w.pr. = cell walls digested by pronase)

Treatment[a]			MST[b]	Survivors after 60 days	Survivors %
Mycobacteria	Doses (μg)	Suspension in			
Controls			20	1/78	1.3
BCG	10	Saline	> 60	7/10	70
	30		> 60	9/10	90
	100		59	23/37	62.2
	300		52	29/50	58
M. kansasii	300	Saline	31	5/39	12.8
M. kansasii (a)	100	Saline	35	1/9	11.1
	300		35	3/18	16.6
M. kansasii (a, ae, c)	10	Saline	> 60	7/10	70
	30		> 60	8/10	80
	100		> 60	8/10	80
	300		> 60	16/20	80
M. kansasii (c.w.)	10	Saline	20	1/10	10
	30		44	8/19	42.1
	100		47	16/40	40
	300		51	23/49	46.9
M. kansasii (c.w.)	10	Oil	40	4/10	40
	30		> 60	6/10	60
	100		> 60	13/18	72.2
	300		> 60	9/10	90
M. kansasii (c.w.pr.)	10	Saline	19	0/10	0
	30		23	0/20	0
	100		37	6/20	30
	300		32	2/19	10.5
M. kansasii (c.w.pr.)	30	Oil	26	3/9	33.3
	100		48	3/10	30
	300		> 60	9/10	90

[a] All mycobacterial immunostimulants were injected i.p. 14 days before inoculation of 10^5 tumor cells by i.p. route.

[b] MST = Median survival time: day at which 50% of mice are dead.

These preparations which do not sensitize to histamine and have lost the capacity to induce hyper-reactivity to endotoxins are still capable of increasing the host's resistance to tumors as effectively as or even better than BCG.

Table 2 represents experiments comparing the activity of BCG and some of the previous preparations against Ehrlich ascites carcinoma. All mycobacterial immunostimulants were injected i.p. 14 days before inoculating 10^5 tumor cells by the same route. Whereas the average survival of the controls is 20 days, mice are very well protected if they have been treated by phenol-killed BCG which also induces tuberculin sensitivity and hyper-reactivity to endotoxins. These effects however, are not a prerequisite since a strong antitumoral activity can be demonstrated under conditions in which the resistance of mice to endotoxins is not decreased. Thus, *M. kansasii*

Table 3. Syngeneic lymphoid leukemia. Comparison between BCG and various mycobacterial immunostimulants (a, ae, c = acetone, alcohol plus ether, and chloroform; c.w. = cell walls; c.w.pr. = cell walls digested by pronase)

Treatment[a]		MST[b]	Survivors after 60 days	Survivors %	Therapeutic index
Mycobacteria	Doses (µg)				
Controls saline		25	1/58	1.7	
Controls oil		24	0/7	0	
BCG	10	35	7/26	27	
	30	51	21/49	43	$\frac{1}{1} = 1$
	100	42	16/48	33.3	
M. kansasii	10	27	1/10	10	
(a, ae, c)	30	44	5/10	50	$\frac{\geqq 1}{0.005} = \geqq 200$
	100	> 60	8/10	80	
M. kansasii	10	28	0/10	0	
(c.w.)	30	29	3/20	15	$\frac{\sim 0.25}{0.005} = \sim 50$
	100	33	2/20	10	
M. kansasii	30	> 60	6/10	60	$\frac{> 1}{0.006} = > 160$
(c.w.) in oil	100	> 60	9/10	90	

[a] All mycobacterial immunostimulants were injected i.p. 8 days before i.p. inoculation of 2×10^2 tumor cells.

[b] MST = Median survival time: day at which 50% of mice are dead.

[c] Therapeutic Index = $\frac{\text{Activity}}{\text{Toxicity}}$. In this case toxicity was evaluated as hyper-reactivity to endotoxin.

preparations obtained by delipidating whole cells with four solvents are all active to a high degree in protecting mice against Ehrlich ascites. Although the *M. kansasii* cell-wall preparations are less active in saline, their activity is fully restored if they are injected with oil at dosages which do not sensitize to endotoxin (see Table 1). This is also the case with the cell walls digested by pronase, a treatment which moreover greatly inhibits tuberculin sensitization.

The same protection can be demonstrated against a syngeneic lymphoid leukemia This leukemia appeared spontaneously in a F_1 (AKR/C 57 BL 6) hybrid. In all experiments, the mycobacterial immunostimulants were injected i.p. 8 days before inoculation by the same route 2×10^2 leukemia cells. As Table 3 shows, delipidated preparations of *M. kansasii* in saline and purified cell walls in oil are more active than BCG although these treatments do not sensitize to endotoxins. Therefore, one can consider these preparations as preferable on the basis of a therapeutic index calculated from BCG activity and toxicity.

Ideally, to increase immune resistance against tumors, an agent should stimulate the host's cell-mediated immunity (T cells) either specifically or by increasing allogeneic inhibition, decrease humoral immunity (B cells) and also modify the antigenic pattern of the tumor cell. All these activities can be demonstrated experimentally with mycobacteria in Freund's complete adjuvant. However, whole mycobacteria produce toxic or undesirable effects. Chemical fractionation may separate and enhance the different activities of mycobacteria. Several biological effects produced by the injection of whole mycobacterial cells can already be induced in full or even reinforced by preparations which have lost many of their pathological effects.

We thank Mrs. F. GUEGUEN and Miss A. DESLANDRES for their technical assistance.

References

1. ADAM, A., CIORBARU, R., PETIT, J. F., LEDERER, E.: Isolation and properties of a macromolecular, water-soluble, immunoadjuvant fraction from cell walls of *Mycobacterium smegmatis*. Proc. nat. Acad. Sci. (Wash.) 69, 851 (1972).
2. ADLAM, C., BROUGHTON, E. S., SCOTT, M. T.: Enhanced resistance of mice to infection with bacteria following pretreatment with *Corynebacterium parvum*. Nature New Biol. **235**, 219 (1972).
3. ASHERSON, G. L., ALLWOOD, G. G.: The biological basis of medicine. Immunological adjuvants (BITTAR, E. E., BITTAR, N., Eds.), p. 327. New York, London: Academic Press 1969.
4. BERMAN, L. B., ALLISON, A. C., PEREIRA, H. G.: Effects of Freund's adjuvant on adenovirus oncogenesis and antibody production in hamsters. Int. J. Cancer **2**, 539 (1967).
5. BONA, C., HEUCLIN, C., CHEDID, L.: Enhancement of mixed human lymphocyte cultures by a water soluble adjuvant. This volume.
6. CANTRELL, J. C., JUTILA, J. W.: Bacteriologic studies on wasting disease induced by neonatal thymectomy. J. Immunol. **104**, 79 (1970).
7. CHEDID, L.: Possible role of endotoxemia during immunological imbalance. J. infect. Dis. (1973) **128**, S. 112 (1973)
8. CHEDID, L., PARANT, M., BOYER, F., SKARNES, R. C.: Bacterial endotoxins. Non-specific host response in tolerance to the lethal effect of endotoxin (LANDY, M., BRAUN, W., Eds.), p. 500. New Brunswick, N.J.: Rutgers Univ. Press 1964.
9. CHEDID, L., PARANT, M., PARANT, F., BOYER, F.: A proposed mechanism for natural immunity to enterobacterial pathogens. J. Immunol. **100**, 292 (1968).
10. CHEDID, L., PARANT, M., PARANT, F., GUSTAFSON, R. H., BERGER, F. M.: Biological study of a non toxic hydrosoluble immuno-adjuvant from mycobacterial cell walls. Proc. nat. Acad. Sci. (Wash.) **69**, 855 (1972).
11. GUYER, R. J., CROWTHER, D.: Active immunotherapy in treatment of acute leukaemia. Brit. med. J. **1969 IV**, 406.
12. HALPERN, B. N., BIOZZI, G., STIFFEL, C., MOUTON, D.: Inhibition of tumour growth by administration of killed *Corynebacterium parvum*. Nature (Lond.) **212**, 853 (1966).
13. HIU, I. J.: MAAF, a fully water soluble lipid free fraction from BCG with adjuvant and antitumor activity. This volume.
14. HOWARD, J. G., BIOZZI, G., HALPERN, B. N., STIFFEL, C., MOUTON, D.: The effect of BCG infection on the resistance of mice to bacterial endotoxin and *Salmonella enteritidis* infection. Brit. J. exp. Path. **40**, 281 (1959).
15. KEAST, D., WALTERS, N. I.: The pathology of murine runting and its modification by neomycin sulphate gavages. Immunology **15**, 247 (1968).
16. LAMENSANS, A., MOLLIER, M. F., LAURENT, M.: Action du BCG sur l'activité catalasique hépatique chez la souris. Rev. franç. Étud. clin. biol. **13**, 871 (1968).

17. LIACOPOULOS, P., BIRIEN, J. L., BLEUX, C., COUDERC, J.: Early recovery of the immune response of a specifically depleted cell population under the influence of WSA. This volume.
18. MATHÉ, G.: Active immunotherapy. Advanc. Cancer Res. **14**, 1 (1971).
19. MIGLIORE, D., SAMOUR, D., JOLLES, P.: An adjuvant-active hydrosoluble substance from mycobacterial cells. This volume.
20. MORTON, D. L., HOLMES, E. C., EILBER, F. R., WOOD, W. C.: Immunological aspects of neoplasia: a rational basis for immunotherapy. Ann. intern. Med. **74**, 587 (1971).
21. OLD, L. J., CLARKE, D. A., BENACERRAF, B.: Effect of Bacillus Calmette-Guérin infection on transplanted tumours in the mouse. Nature (Lond.) **184**, 291 (1959).
22. PARANT, M., CHEDID, L.: Biological properties of non toxic water-soluble immuno-adjuvant from mycobacterial cells. This volume.
23. PARFENTJEV, I. A., GOODLINE, M. A.: Histamine shock in mice sensitized with *Hemophilus pertussis* vaccine. J. Pharmacol. exp. Ther. **92**, 411 (1948).
24. SHILO, M.: Non specific resitance to infections. Ann. Rev. Microbiol. **13**, 255 (1959).
25. SUTER, E., KIRSANOW, E. M.: Hyperreactivity to endotoxin in mice infected with mycobacteria. Induction and elicitation of the reactions. Immunology **4**, 354 (1961).
26. SUTER, E., MUNOZ, J. J.: Effect of BCG infection on sensitivity of mice to histamine, serotonin and passively induced anaphylaxis. Proc. Soc. exp. Biol. (N.Y.) **114**, 211 (1963).
27. SUTER, E., ULLMAN, G. E., HOFFMAN, R. G.: Sensitivity of mice to endotoxin after vaccination with BCG. Proc. Soc. exp. Biol. (N.Y.) **99**, 167 (1958).
28. WHITE, R. G., JOLLES, P., SAMOUR, D., LEDERER, E.: Correlation of adjuvant activity and chemical structure of wax D fractions of *Mycobacteria*. Immunology **7**, 158 (1964).
29. WISSLER, R. W., CRAFT, K., KESDEN, D., POLISKY, B., DZOZA, K.: Inhibition of the growth of the Moris hepatoma (5123) in Buffalo rats using a mixture of *Pertussis* vaccine and irradiated tumor. Adv. Transplant. **1**, 539 (1968).
30. YASPHE, D. J.: Immunological parameters of host-tumor relationships. Immunological factors in non specific stimulation of host resistance to syngeneic tumors (WEISS, D. W., Ed.), p. 90. New York, London: Academic Press 1971.
31. ZBAR, B., BERNSTEIN, I., TANAKA, T., RAPP, H. J.: Tumor immunity produced by the intradermal inoculation of living tumor cells and living *Mycobacterium bovis* (strain BCG). Science **170**, 1217 (1970).

Chemical Structure of Mycobacterial Cell Walls

J. F. Petit, A. Adam, R. Ciorbaru, J. Wietzerbin-Falszpan, and E. Lederer

Institut de Biochimie, Université de Paris XI, Centre d' Orsay, Orsay

Many of the immunostimulant effects of living or killed cells of mycobacteria can be obtained with isolated cell walls: protection against tuberculosis [25, 26], stimulation of nonspecific resistance against infections [14, 22], adjuvant activity [4, 11], stimulation of resistance to tumors [12] and tumor suppression [34].

Owing to the different enzymatic and chemical treatments to which cell walls had been submitted, the various authors have in fact studied different materials. In our examination of the chemical structure of mycobacterial cell walls, we shall attempt to determine what chemical changes are induced by the various treatments of mycobacterial cell walls. The way in which these cell walls are prepared for injection, especially the presence of mineral oil in the suspension and the method used to obtain the suspension also seem very important [12, 26, 27, 34].

Preparation of Cell Walls

Cell walls are obtained by disruption of mycobacterial cells followed by differential centrifugation to remove unbroken cells and cytoplasm. Disruption is often performed with a French pressure cell. Cell rupture can also be obtained by ultrasonic waves or by shaking a cell suspension with glass beads: these processes are suitable to disrupt delipidated cells or cells killed by heat or chemicals [17, 33].

The cell walls obtained by disruption of intact cells have the following composition: free lipids (i.e. lipids which can be removed by neutral solvents) 20—25%; bound lipids: 25—30%; neutral sugars (mainly arabinose and galactose, usually in a ratio of 5:2): 25—30%; amino acids (half of these belonging to the peptidoglycan): 20—25%; amino sugars (mainly glucosamine and muramic acid in equimolar amounts; the latter are acylated before hydrolysis): 7—9%; phosphorus 0.05—0.2%. Cell walls of human strains of *M. tuberculosis* contain large quantities of glutamic acid [21] which forms a polyglutamic acid polymer [2].

Treatment of these crude cell walls with proteolytic enzymes (trypsin, trypsin and chymotrypsin, pronase) solubilizes most of the amino acids which do not belong to the peptidoglycan, except for the excess glutamic acid in strains which contain a "polyglutamic acid" [21]. Removal of most of the non-peptidoglycan amino acids renders cell walls unable to elicit a delayed-hypersensitivity response in animals sensitized to tuberculin [22].

When cell walls treated with proteolytic enzymes are delipidated with neutral solvents (usually: acetone, alcohol-ether 1:1, and chloroform) one obtains the "basic structure" of the mycobacterial cell wall. This basic structure is made up of two covalently linked polymers: the peptidoglycan, and a mycolate of an arabinogalactan [6, 17, 20].

The Peptidoglycan

The linkage between the peptidoglycan and the arabinogalactan mycolate can be hydrolyzed by mild acid treatment (0.1 N HCl for 12 h at 60°), which does not substantially alter the peptidoglycan [31]. Most of the arabinogalactan is solubilized by such a treatment and most of the mycolic acid becomes either free or at least extractable by chloroform. However, in the BCG strain which we have studied, some polysaccharides, lipids and part of the glutamic acid remain insoluble in water or chloroform [32].

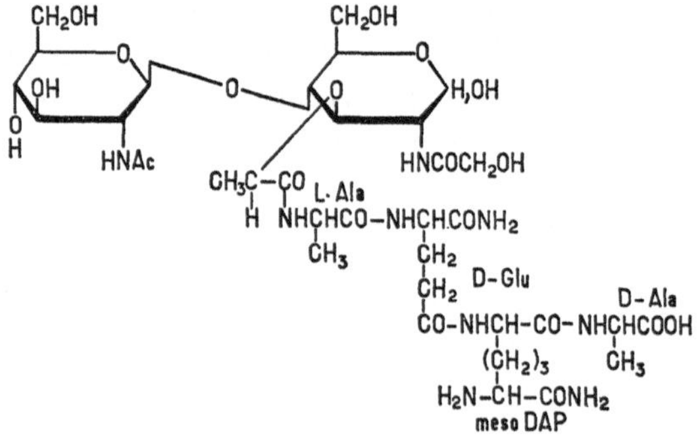

Fig. 1. Structure of the monomer of the peptidoglycan of mycobacterial cell walls [20]

Partial acid hydrolysis makes the peptidoglycan sensitive to bacteriolytic enzymes: in the cell walls which we have studied in detail, namely those of *M. smegmatis* and *M. tuberculosis*, strain BCG, more than 90% of this polymer can be solubilized by lysozyme, by *Myxobacter AL 1* enzyme, or by the *Chalaropsis* muramidase [24, 32].

Sephadex filtration of the products solubilized by *Myxobacter AL 1* enzyme enabled us to isolate the repeating tetrapeptide unit of the peptide moiety of the peptidoglycan of four mycobacteria [24, 31]. After further purification on an ion-exchange resin, its structure has been established, mainly by mass spectrometry [31]: it is a classical peptidoglycan tetrapeptide L-Ala-γ-D-Glu-meso-DAP-D-Ala with two amide groups, one on the α-carboxyl group of Glu and the other on DAP (Fig. 1)[1]. These monomeric peptide units are cross-linked. Most of the cross-linkages occur by direct linkage between the terminal D-Ala of one tetrapeptide and the DAP of another [19, 20, 24, 30] (Fig. 2). One cannot, however, rule out the possible existence of other linkages [32]. The glycan is made up of linear strands where N-acetylglucosamine and N-glycolylmuramic acid, linked by $\beta 1 \rightarrow 4$ linkages, alternate regularly. The repeating disaccharide unit has been obtained by lysozyme treatment of the hexosamine-containing peak of the *Myxobacter AL 1* lysate, followed

[1] DAP = 2,6-diaminopimelic acid.

by Sephadex filtration. Its structure (Fig. 1) has been established by mass spectrometry [3]. The presence of N-glycolylmuramic acid instead of the N-acetyl derivative found in most bacteria seems to be characteristic of mycobacteria [10] and of the closely related genus *Nocardia* [15]. It is not found in corynebacteria.

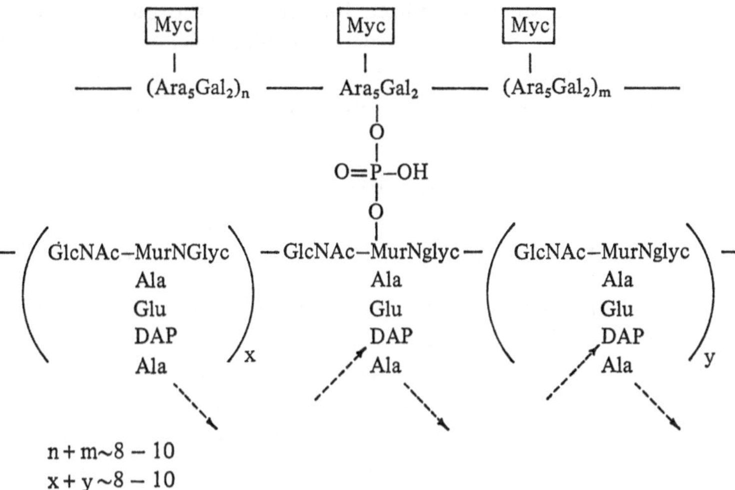

Fig. 2. Hypothetical structure of mycobacterial cell walls. "Myc" indicates a molecule of mycolic acid esterified to arabinose. Dashed arrows indicate cross-linkages between peptide chains [20]

The Arabinogalactan Mycolate

The arabinogalactan is a branched polymer of arabinose and galactose in a molar ratio of about 5 to 2 [9, 23]. The arabinogalactan of BCG cell walls has been isolated by Misaki *et al.* [23] by alkali treatment of delipidated cell walls; its molecular weight is about 30,000. Other polysaccharides, e.g. a glucan [7] might be linked to the arabinogalactan. The detailed structure of the arabinogalactan is discussed by Vilkas (this volume). The linkage between the peptidoglycan and the arabinogalactan is supposed to be a phosphodiester bond between 6-phosphomuramic acid and an arabinofuranose residue of the arabinogalactan: this hypothesis, however, rests only on the isolation of 6-phosphomuramic acid by acid hydrolysis of the cell walls of various mycobacteria [17]; another kind of linkage has been suggested by Kanetsuna [18].

About one in five of the arabinose residues is esterified (C-5) with a molecule of mycolic acid: this structural feature is consistent with the isolation of an arabinose mycolate and a diarabinose mycolate after mild acid hydrolysis of cell walls, whole bacilli or wax D [1, 7, 8, 19] (Fig. 2).

The "Non-Peptidoglycan" Amino Acids

We have recently investigated the non-peptidoglycan amino acids of BCG cell walls. Our starting material was crude delipidated cell walls which had been washed with 8 M urea. These cell walls were then submitted to partial acid hydrolysis (HCl 0.1 N, 12 h, 60°); after this treatment, *Myxobacter AL 1* enzyme or lysozyme almost completely solubilize the peptidoglycan, leaving an insoluble residue which contains about 20% of neutral sugars, 50% of lipids and 30% of aminoacids but only traces of DAP and hexosamines. When this residue was digested with trypsin, most of the amino acids were solubilized but most of the glutamic acid (poly-α-L-glutamic acid) remained insoluble; nearly all could, however, be solubilized by partial acid hydrolysis after alkaline treatment. Its relative importance compared to the other constituents is less than in human strains of *M. tuberculosis* [1, 21, 29, 30, 32].

Conclusion

The chemical structure of mycobacterial cell walls is probably as follows (for a detailed review see [20]):

1. a basic covalent structure made up of a peptidoglycan to which is attached an arabinogalactan esterified by mycolic acids;
2. peptides or proteins which can be removed by proteolytic enzymes; they are linked to sugar or lipids which make them insoluble. The problem of their possible covalent attachment to the basic structure does not seem to have been solved yet;
3. a polyglutamic acid polymer in human strains of *M. tuberculosis* and BCG. In BCG at least, it is composed of L-glutamic acid. We do not know to what other part of cell wall this polyglutamic acid is attached.
4. free lipids which are not covalently attached to the basic structure and which can be removed by neutral solvents (in particular wax D, cord factor and mycosides);
5. glucans and other polysaccharides which may be part of the basic structure.

We have very few data on the topological position of these various compounds in the cell wall. The relationship between the picture seen in an electron microscope and chemical structure is uncertain [13, 16, 28].

For clinical applications, one would require cell walls treated so as to retain the beneficial properties, the harmful components being removed by chemical or enzymatic treatments. One should then try to define the chemical structure(s) responsible for the biological activities. This part of the work has already been started with the isolation of relatively simple adjuvants [5].

References

1. ACHARYA, N., SENN, M., LEDERER, E.: Sur la présence et la structure de mycolates d'arabinose dans les lipides liés de deux souches de Mycobactéries. C.R. Acad. Sci. (Paris) **264** C, 2173 (1967).
2. ACHARYA, N.: Doctoral Thesis, Paris 1967.
3. ADAM, A., PETIT, J. F., WIETZERBIN-FALSZPAN, J., SINAY, P., THOMAS, D.W., LEDERER, E.: L'acide N-glycolyl-muramique, constituant des parois de *Mycobacterium smegmatis*: identification par spectrométrie de masse. FEBS Letters **4**, 87 (1969).
4. ADAM, A., CIORBARU, R., PETIT, J. F., LEDERER, E.: Isolation and properties of a macromolecular water soluble immunoadjuvant fraction from the cell wall of *Mycobacterium smegmatis*. Proc. nat. Acad. Sci. (Wash.) **69**, 851 (1972).
5. ADAM, A., CIORBARU, R., PETIT, J. F., LEDERER, E.: Water-soluble immuno-adjuvants from the cell wall of *Mycobacterium smegmatis*. This Symposium.

6. Amar-Nacasch, Cl., Vilkas, E.: Etude des parois d'une souche humaine virulente de *Mycobacterium tuberculosis* (1). Préparation et analyse chimique. Bull. Soc. Chim. biol. (Paris) **51**, 613 (1969).
7. Amar-Nacasch, Cl., Vilkas, E.: Etude des parois de *Mycobacterium tuberculosis* (2). Mise en évidence d'un mycolate d'arabinose et d'un glucane dans les parois de *M. tuberculosis* H 37 Ra. Bull. Soc. Chim. biol. (Paris) **52**, 145 (1970).
8. Azuma, I., Yamamura, Y.: Studies on the firmly bound lipids of human tubercle Bacillus. I. Isolation of arabinose mycolate. J. Biochem. (Tokyo) **52**, 200 (1962).
9. Azuma, I., Yamamura, Y., Fukushi, K.: Fractionation of mycobacterial cell wall. Isolation of arabinose mycolate and arabinogalactan from cell wall fraction of *Mycobacterium tuberculosis* strain Aoyama B. J. Bact. **96**, 1885 (1968).
10. Azuma, I., Thomas, D. W., Adam, A., Ghuysen, J. M., Bonaly, R., Petit, J. F., Lederer, E.: Occurrence of N-glycolylmuramic acid in bacterial cell walls. A preliminary Survey. Biochim. biophys. Acta (Amst.) **208**, 444 (1970).
11. Azuma, I., Kishimoto, S., Yamamura, Y., Petit, J. F.: Adjuvanticity of Mycobacterium cell walls. Japan J. Microbiol. **15**, 193 (1971).
12. Chedid, L., Lamensans, A., Parant, F., Parant, M., Adam, A., Petit, J. F., Lederer, E.: Protection effect of delipidated mycobacterial cells and purified cell walls against a syngeneic lymphoid leukemia in mice. Cancer Res. **33**, 2187 (1973).
13. Draper, P.: The walls of *Mycobacterium lepraemurium*: chemistry and ultrastructure. J. gen. Microbiol. **69**, 313 (1971).
14. Fox, A., Anschel, J., Evans, G. L., Mohan, R. R., Schwartz, B. S.: Isolation of a soluble resistance enhancing factor from *Mycobacterium phlei*. J. Bact. **92**, 285 (1966).
15. Guinand, M., Vacheron, M. J., Michel, G.: Structure des parois cellulaires des *Nocardia*. I. Isolement et composition des parois de *Nocardia kirovani*. FEBS Letters **6**, 37 (1970).
16. Imaeda, T., Kanetsuna, F., Galindo, B.: Ultrastructure of cell walls of genus *Mycobacterium*. J. Ultrastruct. Res. **25**, 46 (1968).
17. Kanetsuna, F.: Chemical analyses of mycobacterial cell walls. Biochim. biophys. Acta (Amst.) **158**, 130 (1968).
18. Kanetsuna, F., San Blas, G.: Chemical analysis of a mycolic acid-arabinogalactan-mucopeptide complex of mycobacterial cell wall. Biochim. biophys. Acta (Amst.) **208**, 434 (1970).
19. Kotani, S., Yanagida, I., Kato, K., Matsuda, T.: Studies on peptides, glycopeptides and antigenic polysaccharide-glycopeptide complexes isolated from an L-11 enzyme lysate of the cell walls of *Mycobacterium tuberculosis* strain H 37 Rv. Biken's J. **13**, 249 (1970).
20. Lederer, E.: The mycobacterial cell wall. Pure Appl. Chem. **25**, 135 (1971).
21. Migliore, D., Acharya, N., Jolles, P.: Caractérisation de quantités importantes d'acide glutamique dans les parois de Mycobactéries de souches humaines virulentes. C.R. Acad. Sci. (Paris) **263** D, 846 (1966).
22. Misaki, A., Yukawa, S., Tsuchiya, K., Yamasaki, T.: Studies on cell walls of Mycobacteria I. Chemical and biological properties of the cell walls and the mucopeptide of BCG. J. Biochem **59**, 388 (1966).
23. Misaki, A., Yukawa, S.: Studies on cell walls of Mycobacteria. II. Constitution of polysaccharides from BCG cell walls. J. Biochem. **59**, 511 (1966).
24. Petit, J. F., Adam, A., Wietzerbin-Falszpan, J., Lederer, E., Ghuysen, J. M.: Chemical structure of the cell wall of *Mycobacterium smegmatis*. I. Isolation and partial characterization of the peptidoglycan. Biochem. biophys. Res. Commun. **35**, 478 (1969).
25. Ribi, E., Larson, C., Wicht, W., List, R., Goode, G.: Effective nonliving vaccine against experimental tuberculosis in mice. J. Bact. **91**, 975 (1966).
26. Ribi, E., Anacker, L., Brehmer, W., Goode, G., Larson, G. L., List, R. H., Milner, K. C., Wicht, W. C.: Factors influencing protection against experimental tuberculosis in mice by heat-stable cell wall vaccines. J. Bact. **92**, 869 (1966).
27. Ribi, E., Anacker, R. L., Barclay, W. R., Brehmer, W., Harris, S. C., Leif, W. R., Simmons, J.: Efficacy of mycobacterial cell walls as a vaccine against airborne tuberculosis in the Rhesus monkey. J. infect. Dis. **123**, 527 (1971).
28. Takeya, K., Hisatsune, K.: Mycobacterial cell walls. I. Methods of preparation and treatment with various chemicals. J. Bact. **85**, 16 (1963).

29. Vilkas, E., Markovits, J.: Sur la présence d'un acide polyglutamique dans les parois d *Mycobacterium tuberculosis*, souche Peurois. C.R. Acad. Sci. (Paris) **275** C, 913 (1972).
30. Wietzerbin-Falszpan, J.: Unpublished observations 1972.
31. Wietzerbin-Falszpan, J., Das, B. C., Azuma, I., Adam, A., Petit, J. F., Lederer, E.: Isolatio and mass spectrometric identification of the peptide subunits of mycobacterial cell walls. Bic chem. biophys. Res. Commun. **40**, 57 (1970).
32. Wietzerbin-Falszpan, J., Das, B. C., Gros, C., Petit, J. F., Lederer, E.: The amino acid of the cell wall of *Mycobacterium tuberculosis* var. *bovis*, strain BCG. Europ. J. Biochem. **32**, 52 (1973).
33. de Wijs, H., Jolles, P.: Cell walls of three strains of Mycobacteria (*Mycobacterium phlei*, *Myco bacterium fortuitum* and *Mycobacterium kanasii*). Preparation, analysis and digestion by lysozyme of different origins. Biochim. biophys. Acta (Amst.) **83**, 326 (1964).
34. Zbar, B., Rapp, H. J., Ribi, E.: Tumor suppression by cell walls of *Mycobacterium bovis* attache to oil droplets. J. nat. Cancer Inst. **48**, 831 (1972).

Water-Soluble Immuno-Adjuvants from the Cell Wall of *Mycobacterium Smegmatis*

A. Adam, R. Ciorbaru, J. F. Petit, and E. Lederer

Institut de Biochimie, Université Paris-Sud, Centre d'Orsay, Orsay

Adjuvant activity is an important property of mycobacteria, commonly used in Freund's adjuvant [4]; the isolation of the "principle" responsible for this activity has been the subject of numerous investigations: it has been demonstrated [9] that wax D from human strains of *M. tuberculosis* can replace whole mycobacteria in increasing precipitin levels and inducing delayed hypersensitivity to an antigen injected in oil emulsion [11]. Wax D is a mycolate of arabinogalactan linked in the active wax D to a peptidoglycan qualitatively similar to the murein of mycobacterial cell walls [7, 8]. The results reported here concern *M. smegmatis*, a saprophytic strain lacking adjuvant-active wax D; similar results can be obtained with *M. kansasii* and *M. tuberculosis* BCG [1, 3].

Adjuvant activity is measured as described by [9]: the product to be tested (10—2000 μg per ml) is suspended in Freund's incomplete adjuvant and emulsified with a saline solution of ovalbumin (50 mg per ml); 0.1 ml of the emulsion is injected in both hind foot pads of guinea pigs; sera are collected 3 weeks after the injection and levels of antibodies are determined by measuring the antigen-antibody complex with the Folin reagent. Sera are submitted to immunoelectrophoresis to detect the presence of γ_2 immunoglobulins; the presence of this class of immunoglobulin is associated with delayed hypersensitivity [10], which is detected by intradermal reaction to ovalbumin 4 weeks after the injection.

Adjuvant Activity of Cell Walls

The cell walls of *M. smegmatis* have adjuvant activity: they increase the level of circulating antibodies as shown in Table 1 and induce delayed hypersensitivity to ovalbumin. Analogous results have been obtained by others [2, 5].

Adjuvant Activity of a Water-Soluble Compound (WSA) from Mycobacterial Cell Walls

Cell walls are hydrolysed with lysozyme; a 1% suspension of cell walls in 0.1 m NH_4 acetate at pH 6.3 is incubated overnight at 37 °C with 2% lysozyme; solubilized compounds are separated from the residue by centrifugation, filtered on sintered glass and lyophilized; 10 to 20% of the cell walls are solubilized [1]. The soluble material retains the adjuvant property of the cell wall and is, even on a weight basis, more active than the starting material.

Table 1. Adjuvant activity of mycobacterial cell walls

Material injected	Dose (μg)	Antibody titers [a]
Freund's incomplete adjuvant	—	212
Freund's complete adjuvant	50	3000
Cell walls of *M. smegmatis*	2.5	2107
in Freund's incomplete	10	3424
adjuvant	25	3944
	75	4040
	200	4672

[a] Mean values for 6 guinea pigs.

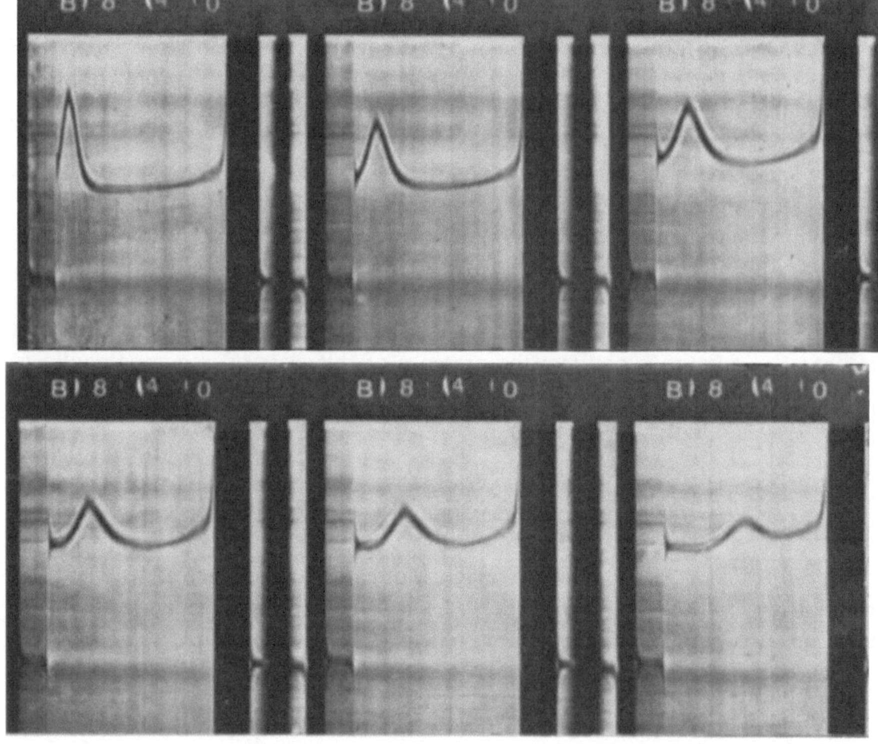

Fig. 1. Sedimentation pattern of WSA in a Beckman ultracentrifuge at 67,770 rpm and 20°C in phosphate buffer, $\mu = 0.1$, pH = 7.0 at a concentration of 5 mg/ml $S_{20} = 2.05$. From left to right, the bar angle and minutes elapsed after reaching speed are: 50°, 16; 50°, 32; 45°, 48; 45°, 64; 45°, 80 and 45°, 96

This crude filtrate contains mainly polymers of the disaccharide tetrapeptide GlcNac—Mur-glycol-L-Ala-D-Glu-meso-DAP-L-Ala, the structure of which has been described for the basal unit of the peptidoglycan of mycobacterial cell wall (for review see [6]). The basal units are linked to the arabinogalactan, probably by

Table 2. Adjuvant activity of a WSA from *M. smegmatis* cell walls

Material injected	Dose (μg)	Antibody titers[a]
Freund's incomplete adjuvant	—	640
Freund's complete adjuvant	50	3164
WSA in Freund's	1	2120
incomplete adjuvant	2.5	3380
	10	4680
	25	4828
	50	6880
	200	7500

[a] Mean values of 6 guinea pigs.

a phosphodiester linkage. These various compounds are free of fatty acids and differ only in their size. The mixture is fractionated on Sephadex G 50; the first peak is excluded from the gel, it behaves as an homogeneous compound on anion exchanger, electrophoresis and ultracentrifugation, where it appears as a slightly polydisperse macromolecule with a sedimentation coefficient of 2.05 S (Fig. 1). This water-soluble adjuvant contains 12—15% of amino sugars (glucosamine and muramic acid in equimolar proportion), 60—70% of neutral sugars (arabinose and galactose in molar ratio 2:1) and 12—15% of amino acids (Ala, Glu, α-ε-diaminopimelic acid in a molar ratio of 1.3 : 1 : 1, traces of other amino acids: Asp 0.04, Ser and Thr 0.015), and 0.2% of phosphorus.

This water-soluble compound has a stronger adjuvant activity than similar amounts of whole bacilli or cell walls; it is able to increase the amount of precipitating antibodies, as shown in Table 2, and to induce hypersensitivity to an antigen (demonstrated by skin test to ovalbumin and by the presence of γ_2 antibodies) at doses as low as 1 μg per animal.

Water-Soluble Adjuvant from Whole Bacilli

WSA is obtained from the mycobacterial cell walls with a 10% yield. We tried to extract this compound from the whole bacilli: cells of *M. smegmatis* are delipidated in a Soxhlet apparatus, washed with water and incubated with lysozyme: 95% of the cell-wall material is solubilized. This crude filtrate obtained with a 10% yield from the whole bacilli has strong adjuvant activity[1]; the "direct" WSA is prepared on Sephadex G 75 in the same way as that from cell walls. It contains 75% of neutral

[1] The adjuvant activity of these compounds has been established by CHEDID *et al.* (Pasteur Institute, Paris).

sugars (arabinose and galactose), 10—12% of amino sugars (glucosamine and muramic acid), 10—12% of murein amino acids: (Ala, Glu, meso-DAP), 3% of non-peptidoglycan amino acids and 0.3% of phosphorus. This compound is very active as an adjuvant, it behaves as a homogeneous compound both on ultracentrifugation with a sedimentation coefficient of 1.95 S, and on anion-exchange chromatography. Similar results have been obtained with cells of *Nocardia opaca* and a water-soluble adjuvant has been isolated from this strain.

Conclusion

Lysozyme can solubilize 10% of mycobacterial cell walls, releasing a lipid-free WSA able to increase the level of antibodies and to induce delayed hypersensitivity to an antigen.

Acting on whole delipidated cells of mycobacteria or nocardia, lysozyme solubilizes most of the cell-wall material, 95% for instance in the case of *M. smegmatis* where 10 times more WSA is obtained than when cell walls are used as starting material. In whole cells, an autolytic enzyme probably splits off the mycolic acid part of the cell wall, allowing solubilisation by lysozyme.

Biological properties of these WSA preparations are reported by CHEDID *et al.* (this volume).

References

1. ADAM, A., CIORBARU, R., PETIT, J. F., LEDERER, E.: Isolation and properties of macromolecular water soluble immunoadjuvant. Proc. nat. Acad. Sci. (Wash.) **69**, 851 (1972).
2. AZUMA, I., KISHIMOTO, S , YAMAMURA, Y , PETIT, J. F.: Adjuvanticity of mycobacterial cell walls. Jap. J. Microbiol. **15**, 193 (1971).
3. CHEDID, L., PARANT, M., PARANT, F., GUSTAFSON, R. H., BERGER, F. M.: Biological study of a non toxic water soluble immunoadjuvant from Mycobacterial cell walls. Proc. nat. Acad. Sci. (Wash.) **69**, 855 (1972).
4. FREUND, J., CASALS, J., HOSMER, E. P.: Sensitization and antibody formation after injection of tubercle bacilli and paraffin oil. Proc. Soc. exp. Biol. (N.Y.) **37**, 509 (1937).
5. LARSON, C. L., BELL, J. F., LIST, R. H., RIBI, E., WICHT, W. C.: Symposium on relationship of structure of microorganisms to their immunological properties. II. Host reactive properties of cell walls and protoplasm from mycobacteria. Bact. Rev. **27**, 341 (1963).
6. LEDERER, E.: The mycobacterial cell wall. Pure and applied chemistry **25**, 135 (1971).
7. MARKOVITS, J., VILKAS, E., LEDERER, E.: Sur la structure chimique des cires D, peptidoglycolipides macromoléculaires des souches humaines de *Mycobacterium tuberculosis*. Europ. J. Biochem. **18**, 287 (1971).
8. MIGLIORE, D., JOLLÈS, P.: Contribution to the study of the structure of adjuvant active wax D from Mycobacteria isolation of a peptidoglycan. FEBS Letters **2**, 7 (1968).
9. WHITE, R. G., BERNSTOCK, L., JOHNS, R. G. S., LEDERER, E.: The influence of components of *Mycobacterium tuberculosis* and other mycobacteria upon antibody production to ovalbumin. Immunology **1**, 54 (1958).
10. WHITE, R. G.: Factors affecting the antibody response. Brit. med. Bull. **19**, 207 (1963).
11. WHITE, R. G., JOLLÈS, P., SAMOUR, D., LEDERER, E.: Correlation of adjuvant activity and chemical structure of Wax D fractions of mycobacteria. Immunology **7**, 158 (1964).

Stimulation of T Cell Activity by a Methanol-Extraction Residue (MER) of BCG

D. Jacobs, D. T. Yashphe, and C. Abraham

Department of Biology, University of California-San Diego, La Jolla, CA
and Department of Immunology, Hebrew University Hadassah Medical School, Jerusalem

A Methanol Extraction Residue (MER) of BCG nonspecifically stimulates resistance to a variety of microorganisms and to spontaneous and transplanted tumors in mice [10, 11]. It also stimulates both primary and secondary circulating antibody responses to several conventional antigens such as sheep red blood cells (SRBC), T 2 phage and bovine gamma globulin [8, 12, 13, 14]. Our interest in the tumor-protective effects of MER has been focused more recently on its ability to stimulate cellular immune responses, since this type of response is held to be mainly responsible for immunity to foreign cell antigens and more particularly to syngeneic tumor cells [5]. We have investigated whether MER can stimulate cellular immunity to defined antigens, and whether it can enhance formation of specifically sensitized thymus-derived lymphocytes (T cells) which are effector cells for specific cellular immunity and cooperate to trigger antibody-forming cell precursors (B cells) [7, 9]. The effect of MER was examined on four different systems: allograft immunity, delayed hypersensitivity to guinea-pig DNP-globulin, θ^+ rosette-forming cells (RFC's), and carrier activity of primed cells. In all cases MER was found to stimulate the given T-cell activities.

Allograft Immunity

Lymph-node cells of C3Hf mice immunized with a BALB/c plasmacytoma will kill the same tumor cells *in vitro*, as measured by release of ^{51}Cr from labeled target cells. When mice had been treated with MER before immunization, lymph-node cells from these animals were more effective in killing labeled allogeneic target cells (Table 1). As indicated, greater killing efficiency could be demonstrated at several lymphoid: target cell ratios. Other experiments showed increased levels of immunity to allogeneic tumor cells in MER-treated C57Bl mice as well, also that the interval between MER treatment and immunization could be varied from days to weeks [6].

Delayed Hypersensitivity

It was of interest to ascertain whether pretreatment of guinea pigs with MER would enable animals to be sensitized with a weak immunogen, namely DNP coupled to a homologous protein, guinea-pig globulin (DNP-GPG) [6]. Induction of delayed hypersensitivity in guinea pigs is very difficult unless the antigen is administered in an emulsion with mycobacteria, usually complete Freund's adjuvant (CFA). However, pretreatment with a saline suspension of MER 2 weeks before sensitization with DNP-GPG enabled guinea pigs to manifest skin reactions to the antigen when subsequently tested (Table 2).

Table 1. Allogeneic cell damage by lymphoid cells taken from mice treated with MER or saline and immunized against a Balb/c plasmacytoma. C 3 Hf mice were treated with MER i.p. 30 days before i.p. immunization with plasmacytoma cells. Assays were done 10 days later using mesenteric lymph-node cells [10]

Ratio lymphoid to target cells	% ^{51}Cr release when cell donor pretreated with	
	MER	Saline
100 : 1	31	5
50 : 1	21	0
20 : 1	25	6
10 : 1	18	1

Table 2. Effect of MER on development of delayed hypersensitivity to DNP-GPG in guinea pigs. FCA = Freund's complete adjuvant; IFA, incomplete Freund's adjuvant. The interval between treatment and sensitization and sensitization and testing was 14 days in each case. Sensitization was by injection of a total of 10 μg DNP-GPG in all 4 footpads. MER in IFA was administered in 4 footpads. Testing was by i.d. injection of 10 μg DNP-GPG and the 24-hour reactions given

Pretreatment	Sensitization	Hypersensitivity reaction	
		Animals positive	Mean lesion diameter (mm)
None	Ag + FCA	5/5	18.2
FCA, i.p.	Ag in saline	0/5	—
2 mg MER in IFC	Ag in saline	0/5	—
None	Ag in saline + 2 mg MER	0/5	—
2 mg MER, i.p.	Ag in saline	4/5	13.2
None	Ag + 2 mg MER in IFA	5/5	13.2

MER could also replace the whole mycobacteria of CFA (IFA + MER + Ag) showing that this material contains the mycobacterial moiety responsible for classical (CFA) adjuvant activity. If pretreatment were the only criterion for activity, CFA and MER in IFA should be as effective as MER in saline. That they were not indicates that the mode of administration is important. However, MER administered simultaneously with antigen was also ineffective, suggesting that the activity of MER administered in saline takes some time to develop. This is in contrast to studies on antibody formation and RFC's in the mouse where MER stimulates the response when given simultaneously with antigen.

Effect on θ^+ Rosette-Forming Cells (RFC's)

Spleens of mice immunized with SRBC contain many lymphoid cells which can bind to the specific antigen *in vitro* to form rosettes (RFC's). A fraction of these RFC's are inhibited by antiserum (anti-θ) to the θ alloantigen, an antigen considered to be a marker for T cells [2, 3].

Table 3. MER stimulation of RFC: Antigen dose-response. 0.4 mg MER administered i.p., SRBC, i.p. Assays from pooled spleen cells from 3 donors, method as in [1]

Treatment		Assay, day 7		
MER (— 14, — 3)	SRBC (0)	Cells/spleen $\times 10^6$	RFC/10^6 cells	RFC/spleen $\times 10^{-2}$
+	5×10^5	187	1400	2,620
—	5×10^5	128	550	700
+	5×10^6	153	7800	11,930
—	5×10^6	113	1500	1,700
+	5×10^7	187	9500	17,760
—	5×10^7	136	8500	11,560

Table 4. MER stimulation of RFC: Interval between treatment and challenge. 0.4 mg MER administered i.p., SRBC, i.p. Assays on pooled spleen cells from 3 donors

Treatment		Immunization		Assay	
Day	MER	Day	SRBC	Day	RFC/10^6 cells
0	+	0	5×10^6	7	8,200
0	none	0	5×10^6	7	3,100
— 6	+	0	5×10^6	7	10,700
	none	0	5×10^6	7	3,700
— 10	+	0	5×10^6	7	7,250
	none	0	5×10^6	7	1,266
— 15, — 4	+	0	5×10^6	7	14,525
	none	0	5×10^6	7	7,400

Mice pretreated with MER respond to immunization by producing a greater number of RFC's than untreated mice. Heightened responses were seen more consistently when stimulation was with low doses of antigen (Table 3). With this standard low dose of SRBC, MER stimulated the RFC response when administered before or simultaneously with antigen (Table 4). When RFC's were examined for their capacity to be inhibited by anti-θ serum, it was apparent that the number of θ^+ RFC's was increased by prior treatment of the animals with MER (Table 5). Although the proportion of θ^+ RFC's was the same under the influence of low doses of antigen in both treatment groups, the absolute number of θ^+ RFC's per spleen

Table 5. MER stimulation of θ^+ and θ^- RFC. 0.4 mg MER administered i.p.; SRBC, i.p. Assays on pooled spleen cells from 3 donors

Treatment		RFC/10^6 cells		RFC/spleen $\times 10^{-2}$	
MER (— 14, — 3)	SRBC (0)	Total	Inhibition by Aθ	θ^+	θ^-
+	5×10^6	10,000	40%	5,500	8,300
—	5×10^6	3,100	45%	2,000	2,300
+	5×10^8	12,900	16%	3,500	19,300
—	5×10^8	2,200	41%	900	1,300

was higher in the MER-treated group. With high doses of antigen, the proportion of θ^+ RFC's in MER-treated mice was less than in controls, but the absolute number of θ^+ RFC's was higher. Thus formation of θ^- RFC's (either B cells or T cells with no detectable θ or both) was preferentially stimulated in the latter case, either because MER directly stimulated B cells or increased the efficiency of T cell-B cell interaction.

It is clear that even under conditions where T-cell activity is increased and there are more θ^+ RFC per spleen, B-cell activity is also increased.

MER Stimulation of Carrier Priming

Another activity of T cells is synergism with B cells in the induction of antibody synthesis [7] of which the "helper" effect is a special example. Animals give a better anti-hapten response to a hapten-antigen stimulus when they have been previously primed with the same carrier [7]. This can be demonstrated clearly in the Mishell-

Table 6. MER effect on SRBC response and on carrier priming for the TNP response. 0.4 mg MER and SRBC were administered i.p. 4 days before removal of spleens. The *in vivo* response is the content of PFC of spleen suspensions just before culturing. Cultures were set up as previously described and stimulated *in vitro* with 0.05 ml 0.1% SRBC-TNP. The *in vitro* response is that of cultures harvested after 4 days [13]

Priming dose		PFC/10^6		
SRBC	MER	SRBC		TNP
		in vivo	*in vitro*	*in vitro*
2×10^5	+	2	1,269	480
	—	1	106	60
6×10^5	+	2	1,754	706
	—	1	564	192
2×10^6	+	17	2,619	1,149
	—	1	844	301
6×10^6	+	53	2,950	424
	—	2	1,007	440
unprimed	—	1	150	34

Dutton system: spleen cells from mice primed with SRBC make more plaque-forming cells to TNP when stimulated *in vitro* with TNP-SRBC than unprimed mice [4], and this increase in TNP-PFC is felt to be attributable to T-cell activity since it is inhibited by anti-θ serum [1].

Cells from mice primed with SRBC in the presence of MER have even greater TNP responses at several priming doses of antigen (Table 6, last column) than cells from normal primed animals. The ability of MER to enhance priming is specific for the priming antigen; other experiments have shown that the *in-vitro* response to noncross-reacting antigens is not elevated. In the antibody response, increased T-cell function would result in increased B-cell activity as measured by increased PFC's to the homologous antigen, and MER would be expected to increase the number of SRBC PFC's, as in fact it does (Table 6) [14]. The secondary response to SRBC as measured *in vitro* is also greater in MER-treated spleen cells, but as "memory" is a function of both T and B cells, these results do not indicate which cell type is affected by MER.

Discussion

In four different systems, activity attributed to T cells has been shown to be stimulated by MER treatment. In conventional systems of cellular immunity (allograft immunity and delayed hypersensitivity), stimulation of T-cell activity is more easily demonstrated, and there is little evidence of antibody formation. However, one cannot conclude that MER preferentially stimulates T cells. Other factors such as the nature of the antigen or the strength of the antigenic stimulus are likely to play a role. For example, MER-treated guinea pigs responded to 10 γ DNP-HSA by increased production of antibody without manifesting delayed hypersensitivity. By reduction of the immunizing dose to 1 γ DNP-HSA, delayed hypersensitivity was induced by MER without increased production of circulating antibody (Ben-Efraim, pers. comm.). Thus, though T cells may be activated, under certain conditions they apparently function instead as helper cells to stimulate B cells to produce antibody. Thus, T-B cell interaction may be improved, B cells themselves may be affected by MER, or macrophages may be responsible for the effect on immunocomponent cells.

Stimulation of B-cell activity is more clearly seen in the other two systems studied. An increased level of θ^- RFC was observed to occur simultaneously with increased numbers of θ^+ RFC, indicating that it was not possible to increase T-cell activity alone with SRBC under the conditions used. Similarly, increased levels of helper or carrier-primed cells enhanced the antibody response to the same antigen or to a hapten on the homologous carrier. Where the conditions of treatment or the nature of the antigen allow antibody formation to take place, MER stimulation of T-cell activity apparently results in increased antibody formation.

How are these observations on MER activity related to other information on nonspecific stimulators? It is clear from the results presented at this meeting that the nature of the complex mycobacterial cell walls is gradually becoming clearer and their subunits defined. As these cell-wall components are tested for biological activity, it is likely that they will be found to affect discrete steps in the immune response by comparison to the whole mycobacterium or MER, i.e. it may be possible to separate the several activities of its component parts. In conjunction with other nonspecific stimulators, such as synthetic polynucleotides, lipopolysaccharides, and plant mitogens, these fractions should enable us to manipulate more effectively the cells participating in the immune response.

Acknowledgements

We are grateful to Professor D. W. Weiss for his interest in this work. These investigators were supported by the Concern Foundation of Los Angeles, the New York Cancer Research Institute, NIH contracts, NIH 70-2208 and NIH 71-2127, Mr. and Mrs. Frank Lautenberg, Mr. and Mrs. Stanley Bogen and Mr. and Mrs. Larry Tisch.

We also wish to thank Professor R. W. Dutton for his interest. Some studies reported here were supported by American Cancer Society research grant IC-1E, and USPHS research grant AI-08795.

One of us (D.J.Y.) is a Fellow of the New York Cancer Research Institute at the University of California, San Diego.

References

1. Dutton, R. W., Campbell, P., Chan, E., Hirst, J., Hoffmann, M., Kettman, J., Lesley, J., McCarthy, M., Mishell, R. I., Raidt, D. J., Vann, D.: Cell cooperation during immunologic responses of isolated lymphoid cells. In: *Cellular Interactions in the Immune Response*, 2nd Int. Convocation Immunol. (McClusky, R. T., Cohen, S., Cudkowicz, G., Mohn, J., Eds), p. 31. Basel: Karger 1971.
2. Greaves, M. F., Möller, E.: Studies on antigen-binding cells. I. The origin of reactive cells. Cell. Immunol. **1**, 372 (1970).
3. Greaves, M. F., Raff, M. C.: Specificity of anti-θ sera in cytotoxicity and functional tests on T lymphocytes. Nature New Biol. **233**, 239 (1971).
4. Kettman, J., Dutton, R. W.: Radioresistance of the enhancing effect of cells from carrier-immunized mice in an *in vitro* primary immune response. Proc. nat. Acad. Sci. (Wash.) **68**, 699 (1971).
5. Klein, G.: Experimental studies in tumor immunology. Fed. Proc. **28**, 1739 (1969).
6. Kuperman, O., Yashphe, D. J., Sharf, S., Ben-Efraim, S., Weiss, D. W.: Non-specific stimulation of cellular immunological responsiveness by a mycobacterial fraction. Cell. Immunol **3**, 277 (1972).
7. Miller, J. F. A. P., Mitchell, G. F., Davies, A. J. S., Claman, H. N., Chaperon, E. A., Taylor, R. B.: Antigen sensitive cells. Trans. Rev. **1**, 1 (1969).
8. Pass, E., Yashphe, D. J.: Stimulation of antibody synthesis to soluble bovine γ-globulin by a methanol-extraction residue of BCG. Israel J. med. Sci. **7**, 609 (1971).
9. Roitt, I. M., Greaves, M. F., Torrigiani, G., Brostoff, J., Playfair, J. H. L.: The cellular basis of immunological responses. Lancet **1969 II**, 367.
10. Weiss, D. W., Bonhag, R. S., Parks, J. A.: Studies on the heterologous immunogenicity of a methanol-insoluble fraction of attenuated tubercle bacilli (BCG). I. Antimicrobial protection. J. exp. Med. **119**, 53 (1964).
11. Weiss, D. W., Bonhag, R. S., Leslie, P.: Studies on the heterologous immunogenicity of a methanol-insoluble fraction of attenuated tubercle bacilli (BCG). II. Protection against tumor isografts. J. exp. Med. **124**, 1039 (1966).

12. YASHPHE, D. J.: Modulation of the immune response by a methanol-insoluble fraction of attentuated tubercle bacilli (BCG). II. Relationship of antigen dose to heightened primary and secondary immune responses to sheep red blood cells. Clin. exp. Immunol. **12,** 497 (1972).
13. YASHPHE, D. J., STEINKULLER, C. B., WEISS, D. W.: Modulation of immunological responsiveness by pretreatment with a methanol-insoluble fraction of killed tubercle bacilli. Israel J. med. Sci. **5,** 259 (1969).
14. YASHPHE, D. J., WEISS, D. W.: Modulation of the immune response by a methanol-insoluble fraction of attenuated tubercle bacilli. Primary and secondary responses to sheep red blood cells and T_2 phage. Clin. exp. Immunol. **7,** 269 (1970).

Biological Properties of Non-Toxic Water-Soluble Immunoadjuvants from Mycobacterial Cells

M. PARANT and L. CHEDID

C.N.R.S. and Institut Pasteur, Paris

The use of mycobacteria in cancer therapy, either as systemic or as local immunoadjuvants, has been proposed [9, 11, 16]. These microorganisms can enhance the resistance of the host to a variety of attacks (bacterial, protozoal, viral or tumoral) by nonspecific mechanisms. Because they are powerful immunoadjuvants, they can also potentiate specifically the immune response to a given antigen. This capacity may be particularly valuable in the case of neoantigens that are weak immunogens. In recent years, both approaches have been used clinically and experimentally [11, 13, 20]. BCG (*Mycobacterium tuberculosis*, bacillus Calmette-Guérin), *Hemophilus pertussis* and *Corynebacterium parvum* are amongst the most popular candidates for clinical and animal experimentation in this field. *H. pertussis* and more recently *C. parvum* have been shown to increase the susceptibility of mice to histamine [3, 14] and may therefore expose the host to a wide variety of allergic and physiological accidents. Although BCG lacks this histamine-sensitizing activity, it is still capable of inducing many of the noxious effects observed after the injection of *H. pertussis* or *C. parvum*. Thus, killed BCG administered in saline sensitizes to tuberculin, produces lymphoid hyperplasia and increases the reactivity of mice to endotoxins [8, 18]. The decreased resistance towards lipopolysaccharides may be the cause of a great number of pathophysiological disturbances. Mycobacteria administered as a water-in-oil emulsion also produce allergic polyarthritis in the rat, a response which has been considered to indicate autoimmune disease [17]. Several investigators have suggested that insoluble Wax D extracted from virulent strains was the immunoadjuvant component of mycobacterial cells and that this substance is also responsible for allergic polyarthritis [17, 19].

Recently [1] have shown that a water-soluble fraction extracted from mycobacteria is capable of increasing the titer of precipitating antibodies and of inducing hypersensitivity to ovalbumin in guinea pigs. We have confirmed this activity and shown that a stronger immune response could be obtained with a viral antigen. In the same series of experiments, it was also observed that the water-soluble adjuvant (WSA) lacks the toxic properties of whole mycobacterial cells. Administration of this preparation induces neither splenomegaly nor hypersensitivity to endotoxins. It was also demonstrated that animals treated with WSA in Freund's incomplete adjuvant (FIA) show no sensitization to tuberculin nor induction of experimental polyarthritis [6]. Rats were treated with 0.1 ml of FIA to which was added either 5 mg/ml of BCG or 5 mg/ml of WSA. A group of controls received FIA alone. The animals were killed 14 days later and the severity of the arthritis was assessed by the increase in weight of the injected paw (Fig. 1). Administration of BCG produced a 100% increase of the volume of the injected paws, a reaction which was accompanied by a lack of gain of body weight and by a reversal of the albumin-to-globulin ratio. Such was not the case for the group which was treated with WSA.

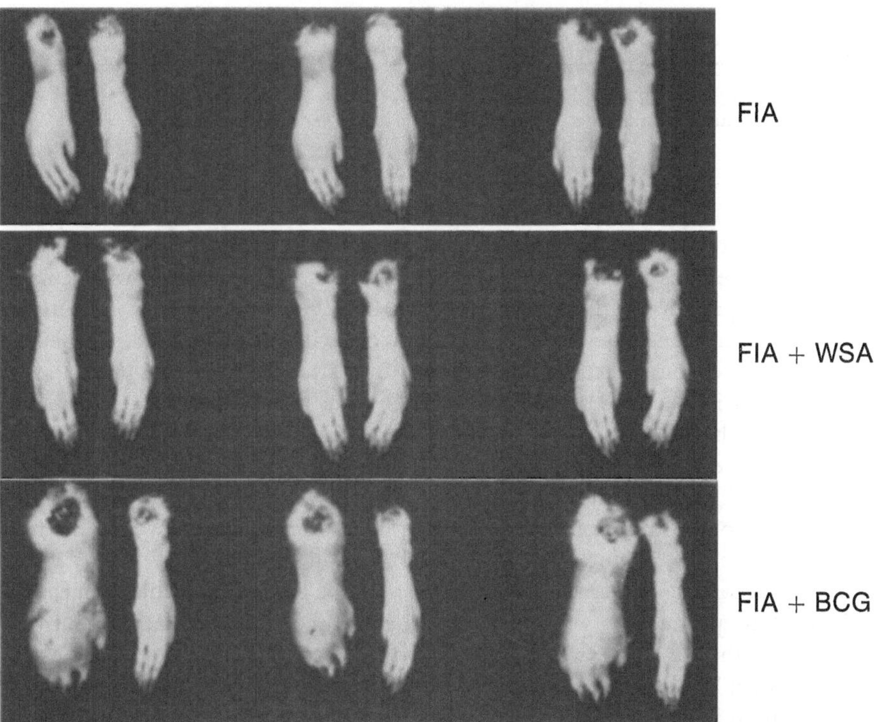

Fig. 1. Experimental polyarthritis in the rat

More recently, [2] have shown that a similar substance can be obtained from mycobacteria and from *Nocardia* by a procedure which has the advantage of being simpler and of giving greater yields. We have observed that these preparations, which we call "neo-WSA", are immunoadjuvants and that they do not display the toxic properties inherent in the use of whole mycobacteial cells (unpublished experiments). The increase of antibodies to ovalbumin is apparent from Table 1, where each figure represents the average of 6 guinea pigs. Ovalbumin (5 mg) was administered to 2 control groups either with Freund's complete adjuvant (FCA) or with FIA. In the other groups, the antigen was added to crude WSA extracted from the cell walls of *Mycobacterium smegmatis*. In the last group, neo-WSA was extracted from whole cells of *M. smegmatis*. In all cases, the fractions were used with FIA. The guinea pigs were bled 21 days after immunization and the antibody titers were evaluated by quantitative precipitation and by passive hemagglutination.

Table 1. Humoral antibody response to ovalbumin. Dose of WSA: 200 μg/guinea pig

	Quantitative precipitation[a]	Passive hemagglutination[b]
FCA	2350	4320
FIA (controls)	< 200	830
FIA + crude WSA (*M. smegmatis*)	2510	5600
FIA + crude WSA (BCG)	3940	5600
FIA + crude WSA (*M. kansasii*)	3950	4640
FIA + WSA (*M. smegmatis*)	5260	8000
FIA + nWSA (*M. smegmatis*)	5020	3840

[a] μg of antigen-antibody complex per ml of serum.
[b] Reciprocal titer of serum.

As can be seen, all preparations of WSA increased the antibody response compared to the FIA controls, giving levels equal to or greater than those obtained with FCA.

In all the previous results the activity of the water-soluble fraction was demonstrated in the presence of FIA. It is possible, however, under certain conditions to increase the immune response by injecting WSA without mineral oil. This effect was first observed on measuring the increase in plaque-forming cells (PFC) after immunization with sheep red blood cells (SRBC) (FUKUI and BERGER, pers. comm.). We confirmed those results *in vivo* and *in vitro* and demonstrated the effect of WSA on soluble antigens.

A. Effect of WSA on immunization by SRBC. 2×10^7 SRBC *suspended in saline* were injected i.p. in groups of 5 mice, alone or in combination with WSA. Controls were not immunized. The number of PFC contained in the spleen was evaluated on day 3 or 4, according to Jerne's technique. As can be seen from Table 2, injection of SRBC alone produced a good response as compared to the untreated controls. Nevertheless, this response was much increased when the erythrocytes were administered with WSA. Similar results were observed when pigeon or horse erythrocytes were used instead of SRBC, but no increase was observed with a heterologous antigen which does not cross-react with the injected red blood cells. Finally, when

Table 2. Influence of water-soluble adjuvant (WSA) on the production of direct plaque-forming spleen cells in mice immuniced with sheep red blood cells. WSA (a) and WSA (b) = 2 batches of water-soluble adjuvants

Treatment	PFC per 10^8 nucleated cells			
	Day 3		Day 4	
	average	increase %	average	increase %
Untreated controls	120		280	
Controls (only SRBC)	22,120		101,600	
SRBC + WSA (a) 20 μg	158,200	615	290,800	185
SRBC + WSA (b) 20 μg	167,000	654	—	—

mice were treated with WSA only, there was no increase in the number of PFC. The increase of PFC can also be shown if SRBC and WSA are incubated *in vitro* with splenocytes [12]. Details of these experiments will be published later.

B. Effect of WSA on immunization by bovine serum albumin (BSA) or BCG. WSA can also increase humoral antibodies to bovine serum albumin in the absence of FIA. Mice were immunized with 0.5 mg of BSA in saline with 0, 25, 50 or 100 μg

Table 3. Influence of WSA on the immune response to injection of bovine serum albumin (BSA) in mice

Treatment	Radioactivity in the blood[a]		ABC ^{125}I-BSA bound/ml II response
	I response day 10	II response Day 35	
Controls	42.6 ± 18.05	37.3 ± 6.72	neg.[b]
WSA	38.0 ± 11.3	—	neg.[b]
BSA	22.6 ± 5.61	17.6 ± 4.67	20 μg
BSA + WSA 25 μg	12.6 ± 7.5	6.7 ± 3.7	30 μg
BSA + WSA 50 μg	7.9 ± 2.8	3.4 ± 2.27	67 μg
BSA + WSA 100 μg	5.0 ± 3.46	—	—

[a] 16 h after injection of 5 μg of ^{125}I-BSA.
[b] Negative at a 1:5 dilution of serum.

Table 4. Influence of WSA on the antigen-elimination test in mice paralysed with centrifuged bovine γ-globulin (BGG)

Treatment	Radioactivity in the blood on day 10 (%)[a]
Controls	71.4 ± 8.9
BGG	63.0 ± 11.8
BGG + WSA 25 μg	62.6 ± 15.3
BGG + WSA 50 μg	46.6 ± 8.7
BGG + WSA 100 μg	41.4 ± 5.9

[a] 16 h after ^{125}I-BGG injection.

of WSA. The animals were challenged 10 days later by injecting 5 μg of ^{125}I-BSA i.p. and measuring the residual radioactivity in the blood 16 h later. As can be seen from Table 3, the level of radioactivity is lower in animals immunized with the immunoadjuvant than in those immunized with the antigen alone. In certain cases, 0.1 mg of cold BSA was injected 30 days later and the animals were challenged with a second dose of radioactive BSA. Animals pretreated with WSA had less radioactivity in the blood than the immunized controls (Table 3).

It is well established that mycobacteria stimulate phagocytosis of colloidal carbon and a large variety of bacteria and antigens [4, 15]. In control experiments we observed that WSA did not increase the blood clearance of BSA by nonspecific stimulation of the RES as did injected cells. Indeed, the blood clearance of BSA was related to a higher titer of antibodies in the serum. This could be demonstrated by bleeding the mice and by measuring the serum antigen-binding capacity *in vitro* by Farr's technique (with radioactive BSA).

The activity of WSA could also be demonstrated by means of Dresser's immune paralysis technique [7]. In this case, a paralysing dose of centrifuged bovine γ globulin (BGG, 4 mg) was injected into mice without or with different doses of WSA. Ten days later, all animals received an injection of 5 μg of ^{125}I-BGG i.p. Table 4 shows that the administration of WSA inhibited the tolerance to BGG. Details of these experiments will be published later.

Conclusion

The findings reported here confirm that water-soluble fractions prepared from purified cell walls (WSA) or from whole cells (neo-WSA) contain the immunoadjuvant component of mycobacteria. These preparations do not produce the toxic effects elicited by the administration of whole cells. More recently, we have observed that adjuvant activity can be demonstrated in the absence of mineral oil. Other experiments concerning the mixed-lymphocyte reaction [5] and the restoration of the immune response in RFC-depleted mice [10] indicate that the activity of WSA may be mediated by thymus-dependent cells.

References

1. ADAM, A., CIORBARU, R., PETIT, J. F., LEDERER, E.: Isolation and properties of a macromolecular, water-soluble, immuno-adjuvant fraction from the cell wall of *Mycobacterium smegmatis*. Proc. nat. Acad. Sci. (Wash.) **69**, 851 (1972).
2. ADAM, A., CIORBARU, R., PETIT, J. F., LEDERER, E.: Water-soluble immunoadjuvant from the cell wall of *Mycobacterium smegmatis*. This volume.
3. ADLAM, C., BROUGHTON, E. S., SCOTT, M. T.: Enhanced resistance of mice to infection with bacteria following pretreatment with *Corynebacterium parvum*. Nature New Biol. **235**, 219 (1972).
4. BIOZZI, G., STIFFEL, C., HALPERN, B., MOUTON, D.: Recherches sur le mécanisme de l'immunité non spécifique produite par les Mycobactéries. Rev. franç. Étud. clin. biol. **5**, 876 (1960).
5. BONA, C., HEUCLIN, C., CHEDID, L.: Enhancement of mixed human lymphocyte cultures by a water soluble adjuvant. This volume.
6. CHEDID, L., PARANT, M., PARANT, F., GUSTAFSON, R. H., BERGER, F. M.: Biological study of a non toxic hydrosoluble immunoadjuvant from Mycobacterial cell walls. Proc. nat. Acad. Sci. (Wash.) **69**, 855 (1972).
7. DRESSER, D. W.: An assay for adjuvanticity. Clin. exp. Immunol. **3**, 877 (1968).
8. HALPERN, B. N., BIOZZI, G., HOWARD, J. G., STIFFEL, C., MOUTON, D.: Exaltation du pouvoir toxique d'*Eberthella typhosa* tué chez la souris inoculée avec le BCG vivant. Relation entre cette augmentation de la susceptibilité et l'état fonctionnel du système réticulo-endothélial. C.R. Soc. Biol. (Paris) **152**, 899 (1958).
9. LAMENSANS, A., MOLLIER, M. F., LAURENT, M.: Action du BCG sur l'activité catalasique hépatique chez la souris. Rev. franç. Étud. clin. Biol. **13**, 871 (1968).
10. LIACOPOULOS, P., BIRIEN, J. L., BLEUX, C., COUDERC, J.: Early recovery of the immune response of a specifically depleted cell population under the influence of WSA. This volume.
11. MATHÉ, G.: Active Immunotherapy. Advanc. Cancer Res. **14**, 1 (1971).
12. MODOLELL, M., LUCKENBACH, G. A., MUNDER, P. G., PARANT, M.: The adjuvant activity of a Mycobacterial water-soluble adjuvant *in vitro*. J. Immunol. In press (1974).
13. MORTON, D. L., HOLMES, E. C., EILBER, F. R., WOOD, W. C.: Immunological aspects of neoplasia: a rational basis for immunotherapy. Ann. intern. Med. **74**, 587 (1971).

14. MUNOZ, J., BERGMAN, R. K.: Histamine-sensitizing factors from microbial agents with special reference to *Bordetella pertussis*. Bact. Rev. **32**, 103 (1968).
15. OLD, L. J., BENACERRAF, B., CLARK, D. A., CARSWELL, E. A., STOCKERT, E.: The role of the reticuloendothelial system in the host reaction to neoplasia. Cancer Res. **21**, 1281 (1961).
16. OLD, L. J., CLARK, D. A., BENACERRAF, B.: Effect of Bacillus Calmette-Guérin infection on transplanted tumours in the mouse. Nature (Lond.) **184**, 291 (1959).
17. PEARSON, C. M., WOOD, F. D.: Studies of polyarthritis and other lesions induced in rats by injection of mycobacterial adjuvant. I. General clinical and pathclogical characteristics and some modifying factors. Arthr. and Rheum. **2**, 440 (1959).
18. SUTER, E., ULLMAN, G. E., HOFFMAN, R. G.: Sensitivity of mice to endotoxin after vaccination with BCG (Bacillus Calmette-Guérin). Proc. Soc. exp. Biol. (N.Y.) **99**, 167 (1958).
19. WHITE, R. G., JOLLES, P., SAMOUR, D., LEDERER, E.: Correlation of adjuvant activity and chemical structure of wax D fractions of Mycobacteria. Immunology **7**, 158 (1964).
20. ZBAR, B., RAPP, H. J., RIBI, E. E.: Tumor suppression by cell walls of *Mycobacterium bovis* attached to oil droplets. J. nat. Cancer Inst. **48**, 831 (1972).

Enhancement of Human Mixed-Lymphocyte Cultures by a Water-Soluble Adjuvant

C. Bona, C. Heuclin, and L. Chedid

C.N.R.S., Institut Pasteur, Paris

Adam *et al.* [1] showed that a water-soluble fraction (WSA) extracted from mycobacteria was a potent adjuvant to various antigens when added to Freund's incomplete adjuvant (FIA). Furthermore, this substance was free of the untoward effects of whole mycobacteria: WSA did not sensitize to tuberculin, did not increase the susceptibility of mice to endotoxin nor did it induce allergic polyarthritis in rats [4]. Under certain conditions, WSA in saline also potentiated the immune response [10].

Therefore, it was of interest to determine the mitogenic activity of this mycobacterial fraction on lymphocytes *in vitro* and its influence on the mixed-lymphocyte reaction (MLR). This was evaluated on human lymphocytes and compared concurrently with tuberculin and lipopolysaccharide (LPS).

Materials and Methods

1. Stimulating Agents

a) WSA prepared from *M. smegmatis* according to the method of [1] was used in a concentration of 50 μg/ml/10^6 cells.

b) *S. enteritidis* (Danysz strain) LPS extracted by the phenol-water procedure of [13] was used also at a concentration of 50 μg/ml/10^6 cells.

c) The Pe fraction of tuberculin prepared from *M. tuberculosis bovis* (Behring strain), according to the method of [5] was used in a concentration of 25 μg, corresponding to 1250 IU.

2. Separation of Lymphocytes

The separation technique was essentially that of [2] with minor modifications. Human blood was drawn into sterile recipients containing 100 units/ml heparin (Liquemin; Roche); 28 ml of the diluted blood (one part venous blood, three parts Hanks medium) was layered over 9 ml of Ficoll-Triosil gradient in siliconized 40 ml centrifugation tubes; care was taken not to disturb the interface.

The tubes were spun for 20 min at 4 °C (400 g at the interface). After centrifugation, the lymphocyte layer was removed with a Pasteur pipette, centrifuged and washed 3 times in Hanks medium.

3. Preparation of Lymphocyte Cultures

a) Blast transformation: 10^6 lymphocytes were transferred to the tubes containing 1 ml MEM (Gibco), supplemented with 10% autologous human serum which had previously been decomplemented by heating at 56 °C for 30 min. The stimulating agents (in 0.1 ml of MEM) were then added to these tubes.

b) Mixed-lymphocyte reaction. For this reaction, the two genetically unrelated populations of lymphocytes were combined and mixed thoroughly. One population had previously been treated for 20 min at 37° with mitomycin C (Sigma Co.) (50 μg/10^7 cells) and washed 3 times in Hanks medium.

The single lymphocyte population was then diluted in MEM supplemented with 10% autologous human serum to a concentration of 10^6 cells per ml.

The tubes were incubated for various times at 37 °C in a container gassed with CO_2.

4. Incorporation of Tritiated Thymidine

24 h before harvest, 1 μCi of ^{3}H-thymidine (1 Ci/m mole) was added to each tube.

5. Processing of Thymidine-labelled Lymphocytes

At the end of the ^{3}H-thymidine pulse, 100 times the amount of cold thymidine was added to each tube, which was centrifuged 450 g for 10 min at 4 °C, and the supernatants discarded. The pellet was precipitated with 2 ml of ice-cold 5% trichloracetic acid (TCA), washed once more with 2 ml TCA, finally resuspended in 0.5 ml Soluene 100 (Packard) and incubated for 30 min at 60 °C.

The dissolved products were transferred to scintillation vials together with 3 washings (1 ml each of isopropanol, Prolabo) of the container; 10 ml of Instagel (Packard) was added to each scintillation vial.

Radioactivity in the bottles was determined in a Tricarb liquid scintillation spectrometer.

6. Statistical Evaluation of the Results

The mitogenic effect of WSA, tuberculin, LPS and unrelated lymphocytes was expressed as index of transformation (IT) representing the ratio of the radioactivity of the treated lymphocytes to the radioactivity of the control lymphocytes.

The stimulatory effect of WSA and LPS on mixed lymphocytes was expressed in a similar way as index of stimulation (IS). This index represents the ratio IT of the treated mixed-lymphocytes culture to IT of the control mixed lymphocytes.

For statistical evaluation (Student's "t" test) experimental and control samples from the same donor were compared in each case.

Results

A. Blast Transformation

As Table 1 shows, very strong stimulation was obtained when the lymphocytes were cultivated with tuberculin. The IT (7.26) is the average of several significant

Table 1. Incorporation of ^{3}H-thymidine by human lymphocytes incubated for 3 days with tuberculin, WSA, LPS and unrelated lymphocytes

Index of transformation (IT)[a] after incubation with			
WSA	Tuberculin	LPS	MLC one way
0.93	7.26	1.45	10.01
No stimulation	(< 0.01)	—	(< 0.01)
No stimulation	(< 0.01)	—	(< 0.01)
No stimulation	(< 0.01)	(0.03)	(< 0.01)
No stimulation	(< 0.01)	N.S.	(< 0.01)
No stimulation	(< 0.01)	N.S.	(< 0.01)
No stimulation	(0.04)	(< 0.01)	(< 0.01)

[a] IT: Radioactivity of treated lymphocytes/Radioactivity of control lymphocytes. In parenthesis, values of p. N.S.: not significant.

Table 2. Influence of WSA and LSP on one-way MLC

Culture in time	Index of stimulation (IS)[a] of one-way MLC after incubation with			
	Controls	WSA	Controls	LPS
	10.02	11.78	7	6.33
		1.17		**0.9**
3 days	(< 0.01)	(0.02)		
	(< 0.01)	N.S.	(< 0.01)	no st.
	(< 0.01)	(< 0.01)	(< 0.01)	no st.
	(< 0.01)	N.S.	(< 0.01)	no st.
	(< 0.01)	no st.		
	(< 0.01)	N.S.		
	19.85	35.65	25.23	23.24
		1.79		**0.92**
5 days	(0.15)	(< 0.01)		
	(< 0.01)	(< 0.01)	(< 0.01)	no st.
	(< 0.01)	(< 0.01)	(< 0.01)	(< 0.01)
	(< 0.01)	(< 0.01)	(< 0.01)	no st.
	(< 0.01)	(< 0.01)	(< 0.01)	no st.
	(< 0.01)	N.S.	(< 0.01)	no st.
	(< 0.01)	no st.		
	15.39	22.66	20.46	22.07
		1.47		**1.07**
7 days	(< 0.01)	(0.03)		
	(< 0.01)	(< 0.01)		
	(< 0.01)	(< 0.01)	(< 0.01)	no st.
	(< 0.01)	(0.05)	(< 0.01)	(< 0.01)
	(< 0.01)	(< 0.01)	(< 0.01)	N.S.
	(< 0.01)	N.S.	(< 0.01)	no st.
	(< 0.01)	N.S.		
	(< 0.01)	(< 0.01)		
	(< 0.01)	(< 0.01)		

[a] IS = IT of treated MLC/IT of control MLC. Figures underlined = IT. Figures in boldface = IS. In parenthesis, values of p. No st. = no stimulation, N.S. = not significant.

($p < 0.01$) experiments. In contrast, WSA did not stimulate the incorporation of ^{3}H-thymidine, the average IT being 0.93. Although LPS induced a slight stimulation, this response was not significant in two cases out of four. Finally, a high response was regularly observed when responder lymphocytes were incubated with genetically unrelated mitomycin C-pretreated lymphocytes (the IT was 10.01).

B. Influence of WSA and LPS on the MLR

The influence of WSA and LPS on the MLR was studied after 3, 5 and 7 days. A very high level of transformation of lymphocytes was observed in all cases. The incorporation of ^{3}H-thymidine was time-dependent with a peak at day 5. All values obtained were highly significant.

The addition of WSA to mixed-lymphocyte cultures (MLC) stimulated the incorporation of ^{3}H-thymidine as compared with MLC controls. Table 2 shows the response was greatest at 5 days, the average index of stimulation being 1.79. The response in 5 of 7 cases was very highly significant. In contrast to WSA, LPS did not stimulate the mixed lymphocyte reaction.

Discussion

In the experiments reported here, tuberculin extracted from *M. tuberculosis bovis* strongly stimulated lymphocytes. We have also observed that tuberculin extracted from *M. smegmatis* produces the same effect (unpublished results). However, WSA was not mitogenic for lymphocytes which responded to the tuberculin extracted from *M. bovis* and *M. smegmatis*. These results confirm that the purified "cell-wall oligomer" was not contaminated with tuberculin and did not contain an antigen which could cross-react with tuberculin protein.

The effect of LPS varies with different animal species. Whereas it has been established that endotoxins behave like a nonspecific mitogenic agent [11] on the B cells of mice [8, 9], using rabbit lymphocytes, obtained only a very weak effect which they considered to be specific; our data were consistent with their results.

WSA, which has previously been shown to increase the humoral antibody response to ovalbumin and to particulate antigens (virus and erythrocytes) [4, 10] can also stimulate MLR. Indeed, thymidine incorporation was significantly increased when mixed-cell lymphocytes were cultured in presence of WSA. In contrast, LPS (which is an adjuvant *in vivo*) had no effect under the same experimental conditions. We recall that neuraminidase treatment is another experimental procedure by which MLR can be enhanced by the use of an external agent. The enzyme augments the antigenicity of the stimulating cells by unmasking some antigenic determinants [7]. In contrast, we have observed that MLR is not enhanced when the mitomycin C-pretreated cells have been exposed to WSA for 30 min and then washed before being mixed with the responding lymphocytes.

The results reported here suggest that the activity of WSA is mediated by the thymus-dependent cells which are responsible for the MLR [3]. Therefore, contrary to what would be expected, the mechanism of this adjuvant response seems to be related to T cells. It was possible to observe this phenomenon because the immunoadjuvant used was water-soluble; to our knowledge such an effect has not previously been reported with either soluble or insoluble adjuvants. These findings seem to be of interest both from a fundamental point of view and also because of their possible clinical application.

We wish to thank Miss Francine Parant for statistical evaluation of data.

References

1. Adam, A., Ciorbaru, R., Petit, J. F., Lederer, E.: Isolation and properties of a macromolecular, water soluble immunoadjuvant fraction from the cell wall of *Mycobacterium smegmatis*. Proc. nat. Acad. Sci. (Wash.) **69**, 851 (1972).
2. Böyum, A.: Separation of leucocytes from blood and bone marrow. Scand. J. clin. Lab. Invest. **97**, 25 (1968).
3. Carlson, M. R., Robson, L., Schwartz, M. R.: The influence of adult thymectomy on immunological competence as measured by the mixed lymphocyte reaction. Transplantation **11**, 465 (1971).
4. Chedid, L., Parant, M., Parant, F., Gustafson, R. H., Berger, F. M.: Biological study of a non toxic, water soluble immunoadjuvant from mycobacterial cell walls. Proc. nat. Acad. Sci. (Wash.) **69**, 855 (1972).
5. Lamensans, A., Grabar, P., Bretey, J.: Fractionnement de la tuberculine purifiée. C.R. Acad. Sci. (Paris) **232**, 1880 (1951).
6. Ling, N. R.: Lymphocyte stimulation. North-Holland. Amsterdam 1968.
7. Lungren, G., Simmons, R. L.: Effect of neuramidase on the stimulatory capacity of cells in human mixed lymphocyte cultures. Clin. exp. Immunol. **9**, 915 (1971).
8. Möller, G.: Immunogenic tolerance and mitogenic properties of lipopolysaccharides. Virginia, USA: Endotoxin Conference Airline House 1972.
9. Oppenheim, J. J., Perry, S.: Effects of endotoxins on cultured lymphocytes. Proc. Soc. exp. Biol. (N.Y.) **118**, 1014 (1965).
10. Parant, M., Chedid, L.: Biological properties of a non toxic water soluble immunoadjuvant from mycobacterial cells. This volume.
11. Peavy, D. L., Adler, W. H., Smith, R. T.: The mitogenic effects of endotoxin and staphylococcal enterotoxin B on mouse spleen cells and human peripheral lymphocytes. J. Immunol. **105**, 1453 (1970).
12. Smith, R. T.: Selective effects of endotoxins on various lymphoreticular cell subpopulations. Virginia, USA: Endotoxin Conference Airlie House 1972.
13. Westphal, O., Lüderitz, O., Bister, F.: Über die Extraktion von Bakterien mit Phenol-Wasser. Z. Naturforsch. **7b**, 148 (1952).

Early Recovery of the Immune Response of a Specifically Depleted Cell Population under the Influence of Water-Soluble Adjuvant

P. LIACOPOULOS, J. L. BIRRIEN, C. BLEUX, and J. COUDERC

Institut d'Immuno-Biologie de l'INSERM et Association Claude Bernard, Hôpital Broussais, Paris

Recently developed methods of studying immunological responses at the cellular level consistently showed cells specifically reacting to various antigens in non-immunized animals [4, 7]. Whatever may be the origin of these cells, they seem to participate actively in the immunological response to the corresponding antigen. It has been shown, indeed, that cell populations depleted of cells of a given specificity become incapable of responding at the usual time interval when transferred with the homologous antigen into lethally irradiated animals [1, 2, 10].

Such specifically unresponsive animals would be suitable tools for studying whether cells of the missing specificity could arise again either spontaneously or after stimulation with the same antigen. Furthermore, one could also see whether a nonspecific stimulation would have an effect on the patterns of specific recovery.

In order to investigate these possibilities spleen cells from normal CBA mice (C.S.E.A.L., 45 — Orléans-La-Source, France) were harvested and used for rosette formation [4] with pigeon erythrocytes (PRBC). Then, rosette and cell suspension were layered on an Isopaque gradient of 9% Ficoll (Pharmacia) and 34% Triosil (sodium metrizoate, Glaxo) and centrifuged for 10 min at 1,000 rpm, according to the method of [6]. The cell population which remained at the top of the gradient was carefully removed, washed with Hank's solution and transferred i.v. with PRBC (50×10^6 cells + 2×10^8 PRBC) into lethally irradiated (950 r) CBA recipients. The anti-PRBC response of these animals was determined by counting the number of rosette-forming cells (RFC) in their spleens 7 days after transfer.

Table 1 shows that a normal spleen-cell population depleted of anti-PRBC natural RFC does not develop an anti-PRBC response the 7th day after transfer into irradiated recipients and stimulation with this antigen. However, when such a population is stimulated with sheep erythrocytes (SRBC), it produces an excellent response. These results confirm previous findings [1, 2, 10] and show that, in the abscence of natural anti-PRBC RFC, the remaining cell population loses its capacity to respond to this antigen. However, it retains its ability to respond to unrelated antigens.

The next point was to investigate how long this specific unresponsiveness lasts. The same procedure of depletion followed by transfer and stimulation was applied

Table 1. Number of RFC in spleens of lethally irradiated recipients on day 7 after transfer of 5×10 donor spleen cells depleted of natural anti-PRBC RFC and stimulation with either PRBC or SRBC

Expt. No.	Stimulation with PRBC (2×10^8)		Stimulation with SRBC (4×10^8)	
	No. of cells examined	Anti-PRBC RFC	No. of cells examined	Anti-SRBC RFC
1	76,923	0	23,620	92
2	24,716	0	36,456	152
3	23,840	0	46,548	126
4	33,256	0	24,625	76
5	33,326	0		
	192,061	0 > $5.5/10^6$ cells	131,249	446 $3{,}400/10^6$ cells

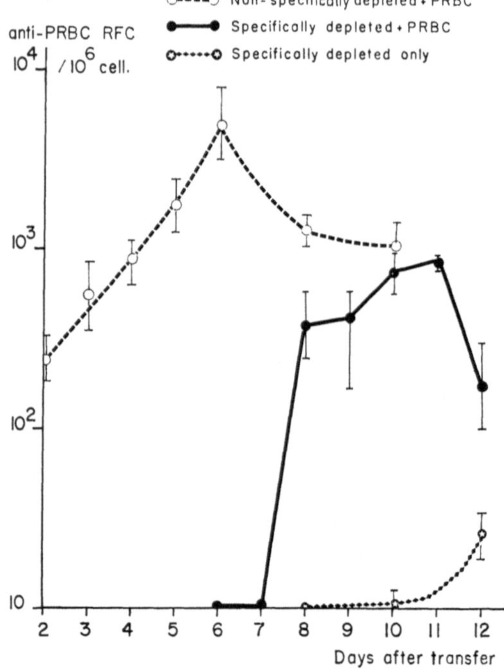

Fig. 1. Numbers of anti-PRBC RFC/10^6 spleen cells of irradiated recipients given on day 0: a) normal donor spleen cells non-specifically depleted and PRBC added; b) cells depleted of natural anti-PRBC RFC and PRBC added; c) same cells without PRBC

to normal CBA spleen cells. Spleen cells of recipients were examined for anti-PRBC RFC every day from day 6 to day 15 after transfer. It can be seen (Fig. 1) that the specifically depleted population, which remained silent until the day 7 after transfer and stimulation, suddenly began to respond on the day 8, reached its peak on the day 11, and progressively declined thereafter. For comparison, Fig. 1 also shows the reactivity to PRBC of a normal spleen cell population similarly centrifuged on an

Isopaque-Ficoll gradient without prior anti-PRBC rosette formation. Both the timing and the kinetics of this response were entirely different: a typical exponential increase in the number of specific RFC was recorded with a peak value on the day 6. Perhaps the most meaningful difference between these two responses is the respective rate of appearance of specific cells: whereas the non-depleted population produced an early exponential response, the specifically depleted population gave a late and sudden response, the kinetics of which suggest simultaneous recruitment by cell differentiation and maturation, similar to that described by [8, 9]. When the depleted

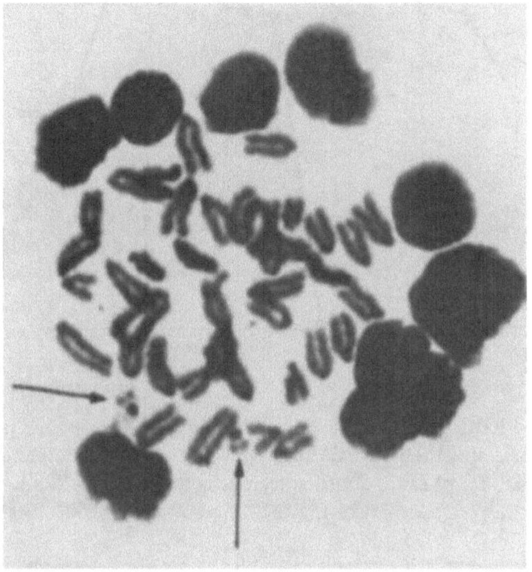

Fig. 2. An anti-PRBC RFC bearing T_6T_6 (↑) chromosome markers. Only nuclei of PRBC are visible

cell population was not stimulated with the specific antigen (PRBC), appearance of low numbers of anti-PRBC RFC was delayed until the day 12. These RFC could therefore be taken as indicating reappearance of natural anti-PRBC.

In a number of experiments, CBA T_6T_6 mice used as donors for CBA recipients to see whether RFC appearing on the day 10 after transfer of depleted populations do indeed belong to the donor population. Out of 148 anti-PRBC RFC found in metaphase, all were positive for T_6T_6 chromosome markers (Fig. 2).

In view of the late and rather weak response produced by specifically depleted populations, we wondered whether the adjuvants could have an effect on the time or the intensity of this response. We chosed the water-soluble adjuvant (WSA) extracted from mycobacteria [3, 5]. A dose of 20 μg of WSA was mixed in the same suspension of spleen cells and PRBC and given i.v. to the recipient mice. The results of these experiments are shown in Fig. 3. By the day 3 a significant number of anti-PRBC RFC was found; on day 4 this number was 2—3 times more, reached its peak value on the 6th day and progressively diminished thereafter. Examination of the sera of these animals for anti-PRBC hemagglutinins showed that serum antibody was produced simultaneously with resurgence of cellular response, although titers remained low (Table 2).

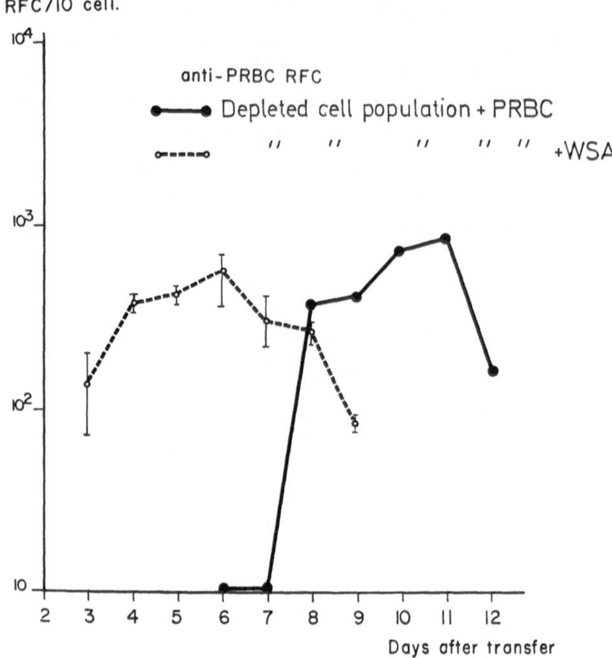

Fig. 3. Numbers of anti-PRBC RFC/10^6 spleen cells of irradiated recipients given on day 0: a) specifically depleted of natural anti-PRBC RFC donor spleen cell population and PRBC (same as b of Fig. 1); b) same donor spleen cells + PRBC + WSA

Table 2. Average reciprocal hemagglutination titers found in sera of irradiated recipients given 50×10^6 spleen cells specifically depleted of anti-PRBC RFC and PRBC (4×10^8)

Treatment of transferred cells	Days after transfer and stimulation with PRBC				
	5	6	7	8	10
Cells only centrifuged on the gradient	64	184	320	220	760
Cells specifically depleted	< 8	< 8	< 8	< 8	54
Cells specifically depleted and WSA added	< 8	12	48	28	64

The origin of anti-PRBC RFC was determined by studying the sensitivity of these cells to the anti-θ antigen serum, kindly offered by J. F. BACH (Fig. 4). For this, spleen cells of recipients were incubated with increasing dilutions of anti-θ serum and guinea-pig complement for 90 min at 37 °C and then used for anti-PRBC rosette formation. These experiments showed that on day 6 RFC are mainly of thymic origin as they are RFC arising on day 10 after stimulation with PRBC. The rarity of bone marrow cells giving rise to RFC would explain why hemmagglutination titers remained low in spite of the appearance of considerable numbers of anti-PRBC RFC.

The above results suggest that: a) Natural rosette and probably hemolytic plaque-forming cells play a very important role in the development of a rapid and intense immunological reaction. However, in their absence, the remaining population could ensure recovery of specific response after a sufficient period of time. The pattern of this recovery suggests that it results from differentiation and maturation

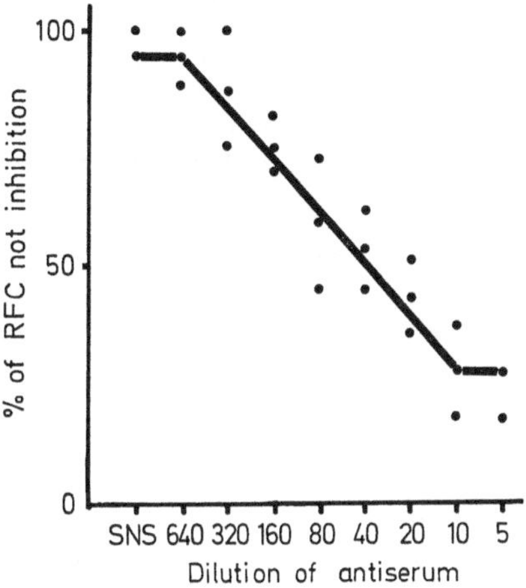

Fig. 4. Sensitivity of spleen RFC of irradiated recipients to increased dilutions of anti-θ-antigen serum. The cells were harvested on day 6 after transfer of specifically depleted spleen cells + PRBC + WSA

of cells in presence of the antigen. b) Stimulation with WSA and antigen greatly accelerates the appearance of the specific response of the depleted population. It seems therefore that WSA enhances recruitment of new cells for the specific response not only by favoring specific cell multiplication but also by promoting cell differentiation and maturation.

Acknowledgements

We wish to thank Dr. LEDERER for kindly supplying the WSA used in these experiments. We are grateful to Mrs. Y. CREPIN for her help in performing the chromosome T_6T_6 analysis.

This work was supported by RCP Grant 290 of the C.N.R.S.

References

1. ABDOU, N. I., RICHTER, M.: Cells involved in the immune response. X. The transfer of antibody-forming capacity to irradiated rabbits by antigen-reactive cells isolated from normal allogeneic rabbit bone marrow after passage through antigen-sensitized glass bead columns. J. exp. Med. **130**, 141 (1969).
2. ADA, G. K., BYRT, P.: Specific inactivation of antigen reactive cells with ^{152}I-labelled antigen. Nature (Lond.) **222**, 1291 (1969).

3. Adam, A., Ciorbaru, R., Petit, J. F., Lederer, E.: Isolation and properties of a macromolecular, water soluble, immuno-adjuvant fraction from the cell wall of *Mycobacterium smegmatis*. Proc. nat. Acad. Sci. (Wash.) **69**, 851 (1972).
4. Biozzi, G., Stiffel, C., Mouton, D., Bouthillier, Y., Decreusefond, C.: A kinetic study of antibody producing cells in the spleen of mice immunized with sheep erythrocytes. Immunology **14**, 7 (1968).
5. Chedid, L., Papant, M., Papant, F., Gustafson, R. H., Berger, F. M.: Biological study of a non toxic, water soluble immuno-adjuvant from mycobacterial cell walls. Proc. nat. Acad. Sci. (Wash.) **69**, 855 (1972).
6. Harris, R., Ukaejiofo, E. O.: Tissue typing using a routine one-step lymphocyte separation procedure. Brit. J. Haemat. **18**, 229 (1970).
7. Jerne, N. K., Nordin, A. A.: Plaque formation in agar by single antibody producing cells. Science **140**, 405 (1963).
8. Perkins, E. H., Sado, T., Makinodan, T.: Recruitment and proliferation of immunocompetent cells during the log phase of the primary antibody response. J. Immunol. **103**, 668 (1969).
9. Tannenberg, W. J. K., Jehn, U. W.: The life cycle of antibody-forming cells. II. Evidence for steady state proliferation of direct haemolytic plaque-forming cells during the primary and secondary responses. Immunology **22**, 589 (1972).
10. Wigzell, H., Makela, O.: Separation of normal and immune lymphoid cells by antigen-coated columns. Antigen-binding characteristics of membrane antibodies as analyzed by hapten-protein antigens. J. exp. Med. **132**, 110 (1970).

An Adjuvant-Active Water-Soluble Substance ("Polysaccharide-Peptidoglycan") from Mycobacterial Cells. Preparation by a Simple Extraction Technique

D. Migliore-Samour and P. Jollès

Laboratory of Biochemistry, University of Paris VI, Paris

1. Adjuvant-Active *Water-Insoluble* Substances from Mycobacteria

Mycobacteria possess several important biological properties, particularly an adjuvant effect in antibody formation (Freund's adjuvant effect; [4]) and induction in rats of experimental arthritis, termed adjuvant arthritis [14]. These reactions can also be provoked [15, 16]:

a) by cell walls from human and non-human mycobacterial strains;
b) by wax D fractions with a nitrogen-containing moiety (peptidoglycolipids).

In the different active substances, a polysaccharide (Poly), mainly an arabinogalactan [8] was linked to a peptidoglycan (PA) [10]. Poly-PA constitutes the water-soluble moiety which can be joined by ester linkages to the lipid part (Lip) consisting of mycolic acids, as in mycobacterial wax D. We studied in detail the chemical structure of the nitrogen-containing part of wax D fractions from human mycobacterial strains [10, 11], and were the first to propose a tentative formula (Fig. 1).

We could thus demonstrate a close relationship between the peptidoglycan of an active wax D and the material which constitutes the backbone of mycobacterial and other cell walls. Fig. 1 also indicates a schematic representation of an active wax D.

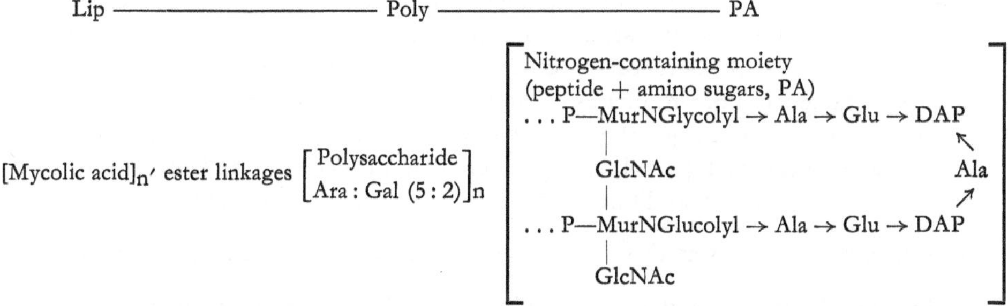

Fig. 1. Tentative formula of an adjuvant-active wax D with its peptidoglycan moiety [10, 11]

Human strains of *Mycobacterium tuberculosis* that contain the nitrogen moiety (PA) are not the only ones which show adjuvant activity [16]. PA was also found in atypical strains (*M. kansasii*) [5]. We extended our biochemical investigations to several Mycobacteria classified as bovine strains [12]. Extracts from *M. tuberculosis* var. *bovis*, strains Behring, LA and BB, gave rise to wax D fractions that did not differ in their constituents and properties from those obtained from human strains.

To extend the possible applications of the adjuvant-active substances isolated from Mycobacteria, we wished to obtain a water-soluble compound devoid of mycolic acids.

2. Water-Soluble Adjuvant Substances from Mycobacteria

A. Water-Soluble Substances Prepared from Wax D.

Wax D can form the starting material for the preparation of water-soluble substances by various techniques

a) Saponification

Asselineau's [2] saponification method yields a water-soluble substance which is not regularly active, probably because the sugars are more or less modified, especially the amino sugars (in which changes were confirmed analytically).

Homogenization of wax D in a buffer medium, gave a "native" Poly-PA, i.e. a water-soluble moiety in which the sugars remained unchanged during the preparative steps [9]; it showed adjuvant activity (Table) but the yield was very low.

B. Water-Soluble Substances Prepared from Mycobacterial Cell Walls

Adam *et al.* [1] quite recently prepared a water-soluble adjuvant from mycobacterial cell walls (*M. smegmatis*). Their procedure required the preparation of purified cell walls which were subsequently submitted to enzymic digestion.

C. Water-Soluble Substances Prepared from Mycobacterial Cells [13]

We tried to obtain a water-soluble adjuvant-active substance by a simple technique which did not require the preparation of complicated intermediate products or the addition of enzymes. Our structural studies [10, 11] and a comparison of the amounts of wax D obtained at different phases of culture with the growth curve (based on the weight of bacilli) strengthened the view that wax D could be a degradation product of mycobacterial cell walls [7, 12]. We considered hat the degradation (autodigestion) might not only produce wax D but give rise to a further water-soluble moiety.

$$\text{Mycobacteria} \xrightarrow{\text{autodigestion}} \text{wax D} \xrightarrow{\text{autodigestion}} \text{water-soluble adjuvant-active substance}$$

This hypothesis was verified, and we have described the preparation and partial purification of such a water-soluble adjuvant-active fraction from mycobacterial

Table. Adjuvant activity [16] and arthrogenicity [3, 6] of wax D of human mycobacterial strains and of their water-soluble moieties, Poly-PA, obtained by different methods

Substance obtained from *M. tuberculosis* var. *hominis*	Adjuvant activity to ovalbumin in guinea pig					Experimental polyarthritis in rat			
	Dose	Number of animals		Cutaneous reaction at 24 h [b]		Dose	Number of animals		Severity [c]
	μg	tested	positive	2 μg	10 μg	μg	tested	with arthritis	
Controls		16	0	0	0				
Wax D_{P35} [a] strain Peurois	200	7	7	17.4	21.1	250	8	8	8+++++
Poly-PA (after saponification) of wax D_{P15} [a], strain Peurois	200	7	7	7.1	9.8				
Poly-PA (after homogenization of wax D_{PT} [a], strain $H_{37}RvSr$)	200	8	8	11.3	15.6				
"Native" Poly-PA from delipidated bacterial residues of strain Peurois	100	8	8	8.8	12.9	250	6	0	

[a] For details see [16].
[b] Mean diameter of papule (mm).
[c] Severity: +++++: arthritis with malformation and ankylosis of the joints.

cells by a simple extraction technique (for details see [13]). Virulent or avirulent mycobacterial strains can be used, provided they contain an active wax D. The bacterial residues from which the lipids had been removed were ground and homogenized in water by means of an Ultra-Turrax. After stirring and centrifugation, the supernatant was treated several times with different amounts of ammonium sulfate, centrifuged, dialyzed and lyophilized. A crude, highly adjuvant-active material was rapidly obtained; further purification could be effected by chromatography on DEAE-cellulose and by filtration on Biogel P 10. About 10 peaks were found in the crude material; only two showed adjuvant activity.

The sedimentation constant S_{20} of our purified water-soluble substance was 1.9, compared to 2 for Poly-PA obtained by saponification. Analysis showed the presence of the characteristic constituents of a Poly-PA (Ala : Glu : DAP : GlcNAc : Mur N-glycolyl, 3 : 2 : 2 : 2 : 2 (molar ratios); presence of Gal and Ara; presence of P). The amino-acid and amino-sugar contents were 6—8% and 6—9%, respectively. On the basis of 3 alanine residues per mole, a molecular weight of 14,800 was calculated. The neutral reducing sugars (Ara, Gal, Man) constituted the remaining part of the active substance, as the lipid content was less than 0.5%. All these analytical data suggest a close relationship between the water-soluble substance described here and the Poly-PA obtained by saponification of wax D.

The table indicates that the "native" water-soluble Poly-PA (polysaccharide-peptidoglycan) obtained by our mild extraction technique possesses adjuvant activity when added to Freund's incomplete adjuvant with an antigen (ovalbumin) [16]. It does not produce arthritis [3, 6]. The purification of active substances of lower molecular weight is in progress.

Acknowledgements

This research was supported in part by C.N.R.S. (ER 102) and I.N.S.E.R.M. (Group U 116 and Research Grant 1972).

References

1. Adam, A., Ciorbaru, R., Petit, J.-F., Lederer, E.: Isolation and properties of a macromolecular, water-soluble, immuno-adjuvant fraction from the cell wall of *Mycobacterium smegmatis*. Proc. nat. Acad. Sci. (Wash.) **69**, 851 (1972).
2. Asselineau, J.: Sur un complexe lipo-polysaccharidique isolé du bacille tuberculeux: constitution de la fraction lipidique. C.R. Acad. Sci. (Paris) **229**, 791 (1949).
3. Bonhomme, F., Boucheron, C., Migliore, D., Jollès, P.: Effet de l'acétylation sur les propriétés arthrogènes d'une fraction de cire D de *Mycobacterium tuberculosis* var. *hominis*. C.R. Acad. Sci. (Paris) Série D **263**, 1422 (1966).
4. Freund, J.: The mode of action of immunologic adjuvants. Advanc. Tuberc. Res. **7**, 130 (1956).
5. Jollès, P., Samour, D., Lederer, E.: Isolement de fractions peptidoglycolipidiques à partir des cires D de Mycobatéries bovines, atypiques, aviaires et saprophytes. Biochim. biophys. Acta (Amst.) **78**, 342 (1963).
6. Jollès, P., Migliore, D., Bonhomme, F.: Wax D, peptidoglycolipid of *Mycobacterium tuberculosis*: further purification and study of an adjuvant arthritis-inhibiting subfraction. Immunology **14**, 159 (1968).
7. Lederer, E.: Mycobacterial cell walls. Pure and Applied Chem. **25**, 175 (1971).

8. MARKOVITS, J., VILKAS, E., LEDERER, E.: Sur la structure chimique des cires D, peptidoglycolipides macromoléculaires des souches humaines de *Mycobacterium tuberculosis*. Europ. J. Biochem. **18**, 287 (1971).
9. MIGLIORE, D., JOLLÈS, P.: Contribution à l'étude de la structure de la partie peptidique des cires D, peptidoglycolipides des mycobactéries: action de quelques enzymes. Bull. Soc. Chim. biol. (Paris) **48**, 829 (1966).
10. MIGLIORE, D., JOLLÈS, P.: Contribution to the study of the structure of adjuvant active waxes D from Mycobacteria: isolation of a peptidoglycan. FEBS Letters **2**, 7 (1968).
11. MIGLIORE, D., JOLLÈS, P.: Sur la structure chimique de la partie azotée des cires D de *Mycobacterium tuberculosis* var. *hominis*. C.R. Acad. Sci. (Paris) D **269**, 2268 (1969).
12. MIGLIORE, D., AUGIER, J., BOISVERT, H., JOLLÈS, P.: Wax D from different bovine strains of Mycobacterium. J. Bact. **107**, 548 (1971).
13. MIGLIORE-SAMOUR, D., JOLLÈS, P.: A hydrosoluble, adjuvant-active mycobacterial "Polysaccharide-peptidoglycan". Preparation by a simple extraction technique of the bacterial cells (strain Peurois). FEBS Letters **25**, 301 (1972).
14. WAKSMANN, B. H., PEARSON, C. M., SHARP, J. T.: Studies of arthritis and other lesions induced in rats by injection of mycobacterial adjuvant. II. Evidence that the disease is a disseminated immunologic response to exogenous antigen. J. Immunol. **85**, 403 (1960).
15. WHITE, R. G., BERNSTOCK, L., JOHNS, R. G. S., LEDERER, E.: Influence of components of *Mycobacterium tuberculosis* and other Mycobacteria upon antibody production of ovalbumin. Immunology **1**, 54 (1958).
16. WHITE, R. G., JOLLÈS, P., SAMOUR, D., LEDERER, E.: Correlation of adjuvant activity and chemical structure of wax D fractions of Mycobacteria. Immunology **7**, 158 (1964).

MAAF: A Fully Water-Soluble, Lipid-Free Fraction from BCG with Adjuvant and Antitumor Activity

I. J. Hɪᴜ

Institut de Cancérologie et d'Immunogénétique, Hôpital Paul-Brousse, Villejuif, France

BCG has been used to influence immune responses [1, 5]. However, the fact that it is not water-soluble and hence difficult to administer has limited its use. Its complex composition and various-side-effects make the resultsdifficult to interpret with both live and killed BCG. This communication reports the isolation from BCG of a water-soluble, lipid free and chemically well-defined fraction called "MAAF" (Mycobacterial Adjuvant and Antitumor Fraction). Animal experiments showed that MAAF is non-toxic and stimulates the delayedhy persensitivity reaction in guinea pigs sensitized with soluble antigen (crystalline eggwhite albumin). It also shows adjuvant activity, stimulating the immune reactions of murine spleen cells against sheep red blood cells. The combined administration of MAAF and killed (by irradiation) leukemic cells to mice receiving 10^4 viable L 1210 leukemic tumor cells induced marked inhibitory effects resulting in 90% survival.

Adjuvant fractions previously isolated from mycobacteria were shown to be lipid-containing fractions which were either water-insoluble [3, 6] or an opalescent solution with water [4]. Completely devoid of lipid. MAAF is fully water-soluble.

Since MAAF enhances cell-mediated and humoral immune responses, its antitumor effects probably involve mechanisms such as increased host reactivity to tumor antigens and non-specific resistance expressed through stimulation of cellular immunity.

The extraction procedure of MAAF and its chemical and biological properties have been described in detail elsewhere [2].

References

1. Bɪᴏᴢᴢɪ, G., Sᴛɪғғᴇʟ, C., Hᴀʟᴘᴇʀɴ, B. N., Mᴏᴜᴛᴏɴ, D.: Effet de l'inoculation du bacillus Calmette-Guérin sur le développement de la tumeur ascitique d'Ehrlich chez la souris. C.R. Soc. Biol. (Paris) **153**, 987 (1959).
2. Hɪᴜ, I. J.: Water soluble and lipid free fraction from BCG with adjuvant and antitumor activity. Nature New Biol. **238**, 241 (1972).
3. Hɪᴜ, I. J., Aᴍɪᴇʟ, J. L.: Fatty acid nature and adjuvant activity of wax D from Mycobacterium tuberculosis. J. gen. Microbiol. **66**, 239 (1971).
4. Hɪᴜ, I. J., Aᴍɪᴇʟ, J. L., Nɪᴋᴅᴊᴏᴜ, K.: Immunochemical study of mycobacterial firmly bound lipids. Europ. J. Clin. Biol. Res. **15**, 887 (1970).
5. Mᴀᴛʜé, G., Pᴏᴜɪʟʟᴀʀᴛ, P., Lᴀᴘᴇʏʀᴀǫᴜᴇ, F.: Active immunotherapy of L 1210 leukaemia applied after the graft of tumour cells. Brit. J. Cancer **23**, 814 (1969).
6. Rᴀғғᴇʟ, S.: Chemical factors involved in the induction of infectious allergy. Experientia (Basel) **6**, 410 (1950).

Comparative Study of the Free Lipids of Eight BCG Daughter Strains

J. Asselineau [1] and V. Portelance [2]

[1] Centre de Recherche de Biochimie et de Génétique cellulaires du C.N.R.S., Toulouse and [2] Institut de Microbiologie et d'Hygiène, Université de Montréal, P.Q.

BCG is widely used for vaccination against tuberculosis and this is its primary use. The initial strain of Calmette and Guérin has been maintained in many laboratories for more than 40 years during which time the original BCG strain has undergone some genotypic changes that are noticeable *in vitro* as well in animal tests and in man [6]. There are now some dozens of BCG daughter strains, differing in particular in the degree of attenuation [5]. It is difficult to compare these daughter strains and to evaluate their immunogenic properties [6].

BCG is increasingly being used as a nonspecific stimulant of immune responses in the treatment of various kinds of cancer [10, 11, 13]. So far little attention seems to have been devoted to the particular daughter strain used. In 1971, positive results against leukemia cells were obtained by means of the strain of the Pasteur Institute, whereas an American daugther strain exhibited little or no activity [17]; however, as there were also differences in the form of bacterial cells used (a living suspension of the Pasteur strain and lyophilized cells of the American strain), no conclusion could be drawn.

BCG lipid components have been shown to influence protection against tuberculosis [14] and tumor cells [8, 9]. We have therefore undertaken a comparative study of the lipid composition of some of the most commonly used daughter strains.

Material and Methods

We used batches of bacterial cells of the following daughter strains, obtained by surface culture on Sauton medium for 28 days:

Danish COP 3	Paris I.P.
Japanese	Russian
Montreal I.M.H.	Swedish D-3
Moreau (Brazil)	Tice 946 BL.

Immediately after harvesting, the lipids were extracted according to the modified Anderson procedure [1]. Each lipid fraction was studied by column or thin-layer chromatography, ir spectroscopy, hydrolysis, and identification of components [2, 7].

Results

The main lipid fractions are given in Table 1, and it is apparent that the total content of free lipids can vary from 21.0—31.6% and the chloroform-extractable lipids from 0.7—3.0%. However, it is difficult to obtain reproducible quantitative results for surface cultures of slow-growing mycobacteria.

Table 1. Content of lipid fractions isolated from 8 BCG daughter strains (expressed as percent of the dry weight of the bacterial cells)

Daughter strains	Total free lipids	Lipid fractions					
		Ehtanol-ether extracts			Chloroform extracts		
		Fats	Phospho-lipids	Wax A	Wax B	Wax C	Wax D
Danish	31.6	17.7	6.7	4.8	0.4	1.8	0.2
Japanese	26.6	9.5	6.7	9.7	0.1	0.6	0.02
Montreal	31.1	18.2	4.3	6.2	0.3	2.0	0.1
Moreau	25.5	13.4	5.7	4.7	0.4	1.2	0.1
Paris (Pasteur Institute)	29.4	9.8	5.1	11.5	0.1	2.7	0.2
Russian	24.3	9.1	5.5	9.5	0.1	0.04	0.1
Swedish	21.01	9.6	5.1	5.5	0.2	0.4	0.2
Tice 946 BL	26.3	16.8	5.9	2.9	0.2	0.4	0.1

In every case, fats were the main lipid fraction. Their content of free fatty acids (as determined by extraction with an aqueous solution of Na_2CO_3) varied from 8.5% for the Danish BCG cells to 49.2% of total fat fraction for the Tice BCG cells. The infrared spectrum of the neutral fat isolated from the Russian strain showed absorption at 6400 nm, characteristic of mycoside B, a typical component of *Mycobacterium bovis* [2, 7].

In view of the known biological activity of some of their components, our study focused mainly on phospholipids and waxes A, C and D.

Phospholipids

Phospholipid samples were analysed by thin-layer chromatography, the mixture chloroform-methanol-water (65 : 25 : 4) being used as the solvent system. Four groups of phospholipids were detected: cardiolipids, phosphatidylethanolamine, lysophosphatidylethanolamine and mannosides of phosphatidylinositol. The general pattern of the thin-layer chromatograms was very similar for the samples isolated from the various daughter strains. However, the cardiolipid spot was easily detected in the Pasteur, Moreau, Montreal, Russian and Japanese strains, but difficult to detect in the Danish, Swedish and Tice strains.

Two-dimensional thin-layer chromatography showed no important difference between the mannosides of phosphatidylinositol: the same spots were detected in all samples.

In a previous communication [15], we have stressed the presence of non-phosphorus-containing components in these phospholipid samples. An ornithine-containing lipid [16] was present in all the daughter strains studied.

Waxes A

Thin-layer chromatography of the wax A samples detected three main groups of constituents:

Group I. Weakly adsorbed substances, consisting of a mixture of esters of phthiocerol and triglycerides. Esters of phthiocerol were characterized by their chromatographic behavior and by the identification of phthiocerol (and related alcohols) as the neutral saponification product.

Group II. Relatively strongly adsorbed substances containing glyceryl monomycolate.

Group III. Strongly adsorbed substances, consisting of cord factor (6,6'-dimycoloyl trehalose) contaminated by unidentified substances which on saponification yielded glycerol and a reducing hexose. Group III substances accounted for 5—10% of waxes A isolated from the Moreau strain and 1—2% of those isolated from the Swedish strain, while only traces were found in the other daughter strains.

The following quantitative differences were found:

a) larger quantities of group I substances were found in the waxes A of the Pasteur strain.

b) group II substances were unevenly distributed. The Tice strain was the richest in Group II substances (about 52% of waxes A); substantial quantities were found in the Swedish, Russian and Japanese strains, while the Pasteur strain was the poorest.

Group II substances were isolated by chromatography of the waxes A of the Tice strain on florisil, and eluted with a mixture of benzene and ether (1 : 1). A waxy solid was obtained, m.p. 38—40°C, $[\alpha]_D^{21} + 7°$; chloroform, c = 3.40. Its i.r. spec-

Table 2. Fatty acid composition of three lipid fractions (expressed as percent of the total fatty acids of each fraction, as determined by gas-liquid chromatography of the methyl esters)

Fatty acids	Tice strain Wax A	"Montreal" strain Wax C	
	Monoesters of glycerol and ethylene glycol	"Petroleum ether-benzene" fraction	"Benzene-ether" fraction
14 : 0		1.3	3.0
16 : 0	4.6	15.5	31.5
18 : 0	3.1	19.8	27.2
20 : 0		9.0	9.4
22 : 0	3.0	5.9	5.3
24 : 0	41.5	11.2	7.7
Unknown I		3.2	
Unknown II (C_{25}?)	4.5	1.3	
26 : 0	35.0	28.8	13.8
Mycocerosic acids		2.7	
		1.4	

trum showed a hydroxyl band at 3000 nm, a carbonyl band at 5850 nm with a shoulder at 5750 nm, and a significant polymethylene band at 13,900 nm. On thin-layer chromatograms, a single elongated spot was detected (approximate $R_f = 0.30$ with chloroform-methanol 95 : 5 as solvent). Saponification gave mycolic acids and a mixture of *n*-tetracosanoic and *n*-hexacosanoic acids (see Table 2). The water-soluble fraction desalted on Amberlite MB-3 was analyzed by paper chromatography; only spots of glycerol and ethylene glycol were detected.

Since the initial product behaved like glyceryl monomycolate on thin-layer chromatograms, we believe that the fraction isolated from the Tice strain is a mixture of glyceryl monomycolate and monoesters of ethylene glycol with saturated fatty acids having 24 or 26 carbon atoms.

Group II substances were simultaneously isolated from waxes A of the Swedish strain. The product obtained (m.p. 44—46 °C; $[\alpha]_D^{21} + 9°$) behaved like pure glyceryl monomycolate (neither ethylene glycol nor tetra- or hexacosanoic acids were found in the saponification products). Ethylene glycol monoesters are not evenly distributed among BCG daughter strains.

Waxes C

Waxes C isolated from 7 of the 8 strains studied were first fractionated by column chromatography on magnesium trisilicate-celite; the Russian daughter strain yielded too little wax C to permit column fractionation. Two main fractions were obtained from wax C isolated from the Montreal strain, three wax-C fractions were isolated from the Danish, Pasteur, Japanese and Tice strains, and four from the Moreau and Swedish strains. Quantitative differences were observed in the proportions of each wax-C fraction in the various daughter strains studied (see Table 3).

The petroleum ether-benzene eluates consisted of triglycerides, which on saponification gave a complex mixture of fatty acids rich in long-chain saturated acids (see Table 2).

The benzene-ether eluates consisted of mixed glycerides containing normal-chain fatty acids and mycolic acids. The presence of mycolic acids explains their slightly stronger adsorption (for an example of fatty acid composition, see Table 2).

The ether-methanol (95 : 5) eluates (absent in the Montreal strain) represented 2.0—53.0% of the waxes C isolates. The main constituent of this fraction was cord factor, as shown by ir spectrometry, behavior on thin-layer chromatography, and saponification giving trehalose and mycolic acids (along with small quantities of glycerol and a reducing hexose).

Ether-methanol (9 : 1) eluates were obtained only from the Moreau and Swedish strains. The product isolated from the Moreau strain contained a major constituent migrating like cord factor (and having the same ir spectrum); more strongly adsorbed glycolipids were also detected. It may be concluded that this fraction was trehalose dimycolate (cord factor) contaminated by more complex glycolipids.

Waxes D

Crude waxes D of mycobacteria are mixtures of an arabinogalactan with mycolic acids (glycolipids) and peptidoglycolipids consisting of mycolate esters of the same

Table 3. Main fractions isolated by chromatography of waxes C (% of waxes C and melting point)

Daughter strains						
Montreal I.M.N.	Danish COP_3	Japanese	Moreau	Pasteur	Swedish D_3	Tice 946 BL
Petroleum ether-benzene 1 : 1						
71.7% 54—56 °C	59.6% 48—56 °C	62.3% 56—59 °C	45.1% 58—62 °C	54.0% 57—59 °C	35.7% 56—59 °C	25.3% 52.5—55 °C
benzene-ether 1 : 1						
28.7% 47—50 °C	22.4% 48—53 °C	21.3% 51—52 °C	15.2% 50—55 °C	32.8% 52—53 °C	17.2% 49—53 °C	20.3% 44—46 °C
ether-methanol 95 : 5						
	5.1% 45—50 °C	2.0% 44—46 °C	21.7% 47—49 °C	3.6% 43—45 °C	31.9% 47.5—49.5 °C	53.1% 46—47 °C
ether-methanol 9 : 1						
			5.3% 47—48 °C		4.4% 48.5—53 °C	

arabinogalactan linked to a glycopeptide moiety made of glucosamine, muramic acid and peptide chains (arising from the peptidoglycan of the cell wall) [3, 12]. Samples rich in glycolipids have a low melting point (about 50 °C) whereas samples rich in peptidoglycolipids have a high melting point (about 200 °C).

All the daughter strains studied, except the Russian and the Japanese ones, gave waxes D in the form of amorphous, yellowish powders having a melting point around 50 °C; those isolated from the Russian and Japanese strains had m.p. 205 to 210 °C. Identification of the products obtained by saponification or by acid hydrolysis gave results in agreement with a structure of the peptidoglycolipid type. Amino acid analysis showed the presence of several amino acids, mainly alanine, glutamic acid and diaminopimelic acid, which are the usual components of high-melting waxes D.

Conclusion

Many small differences have been observed between the lipid fractions isolated from the 8 BCG daughter strains studied, though the significance of most of them is not yet clear. However, two important differences have been found, concerning cord factor and waxes D.

Among the daughter strains studied, Moreau had the highest content of cord factor (about 0.6% of the dry weights of the cells, calculated from the amounts isolated from waxes A and C), while only traces of cord factor were detected in the Montreal strain. Injection of cord factor into the foot-pads of mice is able to induce histological changes similar to those provoked by living BCG [4]. The granuloma induced by this treatment seems to play an important role in the host resistance to infection with heterologous bacteria and tumor cells [4]. No simple relation seems to exist between the content of cord factor and the immunogenic properties of a

BCG daughter strain; both the Moreau and the Montreal strains appear to give good results in tuberculosis vaccination whereas the Tice strain (with about 0.2% cord factor) is definitely less effective [6].

Human strains of *M. tuberculosis* contain high-melting waxes D and are rich in peptidoglycolipids, whereas waxes D isolated from *M. bovis* are rich in glycolipids and have a low melting point. It is well established that the peptide moiety is essential for the adjuvant activity of these compounds [18]. All wax-D samples isolated from the BCG daughter strains studied had a low melting point except the Russian and Japanese isolates which had the properties of peptidoglycolipids and contained the amino acids usually found in the peptide part. The Russian strain has retained a bovine character, as the neutral fats showed bands characteristic of mycoside B in their ir spectrum.

The production by a particular BCG daughter strain of large amounts of cord factor and of waxes D rich in peptidoglycolipid might be a factor to consider in the choice of strain for tumor immunotherapy. This circumstance may also shed light on the phenomena involved in host resistance to tumor cells.

References

1. Aebi, A., Asselineau, J., Lederer, E.: Sur les lipides de la souche *Brévannes* de *Mycobacterium tuberculosis*. Bull. Soc. Chim. biol. (Paris) **35**, 661 (1953).
2. Asselineau, J.: The bacterial lipids. Paris: Hermann. San Francisco: Holden-Day 1966.
3. Asselineau, J., Buc, H., Jolles, P.: Lederer, E.: Sur la structure chimique d'une fraction peptido-glycolipidique (cires D) isolée de *Mycobacterium tuberculosis* var. *hominis*. Bull. Soc. Chim. biol. (Paris) **40**, 1953 (1958).
4. Bekierkunst, A., Levij, I. S., Yarkoni, E., Vilkas, E., Lederer, E.: Suppression of urethane-induced lung adenomas in mice treated with trehalose-6,6'-dimycolate (cord factor) and living Bacillus Calmette-Guérin. Science **174**, 1240 (1971).
5. Dubos, R. J.: Biochemical determinants of microbial diseases, p. 97. Cambridge, Mass.: Harvard University Press 1954.
6. Frappier, A., Portelance, V., St. Pierre, J., Panisset, M.: Conference on immunization in tuberculosis. Progress to date and future trends and research needs. Washington 1971.
7. Goren, M. B.: Mycobacterial lipids: selected topic 'sBact. Rev. **36**, 33 (1972).
8. Hiu, I. J., Amiel, J. L.: Isolation of immunological adjuvant component from BCG cells. Rev. Europ. Etud. clin. biol. **16**, 55 (1971).
9. Hiu, I. J., Amiel, J. L., Nikdjon, K.: Immunochemical study of mycobacteria firmly bound lipids. Rev. Europ. Etud. clin. biol. **15**, 887 (1970).
10. Lemonde, P., Clode, M.: Effect of BCG infection on leukemia and polyoma in mice and hamsters. Proc. Soc. exp. Biol. (N.Y.) **111**, 739 (1962).
11. Lemonde, P., Clode, M.: Influence of Bacillus Calmette-Guérin infection on polyoma in hamsters and mice. Cancer Res. **26**, 585 (1966).
12. Markovits, J., Vilkas, E., Lederer, E.: Sur la structure des cires D, peptidoglycolipides macromoléculaires des souches humaines de *Mycobacterium tuberculosis*. Europ. J. Biochem. **18**, 287 (1971).
13. Mathé, G.: Active immunotherapy of leukemia L-1210 administered after tumor grafting. Rev. franc. Etud. clin. biol. **13**, 881 (1968).
14. Pigretti, M., Vilkas, E., Lederer, E., Bloch, H.: Propriétés chimiques et biologiques de fractions phosphatidiques isolées de l'antigène méthylique de *Mycobacterium tuberculosis*. Bull. Soc. Chim. biol. (Paris) **47**, 2039 (1965).

15. Portelance, V., Asselineau, J.: Non-phosphorus contaminants of mycobacterial phospholipid preparations. Amer. Rev. resp. Dis. **103**, 853 (1971).
16. Promé, J. C., Lacave, C., Lanéelle, M. A.: Sur les structures des lipides à ornithine de *Brucella melitensis* et de *Mycobacterium bovis* (BCG). C.R. Acad. Sci. (Paris), Ser. C **269**, 1664 (1969).
17. Reif, A. E., Kim, C. A. H.: Leukemia L-1210 therapy trials with antileukemia serum and Bacillus Calmette-Guérin. Cancer Res. **31**, 1606 (1971).
18. White, R. G., Jolles, P., Samour, D., Lederer, E.: Correlation of adjuvant activity and chemical structure of wax D fractions of Mycobacteria. Immunology **7**, 158 (1964).

A Galactose Disaccharide from Immunoadjuvant Fractions of Mycobacterium Tuberculosis (Cell Wall and Wax D)

E. VILKAS, C. AMAR-NACASCH, and J. MARKOVITS

Institut de Chimie des Substances Naturelles, C.N.R.S., Gif sur Yvette

The cell walls and wax D of *Mycobacterium tuberculosis* var. *hominis* contain an acylated arabinogalactan with D-arabinose and D-galactose in a molar ratio of about 5 : 2 [14].

[1] have proposed the following structure for the arabinogalactan of mycobacterial cell walls (Fig. 1). This structure was consistent with our first results obtained with

$$\left(\begin{array}{l} \rightarrow 5)\text{-}\alpha\text{-D-Ara}_f\text{-}(1 \rightarrow 5)\text{-}[\alpha\text{-D-Ara}_f]_x\text{-}(1 \rightarrow 4)\text{-}[\text{D-Gal}_p]_2\text{-}(1 \rightarrow \\ \qquad\quad 3 \\ \qquad\quad \uparrow \\ \qquad\quad 1 \\ \qquad [\alpha\text{-D-Ara}_f]_y \\ \qquad\quad 5 \\ \qquad\quad \uparrow \\ \qquad\quad 1 \\ \text{R-CO} \rightarrow 5\text{-}\alpha\text{-D-Ara}_f \quad (x = 1\text{—}3,\ y = 2\text{—}0) \end{array}\right)$$

D-Ara_f = D-arabinofuranose, D-Gal_p = D-galactopyranose.

Fig. 1. Arabinogalactan from mycobacterial cell walls

the human strain of *M. tuberculosis* Peurois [8]. Recently we isolated a disaccharide which contains only D-galactose from the products of partial acid hydrolysis of cell walls and of wax D from Peurois and $H_{37}Ra$ strains; this material appeared to be a D-galactofuranose disaccharide [15].

The optical rotation of our galactobiose ($[\alpha]_D$ = —26° ± 2) differs from that of 4-O-β-D-galactopyranosyl-D-galctopyranose ($[\alpha]_D$ = +67°) and from that of its α isomer ($[\alpha]_D$ = +186° → 173°) [13]. Tests with α- and β-galactoside were negative. Chromatographic mobility differed from that of 1—4 galactopyranose disaccharide [6, 9, 17]. The disaccharide also migrates more rapidly than lactose and maltose. With aniline hydrogen phthalate the galactobiose gives an yellow-brown spot indistinguishable from those of galactose, lactose and maltose. With the aniline-diphenylamine-phosphoric acid reagent [2] the spot is greyish-green, whereas the spots of lactose and maltose (1—4 linked hexopyranoses) are blue. These results seem to exclude the structure 4-O-galactopyranosyl galactose for the disaccharide isolated from cell walls and wax D.

Proof for the Existence of the Furanose Ring

The galactobiose contains a non-reducing furanose end unit since the sugar is rapidly hydrolysed with 0.01 *N* sulphuric acid at 85°. The mass spectra of per-acetylated and pertrimethylsilyl derivatives confirm the occurrence of a non-reducing furanose ring:

peracetylated derivative

m/e 145 CH_2—CH (| OAc | OAc)

m/e 533 M-145

permethylsilyl derivative[1]

m/e 583 indicative for a (1 → 5) or (1 → 6) linkage

m/e 623 m/e 713-TMSOH.

The ratio of the peak intensities m/e 217 : 204 is greater than unity, therefore at least one furanose ring must be present in the molecule.

The PMR experimental results indicate that the reducing unit of the disaccharide must also be present in furanose form, and that the glycosidic linkage has a β configuration.

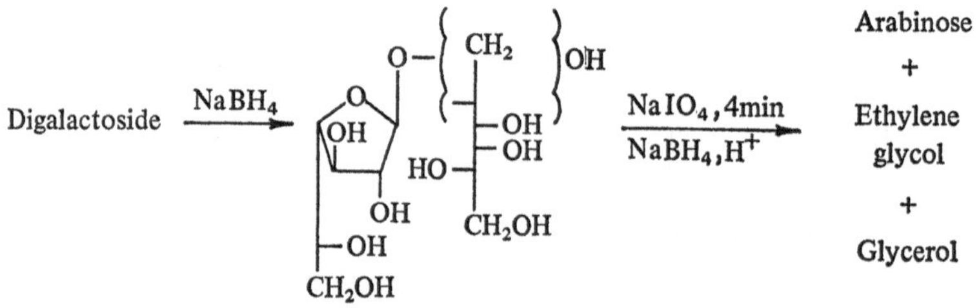

Fig. 2. Degradation of the digalactoside

The procedure used to degrade the galactobiose is summarized in Fig. 2. The same sequence of reactions was used by [5] to characterize 5-O-β-D-galactofuranosyl-D-galactose from galactocarolose and by [11] to study 6-O-β-D-galactofuranosyl-D-galactose from *Mycoplasma mycoides*.

The only reducing sugar obtained is arabinose, but both ethylene glycol and glycerol are formed. The ethylene glycol suggests a 1—6 linkage; glycerol could result from a 1—5 linkage or from incomplete oxidation of galactitol. The 1—6 linkage is not consistent with formation of the 2, 3, 6-tri-O-methyl derivative of galactose [1, 8] after permethylation and hydrolysis of the polysaccharide. The retention times of 2, 3, 6 tri-O-methyl-galactose and 2, 3, 5 tri-O-methyl-galactose in gas-liquid chromatography have been found to be almost identical [10]. We hope to elucidate this point soon by synthesis.

---

[1] We are indebted to Dr. J. F. G. VLIEGENTHART, Rijksuniversiteit of Utrecht, for this measurement, for the PMR spectra and their interpretation.

From our results it can be concluded that the digalactoside isolated from the arabinogalactan of cell walls and wax D is a digalactofuranoside with a 1—6 or 1—5 linkage, but we are not yet able to say whether all the galactose units present in the polysaccharide are in furanose form [2].

D-galactofuranoside are not very frequent in nature. It is noteworthy that several of the type-specific substances of *Pneumococcus* spp. contain this unit [4]. More recently a galactofuranosyl residue has been found in the T_1-specific chain of a lipopolysaccharide from *Salmonella friedeneau* [3]. Other microorganisms known to produce polysaccharides containing D-galactose in the furanose ring form include *M. mycoides*, [11], *Gibberella fujikuroi* [12], *Peltigera horizontalis* [7] and *Penicillium charlesii* [5].

References

1. Azuma, J., Yamamura, Y., Misaki, A.: Isolation and characterization of arabinose mycolate from firmly bound lipids of mycobacteria. J. Bact. **98**, 331 (1969).
2. Bailey, R. W., Bourne, E. J.: Colour reactions given by sugars and diphenylamine-aniline spray reagents on paper chromatography. J. Chromat. **4**, 206 (1960).
3. Berst, M., Hellerquist, C. G., Lindberg, B., Luderitz, O., Svensson, S., Westphal, O.: Structural investigations on T_1 Lipopolysaccharides. Europ. J. Biochem. **11**, 353 (1969).
4. Chittenden, G. J. F., Roberts, W. K., Buchanan, J. G., Baddiley, J.: The specific substance from Pneumococcus type 34 (41). Biochem. J. **109**, 597 (1968).
5. Gorin, P. A., Spencer, J. F. T.: 5-O-β-galactofuranosyl-D-galactose from galactocarolose. Canad. J. Chem. **37**, 499 (1959).
6. Jones, J. K. N., Reid, W.: The structure of the oligosaccharides produced by the enzymic breakdown of peptic acid. J. chem. Soc. 1890 (1955).
7. Lindberg, B., Silvaner, B. G., Wachmeister, C. A.: Studies on the chemistry of lichens. Mannitol Glycosides in Peltigera Species. Acta chem. scand. **18**, 213 (1964).
8. Markovits, J., Vilkas, E., Lederer, E.: Sur la structure chimique des Cires D Peptido-glycolipides macromoléculaires des souches humaines de *Mycobacterium tuberculosis*. Europ. J. Biochem. **18**, 287 (1971).
9. Meier, H.: Studies on a galactan from tension wood of beech. Acta chem. scand. **16**, 2275 (1962).
10. Ovodov, J. S., Pavlenko, A. F.: Gas-liquid chromatography of methylated D-galactose derivatives. J. Chromat. **36**, 531 (1968).
11. Plackett, P., Buttery, S. H.: A galactofuranose disaccharide from the galactan of *Mycoplasma mycoides*. Biochem. J. **90**, 20 (1964).
12. Siddiqui, J. R., Adams, G. A.: An extracellular polysaccharide from *Gibberella fujikuroi* (*Furarium moniliforme*). Canad. J. Chem. **39**, 1683 (1961).
13. Stanek, J., Cerny, M., Pacak, J.: The oligosaccharides, p. 252. Prague: Csechoslovak Academy of Sciences 1965.
14. Vilkas, E., Delaumeny, J. M., Nacasch, C.: Sur la structure du Polysaccharide des Cires D d'une souche humaines virulente de *Mycobacterium tuberculosis*. Biochim. biophys. Acta **158**, 147 (1968).
15. Vilkas, E., Markovits, J., Amar-Nacasch, C., Lederer, E.: Sur la présence d'unités de D-galactofuranose dans l'arabinogalactane des parois et des Cires D de souches humaines de *Mycobacterium tuberculosis*. C.R. Acad. Sci. (Paris) **273**, 845 (1971).
16. Vilkas, E., Amar, C., Markovits, J., Vliegenthart, J. F. G., Kamerling, J. P.: Occurrence of a galactofuranose disaccharide in immunoadjuvant fractions of *Mycobacterium tuberculosis* (cell walls and wax D). Biochim. biophys. Acta (Amst.) **297**, 423 (1973).
17. Whistler, R. L., Conrad, H. E.: A cristalline galactobiose from acid hydrolysis of okna mucilage. J. Amer. chem. Soc. **76**, 1673 (1954).

---

[2] (Note added May 2nd, 1973.) Our recent results indicate that the digalactoside is 6-O-β-D-galcatofuranosyl-D-galactose. See [16].

Summary of Working Session on the Mechanism of Action of Immunological Adjuvants

B. Benacerraf

Department of Pathology, Harvard Medical School, Boston, Mass.

It has been known since the early observations of Old and Benacerraf and of Biozzi and Halpern that treatment with mycobacteria or corynebacteria or their products could enhance resistance to tumor growth as well as tumor immunity. Several reports have described this type of phenomenon.

Zbar reported that, in guinea pigs and mice, injection of live BCG at the site of a syngeneic tumor transplant would cause its rejection. Moreover, the inoculation of tumor cells with BCG could result in the rejection of the inoculum and, particularly in guinea pigs, in the establishment of lasting immunity to the tumor-specific transplantation antigen (TSTA). More dramatically, when local treatment with BCG was started soon after inoculation of the tumor in guinea pigs, even when the local lymph nodes were already involved, regression of the tumor occurred at its metastatic sites in the draining lymph-nodes. Zbar claimed he had clear evidence of enhancement of immunity of his guinea-pig system but that, in the mouse, the rejection observed was attributable to the immune inflammatory reaction elicited by the reaction to the microorganism; this reaction itself is able to destroy the tumor. Zbar emphasized that inoculation of BCG in combination with the tumor cells was required for the best results, and also that treatment must be initiated not too long after inoculation of the tumor, or the tumor mass is too large to permit rejection.

Similar results were reported by Baldwin with chemical carcinogen-induced syngeneic tumors in the rat. He succeeded in provoking the rejection of metastatic tumor nodules in the lung, which follow intravenous injection of tumor cells, by local inoculation of the sarcoma cells with live BCG. The results were quite dramatic, though depended upon the strength of the TSTA of the tumor. Thus, the result of BCG and live tumor cells for each tumor could be predicted from the degree to which one could immunize a normal recipient with irradiated tumor cells alone.

Treatment with corynebacteria was also able to enhance the ability to suppress tumor growth, as reported by Herman and Raymond, and by Stiffel in syngeneic tumor systems. In these cases the mycobacteria had a systemic effect and were most effective when administered before tumor implantation. Thus, systemic treatment appears to be effective in some systems, but, generally, administration of the adjuvant with the tumor cell or at the site of tumor inoculation proved more effective when BCG was used.

There was very little reported about the precise nature of the mycobacteria or corynebacteria fractions with power to enhance tumor rejection and tumor immunity. However, YASPHE reported that the solid residue from methanol extraction of mycobacteria was very active in promoting tumor rejection. LEDERER pointed out that this was a poorly characterized fraction containing many bacterial products.

It was obvious to most of the participants that many biological properties could be attributed to the crude bacterial products. Indeed, the cruder the product, the more activities it possesses. Thus, YASPHE's fraction was able to enhance all forms of cellular immunity, allograft immunity, delayed sensitivity, carrier function, and also humoral immunity. YASPHE presented evidence, however, that most of the activity of the fraction could be attributed to its action on T cells. Similarly, treatment with corynebacteria, as shown by HERMAN and by HOWARD, is also able markedly to enhance humoral immunity even to a thymus-dependent antigen such as pneumococcus polysaccharide type III. However, HOWARD demonstrated that, in the pneumococcus polysaccharide system, the antibody enhancement caused by corynebacteria was abolished by prior thymectomy, demonstrating that the adjuvant effect of the preparation required T-cell activity even in humoral activity. It would appear, therefore, that many adjuvants of humoral immunity enhance the helper function of T cells on B cells.

This situation raises a serious problem, since it is well known that cellular immunity must be enhanced and humoral antibodies should be suppressed to obtain the most effective tumor immunity and tumor rejection. There is no preparation at present available which is able to achieve such a result. However, we are only beginning to explore the problem and with the combined efforts of the bacterial chemists and tumor immunologists, there is considerable hope of improving what is available today for experimental and clinical use.

The harmful effect of antibodies on tumor immunity was dramatically demonstrated in the experiment presented by STIFFEL. In collaboration with BIOZZI, they selected 2 lines of mice for their ability to produce antibodies against sheep erythrocytes. After 20 generations of such a selection, the lines established had remarkable properties. The low antibody-producing line was a low responder to all antigens, and was hypogammaglobulinemic, in contrast to the high antibody-producing line. It had, therefore, a profound defect in all humoral antibody responses. In contrast to this difference, both high low lines were equally able to reject skin grafts and to display contact sensitivity. They had, therefore, identical levels of cellular immunity. The low and high lines were crossed with the inbred AKR mouse strain to permit implantation of AKR leukemia. The F_1 of the high and low line with AKR displayed the antibody responses of the parental line. Thus, the F_1 of the low line and AKR was a poor antibody producer. Both F_1 generations died of leukemia when injected with an appropriate number of AKR leukemia cells. However, the effect of *Corynebacterium parvum* was much more dramatic in the (low line-AKR) F_1 than in the (high line-AKR) F_1, indicating that the best stimulation of tumor rejection is obtained if antibody response is interfered with.

Although a product which enhances cellular immunity solely or predominantly is not available at the present time, several investigators described the very interesting properties of a well-defined water-soluble adjuvant (WSA) extracted from *Mycobacterium smegmatis* by LEDERER. PARANT showed that this product was totally devoid of toxicity, did not possess tuberculin-sensitizing properties, did not cause polyarthritis, but was extremely effective as a stimulant of antibody synthesis, even when injected in saline with an antigen.

The adjuvant activity of this compound for antibody synthesis seemed again to depend upon its effect on T cells, since Bona showed that WSA stimulated significantly both the MLC *in vitro* and the response of sensitized lymphocytes to tuberculin, both known to be T-cell responses. Liacopoulos showed that WSA greatly increases the rate at which a specifically depleted spleen-cell population regenerates an immune response in an irradiated host. There was no report, however, of any effect of this interesting WSA fraction on tumor immunity.

Besides bacterial adjuvants, there are other biological products which enhance cellular and humoral immune responses and which stimulate tumor immunity. Gresser reported that mouse interferon is able to cause the rejection of transplanted tumors in the mouse. He showed that 2 mechanisms were probably involved in this protection. Interferon at very low concentrations was able to inhibit the growth of tumor cells *in vitro* and had, therefore, a direct suppressive effect. Interferon also enhanced the specific cytotoxicity of sensitized lymphocytes for target cells *in vitro*. The degree to which this system was effective in natural tumor rejection was not discussed.

The last paper which I would like to summarize was the contribution of W. Braun, who demonstrated the effect of poly A-poly U (poly A : U) in mice on the rejection of syngeneic tumors. Treatment with this polymer had a very favorable effect on the rejection of such tumors. This polynucleotide is known to activate adenyl cyclase and to cause an increase in intercellular cyclic AMP. Poly A : U has been shown to have a strong adjuvant effect on antibody synthesis; this is also believed to depend on the effect of this compound on T cells and their helper function, as shown by Johnson. However, according to Braun, the effect of poly A : U on the rejection of tumor cells may also depend upon the direct action of the polynucleotide on tumor cells. Poly A : U was able to inhibit *in vitro* the growth of the very tumor cells whose rejection is enhanced by systemic treatment with poly A : U. Braun proposes that all these effects are attributable to the action of the polynucleotide on adenyl cyclase.

What conclusions can we draw from the data presented and the discussions that took place? The most effective adjuvants of tumor immunity to date are the crude bacterial products of mycobacteria and corynebacteria. These agents act by enhancing cellular immunity to the TSTA and by promoting graft rejection. Although these agents can act systemically and generally prophylactically if administered before tumor implantation, in many instances the best results are obtained, particularly with mycobacteria, if they are administered with the tumor cells themselves or at a site of tumor implantation. This is understandable, since all adjuvant effects are most efficient when the antigen is administered with the adjuvant. Moreover, there is clear evidence that a local immune inflammatory reaction of the tuberculin type, which induces mononuclear infiltration, is able to destroy accompanying tumor, even when the immune response is not directed against the tumor cells. However, it seems to me that the most promising therapeutic approach is enhancement of cellular immunity against TSTA. When this occurs, as in Zbar and Baldwin's experiments, metastases at distant sites were resolved by the immune response and lasting immunity was achieved. In order for this to occur, the tumor must have sufficient antigenicity and the treatment must be initiated sufficiently early when the tumor mass is not too large for the immune system to eradicate. Instances have been recorded where immunity resolved some tumor sites but not others when treatment was initiated later.

Two other serious problems to consider are: 1. selective enhancement of cellular immunity to achieve optimal tumor rejection. We do not at present possess selective adjuvants. All factors which increase cellular immunity of T cells also enhance antibody responses. This is understandable, since it has been shown that the antibody response of B cells is regulated by the activity of specific T cells, a phenomenon known as helper function. In addition, most effective adjuvants have been shown to act on antibody synthesis through their effect on T-cell activity. The problem is therefore complex, but not insoluble. The possibility exists that T cell-mediating cellular immunity and helper function are properties of different lines of T cells and that adjuvants will be found that act on the first and not the second postulated line of T cells.

However, more promising are the findings that antibody synthesis may be suppressed, as in antigenic competition, by a physiological mechanism involving the regulating activity of some type of T cells on antibody synthesis or, in other words, that some activity of T cells may suppress humoral immune responses. As our knowledge of the biological phenomena concerning T cell regulation of antibody improves, it is reasonable to expect that we will be able to develop factors that both enhance cellular immunity and, through regulation of T cell function, suppresses humoral immunity.

2. The other promising avenue to consider is fractionation of the bacterial products to identify and isolate factors with activity exclusively enhancing cellular immunity. The combined efforts of the microbial chemists and tumor immunologists should prove very fruitful, as indicated by the exciting early results.

It is fair to state that the future for clinical application of immunotherapy in cancer is very favorable and depends primarily on identification of agents and appropriate procedures to monitor, enhance, and control the natural immune responses to the TSTA by the use of experimental models in the laboratory.

I want to emphasize again, however, that, as in all forms of therapy in cancer, early detection and treatment (as demonstrated in experimental models) is essential for successful results. When the tumor mass is large and the lymphoid system has been extensively invaded by tumor metastases, the task may be unreasonable, even for the immune system. It is unfortunate that immunotherapy has been initiated in many cases at this late stage, when all is lost.

BCG and the Lympho-Reticuloendothelial System

S. R. Rosenthal

University of Illinois and Research Foundation, Chicago, Ill

It is generally agreed that a stimulated and active immune system is operative in the suppression of neoplastic cells. BCG is one of the most active stimulators of the immune system, as indicated by its effects on the lymphoreticuloendothelial system (RES) [4, 8]. Its activity, both specific [7] and nonspecific [4], depends on the physiological state of the organism, the route of administration, the species of animal and the dose. In some species of animals (mouse, monkey) the dermal route of administration of BCG is relatively ineffective, but the intravenous or aerosol routes are highly effective [1]. In the guinea pig and in man the dermal route is effective but to a lesser degree than the intravenous or aerosol routes [2, 10].

The dose of BCG for a specific immunizing effect can be small (10^{-6} mg in the mouse, 5—20 clones in the guinea pig) but to obtain a nonspecific effect, for example as against S-180, relatively large doses (1 mg) are needed [5]. The specific effect may last for years and can be activated very quickly on stimulation by a specific antigen; on the other hand, the nonspecific effect is of short duration and cannot be stimulated by nonspecific agents such as neoplastic cells. Large doses of the specific antigen must be constantly present to maintain the nonspecific effect [4].

This study was undertaken to determine how a large dose of BCG, administered by the intravenous, aerosol, intradermal or oral route, effects nonspecific stimulation of the RES in the guinea pig [8, 9].

Methods

Guinea pigs weighing 300—400 g (suckling animals 2—7 days old for the oral route) were inoculated with BCG intravenously (through the right ventricle 1/M 10—15 mg), by aerosol (in a chamber—3000 clones), intracutaneously (10 mg) and orally (5 mg doses daily for 3 days = 15 mg). The animals were sacrificed at regular intervals (10 min to 14 months). The lungs were fixed *in situ* with Zenker's reagent before the chest was opened. Histological examinations were made of the lung, lymph nodes, liver, spleen, kidney and, for orally treated animals, the intestines as well. The tissues were fixed with paraffin and stained with hematoxylin and eosin and carbolfuchsin-methylene blue.

Control animals of different ages (2 days to 1½ years old) were studied histologically as above. Blood counts and differential cell counts as well as tuberculin testing at specific intervals were also carried out.

Results

Intravenous route. Swelling of the septal cells throughout the lung began almost at once and was pronounced by the third hour. The cells were swollen and protruded into the alveoli as small nodules (Fig. 1). A similar histiocytic swelling was seen about the small blood vessels. This nonspecific process remained very active during the formation of the tubercle (3-15 days) and then gradually subsided (1 month). However, at age 1 month, 3 months, and 1 year, if large doses of tuberculin were

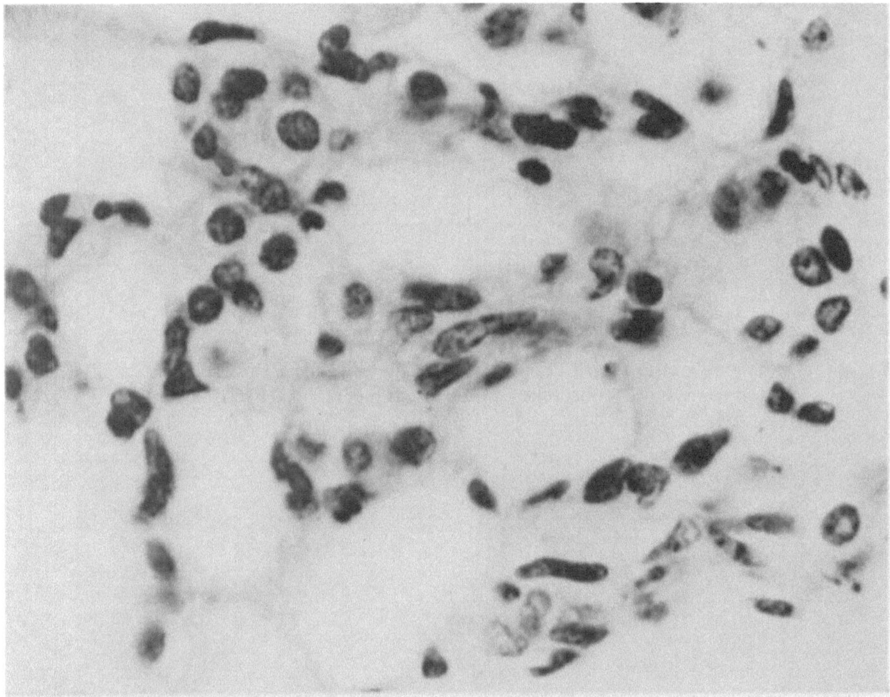

Fig. 1. Lung (1¼ h after i.v. BCG; guinea pig). The septal cells are swollen and arranged along the inner aspect of the alveolar walls. Note the contrast with the flat, dark-staining nuclei of the capillary endothelium (H & E × 500)

injected intradermally (1000 TU-OT), and where a Koch's phenomenon was manifest, there was a marked swelling of the alveolar walls characterized by hyperemia, septal cell swelling, intracapillary lymphocytes and polymorphonuclear leukocytes (Fig. 2). This pronounced anamnestic reaction did not occur if the tuberculin-test area was small (5 × 5 mm). By the time that allergy appeared (9—15 days) there was a marked infiltration of lymphocytes around the tubercles (Fig. 3).

The reaction of the Kupffer cells and the perivascular histiocytes in the liver occurred very early, as they did in the lung. The cells became swollen, the nuclei vesicular and the cytoplasm basophilic and phagocytosis increased. The Kupffer cells increased in number, forming small nodules (Fig. 4). The reticulum cells of the spleen,

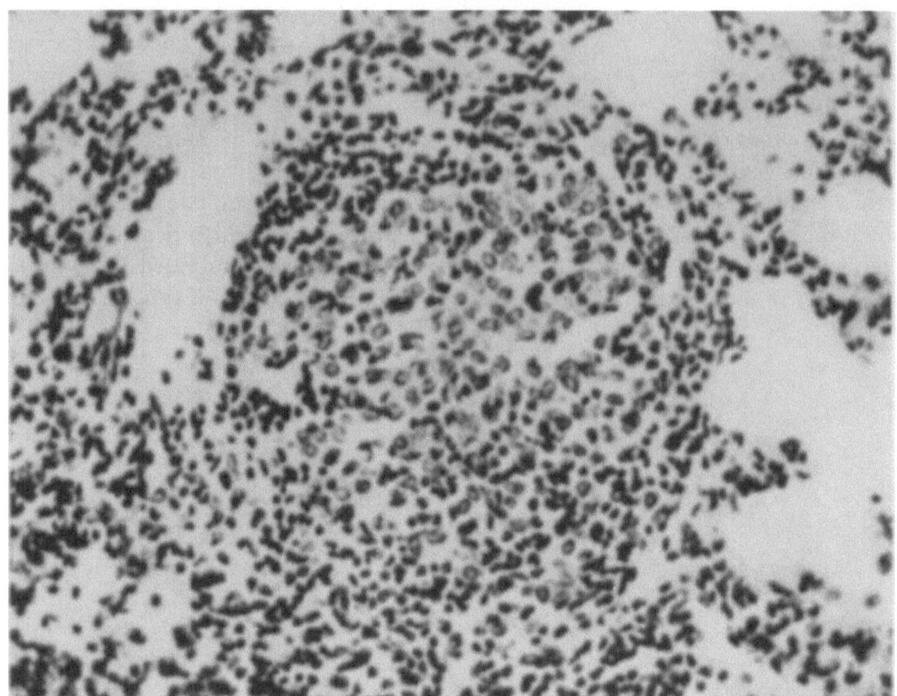

Fig. 2. Lung (3 months after i.v. BCG; guinea pig). Moderate hyperemia and septal cell swelling following Koch's phenomenon due to old tuberculin (H & E $\times$ 125)

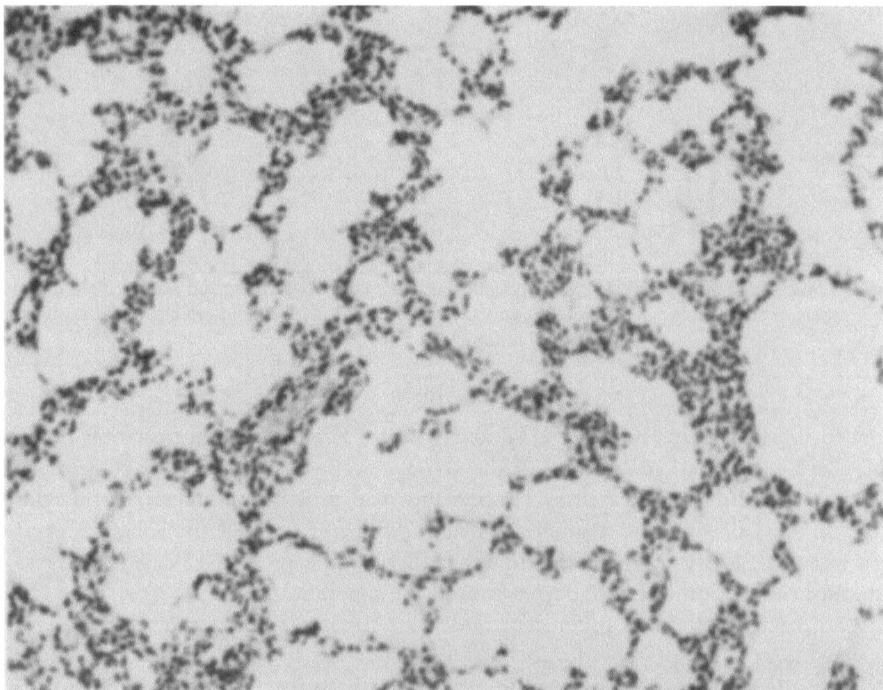

Fig. 3. Lung (15 days after i.v. BCG; guinea pig). Tubercle composed of epithelioid cells, surrounded and invaded by lymphocytes (H & E $\times$ 250)

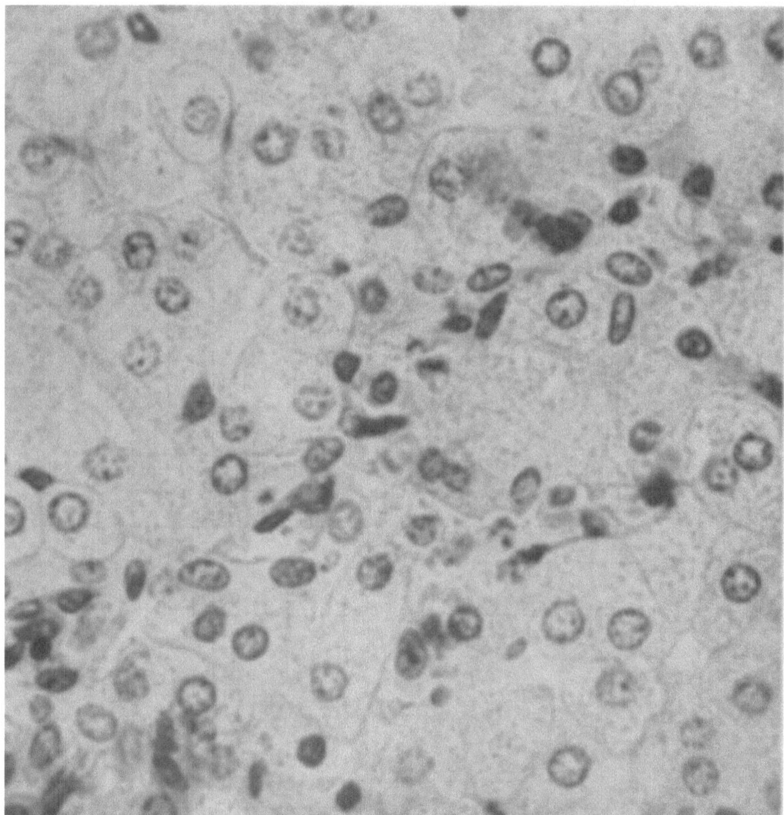

Fig. 4. Liver (16 h after i.v. BCG; guinea pig). Proliferation of the Kupffer cells and their grouping into small nodules. Some of the cells contain tubercle bacilli (H & E $\times$ 500)

the perivascular histiocytes in the hilus of the kidney, and the interstitial cells in the kidney similarly became swollen and increased in number. In general the pattern and duration of reactions before and after stimulation by the specific antigen (OT) followed that of the lung.

The blood responses mirrored the responses of the tissues. The monocytes reached their maximum after 3 days, thus lagging behind the response noted in the tissue. The lymphocytes first fell and then rose, reaching their maximum by day 11 or 12. The M/L (monocyte/lymphocyte) ratio was high after 3 days and again after 15 days. After 8—10 weeks, a large dose of tuberculin given intradermally produced a peak in the M/L ratio, indicating a stimulation of the RES, particularly the monocytes (Fig. 5).

Aerosol Route. The histological picture showed a similar pattern to that of the intravenous group. Our studies here were less extensive than with the intravenous group. One month following exposure and 48 hours after tuberculin testing (with large reactions — 25 $\times$ 25 mm to 100 TU) there was a marked stimulation of septal cells of the alveoli and a monocytic-lymphocytic infiltration in the walls, making

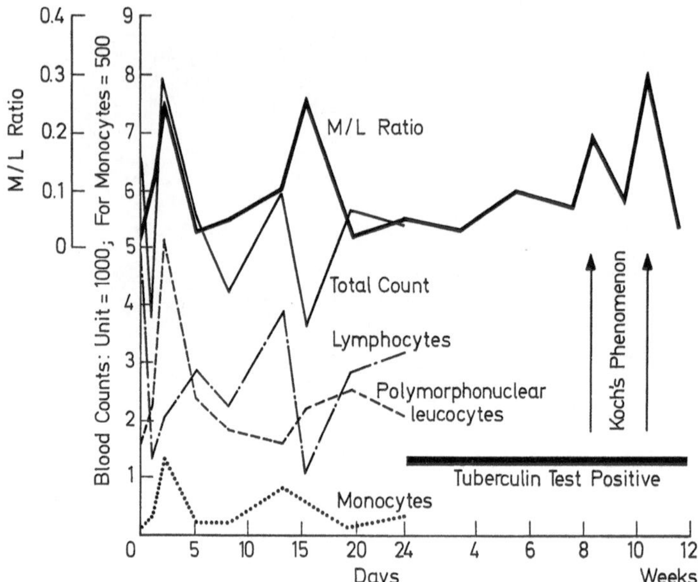

Fig. 5. Peripheral blood changes after i.v. BCG; guinea pig

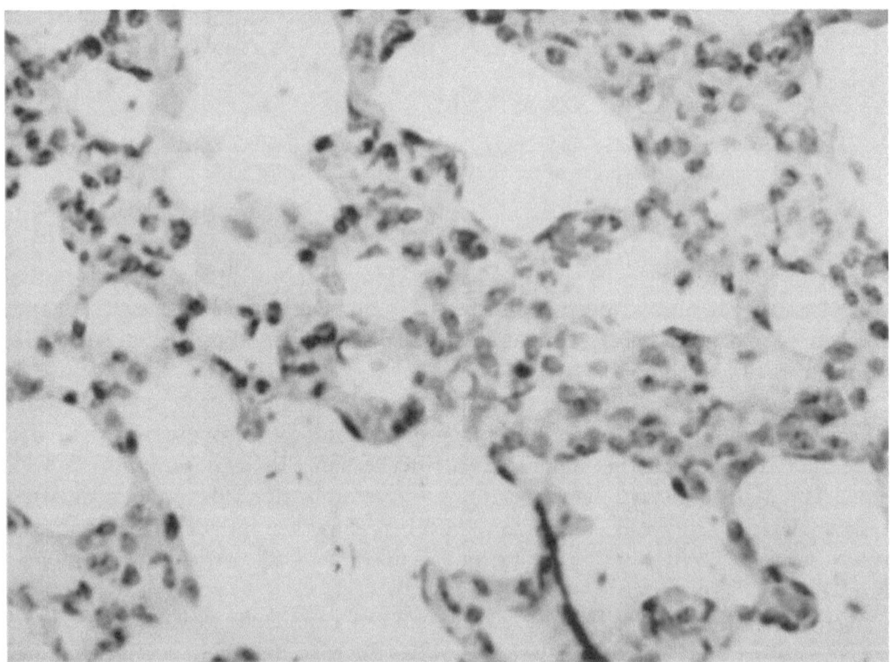

Fig. 6. Lung (1 month after BCG by the aerosol route; guinea pig). The capillary walls are swollen as a result of swelling of the septal cells and intraseptal cellularity; 48 hours after tuberculin testing (H & E $\times$ 250)

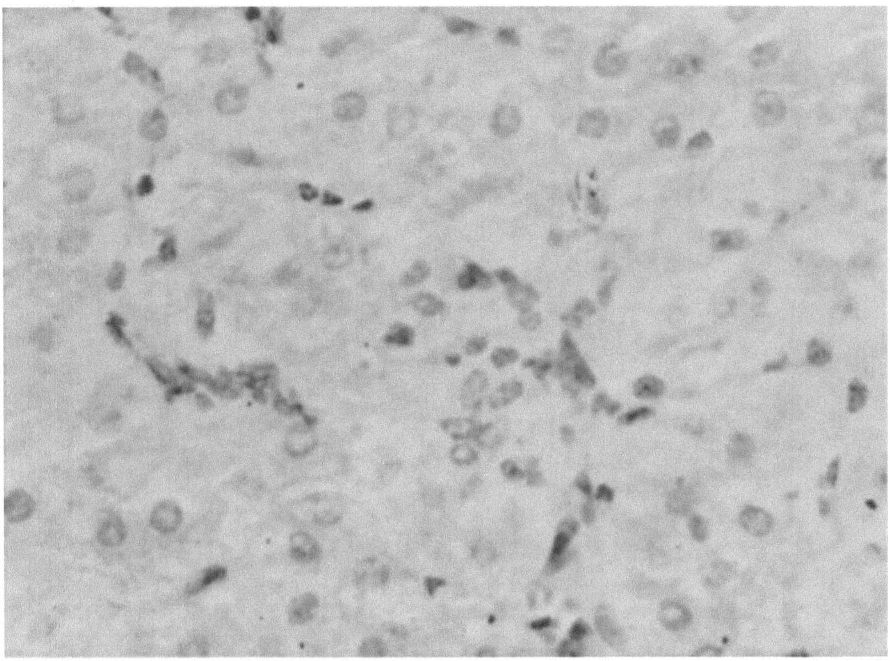

Fig. 7. Liver (1 month after BCG by the aerosol route; guinea pig). The Kupffer cells have increased in number and show increased phagocytosis (H & E $\times$ 500)

them 3 to 5 times the normal thickness (Fig. 6). In the liver there was marked proliferation of the Kupffer cells with increase in their number (Fig. 7).

Intradermal Route. There was a slight to moderate swelling of the septal cells of the lung which was most noticeable at 24 hours (Fig. 8). For the next 6 days the condition remained unchanged. At 8—14 days (after intradermal tuberculin and a positive reaction) there was capillary hyperemia and septal cell swelling as well as an increase in intracapillary cellularity (Fig. 9). At 1 year in the presence of a positive tuberculin reaction there was moderate hyperemia with thickening of the septal walls mainly as a result of intracapillary cellularity of lymphocytes and monocytes.

The Kupffer cells of the liver were not prominent until day 3 (Fig. 10). Increased phagocytosis of red cells and granules was noted at 17 hours. The increased cellularity persisted for about one month and then receded. However, after a positive tuberculin test the cellular reaction was augmented (up to 1 year). A similar pattern of reaction was noted in the spleen, interstitial cells in the kidney, etc.

The blood monocytes, polymorphonuclear leukocytes and lymphocytes paralleled the activity in the tissues.

Oral Route. There was a transitory thickening of the septal cells of the lung (Fig. 11) which disappeared by day 13—14. None of these animals developed positive tuberculin tests so that after testing (observed to 9½ months) there was no hyperemia or proliferation of the septal cells. There was a slight rounding of the Kupffer cells at 5 hours and some increase in their number at 4 days along with increased phagocytosis and basophilia of the cytoplasm. After 13 days these reactions subsided.

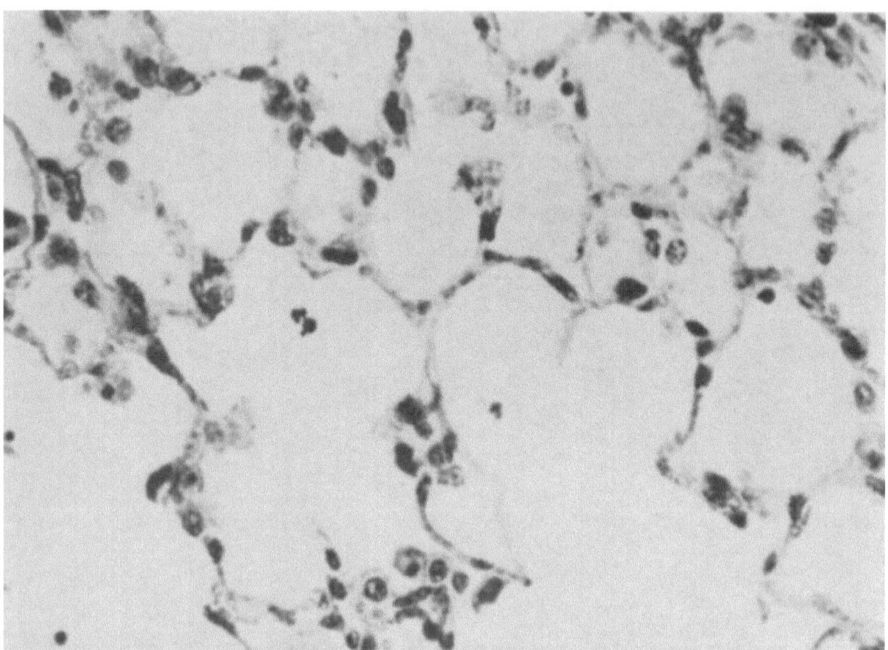

Fig. 8. Lung 24 hours after i.d. BCG (guinea pig). The alveolar walls are thickened as a result of septal cell swelling (H & E × 360)

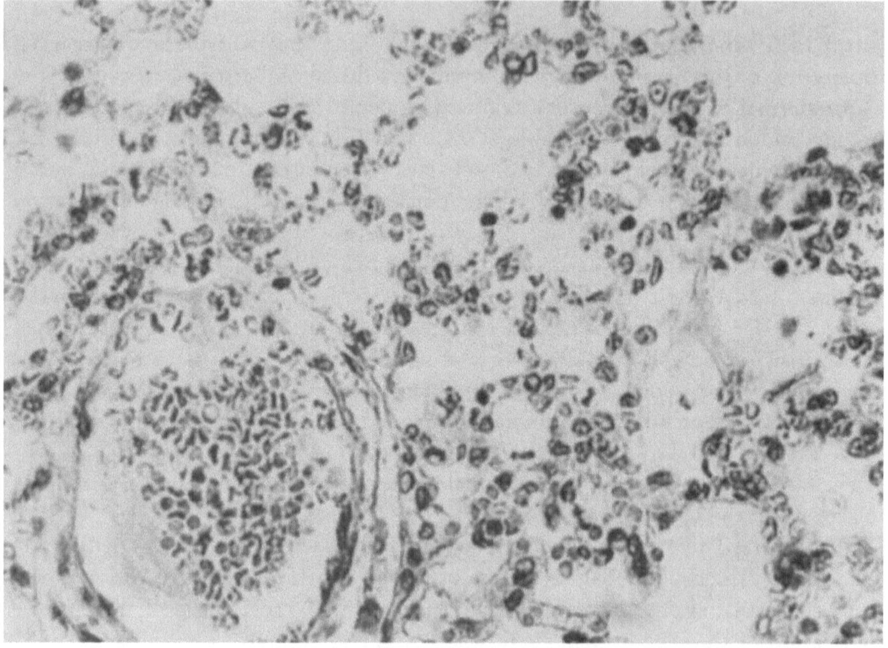

Fig. 9. Lung 14 days after i.d. BCG (guinea pig). The capillaries are diffusely dilated and filled with blood. The tuberculin test was positive on the day of sacrifice (H & E × 360)

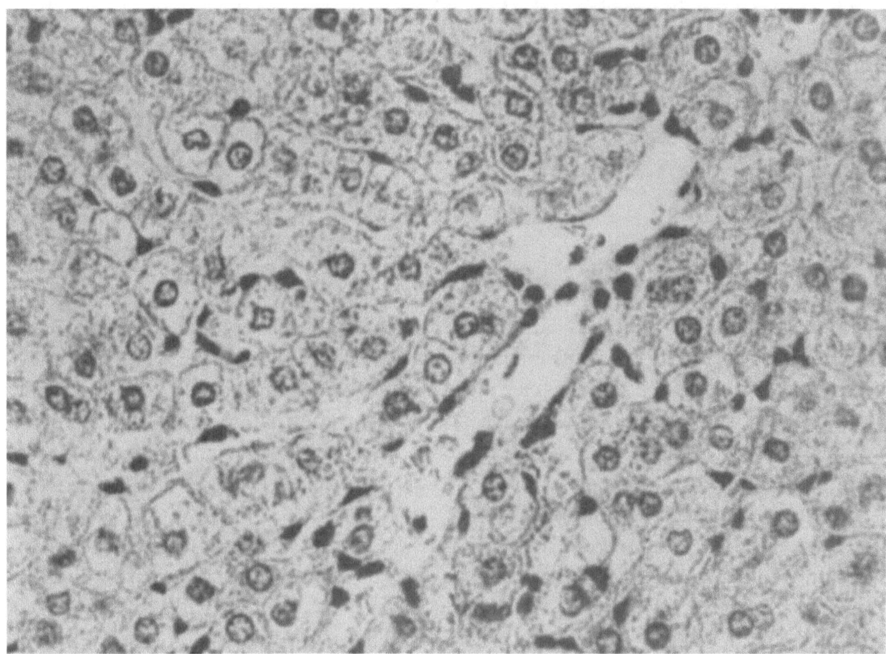

Fig. 10. Liver 3 days after i.d. BCG (guinea pig). The prominence of the Kupffer cells is striking. Clusters of histiocytic cells are common (H & E × 360)

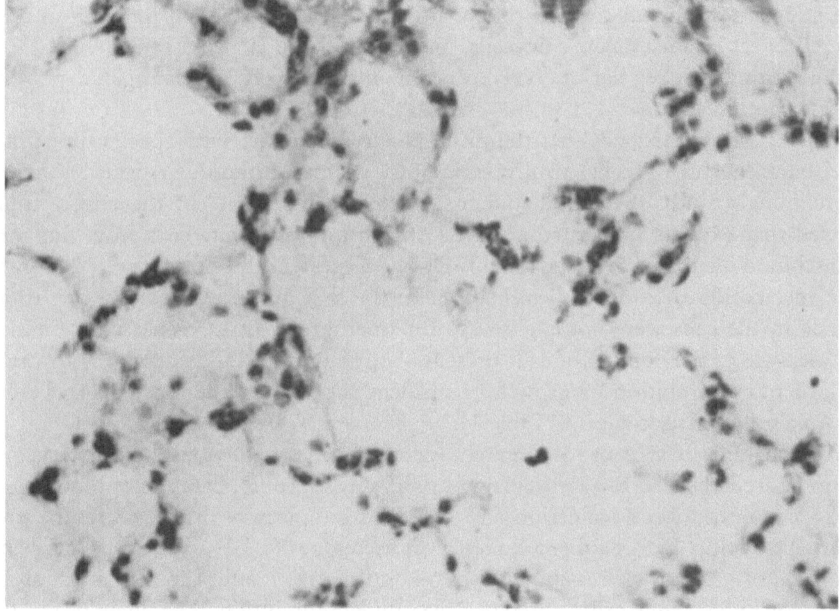

Fig. 11. Lung 48 hours after third daily p. o. dose of BCG (guinea pig). There is a slight increased cellularity that is extracapillary (H & E × 360)

There was some increase in reticulum cell phagocytosis in the spleen plus swelling of the interstitial cells of the kidneys. The sections of the jejunum and ileum were similar to those of normal animals.

Following the ingestion of BCG there was a moderate increase in all cellular elements of the blood. From the fourth to the sixth week the M/L ratio was higher than that of the controls.

Discussion

In the guinea pig, relatively large doses of BCG administered by the intravenous (i.v.) and the aerosol routes resulted in very strong stimulation of the lymphoreticulo-endothelial system in the lung, liver, spleen, kidney and lymph nodes. The oral route gave the least stimulation of the RES and the intradermal route (i.d.) was intermediate between the i.v., aerosol and oral routes. The tuberculin reactions were strongly positive in the i.v., aerosol, and i.d. routes but negative following oral vaccination of suckling guinea pigs.

The generalized response of the RES was manifest for several weeks only. However, after a local severe skin reaction following tuberculin injection there was again a marked general activity of the RES, as indicated by swelling of the septal cells of the lung, Kupffer cells of the liver, reticulum cells of the spleen, lymph nodes, etc. This anamnestic reaction was produced after 1 month, 3 months, 1 year and 14 months (duration of experiment) following BCG vaccination. It is only when the host is in this highly stimulated state that a nonspecific effect is manifest. It is, therefore, of utmost importance to determine the most effective routes of administration in a given species of animal and the proper dosage of BCG to obtain the desired nonspecific effect against neoplastic cells. Furthermore, it is necessary to repeat the specific stimulus at regular intervals to maintain a relatively large antigen depot and the nonspecific effect.

There is now evidence that the macrophages cooperate with specifically stimulated lymphocytes (T cells) to give immunity against intracellular parasites [4, 7]. A preliminary study of medical students vaccinated with BCG by the aerosol route showed that extracts (sonicated at 10 Kc for 10 min) of white cells from the peripheral blood incubated *in vitro* with H37Rv had a greater inhibitory activity 3 months after vaccination than before vaccination. In the first group of students, due to an oversight, the cells were not counted so the micrograms of DNA were determined as a measure of the number of cells present. The amount of DNA necessary to cause 50% or more inhibition of growth of virulent tubercle bacilli was 44.6 μg before and 16.5 μg after vaccination (Table 1).

The anamnestic type of reaction to a specific antigen is demonstrated in a second group of students also BCG-vaccinated by the aerosol route. Samples of blood were taken 3 months after vaccination and a second sample was drawn 48 hours after tuberculin testing. Before tuberculin testing, an average of 29,700 white cells caused no inhibition of growth whereas in 4 out of 6 samples drawn after tuberculin testing an average of 15,500 white cells caused nearly complete inhibition. The difference in the number of cells causing inhibition before and after tuberculin testing is statistically significant ($p = 0.012$) [9] (Table 2). All *in vitro* studies were done as blind tests.

There have been many experimental studies indicating that BCG given prophylactically before challenge will inhibit or completely retard leukemic or tumor grafts [3, 5, 6]. Clinically, as reported elsewhere in this symposium, we have shown that in 1964—1969 in Chicago a sample of 54,514 black infants observed from birth to 6 years

Table 1. Inhibition of virulent tubercle bacilli (H 37 Rv) by disrupted white cells (before and after aerosol vaccination)

Pre-vaccination			Post-vaccination		
Case number	µg DNA	% Growth (controls = 100%)	Case number	µg DNA	% Growth (controls = 100%)
			(Matched)		
—	—	—	151	5.6	51
99	18.5	45	—	—	—
113	39.1	56	149	31.0	57
92	29.3	56	143	8.5	15
94	98.0	56	141	21.0	0
95	63.0	45	—	—	—
108	20.0	51	—	—	—
110	78.2	38	—	—	—
111	11.2	32	—	—	—
Average µg DNA for 50% or more inhibition		44.6		16.5	

Table 2. Inhibition of H 37 Rv by disrupted white cells 3 months after vaccination with BCG aerosol

Before tuberculin test		After tuberculin test	
Number cells in 0.2 ml test mixture	% Growth (control = 100%)	Number cells in 0.2 ml test mixture	% Growth (control = 100%)
30,000	88.63	22,500	104.59
27,000	102.66	11,428	0
28,000	67.59	14,000	93.11
32,000	99.93	25,000	0
35,000	90.99	11,111	0
25,000	99.51	10,322	2.23
31,000	105.32		

of age and vaccinated with BCG at birth suffered only one death due to leukemia. In the non-vaccinated population of Chicago comprising 172,986 infants of the same age and race, 21 leukemic deaths were reported. The annual death rate was 0.31/100,000 for the vaccinated versus 2.02/100,000 for the non-vaccinated. This difference is statistically significant ($p = 0.04$) and represents reduction of 85% in the expected mortality due to leukemia in the vaccinated group.

References

1. Anacker, R. L., Barclay, W. R., Brehmer, W., Goode, G., List, R. H., Ribi, E., Tarmina, D. F.: Effectiveness of cell walls of *Mycobacterium bovis* strain BCG administered by various routes and in different adjuvants in protecting mice against airborne infection with *Mycobacterium tuberculosis* strain H 37 Rv. Amer. Rev. resp. Dis. **99**, 242 (1969).
2. Barclay, W. R., Busey, W. M., Dolgard, D. W., Good, R. C., Janecki, B. W., Kasik, J. L., Ribi, E., Ulrich, C. E., Wolinsky, E.: Protection of monkeys against airborne tuberculosis by aerosol vaccination with Bacillus Calmette-Guérin. Amer. Rev. resp. Dis. **107**, 351 (1973).
3. Halpern, B., Biozzi, G., Stiffel, C., Morton, D.: Effet de la stimulation du système réticulo-endothélial par l'inoculation du Bacille de Calmette-Guérin sur le dévelopment de l'épithéliome atypique T-S de Guérin chez le rat. C.R. Soc. Biol. (Paris) **153**, 919 (1959).
4. Mackaness, G.: The immunology of anti-tuberculous immunity. Amer. Rev. resp. Dis. **97**, 337 (1968).
5. Old, L., Benacerraf, B., Clarke, D., Carswell, E., Storkert, E.: The role of the reticulo-endothelial system in the host reaction to neoplasia. Cancer Res. **21**, 1281 (1961).
6. Old, L., Clarke, D., Benacerraf, B., Goldsmith, M.: The reticuloendothelial system and the neoplastic process. Ann. N.Y. Acad. Sci. **88**, 264 (1960).
7. Patterson, R., Youmans, G.: Multiplication of *Mycobacterium tuberculosis* within normal and "immune" mouse macrophages cultivated with and without streptomycin. Infect. Immunol. **1**, 30 (1970).
8. Rosenthal, S. R.: The general tissue and humoral response to an avirulent tubercle bacillus. Illinois Medical and Dental Monographs. Urbana: University of Illinois Press 1938.
9. Rosenthal, S. R., McEnery, J. T., Raisys, N.: Aerogenic BCG vaccination against tuberculosis in animal and human subjects. J. Asthma Res. **5**, 309 (1968).
10. Schmidt, L., Good, R. C.: Conference on the laboratory evaluation of immunization against tuberculosis. Airlie House, Washington, D. C., Nov. 16—19, 1966. Ann. N.Y. Acad. Sci. **154**, 200 (1968).

Effect of Corynebacterium Parvum on Resistance to Experimental Leukemia in Relation to Genetic Modification of Immunoresponsiveness

C. STIFFEL, D. MOUTON, and G. BIOZZI

Equipe de Recherches n° 70 du C.N.R.S. Fondation Curie,
Institut du Radium, Section de Biologie, Paris

The administration of *Corynebacterium parvum* to experimental animals produces strong and complex modifications of both specific and nonspecific mechanisms of defence against invading bacteria or tumor cells [4, 17]. These modifications are essentially:

1. Stimulation of production of humoral antibody [15].
2. Induction of cell-mediated immunity [15].
3. Stimulation of the phagocytic function of reticuloendothelial phagocytes [9, 16, 17].

The same treatment enhances resistance to allogeneic and syngeneic tumors in the mouse [10, 12, 14]. We discuss here the protective effect of *C. parvum* against the development of experimental leukemia in the mouse. The degree of protection depends on the dose, time and route of inoculation of *C. parvum* in relation to the number of leukemic cells administered. An example of the protective effect of *C. parvum* against AKR leukemia is presented in Table 1.

In our laboratory, "high" and "low" responder lines of mice have been developed by selective breeding for the character "agglutinin production to heterologous

Table 1. Protection induced by *C. parvum* treatment against AKR leukemia transmitted in (CBA × AKR) F_1 (from [12])

	Number of leukemic cells transmitted [b]	Mortality %
Control	1,000	100
	100	100
C. parvum [a]	1,000	47
	100	17

[a] 1 mg *C. parvum* injected i. p. 7 days before leukemia.
[b] Intraperitoneal injection of AKR spleen cells from leukemic donors.

erythrocytes" [1, 2, 4, 5]. After 20 consecutive generations the two lines of mice are homozygous for the character investigated. The difference in humoral responsiveness of the two lines is extremely large, as indicated in Fig. 1. The peak level of anti-sheep erythrocyte agglutinin production in "low" responder mice is 1/80 and in "high" responders about 1/5000. *C. parvum* treatment markedly increases the peak level of agglutinins in "high" responders (1/160,000) but has only a small effect on "low" responder mice. The "high" and "low" responder animals also differ in their

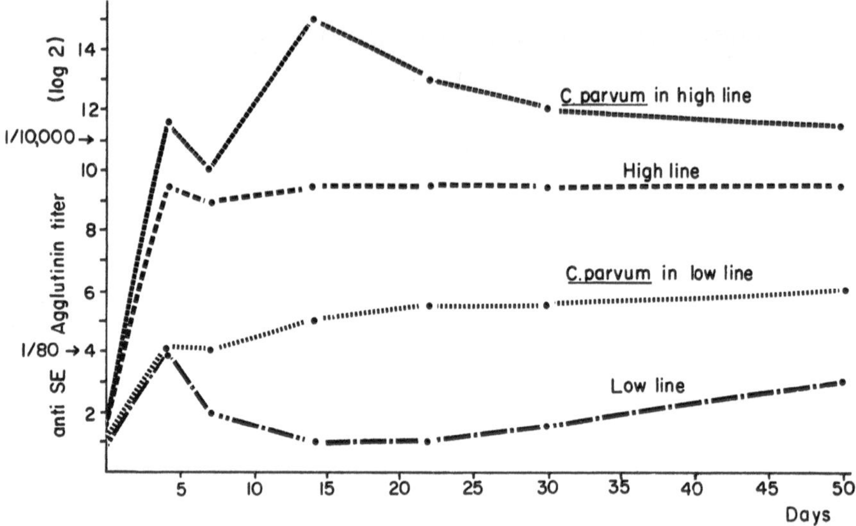

Fig. 1. Effect of *C. parvum* on the kinetics of anti-sheep erythrocyte agglutinin production in "high" and "low" responder mice. *C. parvum* treatment: 500 μg i.v. 4 days before 5 $\times$ 10^8 SE i.v. (from [5])

humoral responsiveness to many other unrelated antigens and haptens [3, 8, 11]. In fact, they differ at the level of a group of genes regulating the rate of proliferation and differentiation of B- derived lymphocytes after antigen stimulation. The potentialities of T- derived lymphocytes, however, were not modified by selective breeding; they are the same in both lines. Skin graft in "high" and "low" responder recipients are rejected in the same time (about 12 days) but the amount of cytotoxic antibody induced by skin grafting is much higher in the "high" responder than in the "low" responder. Other types of cell-mediated immunity such as induction of graft-versus-host reaction [6], PHA stimulation [13] and delayed hypersensitivity responses are of the same intensity in "high" and "low" responders.

Selective breeding for the character "antibody production" has therefore induced a clearcut dissociation between humoral responsiveness, which is very different, and cell-mediated immunity which is of the same intensity in both lines. These animals therefore are useful for measuring the relative importance of humoral and cellular immunity in mechanisms of defence against tumors and infections [4, 7].

The "high" and "low" mice ace derived from random-bred albino mice. Therefore, the leukemia specificity of inbred strains cannot be transmitted in these animals.

The results presented in Table 2 demonstrate that the ability to synthesize antibody characteristic of "high" and "low" responders can be inherited to a large extent by F_1 hybrids of "high" and "low" lines with various inbred strains of mice. The difference in immune responsiveness of F_1 hybrids of "high" and "low" lines is strong enough to justify a study of the resistance to isogenic leukemia transmitted in these hybrids.

Table 2. Peak level of anti-sheep erythrocyte (SE) agglutinin after immunization with 5×10^8 SE i. v.

	Peak anti-SE agglutinin
High responder line	1/10,000
Low responder line	1/100
AKR	1/300
DBA/2	1/1,280
C_{57}Bl	1/1,280
(AKR × high) F_1	1/2,000
(AKR × low) F_1	1/100
(DBA/2 × high) F_1	1/3,840
(DBA/2 × low) F_1	1/480
(C_{57}Bl × high) F_1	1/2,560
(C_{57}Bl × low) F_1	1/240

Table 3. Susceptibility of ("high" × DBA/2) F_1 hybrids and ("low" × DBA/2) F_1 hybrids to DBA/2 leukemia (from [4])

	No. of ascitic cells injected	Mortality %	Mean survival time (days)
(high × DBA/2) F_1	10^3 i. v.	100	10
	10^4 i. p.	100	10.4
(low × DBA/2) F_1	10^3 i. v.	100	10
	10^4 i. p.	100	9.8

No marked difference between "high" and "low" responders hybrids is found in the resistance to DBA/2 leukemia (Table 3) and AKR leukemia (Table 4). However, a slightly higher resistance of "low" responder hybrids in terms of survival time is observed in AKR leukemia.

As Table 1 shows, the administration of *C. parvum* markedly increases the resistance of isogenic animals to AKR leukemia. Similar results are obtained in ("high" or "low" × AKR) hybrids (Fig. 2). This treatment produces a definitive increase in survival in both hybrids, but the protective effect is stronger in ("low" × AKR) F_1.

The similarity in the resistance of "high" and "low" responder hybrids to AKR and DBA/2 leukemia in spite of their different humoral responsiveness suggests that, if specific immunological defence is mounted against these leukemia it should be of cellular nature. Indeed, the fact that they produce more facilitating antibody, renders the "high" responder mice more vulnerable to some infections and tumors that are susceptible to the enhancement phenomenon [4, 7].

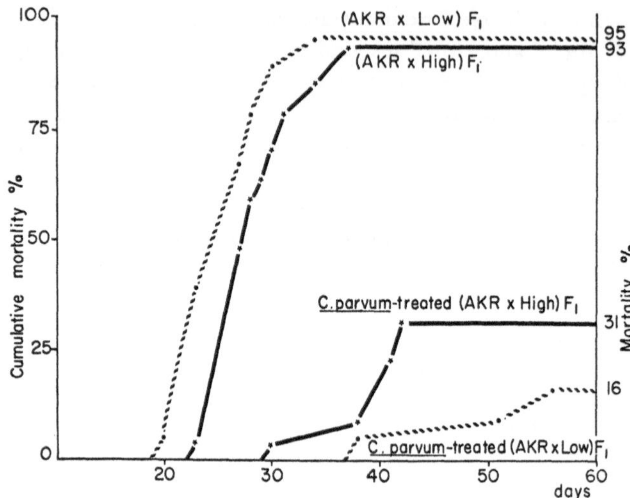

Fig. 2. Effect of *C. parvum* on the resistance of ("high" × AKR) F_1 hybrids and ("low" × AKR) F_1 hybrids to AKR leukemia. *C. parvum* treatment: 1 mg i. p. 6 days before i. p. injection of 100 spleen cells from leukemic AKR mice (from [4])

Table 4. Susceptibility of hybrids ("high" × AKR) F_1 and ("low" × AKR) F_1 to i. p. injection of various doses of spleen cells form leukemic AKR mice (from [4])

No. of spleen cells injected	("high" × AKR) F_1		("low" × AKR) F_1	
	Mortality %	Mean survival time (days)	Mortality %	Mean survival time (days)
10^2	93	29.4	95	27
10^3	100	22	80	30
10^4	98	14.4	100	19.4

References

1. BIOZZI, G., STIFFEL, C., MOUTON, D., BOUTHILLIER, Y., DECREUSEFOND, C.: Genetic selection for antibody production in mice. In: Protides of the Biological Fluids, p. 161 (PEETERS, H., Ed.). Oxford: Pergamon Press 1970.
2. BIOZZI, G., ASOFSKY, R., LIEBERMAN, R., STIFFEL, C., MOUTON, D., BENACERRAF, B.: Serum concentrations and allotypes of immunoglobulins in two lines of mice genetically selected for "high" and "low" antibody synthesis. J. exp. Med. **132**, 752 (1970).
3. BIOZZI, G., STIFFEL, C., MOUTON, D., BOUTHILLIER, Y., DECREUSEFOND, C.: Genetic regulation of the function of antibody producing cells. Progr. Immunol. **1**, 529 (1971).
4. BIOZZI, G., STIFFEL, C., MOUTON, D., BOUTHILLIER, Y., DECREUSEFOND, C.: Importance de l'immunité spécifique et non spécifique dans la défense antitumorale. Ann. Inst. Pasteur **122**, 685 (1972).
5. BIOZZI, G., STIFFEL, C., MOUTON, D., BOUTHILLIER, Y., DECREUSEFOND, C.: Cytodynamics of the immune response in two lines of mice genetically selected for "high" and "low" antibody synthesis. J. exp. Med. **135**, 1071 (1972).
6. BYFIELD, P. E., HOWARD, J. G.: Equivalent graft-versus-host reactivity of spleen cells from two lines of mice genetically selected for "high" and "low" humoral antibody formation. Transplantation **14**, 133 (1972).

7. Dodin, A., Wiart, J., Stiffel, C., Bouthillier, Y., Mouton, D., Decreusefond, C., Biozzi, G.: Paris: Communication à la Société Française d'Immunologie 1972 (in press).
8. Del Guercio, P., Zola, H.: A comparison of the immune response to DNP in mice genetically selected for "high" and "low" antibody synthesis. Immunochemistry **9**, 768 (1972).
9. Halpern, B. N., Prevot, A. R., Biozzi, G., Stiffel, C., Mouton, D., Morard, J. C., Bouthillier, Y., Decreusefond, C.: Stimulation de l'activité phagocytaire du système reticuloendothelial provoquée par *Corynebacterium parvum*. J. reticuloendoth. Soc. **1**, 77 (1964).
10. Halpern, B. N., Biozzi, G., Stiffel, C., Mouton, D.: Inhibition of tumor growth by administration of killed *Corynebacterium parvum*. Nature **212**, 853 (1966).
11. Howard, J. G., Christie, G. H., Courtenay, B. M., Biozzi, G.: Studies on immunological paralysis. VIII. Pneumococcal polysaccharide tolerance and immunity differences between the Biozzi "high" and "low" responder lines of mice. Europ. J. Immunol. **2**, 269 (1972).
12. Lamensans, A., Stiffel, C., Mollier, M. F., Laurent, M., Mouton, D., Biozzi, G.: Effet protecteur du *Corynebacterium parvum* contre la leucémie gréffée AKR. Relations avec l'activité catalasique hépatique et la fonction phagocytaire du Système Reticulo-endothélial. Rev. franç. Etud. clin. biol. **13**, 773 (1968).
13. Liacopoulos-Briot, M., Bouthillier, Y., Mouton, D., Lambert, F., Decreusefond, C., Stiffel, C., Biozzi, G.: Comparison of skin allograft rejection and cytotoxic antibody production in two lines of mice genetically selected for "high" and "low" antibody synthesis. Transplantation **14**, 590 (1972).
14. Mathe, G., Pouillart, P., Lapeyraque, F.: Active immunotherapy of L 1210 leukaemia applied after the graft of tumor cells. Brit. J. Cancer **23**, 814 (1969).
15. Neveu, T., Branellec, A., Biozzi, G.: Propriétés adjuvantes de *Corynebacterium parvum* sur la production d'anticorps et sur l'induction de l'hypersensibilité retardée envers les protéines conjuguées. Ann. Inst. Pasteur **106**, 771 (1964).
16. Stiffel, C., Mouton, D., Biozzi, G.: Kinetics of the phagocytic function of reticulo-endothelial macrophages *in vivo*. In: Mononuclear Phagocytes. p. 335 (Van Furth, Ed.). Oxford: Blackwell 1970.
17. Stiffel, C., Mouton, D., Biozzi, G.: Rôle des macrophages dans l'immunité non spécifique. Ann. Inst. Pasteur **120**, 412 (1971).

The Influence of Mycobacterium Bovis and Corynebacterium Parvum on the Phospholipid Metabolism of Macrophages

P. G. MUNDER and M. MODOLELL

Max-Planck-Institut für Immunbiologie, Freiburg

The more than 300 organic and inorganic substances that have been used as immunological adjuvants exhibit a wide range of physical or physicochemical characteristics. For instance, SiO_2 [9], vitamin A [1] and FREUND's adjuvant [3] appear to have nothing in common, but all are adjuvants. Since it seems rather difficult to find a common physical or chemical property which could possibly explain the action of adjuvants, one is inclined to speculate that perhaps all immunological adjuvants act via a common pathway in the organism. As early as 1925, RAMON [10] proposed an inflammatory reaction as a necessary prerequisite for immunostimulation by a substance like tapioca. Many powerful adjuvants, like FREUND's adjuvant, induce an inflammatory reaction and local and systemic formation of granulomas [7]. Macrophages are usually the predominant cells in these granulomas (for review see [4]) and seem to play an important role in mediating the immunostimulating action of an adjuvant. We studied various biochemical parameters during phagocytosis and observed a distinct alteration of the phospholipid metabolism of macrophages after the ingestion of silica (which has been shown to be an adjuvant; [9]). The crystalline silica particles activate an intracellular phospholipase A [5] which breaks down cellular phospholipids and causes accumulation of free fatty acids and lysophosphatides. We obtained similar results when other well-known adjuvants (FREUND's adjuvant and $Al(OH)_3$) were phagocytosed by macrophages [6]. Large numbers of cells were needed for these studies and a method had to be developed to enable the most important cellular phospholipids to be prelabeled with 1-^{14}C-oleic acid. We then studied the following adjuvants in their influence on the phospholipid metabolism of macrophages: FREUND's complete adjuvant, *Bordetella pertussis*, *Mycobacterium bovis*, *Corynebacterium parvum*, *Salmonella minnesota* R 595, endotoxin, vitamin A bentonite, $Al(OH)_3$, saponin and some unusual ones like $Ca_3(PO_4)_2$ and $BeSO_4$. This report deals in particular with the results obtained when mouse peritoneal exudate cells (PEC) were incubated with BCG and *Corynebacterium parvum*.

Methods

Prelabeling of PEC with 1-^{14}C-oleic Acid

Mice were injected intraperitoneally with 2 mg lysolecithin (1-acyl-glycero-3-phosphorylcholine), dissolved in 0.5 ml 0.155 M NaCl. 4 days later the animals were killed by N_2, the peritoneum exposed and the cells washed out by injecting 5 ml Eagle's medium + 10 mM HEPES, pH 7.1. Usually 20—30 × 10^6 PEC per animal were collected; of these 70—80% were macrophages and the rest small and medium-sized lymphocytes. These cells were centrifuged once (200 g), resuspended in the same serum-free medium and incubated with ultrasonicated 1-^{14}C-oleic acid (2 nM per 2 × 10^7 PEC) for 2 hours at 37 °C. After 2 hours the 1-^{14}C-oleic acid is incorporated into the cellular phospholipids and lipids with the following proportions: 0.5—1% lysolecithin, 4—6% sphingomyelin, 55—60% lecithin, 8—12% cephalin, 2—4% oleic acid and 15—20% neutral lipids. These prelabeled cells were the incubated with the adjuvants as indicated.

The phospholipids and lipids were extracted and separated by thin-layer silicic acid chromatography as previously described [5]. The separated compounds were scraped off and measured in a scintillation counter (Packard Tri-Carb Liquid Scintillation Spectrometer).

Results

PEC and Corynebacterium Parvum

Figs. 1 and 2 show the results of a typical experiment. The same quantity of PEC (25 × 10^6) was incubated with three different concentrations of *C. parvum*.

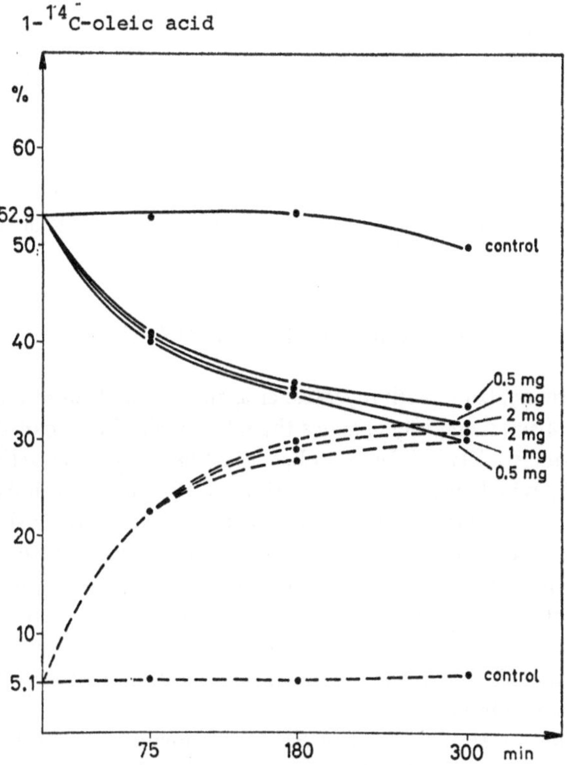

Fig. 1. PEC and *Corynebacterium parvum*. 25 × 10^6 peritoneal exudate cells (PEC) prelabeled with 1-^{14}C-oleic acid and incubated with different amounts of *C. parvum*. Lecithin (solid line) and free 1-^{14}C-oleic acid (dashed line) as percent of total recovered radioactivity

During the first hour after addition of the adjuvant the labeled cellular lecithin is rapidly degraded and 1-^{14}C-oleic acid accumulates. This indicates activity of a cellular phospholipase A, as further confirmed by the findings in Fig. 2.

With all concentrations of *C. parvum* there is a significant increase in labeled lysolecithin.

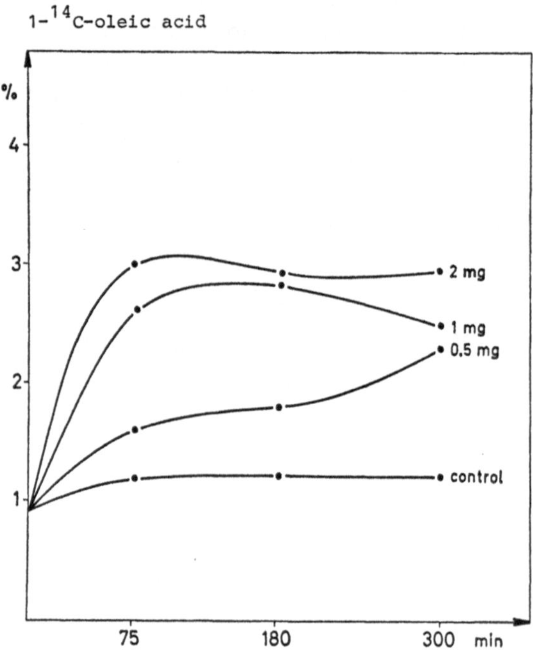

Fig. 2. PEC and *Corynebacterium parvum*. Accumulation of labeled lysolecithin (further results of the experiment described in Fig. 1)

PEC and Mycobacteria (BCG)

When PEC are incubated with mycobacteria, almost identical results are obtained. Addition of mycobacteria rapidly changes the relative distribution of the 1-^{14}-C-oleic acid in the prelabeled PEC. The mycobacteria like *C. parvum* activate a cellular phospholipase A, which leads to degradation of the labeled cellular lecithin and cephalin with a corresponding increase in free 1-^{14}C-oleic acid, as shown in Fig. 3.

These changes are more pronounced after 24 hours (Fig. 4). In addition to the degradation of the diacylphospholipids lecithin and cephalin, prelabeled neutral lipids are also broken down after 24 hours. Lysolecithin (not shown) rose from 0.8% in the control to 2.9% with added mycobacteria. These changes in the relative distribution of phospholipids and neutral lipids have been observed with all the adjuvants mentioned above.

No such changes were found when PEC were incubated with bacteria without known adjuvant activity, e.g. *Staphylococcus albus* (Fig. 5).

There was no significant difference in the relatice distribution of 1-^{14}C-oleic acids as compared to the control even when PEC were incubated with 5 mg *Staph. albus* for 24 hours. A similar result was obtained when titaniumdioxide or starch granules were phagocytosed by PEC. Thus, the activation of a cellular phospholipase A, resulting in the degradation of lecithin and cephalin and accumulation of free fatty acids and lysolecithin, seems to be a specific effect of adjuvants and not of phagocytosis.

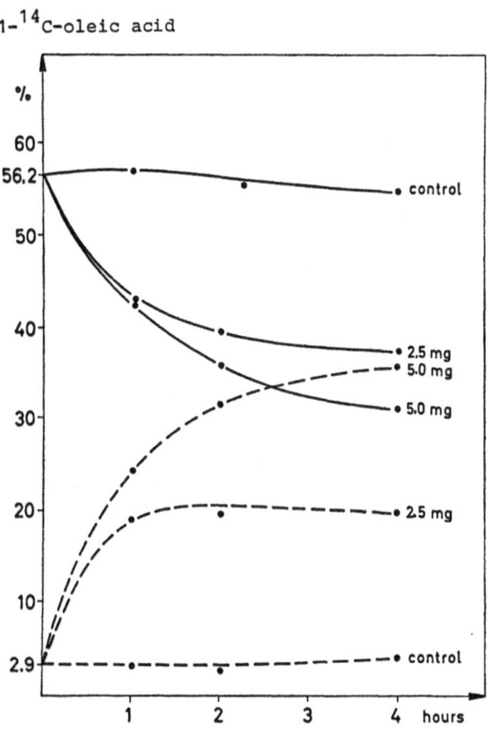

Fig. 3. PEC and BCG. 25 × 10^6 PEC prelabeled with 1-^{14}C-oleic acid and incubated with different amounts of BCG. Lecithin (solid line) and free 1-^{14}C-oleic acid as percent of total recovered radioactivity

If activation of phospholipase A in macrophages after phagocytosis or contact with adjuvants were a common mechanism for mediating the immunostimulating activity of a given substance, the products of this enzyme activity should themselves show adjuvant activity. Free fatty acids were indeed found by Dresser [2] to act like adjuvants. Using his system for studying "adjuvanticity", we found that the other reaction product, lysolecithin, indeed acts as an adjuvant *in vivo*, as shown by the results of a typical experiment (Fig. 6). In this experiment groups of 10 mice were injected intraperitoneally with 2 mg lysolecithin per animal. 4 days later 4 mg bovine gamma globulin was injected by the same route. After 10 days, the primary immune response was measured by injecting about 10 μg ^{125}I-BGG and determining the radioactivity remaining in the circulation 24 and 72 hours later.

The elimination of ^{125}I-BGG is greatly enhanced when the animals are pretreated with 0.2—2 mg lysolecithin. The adjuvant effect is even more evident with synthetic analogous of lysolecithin which cannot be metabolized in the organism [11].

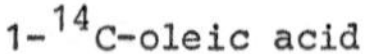

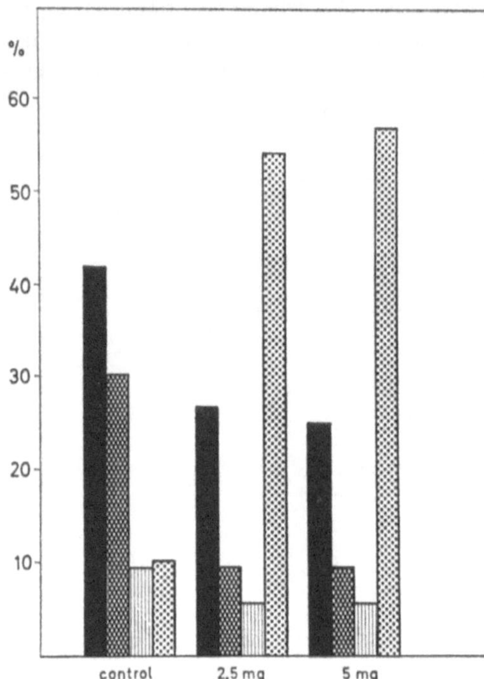

Fig. 4. PEC and BCG. Relative distribution of 1-^{14}C-oleic acid-labeled phospholipids and neutral lipids 24 hours after incubation with BCG (for details see Fig. 3). lecithin, neutral lipids, cephalin, free fatty acids

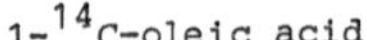

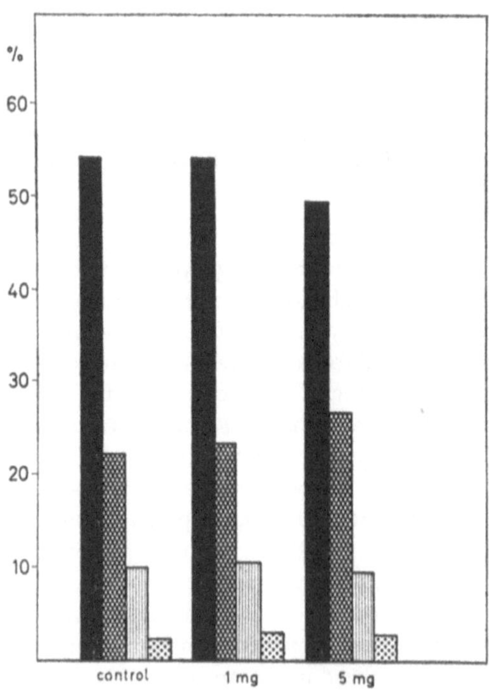

Fig. 5. PEC and *Staphylococcus albus*. Relative distribution of 1-^{14}C-oleic acid-labeled phospholipids and neutral lipids in 25 $\times$ 10^{6} PEC, 25 hours after incubation with 1—5 mg *Staph. albus*. lecithin, neutral lipids, cephalin, free fatty acids

The fact that lysolecithin and its analogous show adjuvant acivity seems to support the hypothesis that adjuvants act by activating a phospholipase A in macrophages. The resulting accumulation of highly surface-active lysophosphatides could in turn influence the membrane-bound process of antigen recognition or the proliferation of antigen-triggered cells [8].

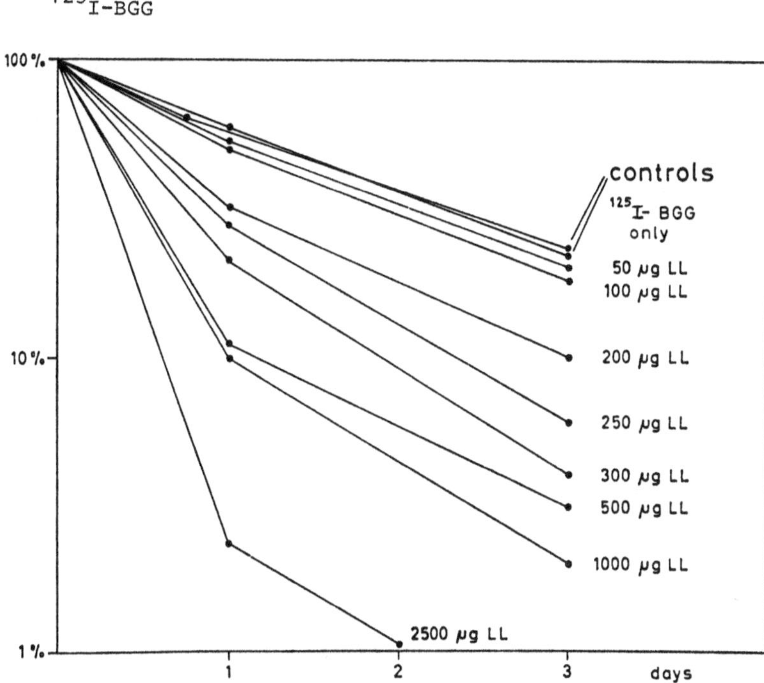

Fig. 6. Adjuvant activity of lysolecithin. Primary BGG-antibody production in the mouse (lysolecithin (LL) given 4 days before the antigen). Immune response measured by elimination of ^{125}I-BGG on day 10. (Protein: 4 mg soluble BGG per mouse)

References

1. Dresser, D. W.: Adjuvanticity of vitamin A. Nature (Lond.) **217**, 527 (1966).
2. Dresser, D. W.: Effectiveness of lipid and lipidophilic substances as adjuvants. Nature (Lond.) **191**, 1169 (1961).
3. Freund, J.: The mode of action of immunologic adjuvants. Fortschr. Tuberk.-Forsch. **7**, 130 (1956).
4. Haas, R., Thomssen, R.: Über den Entwicklungsstand der in der Immunologie gebräuchlichen Adjuvantien. Ergebn. Mikrobiol. **34**, 27 (1960).
5. Munder, P. G., Ferber, E., Modolell, M., Fischer, H.: The influence of various adjuvants on the metabolism of phospholipids in macrophages. Int. Arch. Allergy **36**, 117 (1969).
6. Munder, P. G., Modolell, M., Ferber, E., Fischer, H.: The relationship between macrophages and adjuvant activity. In: Mononuclear Phagocytes, p. 445 (van Furth, Ed.). Oxford: Blackwell 1970.

7. MYRVIK, Q. N., LEAKE, E. S., OSHIMA, S.: A study of macrophages and epitheloid-like cells from granulomatous (BCG-induced) lungs of rabbits. J. Immunol. **89**, 745 (1962).

8 NILAUSEN, K.: Growth promoting effect of lysolecithin in Chinese hamster cells *in vitro*. Nature (Lond.) **217**, 268 (1968).

9. PERNIS, B., PARANETTO, F.: Adjuvant effect of silica (tridymite) on antibody production. Proc. Soc. exp. Biol. (N.Y.) **110**, 390 (1962).

10. RAMON, M.: Sur la production des antitoxines. C. R. Acad. Sci. (Paris) **181**, 157 (1925).

11. WESTPHAL, O., FISCHER, H., MUNDER, P. G.: Adjuvanticity of lysolecithin and synthetic analogues, Abstracts p. 319. Interlaken, Switzerland: 8th Internat. Congr., 3—9th Sept. 1970.

Separation and Purification of Cord Factor (6,6' Dimycoloyl Trehalose) from Wax C or from Mycolic Acids

M. B. Goren [1] and Olga Brokl [2]

Department of Microbiology [1] and
Division of Research, National Jewish Hospital and Research Center [2]
University of Colorado School of Medicine, Denver, Colorado

Mycolic acids are among the most persistent contaminants of the toxic mycobacterial glycolipid 6,6' dimycoloyl trehalose (cord factor). In the past, alternating multiple silicic acid and magnesium silicate column chromatography has been employed, not always successfully, to purify the glycolipid [5]. An ancillary problem which required a rapid method for bulk separation of certain derivatives of mycolic esters from the *free acids* led us to a disarmingly simple solution to both problems and ultimately to an improved method for isolation and purification of cord factor from wax C. Neutral lipids can be separated from quite large amounts of contaminant *free* carboxylic acids by adsorption chromatography on the free base form of diethylaminoethylcellulose (DEAE). The present paper describes the rationale and methods developed for cord factor purification.

Rationale

In appropriate, sufficiently polar solvents, such as ether or mixtures of ether and methanol (9 : 1, or 7 : 3), neutral lipids are quickly eluted from a DEAE column. Free carboxylic acids are retained by apparently reversible salt formation but salts of carboxylic acids are not adsorbed. With continued elutriation the adsorbed carboxylic acids move slowly down the column, more rapidly when the solvent contains minute quantities (much less than a column equivalent) of, for example, acetic acid. These slow elutions can lead to separations of carboxylic acid mixtures. On the other hand, bulk elution of the acids is rapidly effected with slightly more concentrated acetic acid solution.

Methods

Column Preparation

Although DEAE may be used alone, we prefer a 2 : 1 mixture of cellulose and DEAE. DEAE (Carl Schleicher and Schuell Co., 0.96 meq/g) was treated and packed according to methods described by [6] (cf. [3]), with some modifications. After soaking overnight in glacial acetic acid, 1.5 g DEAE was pressed gently with a thick Teflon rod to break up larger pieces. Whatman cellulose powder (3 g) was well mixed into the acetic acid suspension of DEAE and the mixture filtered and washed with $CHCl_3$ to eliminate most of the acetic acid. A chromatography column 11 mm in diameter was then loaded in $CHCl_3$ to give a column about 22 cm in height. It is usually kept in the acetate form, and in methanol.

For use in bulk separation of neutral lipids from carboxylic acids, the column is converted to the free base form with 50 ml of methanol containing 2 ml C.NH_4OH, washed with 100 ml methanol and then with the loading solvent (ether or mixtures of ether and methanol). For larger columns, the same proportions of solvents were used. Column effluents were examined by ir spectrophotometry and by thin-layer chromatography.

Thin-Layer Chromatography (TLC)

Samples were examined on silica gel with magnesium silicate as binder [6]. For rapid identification of less polar contaminants in cord factor samples, or for simplified initial preparative TLC, a mixture of benzene and ethanol (30/2-4) may be used. Cord factor moves only very slightly from the origin, and does not separate satisfactorily from mycolic acids. For separation of mycolic acids and a more rigorous detection of small amounts of impurities in cord factor, a silica gel plate is first developed to the top in a 2 : 1 mixture of $CHCl_3$ and acetic acid and dried at about 35° for 30 min; the samples are then applied and 15 cm of plate developed in a 100:7:0.7 mixture of $CHCl_3$, CH_3OH and acetic acid. In this system, cord factor has an R_f value of about 0.24 whereas the R_f for mycolic acid is 0.77.

Experimental [1]

Separation of Cord Factor and Mycolic Acid

For examining bulk separation of cord factor from contaminant mycolic acids, an extensively chromatographed but still slightly impure sample of cord factor (about 3.5 mg) was mixed with 1.5 mg of mycolic *acid*. (Note: if present in the mixture as a salt, mycolic acid must be transformed into the free carboxylic acid by HCl in ethereal solution, or by a modification of [1] (lipid extraction procedure.) The mixture was dissolved with a few drops of $CHCl_3$, diluted with a 70:30 mixture of ether and CH_3OH, applied to a small column of cellulose-DEAE (1 g : 0.5 g) in the free base form, and washed with the ether-methanol. All of the cord factor, entirely freed from mycolic acid, was recovered in the first 20 ml of effluent. The mycolic acid was then rapidly eluted with ether –CH_3OH–acetic acid (70 : 30 : 1). The ir spectra of Fig. 1 show that the characteristic carboxylic acid peaks (ca. 1700 cm^{-1}) due to free mycolic acid in the mixture (Fig. 1a) are no longer present in the spectrum of the cord factor product (Fig. 1b).

---

[1] In the succeeding sections, the following abbreviations will be used: E ether, M methanol, HAc acetic acid, C chloroform.

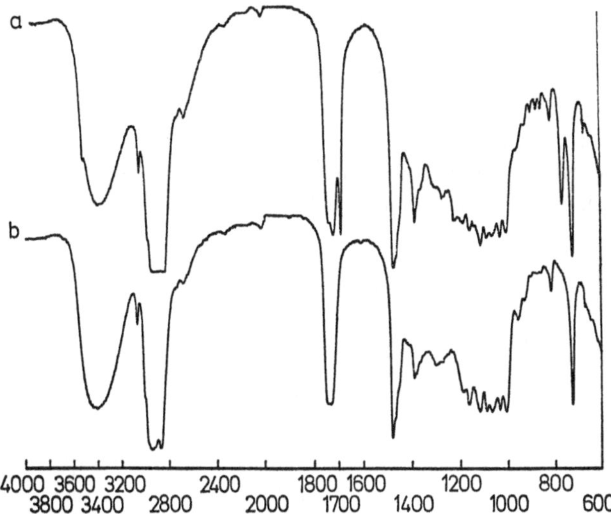

Fig. 1a and b. Separation of a synthetic mixture of cord factor and mycolic acid: ir spectra, a mixture, b recovered cord factor

Purification of Cord Factor "Concentrates"

In examining many cord factor products currently used in various laboratories, we have usually detected (by TLC) four or five additional components, some major, usually including mycolic acid (and its salts), so that the trehalose glycolipid constitutes perhaps no more than one third of the mixture. Similar conclusions were reached by Ribi *et al.* (personal communication). We were able to separate the cord factor along with other neutral lipids (including glycolipids) from the mycolic acid by the procedure described above. Separation of the cord factor from both more and less polar neutral glycolipids was a more difficult task.

Our initial efforts to separate all the constituents in one cellulose-DEAE (free base) chromatography were partly successful. However, slow methanolysis was occurring during the prolonged elution, with resultant partial destruction of glycolipids. This solvolysis, catalyzed by the free-base form of DEAE, is genuine and gentle, and we have subsequently employed this method for a somewhat selective partial deacylation of mycobacterial sulfatide derivatives (Goren and Brokl, in preparation).

Employment of the cellulose-DEAE adsorbent as the *acetate* eliminated solvolysis problems and retained the high-resolving efficiency of the DEAE in separating the neutral (and glyco) lipids. Thus a dual column operation is required: 1. a rapid adsorption of mycolic and other contaminant acids from an ether-methanol (80 : 20) solution of the cord factor "concentrate" charge by passage through cellulose-DEAE (free base form). This allows total recovery of the neutral components (including the glycolipids) and later of the mycolic acids. 2. Selective, stepwise chromatography of the mycolic acid-free, neutral, cord factor-containing lipids on cellulose-DEAE acetate. We have subsequently found that a cellulose column alone can be used in the latter separations, but the capacity and resolving efficiency are poorer than with the DEAE acetate. The cellulose-DEAE acetate separation of a glycolipid-neutral lipid mixture as derivable from step 1. above is detailed in Table 1, supplemented by the ir spectra of Fig. 2.

TLC patterns assessed against relatively pure cord-factor preparations and the ir spectra of Fig. 2 support the assignments given in Table 1. Fig. 2a shows the ir spectrum of the cord-factor concentrate as received. The broad band (1500—1600) is attributable to carboxylate absorption[2] and is eliminated by mixing an ether solution of the sample with dilute aqueous HCl to convert these to the free acids. A new

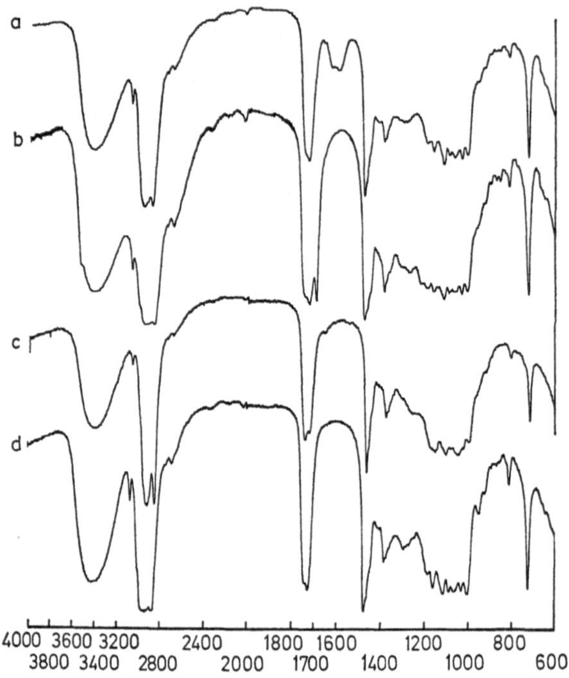

Fig. 2a—d. Purification of cord factor "concentrates" on cellulose-DEAE (acetate): ir spectra, a initial cord factor concentrate, b same after acid wash to convert mycolate salts to free acids, c cord factor-like glycolipid (CF II), d purified cord factor

band appears at about 1700 cm^{-1} due to the free carboxylic acid generated (Fig. 2b). After DEAE (free base) adsorption in E-M (80 : 20) this peak disappears. Fig. 2c shows the fractions rich in glycolipid, provisionally designated CF II. The small peak at about 808 cm^{-1} we have found consistently in every trehalose derivative so far examined [3]. In most other respects this spectrum resembles but does not coincide exactly with that of the purified cord factor itself (Fig. 2d) and includes peaks attributable to mycolate moieties (1025, 3070 cm^{-1}) [2].

---

[2] The carboxylates may be generated when wax C is chromatographed on Mg silicate or on silicic acid, which ordinarily results in partial hydrolysis of cord factor (Noll and Bloch, 1955). DEAE-acetate chromatography seems to be free of this degradative activity.

Table 1. Separation on cellulose-DEAE (acetate) of neutral lipids derived from cord factor "concentrates". Charge: about 4 mg mixture on 1.0 g cellulose — 0.5 g DEAE acetate [a]

Step	Solvent	Volume	Contents
1	E/M 98/2	50 ml	About 1 mg mixed neutral and glycolipids with traces of cord factor
2	E/M 98/2	15 ml	Traces (cord factor + Cord Factor II [b])
3	E/M 98/2	20 ml	Cord factor with trace of CF II
4	E/M 98/2	20 ml	Uncontaminated cord factor (trace)
5	E/M 95/5	100 ml	2.3 mg uncontaminated cord factor
6	E/M 90/10	100 ml	0.7 mg: cord factor + polar glycolipid [c]
7	E/M 85/15	75 ml	0.2 mg: cord factor + polar glycolipid

[a] We have not yet determined the maximum charge of lipids applicable to any individual column of this type. Ether loading and elution before setting up any ether-methanol gradients seems advisable to prevent slight losses of cord factor in early fractions.

[b] Provisional designation of an incompletely characterized trehalose mycolate of higher mobility in TLC than cord factor.

[c] Probably trehalose monomycolate.

Isolation and Purification of Cord Factor from Wax C

These experiments indicated that utilization of the principles developed should permit isolation of pure cord factor preparations from the usual starting material, wax C. At our institution a wax C sample of presently unknown origin but of excellent quality was prepared several years ago by a visiting scientist, Dr. L. T. Rzucidlo (Medical School, Warsaw). Its content of cord factor is unfortunately meager (about 1—1.5%).

One gram of this wax C was dissolved in $CHCl_3$ and recovered after Millipore filtration, redissolved in about 45 ml anhydrous ether and filtered through a sintered glass funnel. The clear ether [3] solution was charged to a cellulose-DEAE (free base) column (12 + 6 g) and the column washed with about 250 ml ether to elute 700 mg of nonpolar components. (TLC indicated no cord factor or mycolic acid leakage.) The remainder of the primary chromatograms are detailed in Table 2.

On the basis of TLC examination, fractions 4—6 were combined as cord factor concentrates. To eliminate possible contamination, the mixture was gently acid-treated by the modified [1] procedure and the recovered glycolipids rapidly passed in 80 : 20 E-M through a small (1.5 : 0.5 g) cellulose-DEAE (free base) column. Essentially all of the glycolipid (43 mg) was recovered in the first 25 ml of effluent. Subsequent fractions contained small amounts of similar components, and finally considerably more polar glycolipids. The principal fraction, judged to contain about 25% cord factor, had significant toxicity for ice, 4 out of 7 dying from 4 injections of oil solutions of the mixture (injections on alternate days; 10 μg per injection). The ir spectrum (Fig. 3) exhibited many of the characteristic features of cord factor (cf. Fig. 2d). A peak at about 1645 (possibly associated with some unsaturated moiety)

[3] An ir spectrum of the wax C showed no carboxylate absorption (ca. 1550 cm^{-1}) but strong carboxylic acid carbonyl absorption (ca. 1700 cm^{-1}). The small glycolipid content was indicated in the shallowness of ordinary broad absorption between 3200—3600 cm^{-1}.

and one at about 750 cm^{-1} are not characteristic of cord factor and were ultimately attributable to a much less polar glycolipid which was separated from this mixture in subsequent purifications.

Table 2. Primary chromatography of wax C on cellulose-DEAE (free base). Charge: 1 g wax C

	Effluent solvent	Volume	Wt. residue	Composition
1	Anhydrous ether	250 ml	700 mg	Non-polar lipids. May be largely phthiocerol dimycocerosate (Noll, 1957)
2	Anhydrous ether	125 ml	4 mg	Non-polar lipids
3	E/M 80/20	75 ml	0.4 mg	Trace glycolipids
4	E/M 80/20	75 ml	43 mg	Mixed glycolipids with cord factor
5	E/M 80/20	30 ml	4 mg	Mixed glycolipids with cord factor
6	E/M 80/20	75 ml	1.5 mg	Mixed glycolipids with cord factor
7	E/M 80/20	45 ml	2.2 mg	Mixed glycolipids plus non-polar
8	E/M/HAc 80/20/2	200 ml	253 mg	Principally mycolic acids
9	$CHCl_3$/MeOH/Acetic 80/20/3	150 ml	1.2 mg	—
10	Wash column with methanol			

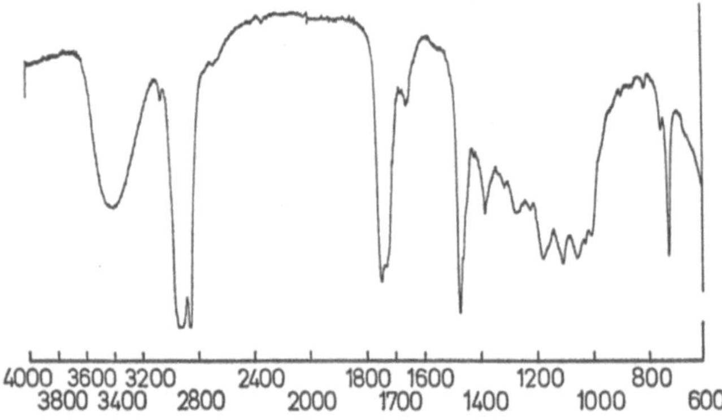

Fig. 3. Toxic cord factor-glycolipid concentrate from chromatography of wax C on cellulose-DEAE (free base): ir spectrum

Final Purification

A variant of the cellulose-DEAE (acetate) chromatography previously described yielded a slightly impure cord factor preparation contaminated only by traces of the less polar "CF II" and of the more polar glycolipid. (Its ir spectrum is essentially indistinguishable from that of our purest preparations). About 8 mg was rechromatographed very carefully on a 7 g column of cellulose powder with slow progression of elutrients: ether containing respectively 2% methanol (150 ml), 2.5% methanol (75 ml), 4% methanol (100 ml), 5% (75 ml), 6% (50 ml) and 7% (50 ml). Fractions (25 ml) were collected throughout and each examined by TLC. The fractions exhibiting no discernible contamination were combined to yield 6.0 mg of the most purified material, obtained as a colorless solid on dissolution in a small amount of ether and precipitation in the cold with methanol.

The product had a melting point of 42—43 °C. Optical rotation was measured in a Rudolph photoelectric polarimeter in 2,2,4 trimethyl pentane solution.

$$\alpha_D^{24} = +32.7° \pm 2° \ (c = 0.0026).$$

Fig. 4 compares the ir spectrum of the present preparation a) with that of a cord factor sample originally prepared by NOLL and BLOCH b) and with a partially purified

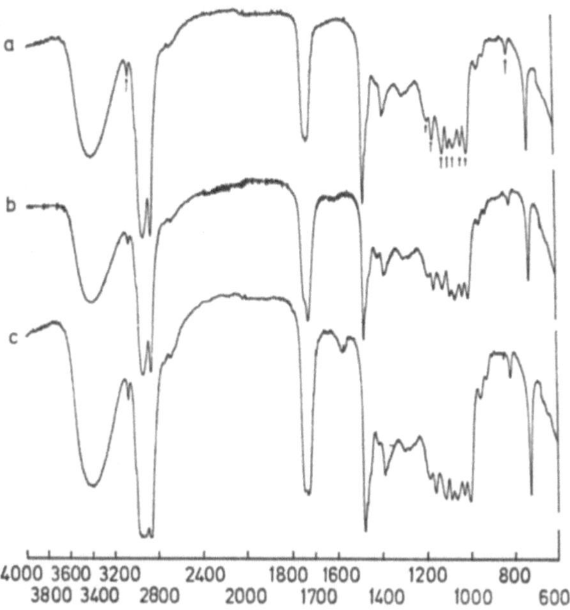

Fig. 4a—c. Infrared spectra of various purified cord factor preparations, a product from present study, b product of NOLL and BLOCH, c product of RIBI (incompletely purified, cf. text)

sample kindly given to us by E. RIBI *et al.* for certain degradative studies. The latter contains a small amount of a mycolate salt detectable by ir spectrophotometry, and by micro-particulate gel chromatography. The NOLL and BLOCH product may be slightly contaminated with the suspected unsaturated component found in the product of Fig. 3 (shallow absorption near 1640 cm^{-1}).

[4] have given the absorption bands which characterized their purest cord factor preparations, and our spectra are generally in excellent agreement with theirs. Beyond the 807 cm^{-1} peak associated with trehalose (arrow) and one at about 3070 cm^{-1} (arrow) associated with cyclopropane methylene groups in the mycolate moieties [2], the cord factor spectrum is uniquely characterized by a group of seven closely spaced major peaks in the "fingerprint region": 997, 1022, 1057, 1079, 1104, 1152 and 1175 cm^{-1} (arrows). We believe these may be used as valid criteria for judging the apparent purity of a cord factor preparation.

Acknowledgements

This investigation was supported by Grant No. AI-08401 of the U.S.-Japan Cooperative Medical Science Program administered by the National Institute of Allergy and Infectious Diseases of the National Institutes of Health, Department of Health, Education and Welfare.

References

1. BLIGH, E. G., DYER, W. J.: A rapid method of total lipid extraction and purification. Canad. J. Biochem. **37**, 911 (1959).
2. GASTAMBIDE-ODIER, M., DELAUMENY, J.-M., LEDERER, E.: Mise en évidence de cycles propaniques dans divers acides mycoliques de souches humaines et bovines de *Mycobacterium tuberculosis*. C.R. Acad. Sci. (Paris) **259**, 3404 (1964).
3. GOREN, M. B.: Sulfolipid I of *Mycobacterium tuberculosis*, strain H 37 Rv. I. Purification and properties. Biochim. biophys. Acta (Amst.) **210**, 116 (1970).
4. NOLL, H.: The chemistry of some native constituents of the purified wax of *Mycobacterium tuberculosis*. J. biol. Chem. **224**, 149 (1957).
5. NOLL, H., BLOCH, H.: Studies on the chemistry of the cord factor of *Mycobacterium tuberculosis*. J. biol. Chem. **214**, 251 (1955).
6. ROUSER, G., KRITCHEVSKY, G., HELLER, D., LIEBER, E.: Lipid composition of beef brain, beef liver, and the sea anemone: two approaches to quantitative fractionation of complex lipid mixtures. J. Amer. Oil Chemists' Soc. **40**, 425 (1963).

Granuloma Induction and Stimulation of the Immune Response in Mice with Trehalose -6,6′-Dimycolate

A. Bekierkunst

Hebrew University, Hadassah Medical School, Jerusalem

It has recently become evident that a chemically defined glycolipid derived from tubercle bacilli, trehalose-6,6′-dimycolate (cord factor) is able to induce a typical granulomatous response in the lungs of mice after an intravenous injection of as little as 1—5 μg. The cellular composition of the tubercles induced by cord factor is indistinguishable from the caused by living BCG. In both cases the granulomas are composed of epitheloid cells, macrophages and lymphocytes. The effect of cord factor seems to be specific, since neither different wax D preparations nor phosphatidyl inositomannosides from mycobacteria were able to induce comparable granuloma formation. Cord factor injected in the foot pad of mice induced histological changes similar to those following injections of living BCG bacilli. Both materials induced in the draining lymph nodes the formation of granulomas, marked hyperplasia of the lymphoid tissue in the paracortical zone and accumulations of macrophages. In some cases the macrophages were very numerous and replaced part of the lymphoid tissue, especially at the periphery of the nodes. Such an accumulation of macrophages was also evident in the draining lymph nodes after injection of emulsion, wax D and Freund's adjuvant, but after emulsion and wax D the macrophages were much less prominent.

I wish to emphasize that after injections of cord factor and BCG bacilli no cellular reaction was seen in the internal organs, such as liver, spleen and lungs, after 28 or 30 days of observation]1, 2].

There is a general consensus that an infection with BCG bacilli causes a change in the immunological apparatus of the host. One of its expressions is an increased antibody response to unrelated antigens. We have assumed that there is a connection between the above activities of BCG bacilli and the local cellular reaction caused by the bacilli in the host tissue. It was conceivable that cord factor, which causes a similar cellular response, would induce a similar change in the immune response of the host. This could be seen from the following experiments. Three groups of mice were injected with 10 μg of cord factor, with Freund's adjuvant and emulsion, and 5 days later challenged with SRBC; the antibody response was strongest in the group pretreated with cord factor. The differences were clearly evident during the 24 days of observation both in hemagglutination and antiglobulin titers. This increased antibody response was related to the cellular reaction in the draining lymph nodes. In mice pretreated with cord factor but with the antigen injected into the contralateral foot pad, the antibody response was much weaker than in the other groups injected with cord factor and antigen in the same foot pad.

The cellular reaction induced by cord factor in the draining lymph nodes of mice after administration into the foot pads persists for at least 30 days, so it was reasonable to expect that the antibody response would be also increased for more than 5 days. Such was the case. The antibody response after intervals of 10, 15 and 20 days was always stronger in the groups pretreated with cord factor.

As mentioned, the reaction in the draining lymph nodes is indistinguishable from that to living BCG bacilli, and in some respects it is very similar to that induced by complete Freund's adjuvant. According to Freund, the adjuvant action of incomplete and complete adjuvants is due to the persistence of antigen at the site of injection, to the slow systemic dissemination of the antigen, and to the cellular reaction involved. In addition, the antigen should be incorporated into the emulsion; an injection of antigen and adjuvant at separate sites is no more effective than injection of antigen alone. We have assumed that the increased antibody response induced by Freund's complete antigen is due mainly to the cellular reaction cause apparently by the cord factor of the mycobacteria. In ordeı to test this assumption, we compared the response to SRBC in groups pretreated with cord factor, living BCG and Freund's complete adjuvant. The hemagglutination titers in the 3 test groups were all much higher than in the emulsion control group and they were quite close and statistically indistinguishable.

As already indicated, no cellular reaction was seen in the internal organs such as liver, spleen and lungs after about 30 days of observation following injection os cord factor and living BCG into the foot pad. A similar lack of cellular response waf also observed by Carter *et al.* [5] after injections of Freund's adjuvant into the foot pads. If the adjuvant effect of Freund's adjuvant and of a BCG infection is due to the cellular reaction evoked in the tissues of the host, there should be no increased antibody response after the injection of the antigen into a site at which no cellular reaction is anticipated. In an experiment in which groups of mice were given living BCG bacilli and Freund's adjuvant in the left foot pad, the hemagglutination titers in the sera of animals injected with SRBC into the contralateral foot pad were at levels resembling those in animals not treated at all with BCG and Freund's adjuvant. The above results also seem to indicate that cord factor is responsible for the adjuvant activity of the mycobacteria present in the mineral oil of the emulsion, as well as for the action of multiplying BCG bacilli. This assumption has been tested in mice injected with SRBC in incomplete Freund's adjuvant, containing cord factor, wax D or mycobacteria. The strongest antibody response to SRBC was in the group treated with the antigen incorpoıated in incomplete Freund's adjuvant containing 5 μg of cord factor [4].

As already mentioned, our basic assumption was that the activity of living BCG is connected with the host cellular reaction induced by the multiplying bacilli at the site of their lodgment. Since cord factor causes a similar cellular reaction, it might be expected to act like BCG under the same experimental conditions. We tested whether the formation of lung adenomas induced by urethane can be affected by an intravenous infection with BCG or by intravenous injections of relatively small amounts of cord factor. Both materials cause a strong granulomatous response in the lungs but urethane is a known inducer of adenomas in the lungs of mice. Six groups of mice were used in the experiment. 17 days after pretreatment of the mice with BCG, cord factor, wax D, and wax D + cord factor, mice of all groups were injected i.p. with urethane. 2 days after injection of urethane, groups pretreated with cord factor, wax D, and cord factor + wax D were injected i.v. with 5 μg cord factor, wax D, or a mixture of both, respectively, twice weekly for 7 weeks. After that time the animals were killed. The presence of the tumors in the lungs and the cellular response was evaluated microscopically. Usually 3 to 5 sections were examined, and their surfaces measured. The granulomas composed of epithelioid cells, macrophages and lymphoid cells were present in lungs of all mice treated with BCG, cord factor, or cord factor + wax D. There was significant suppression of urethane-induced tumors in the groups treated with BCG, cord factor, or a mixture of cord factor and wax D. The differences between these groups and the control groups were statistically significant. The suppression of urethane-induced emerging tumor cells in the lung tissue is apparently due to the encounter with host cells produced during infection with BCG bacilli or treatment with cord factor. These results seem to indicate the importance of the local cellular reaction in suppression of the tumor cells [3].

Our interpretation is supported by recent reports that injection of living BCG bacilli into established intradermal tumors in guinea pigs caused tumor regression and prevented the development of metastases. Our results demonstrate the possibility of suppressing primary tumor formation in mice through induction of a granulomatous cellular response with a chemically defined substance.

References

1. Bekierkunst, A., Levij, I. S., Yarkoni, E., Vilkas, E., Adam, A., Lederer, E.: Granuloma formation induced in mice by chemically defined mycobacterial fractions. J. Bact. **100**, 95 (1969).
2. Bekierkunst, A., Levij, I. S., Yarkoni, E., Vilkas, E., Lederer, E.: Cellular reaction in the foot pad and draining lymph nodes of mice induced by mycobacterial fractions and BCG bacilli. Infect. Immun. **4**, 245 (1971).
3. Bekierkunst, A., Levij, I. S., Yarkoni, E., Vilkas, E., Lederer, E.: Suppression of urethane-induced lung adenomas in mice treated with trehalose-6,6′-dimycolate (cord factor) and living bacillus Calmette-Guérin. Science **174**, 1240 (1971).
4. Bekierkunst, A., Yarkoni, E., Flechner, I., Morecki, S., Vilkas, E., Lederer, E.: Immune response to sheep red blood cells in mice pretreated with mycobacterial fractions. Infect. Immun. **4**, 256 (1971).
5. Carter, R. L., Jamison, D. G., Vollum, R. L.: Histological changes evoked in mice by Freund's complete adjuvant. J. Path. Bact. **97**, 503 (1969).

Corynebacterium Parvum: An Immunomodulator

B. Halpern

Institut d'Immunobiologie, INSERM U 20, Association Claude Bernard, Laboratoire Associé au C.N.R.S. et E.P.H.E. Hôpital Broussais, Paris

My interest in anaerobic corynebacteria as an activator of the reticuloendothelial system (RES) was a natural extension of investigations on the role of the RES in immunity, carried out since 1950 in collaboration with Biozzi, Benacerraf, Stiffel, and some other coworkers [8]. There is evidence that some microbial products, e.g. endotoxins, or infective agents such as mycobacteria, whether pathogens, e.g. *Mycobacterium tuberculosis*, BCG, or saprophytes, e.g. *M. phlei*, are potent RES activators. Animals injected with such substances usually develop resistance to a variety of unrelated infections [14] and also to tumor invasion [10]. Excellent results have been obtained with a water-soluble extract of *M. phlei* [9], indicating clearly that such biological effects are attributable to chemical constituents of the bacterial membranes.

Such results suggest that RES stimulants are widely distributed in the microbial world, and that the resistance-enhancing properties are non specific and closely related to the stimulation of the RES.

In quest of new and possibly more potent substances, I turned in 1962 to *Corynebacterium parvum*. Nothing was then known about the biological properties of anaerobic *Corynebacteria*, except that they possess neither endotoxins nor exotoxins, display an affinity for the lymphoid organs and, when injected into rabbits, produce an intense but reversible hyperplasia of the reticuloendothelial organs [19, 20].

We reported first in 1963 [13] the powerful and long lasting proliferation and stimulation of the RES induced by killed *C. parvum* and the concomitant low toxicity then the protective effects of *C. parvum* against bacterial infections [7] and its enhancement of resistance to malignant tumors [11]. Thus, we established the main biological properties of *C. parvum*, which are rather similar to those previously described for mycobacteria.

Other workers soon confirmed our findings on its protective action against bacterial infection [21] and the enhancement of resistance to tumor invasion [24, 17]; the latter property has since been confirmed in man by Israel and myself [16, 12].

The number of recent publications suggests that interest in the biological and possible therapeutic properties of *C. parvum* is growing. I review here briefly, in the light of recent developments, the main properties of *C. parvum* as an immunostimulant of a new type, and the possible mechanisms of its action in immunological and tumoral processes.

Stimulation of the RES

The fact that *C. parvum* is a potent RES stimulant can be roughly evaluated by the increase in the relative weight of the liver and spleen which, with appropriate doses, can increase two- and ten-fold, respectively [13, 21]. Histologically, both organs show an intense granulomatous reaction, involving proliferation of macrophages and other mononuclear cells which may differentiate into lymphocytes and plasma cells [22].

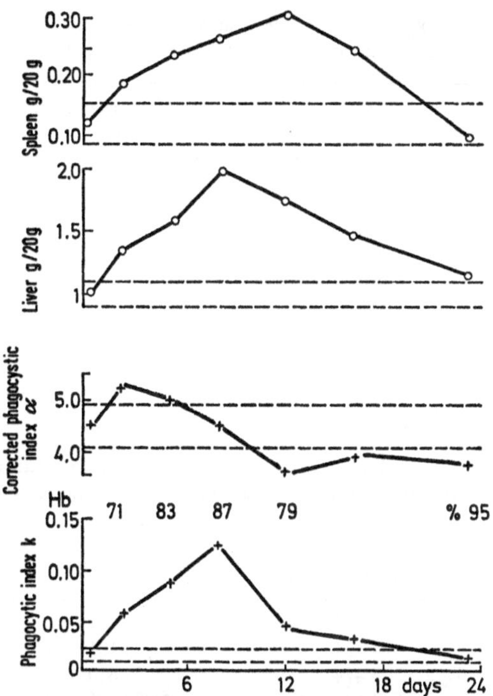

Fig. 1. Effect of intravenous injection of 255 µg of *C. parvum* (dry weight) on the reticuloendothelial system in mice. From top to bottom: relative weight of the spleen; relative weight of the liver; corrected phagocytic index α; percentage of hemoglobin; phagocytic index K. Dotted lines indicate range of standard deviation of the index K in controls

The induced histological changes are generally reversible. A more quantitative technique is to measure the clearance of colloidal carbon particles, as this indicates a significant and longlasting increase in the phagocytic activity of the RE cells [13].

Fig. 1 is a typical example of this phenomenon in mice. Following intravenous injection of 500 µg of *C. parvum*, an increase in the phagocytic index (K) is discernible 48 hours later. The increase in K is roughly linear until day 8, when it reaches its peak at about 9 to 10 times the basal level. K then begins to decline and reaches normal level on about day 25. One of the remarkable features of action of *C. parvum* action on the RES is the absence of the negative phase regularly observed with endotoxin-containing bacteria.

Effect on Antibody Synthesis

In these experiments [7], rabbits were immunized with BSA administered intravenously at a dose of 2.5 mg. The animals were divided into two groups of six; the control group received only the antigen; the treated group received an intravenous injection of 2 mg/kg of *C. parvum* on day 4, followed on day 0 by the injection of 2.5 mg of BSA. The animals of both groups received a booster dose of 2.5 mg BSA on day 21.

Table 1. Rate of antibody synthesis in rabbits immunized with BSA (2.5 mg/kg i.v.) in control and in *C. parvum*-treated groups [a]

Days	Control antibody titer	*C. parvum* treated group antibody titer
5	2 [b]	2
7	44	2 048
10	172	2 752
13	1 429	4 181
17	810	5 546
21	554	5 546

[a] *C. parvum* was given i.v. 2 mg/kg 4 days before
[b] Expressed as the reverse of the dilution giving a positive reaction.

Table 2. Rate of antibody synthesis in rabbits immunized with BSA in control and in *C. parvum*-treated groups: anamnestic response

Days	Control antibody titer	*C. parvum*-treated group antibody titer
1	117 [a]	4 106
2	24	4 101
3	5 474	32 810
5	744 106	1 070 421
8	395 946	1 070 421
12	101 034	447 829
17	49 834	202 069
23	27 648	114 688
31	12 458	111 957
40	6 229	68 266

[a] Expressed as the reverse of the dilution giving a positive reaction.

Antibody titers were determined at regular intervals by the classical BDB passive haemagglutination technique. The respective proportions of IgM and IgG in the induced antibody were determined by treatment with 2-mercaptoethanol. The results are summarized in Tables 1 and 2.

Striking differences were observed in the response of the two groups of animals: 1. In the *C. parvum*-treated group, antibody rose rapidly to levels about 50—100 times those of the controls. 2. At its peak level, the amount of antibody synthesized by the treated animals was about 400% of normal. 3. When antibody synthesis was almost at its peak in the *C. parvum* treated animals, it was declining sharply in the control group. Similar differences were observed in the secondary response.

IgM-type antibody was prevalent during the early primary response, while IgG antibody formed the bulk of immunoglobulins during the secondary response in both group of animals.

Enhanced Resistance to Bacterial Infections

Previous investigations with mycobacteria showed significantly increased resistance of the treated animals to experimental infection with various *Salmonella* [14]. Other authors reported similar protective action of mycobacteria (or their extracts) against a variety of bacteria, e.g. *Klebsellia pneumoniae*, *Staphylococcus aureus* [23].

Table 3. Number of *Brucella* in the spleen of control and *C. parvum*-treated animals at various times after the injection of *C. parvum*. Animals sacrificed 10 days after the infective inoculumm (30,000 live *Brucella abortus*)

Animal No.	Group A (14 days)		Group B (21 days)		Group C (28 days)	
	control	*C. parvum*	control	*C. parvum*	control	*C. parvum*
1	> 10 000	48	5 000	43	> 10 000	15
2	> 10 000	17	± 1 500	41	± 1 000	1
3	> 10 000	12	± 1 225	0	± 625	1
4	> 10 000	0	± 1 200	0	316	0
5	> 5 000	0	± 1 200	0	225	0
6	> 5 000	0	± 1 100	0	217	0
7	> 5 000	0	± 1 050	0	187	0
8	± 2 000	0	± 1 000	0	110	0
9	± 1 200	0	± 950	0	66	0
10	± 1 200	0	± 875	0	67	0
11	664	0	452	0	46	0
12	565	0	276	0	39	0

In a recent study [7], we investigated the effect of *C. parvum* on experimental *Brucella abortus* infections in mice. The treated groups received a single dose of 0.25 mg (dry weight) of *C. parvum* administered intraperitoneally 14, 21 or 28 days before the infective inoculum. All animals were injected intraperitoneally with about 30.000 live *Brucella* (strain 544). The animals were sacrificed 10 days after the infection, and the bacteria in the spleen counted. The results are summarized in Table 3.

All the control groups had a high level of infection, the bacteria often exceeding 10.000 per spleen, while in the treated groups the majority of animals were sterile.

These results have been confirmed by Adlam *et al.* [1], who reported that *C. parvum* afforted considerable protection in animals challenged with a lethal dose of *Brucella*. The maximum effect was observed when *C. parvum* was given 4 days before infection.

The protective action of *C. parvum* against *Brucella abortus* infection merits some discussion. With the strain used in our experiments, mice develop a chronic infection with low mortality. Bacteremia is rare as the infection is mainly intracellular. The RE cells are the main repository of the bacteria, which are mostly located in the spleen. It is generally accepted that humoral antibodies are of little importance in Gram-negative infections and that recovery results from destruction of the bacteria by phagocytes. The protective effect of *C. parvum* may be due to the increased number of phagocytes. Treatment with BCG [2] or with *C. parvum* [6] increases also the proteolytic and bactericidal activity of the stimulated macrophages. This is probably the mechanism by which the *C. parvum*-stimulated animals destroy the infecting bacteria.

Protection against infection with *Staphylococcus aureus* in mice receiving *C. parvum* was reported recently by ADLAM *et al.* [1]. More surprising is the observation reported by the same authors that pretreatment with *C. parvum* resulted in marked resistance of mice to intracranial challenge with approximately 400 LD_{50} of *Bordetella pertussis*. The mechanism of this protective action remains to be explained more particularly since *C. parvum* (like *B. pertussis*) increases the susceptibility of mice to histamine.

Enhancement of Resistance to Viral Infection

CERUTTI [4] has recently shown protective action of *C. parvum* against infections with Mengo virus. The experiments were carried out with Swiss mice, known to be good producers of interferon. The virus was administered intraperitoneally at a dose of 100 LD_{50}. *C. parvum* was administered, at various dosages 7 days before the infective inoculum.

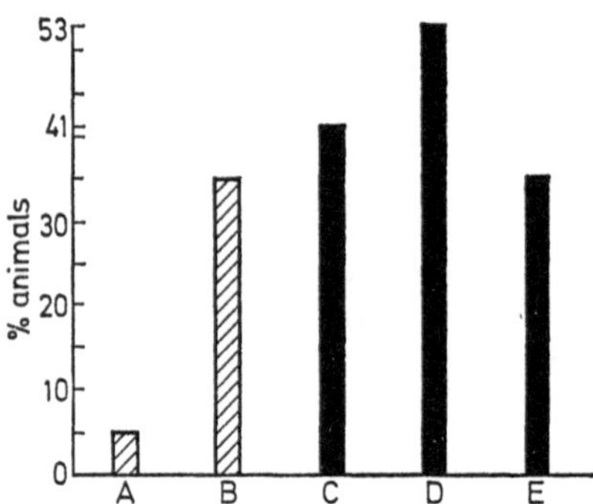

Fig. 2. Effect of *C. parvum* on survival rate (after 1 month) of Swiss mice inoculated with Mengo virus (EMC). A Control EMC, B Control receiving interferon (NDV) + EMC, C *C. parvum* 250 μg + EMC, D *C. parvum* 500 μg + EMC, E *C. parvum* 1,000 μg + EMC

Fig. 2 summarizes the main results. Comparison was made with a virus (NDV) known to be a good interferon producer. On the thirtieth day of observation, survival was 5% in the control group and 53% in the group which had received 500 μg of *C. parvum*. The lower and higher doses were less effective. In the control group which received the interferon-inducing virus survival was only 35%.

It is logical to suppose that *C. parvum* exerts its antiviral activity by inducing interferon, but several attempts to show this have failed, so we must assume that another mechanism is involved.

Enhancement of Resistance to Malignant Tumors and Leukemia

There is increasing evidence that bacterial immunostimulants consistently enhance host resistance to malignant tumors, as first reported by us [10] and subsequently confirmed both in laboratory animals and in cancer patients. In our first experiments in mice [11] two types of tumors were used: A Betz sarcoma, grafted subcutaneously, and Ehrlich's ascites tumor grafted intraperitoneally. Treatment with *C. parvum* significantly reduced the growth rate of the Betz sarcoma and lowered mortality by about 40%. The best results were obtained when *C. parvum* was given intravenously on the day of tumor grafting or 2 days previously. Even more striking effects were

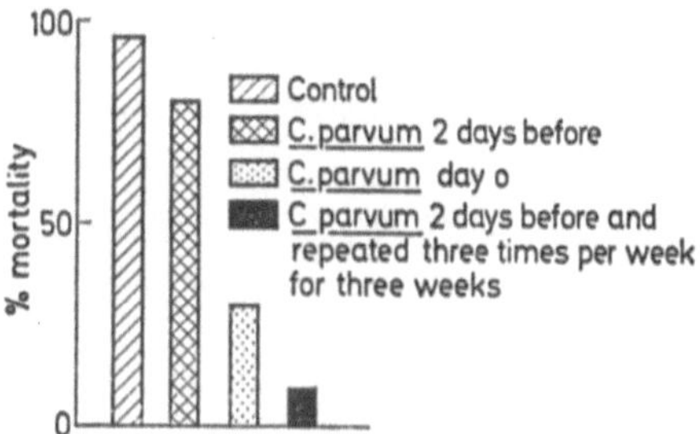

Fig. 3. Effect of *C. parvum* administered intraperitoneally on development of Ehrlich's ascites in Swiss mice

observed in mice infected by Ehrlich's ascites. In appropriate experimental conditions, treatment with *C. parvum* reduced mortality from 90% to 10% (Fig. 3). The best results were obtained when *C. parvum* was administered intraperitoneally on day 0 with repeat injections 3 times a week for 3 weeks.

The tumors used in these experiments were not strain-specific and histocompatibility factors might have been involved in the mechanism of inhibition by *C. parvum*. However, WOODRUFF and BOAK [24] obtained significant protection with *C. parvum* in autologous 3-methylcholanthrene induced sarcoma, and LAMENSANS *et al.* [17] in isogenic and semiallogenic AKR leukemia, so that clearly histocompatibility antigens do not play an essential role, and perhaps none at all, in the mechanisms of the protection against tumors afforded by *C. parvum*.

Stimulation by C. Parvum of "*in vitro*" Cytotoxic Properties of Lymphocytes towards Syngeneic Tumor Cells in Tumor-Bearing Animals

Using the technique of BRUNNER *et al.* [3], we recently studied the effect of *C. parvum* on the cytotoxic properties of lymphocytes towards tumor cells "*in vitro*".

An isologous tumor YC8 was implanted subcutaneously in Balb/c mice. Cells were obtained from spleen, lymph node, and peritoneal exudate of these animals 7 to 18 days after tumor implantation and incubated with ^{51}Cr-labeled tumor cells. The target tumor cells were obtained from syngeneic animals in which the same tumor had been induced in ascitic form. The peritoneal exudate cells were obtained after injection of NaCl from control animal which had received *C. parvum* intraperitoneally 7 days previously. The cytotoxicity of the lymphocytes from *C. parvum*-treated mice is indicated by the percentage of ^{51}Cr released in the medium after 18 hours of culture.

The proportion of lymphocytes to tumor cells used in our experiments was usually 100 : 1. Controls were performed with normal lymphocytes. The results are summarized in Fig. 4. It is clear that treatment with *C. parvum* increased the cyto-

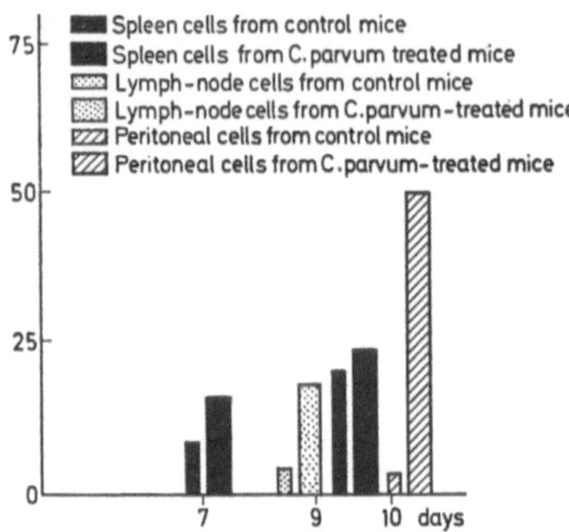

Fig. 4. Cytotoxic effects on tumor cells of lymphocytes from control and from *C. parvum*-stimulated tumor-bearing mice. *C. parvum* was injected intraperitoneally on the day of tumor graft

toxicity of lymphocytes towards autologous tumor cells. Spleen and lymph-node cells were able to destroy tumor cells at various rates depending on the time interval between tumor grafting and challenge.

The remarkable increase in cell mortality observed with peritoneal exudate cells obtained after intraperitoneal injection of *C. parvum* is presently under study. Detailed data will be reported elsewhere.

Mechanism of Action of C. Parvum

C. parvum treatment produces a wide variety of biological and immunological effects in mammals. It is a potent RES stimulant. It enhances antibody synthesis and acts as an adjuvant for induction of cellular immunity [18]. It increases resistance to bacterial and viral infections. It further protects against tumor invasion and inhibits the graft-versus-host (GVH) reaction [15]. Scott [21] has reported that spleen and blood lymphocytes from mice pretreated with intravenous *C. parvum* were found to be markedly depressed in their response to stimulation by PHA or in mixed-lymphocyte reaction, whereas lymph-node lymphocytes from the same animals retained full immunological competence.

According to SCOTT, the inhibitory effect of *C. parvum* on responsiveness of T lymphocytes to PHA is not a direct effect but is mediated by macrophages which have themselves been modified by the immunostimulant. It is unlikely that the inhibition of the lymphocytes is due to release of some toxic material from the stimulated macrophage, as the supernatant is not inhibitory. This leads to the conclusion that the inhibition reflects a qualitative change in the macrophage population similar to that produced in a GVH reaction. The inhibitory effect appears to be mediated through cell–cell contact. Even if this interpretation is accepted, it still remains to be explained why the lymphocyte population of lymphnodes, which includes a high percentage of T cells is unaffected.

DEL GUERCIO and LEUCHARS [5] have recently shown that a thymus-independent antigen, levan, can function as a carrier and induce synthesis of antibody to the haptenic determinant DNP. The DNP-levan conjugate is able to elicit only 19S antibody to the hapten. This immune response is not affected by thymectomy but is abolished in mice tolerant to levan. A mechanism involving cooperation between hapten-specific B lymphocytes and carrier-specific B lymphocytes is suggested to account for this phenomenon.

The most striking finding is that *C. parvum* behaves differently in this system from other so-called adjuvants. By using either bovine gamma-globulin (BGG) or levan coupled with DNP in parallel experiments, DEL GUERCIO has investigated the effect on the antibody synthesis of various adjuvants, namely Freund's complete and incomplete adjuvants, *Bordetella pertussis* and *C. parvum*. It was found that while the Freund adjuvants and *Bordetella pertussis* increased the antibody response to BGG-DNP, they did not affect the response to levan-DNP. Only *C. parvum* injected 4 days before the antigen increased the anti-levan-DNP titers.

On present evidence the immune response to many antigens involves cooperation between two lymphocytes. The protein-carrier and haptenic determinants react specifically with different cells, and cooperation between the carrier-specific cells, supposedly a T cell, and the hapten-specific cell, supposedly a B cell, is required to activate synthesis of antibodies to the haptenic determinant. A different mechanism has to be postulated to explain the immune response to DNP coupled to levan, which is a thymus-independent carrier. In this case, a carrier-specific T-independent cell (i.e. a B cell) interacts with a hapten-specific cell, also a B cell, to elicit the response to DNP. Thus, two cooperative systems, T-B and B-B, can induce a humoral response to haptenic determinant. The BGG-DNP response involves T-B cell cooperation, while the response to levan-DNP is an example of B-B cell cooperation. Adjuvants such as Freund's adjuvant or *B. pertussis* appear to potentiate only T-B cell cooperation. *C. parvum* seems at present the only immunostimulant known to promote B-B cooperation.

It is quite impossible at the moment, to propose a wholly satisfactory hypothesis which would explain all the available data on *C. parvum*, some of which is apparently contradictory. Moreover, much confusion is engendered by the term "adjuvant", which is inappropriate and misleading. The term adjuvant was introduced by FREUND to define certain mineral and biological substances which, when administered with the antigen, enhance antibody synthesis and promote delayed hypersensitivity. FREUND considered that adjuvants active mainly because of their physical properties as emulsifying agents and because they form a depot from which the antigen diffuses to the lymphoid organs at slow and sustained rate. FREUND's main argument was that the adjuvant effect is observed only when the antigen is physically incorporated in the ingredients prior to injection.

There are however, other agents which produce an enhanced immune response, stimulate delayed hypersensitivity, and profoundly modify the immune reaction of the individual to unrelated infections or tumor invasion, and which modify the graft-versus-host reaction. These apparently stimulate not the T cells but the B cells. They also deeply affect macrophage-lymphocyte interactions, do not require emulsifying agents, and are fully effective when administered independently several days or even weeks before the antigen.

It is obvious that we are dealing with two different types of agents. Even though they have certain effects in common, the differences are so great that we need a different name for each group.

My suggestion is that the term adjuvant should be kept for substances which modify antigenicity as a result of their physical properties. Another term should be found for substances which modulate the immune response by their effect on immunocompetent cells, macrophages as well as lymphocytes. I propose the term "immunostimulins" or, even better "immunomodulators", for this group of substances.

References

1. ADLAM, C., BROUGHTON, E. S., SCOTT, M. T.: Enhanced resistance of mice to infection with bacteria following pretreatment with *C. parvum*. Nature (Lond.) New Biology **235**, 219 (1971).
2. BIOZZI, G., STIFFEL, C., HALPERN, B., MOUTON, D.: Étude de la fonction métabolique des cellules de Kuppfer. Rev. franç. Étud. clin. biol. **4**, 427 (1959).
3. BRUNNER, K. T., MAUEL, J., CEROTTINI, J. C., CHAPUIS, B.: Quantitative assay of the lytic action of immune lymphoid cells on ^{51}Cr-labeled allogeneic target cells "*in vitro*". Inhibition of isoantibody and by drugs. Immunology **14**, 181 (1968).
4. CERUTTI, I.: (Unpublished results).
5. DEL GUERCIO, P., LEUCHARS, E.: The immune response in mice to the haptenic determinant DNP coupled to a thymus-independent carrier (levan). J. Immunol. **109**, 951 (1972).
6. FAUVE, R. M., HEVIN, M. B.: Pouvoir bactéricide des macrophages spléniques et hépatiques de souris envers *Listeria monocytogenes*. Ann. Inst. Pasteur **120**, 399 (1971).
7. HALPERN, B.: Immunité nonspécifique — Facteurs cellulaires. Bull. Ass. franç. vet. Microbiol. Immunol. **7**, 3 (1971).
8. HALPERN, B., BENACERRAF, B., DELAFRESNAYE, J. F.: Physiopathology of the reticuloendothelial system. Symposium Oxford: Blackwell Scientific Publ. 1957.
9. HALPERN, B., BIOZZI, G., STIFFEL, C.: Action de l'extrait microbien Wxb 3148 sur l'évolution des tumeurs expérimentales In: Rôle du système réticuloendothélial dans l'immunité antibactérienne et anti-tumorale (HALPERN, B., Ed.), p. 221. Symposium. Paris: C.N.R.S. 1963.
10. HALPERN, B., BIOZZI, G., STIFFEL, C., MOUTON, D.: Effet de la stimulation du système réticuloendothélial par l'inoculation du bacille Calmette-Guérin sur le développement de l'épithélioma atypique T-8 de Guérin chez le rat. C.R. Soc. Biol. (Paris) **153**, 919 (1959).
11. HALPERN, B., BIOZZI, G., STIFFEL, C., MOUTON, D.: Inhibition of tumour growth by administration of killed *C. parvum*. Nature (Lond.) **212**, 853 (1966).
12. HALPERN, B., ISRAEL, I.: Etude de l'action d'une immunostimuline associée aux Corynébactéries anaérobies dans les néoplasies expérimentales et humaines. C. R. Acad. Sci. (Paris) **273**, 2186 (1971).
13. HALPERN, B., PREVOT, A. R., BIOZZI, G., STIFFEL, C., MOUTON, D., MORARD, J. C., BOUTHILLIER, Y., DECREUSEFOND, C.: Stimulation de l'activité phagocytaire du système réticuloendothélial provoquée par *Corynebacterium parvum*. J. Reticuloendoth. Soc. **1**, 77 (1964).

14. Howard, J. G., Biozzi, G., Halpern, B., Stiffel, C., Mouton, D.: The effect of *Mycobacterium tuberculosis* (BCG) infection on the resistance of mice to bacterial endotoxin and *Salmonella enteritidis* infection. Brit. J. exp. Path. **40**, 281 (1959).
15. Howard, J. G., Biozzi, G., Mouton, D., Liacopoulos, P.: An analysis of the inhibitory effect of *C. parvum* on graft-versus-host disease. Transplantation **5**, 1510 (1967).
16. Israel, I., Halpern, B.: Le Corynebacterium dans les cancers avancés. Première évaluation de l'activité thérapeutique de cette immunostimuline. Nouv. Presse Méd. **1**, 19 (1972).
17. Lamensans, A., Stiffel, C., Mollier, M. F., Laurent, M., Mouton, D., Biozzi, G.: Effet protecteur de *C. parvum* contre la leucémie greffée AKR. Relations avec l'activité catalasique hépatique et la fonction phagocytaire du système réticuloendothélial. Rev. franç. Étud. clin. biol. **13**, 773 (1968).
18. Neveu, T., Branellec, A., Biozzi, G.: Propriétés adjuvantes du *C. parvum* sur la production d'anticorps et sur l'induction de l'hypersensibilité retardée envers les antigènes conjugués. Ann. Inst. Pasteur **106**, 771 (1964).
19. Prevot, A. R.: Les Corynébactéries anaérobies. Ergebn. Mikrobiol. **33**, 6 (1960).
20. Prevot, A. R., Levaditi, J. C., Nazimoff, O., Thouvenot, H.: Circonstances d'apparition et évolution de la réticulose plasmodiale qui caractérise certaines formes de la Corynebactériose expérimentale du lapin. Ann. Inst. Pasteur **94**, 405 (1958).
21. Scott, M. T.: Biological effects of the adjuvant *C. parvum*. I. Inhibition of PHA, mixed lymphocyte and GVH reactivity. II. Evidence for macrophage T-cell interaction. Cell. Immunol. **3**, 459 (1972).
22. Stuart, A. E.: In: The reticuloendothelial system (Livingstone, E. D., Ed.), vol. 1. London 1970.
23. Weiss, D. W., Bonhag, R. S., Park, J. A.: Studies on the heterologous immunogenicity of a methanol-insoluble fraction of attenuated tubercle bacilli (BCG). I. Anti-microbial protection. J. exp. Med. **119**, 53 (1964).
24. Woodruff, M. F. A., Boak, J. L.: Inhibitory effect of injection of *C. parvum* on the growth of tumour transplants in isogenic hosts. Brit. J. Cancer **20**, 345 (1966).

Nonspecific Effects of Corynebacteria on Systemic Immunity Responses

M. F. A. Woodruff

Department of Surgery, University of Edinburgh, Scotland

My interest in *Corynebacterium parvum* as a possible anti-tumor agent goes back to 1965 when a colleague, Dr. James Howard, drew my attention to the work of Halpern *et al.* on the remarkable capacity of killed *C. parvum* vaccine to stimulate reticuloendothelial (RE) activity.

It had been known for some years that the growth of various transplanted tumors in rodents could be inhibited by prior treatment of the host with BCG, and certain other agents known to stimulate RE activity, but there did not appear to be any reports of the use of *C. parvum* in this context and, with one exception [4], all this work appeared to have been done with allografted tumors, i.e. tumors transplanted to animals non-isogenic with the animal in which the tumor originated. It seemed worthwhile therefore to examine the effect of *C. parvum* on isogenic tumor transplants. We did this with a heat-killed *C. parvum* vaccine kindly supplied by Halpern [7]. We found that i.v. injection of 0.5 mg wet weight of killed *C. parvum* suspension either 2 days before or 8—12 days after subcutaneous inoculation of 10^5 or 10^4 viable mammary carcinoma cells in A-strain female mice significantly delayed the appearance of the tumor. The effect was comparable to reducing the number of cells injected into untreated mice by a factor of 10; once the tumor had become palpable, however, the rate of growth was much the same in treated and untreated animals. Injection of *C. parvum* also delayed the appearance of a palpable tumor in (CBA $\times$ A) F_1 hybrid mice following s.c. inoculation of 10^4 or 10^5 cells of a sarcoma induced with methylcholanthrene in similar hybrids, though the effect was less marked than in the case of the A-strain carcinoma.

Following this work we and others have been concerned with six main questions:

1. Do other strains of *C. parvum* and other species of bacteria (or other corynebacteria) have similar properties to Halpern's organism? If so, are there any identifiable morphological or other characteristics common to all such organisms?
2. How is the anti-tumor effect of *C. parvum* (and other agents with similar properties) mediated?
3. Do tumors differ significantly in their response to treatment with a particular preparation of *C. parvum*? If so, does the response correlate with identifiable features of the tumor or of the immunological response of untreated hosts to the tumor?
4. What are the most effective methods of preparing and administering *C. parvum* vaccine, or material derived therefrom, as judged by the effect on a variety of tumors?

5. Is it therapeutically advantageous to combine *C. parvum* administration with a) other forms of immunotherapy, and b) other methods of treating cancer, including surgical excision and chemotherapy?

6. Is active non-specific immunotherapy with *C. parvum* or related organisms, or with substances derived therefrom, applicable in the treatment of human cancer? In particular, is the time ripe for a clinical trial? If so, what type of patient should be treated and what are the safeguards to be observed?

Some partial and preliminary answers to some of these questions have already been published (see e.g. [1, 2, 3, 8]), and work is in progress in various laboratories, including our own.

So far as our work is concerned the following conclusions emerge:

1. Different strains of *C. parvum* differ markedly in their anti-tumor activity.

2. Anti-tumor activity shows a rough but not precise correlation with capacity to stimulate phagocytosis.

3. The four transplantable mouse tumors we have studied, i.e. a mammary carcinoma in A/HeJ mice and fibrosarcomas in A/HeJ, CBA/H and (CBA $\times$ A) F_1 mice, all respond (though in different degrees) to treatment with *C. parvum*.

4. Despite some views expressed to the contrary, we have some recent evidence (in collaboration with Dr. W. McBride) that heat-killed and formalin-killed preparations of the same strain of *C. parvum* are about equally effective. The optimum time for administration of a single injection of *C. parvum* with the tumors we have studied is a few days after tumor inoculation. Intravenous injection is a little more effective than i.p. injection which, in turn, is decidedly more effective than s.c. injection.

5. Injection of anti-tumor globulin (ATG) in our experiments did not potentiate M, and indeed appeared to reduce the effect of treatment of two fibrosarcomas with *C. parvum*, although preincubation of the tumor cell suspension with ATG in the absence of complement prior to inoculation did have a potentiating effect.

On the other hand we have confirmed and extended the observation of [1] that visible, growing tumor transplants in mice may be powerfully inhibited and sometimes destroyed by a combination of chemotherapy (a single dose of 200 mg/kg cyclophosphamide) and immunotherapy with *C. parvum*.

6. We have not as yet used *C. parvum* in patients, but in my view the time is ripe for clinical trial of *C. parvum* in combination with standard therapy for the tumor in question. The toxicity of the vaccine should first be studied in non-human primates, and then tried cautiously in patients with advanced cancer. It seems unlikely to result in cures in such patients but if the procedure were shown to be of any benefit, and at the same time safe, the possibility of undertaking a trial in patients exhibiting what I have referred to elsewhere as *minimal residual cancer* [5, 6] would merit serious consideration.

References

1. Currie, G. A., Bagshawe, K. D.: Active immunotherapy with *Corynebacterium parvum* and chemotherapy in murine fibrosarcomas. Brit. med. J. **1970 I**, 541.
2. Halpern, B.: *Corynebacterium parvum*: An immunomodulator. This volume, p. 262-271.
3. Smith, L. H., Woodruff, M. F. A.: Comparative effect of two strains of *C. parvum* on phagocytic activity and tumour growth. Nature (Lond.) **219**, 197 (1968).

4. Weiss, D. W., Bonhag, R. S., de Ome, K. B.: Protective action of fractions of tubercle bacilli against isologous tumours in mice. Nature (Lond.) **190**, 889 (1961).
5. Woodruff, M. F. A.: Le cancer residuel. Immex **5**, 621 (1969).
6. Woodruff, M. F. A.: Residual cancer. Harvey Lect. **66**, 161 (1972).
7. Woodruff, M. F. A., Boak, J. L.: Inhibitory effect of injection of *C. parvum* on the growth of tumour transplants in isogeneic hosts. Brit. J. Cancer **20**, 345 (1966).
8. Woodruff, M. F. A., Inchley, M. P., Dunbar, N.: Further observations on the effect of *C. parvum* and antitumour globulin on syngeneically transplanted mouse tumour. Brit. J. Cancer **26**, 67 (1972).

Immunostimulating Activity of Whole Cells, Cell-Walls and Fractions of Anaerobic Corynebacteria

B. Kouznetzova, B. Bizzini, J.-C. Chermann, F. Degrand, A.-R. Prevot, and M. Raynaud

Service Immunochimie, Institut Pasteur, Garches

Heat-killed whole cells of *Mycobacterium* (Myc. butyricum and Myc. tuberculosis H 37 Ra) have been used as immunostimulants for many years. The studies of [11, 23] have shown that anaerobic corynebacteria display immunostimulant activity similar to or even stronger than that of mycobacteria. Most adult humans exhibit a delayed-hypersensitivity reaction towards mycobacteria, so that repeated injections may be hazardous. However, repeated inoculations by scarification of living BCG cells of appropriate strains have been employed by [18] in leukemic patients. Although a positive cutaneous reaction to anaerobic corynebacteria is present in most adults [30], the delayed-hypersensitivity directed to the latter does not elicit the same general effects as tuberculin hypersensitivity. Large-scale testing has demonstrated that heat-killed cells of anaerobic corynebacteria can be repeatedly injected into humans without serious harm.

We set out to compare the effects of administering anaerobic corynebacteria as whole cells or as their soluble and insoluble fractions, with a view to obtaining an injectable preparation which might be used for nonspecific stimulation of immune functions in man.

For clarity, the effects observed after the injection of mycobacteria or corynebacteria will be discussed separately.

1. Increased Vascular Clearance of Colloidal Carbon

The relationship between an overall increase in phagocytic activity and immunity (comprising all the means an animal organism deploys to withstand microbial or viral infections, as well as oncogenic processes) are problematical.

Some authors [11, 23] now consider that the stimulant effect on the reticulo-endothelial system measured by the clearance test is followed by increased resistance to infections or pathological processes.

[3] showed that certain substances which enhance overall phagocytic activity have no effect on resistance to particular infections, whereas mycobacteria or corynebacteria increase both vascular carbon clearance and the nonspecific resistance.

2. Increased Resistance to Bacterial Infection

Intravenous injection of mycobacteria or corynebacteria enhances resistance to subsequent infection with bacteria. Most reported investigations were carried out with mice and *Enterobacteriaceae*. [3] use BCG cells for protection against *Salmonella* enteritidis and [1] corynebacteria against various bacteria. With a suitably selected strain of mouse and appropriate bacteria, it is possible to demonstrate the protective effect under conditions where 100% of the controls die and most of the "stimulated" animals survive. However, this is not typical. The nonspecific protection induced by mycobacteria or by corynebacteria is generally effective only when a reduced number of infecting bacteria is inoculated.

If the infecting dose of a bacterial strain of low virulence for mice, e.g. E. coli 0111-B4, is increased or if strain known to be very virulent for mice is used, nonspecific protection is then difficult to demonstrate experimentally.

[9] found that heat-killed *Corynebacterium parvum* can enhance the bactericidal capacity of hepatic and splenic macrophages.

3. General Immunostimulating Effect on the Immune Circulating Antibody Response

Mycobacteria and corynebacteria injected intravenously a few days before exposure to a given antigen enhance the intensity of the primary response. We call this the "general immunostimulating effect". It does not depend upon the local combination of the antigen with mycobacteria or with corynebacteria at the site of injection. Therefore, its experimental observation is facilitated. The effect was investigated by [5] in mice and by [20, 21] and by [22] in rabbits.

4. Local Immunostimulating Effect on Antibody Response

The local immunostimulating effect on the antibody response resembling that of Freund's adjuvant is difficult to observe when sheep erythrocytes are used as the antigen [6]. Sheep erythrocytes given intradermally exhibit a relatively high immunogenic potency related to their physical state.

5. Local Immunostimulating Effect with Delayed-Hypersensitivity Reaction

The experimental use of complete Freund's adjuvant in investigating the delayed hypersensitivity response to protein antigens is well known. In the most usual type of study carried out in this field, delayed hypersensitivity was artificially induced by intradermal injection into the footpads of guinea pigs of the protein emulsified in complete Freund's adjuvant. With many protein antigens, an immune reaction with circulating antibody is initiated shortly after the delayed-hypersensitivity reaction is demonstrable. To avoid this complication, we used a simple antigen: azobenzenearsonate-N-acetyl-tyrosine (ABA-TYR).

[15] showed that ABA-TYR was immunogenic when injected in combination with complete Freund's adjuvant. The delayed hypersensitivity can be studied by cutaneous testing with a complex of azobenzenearsonate and guinea pig serum albumin (ABA-GpSA).

[19] have been studying an immune reaction that appears to be of the "pure" delayed type. Doses of antigen (100 μg ABA-TYR) which elicit a delayed-hypersensitivity reaction in 100% of immunized guinea pigs produce no or very few anti-ABA antibodies. The delayed reaction is pronounced with lesions of diameter 10 to 15 mm. Other features of the delayed-hypersensitivity reaction were shown to be present by tests of

a) inhibition of macrophage migration under the influence of the specific antigen ABA-TYR;
b) initiation of blast transformation under the influence of ABA-TYR.

Induction of a delayed-hypersensitivity reaction to ABA-TYR is particularly suitable for demonstrating the specific activity of immunostimulating substances originating from mycobacteria or corynebacteria, because in their absence no reaction is observed.

6. Increased Resistance of Mice or Rats to Certain Grafted Tumors and Leukemias

This effect has been extensively studied [2, 12, 14, 17, 29, 32] but the underlying mechanism is still not understood. It is postulated that substances which stimulate nonspecific defences do so by increasing the cell-mediated immune response (T lymphocytes).

7. Modification of Graft-Versus-Host Reaction

The protection of F_1 hybrid mice against the homologous disease elicited by injection of parental spleen cells by pretreatment with mycobacteria or corynebacteria was observed by [4]. Here too, the mechanism of protection is still to be elucidated.

Material and Methods

All investigations reported in this paper were conducted with *Corynebacterium granulosum*, strain 5196 (cf. [22, 25]).

1. Cultivation and Preparation of Bacterial Suspensions

Bacteria were cultivated in fermentors (150—300 liters or 700 liters). The medium consisted of: 40 g freeze-dried VF medium (Organotechnie, France); 4 g yeast-extract (Difco); 2.5 g NaCl; 10 g glucose in 1 liter distilled water; pH was adjusted to 7.2—7.3. Cultures were incubated at 37 °C and bacteria were harvested after 48—72 hours by centrifugation with a Sharples centrifuge (Type MV 12-RV 5 P1). Collected bacteria were then weighed (wet weight). The yield varied from run to run within a range of 0.5 g to 5 g wet bacteria per liter of medium.

Bacterial cells were subsequently washed three times with saline (0.9% NaCl) in the proportion of 1000 ml saline for 100 g wet weight. The supernatants from the two last washings were dialyzed against distilled water and freeze-dried. The dry product so obtained (solubilized fraction in saline; SFS) was used in some experiments after redissolution in saline.

Washed bacteria were resuspended in saline by means of an Omni-Mixer (Sorvall) and the suspension was heated in a water bath at 60 °C for 1 hour. After cooling at room temperature, 40% formaldehyde was added to a total of 0.2% (v/v). Sterility of the suspension was thereby achieved and the dry weight of bacteria then determined. Suspensions were stored as such at 4 °C or distributed in vials after adjustment of their concentrations to 10; 2; 1 or 0.25 mg per ml and readjustment of the concentration in formaldehyde.

2. Preparation of Cell Walls

Three types of preparations were used:

a) Partly Purified Cell Walls (CW)

Heat-killed and formaldehyde-treated bacteria or thawed unprocessed bacteria were suspended in distilled water at a concentration of about 100 mg dry weight per ml. Cells were then disrupted by means of a cell-fractionator (Sorvall: type RIBI, model RF 1) [27].

This treatment was repeated if indicated by carbon clearance activity determinations. The disrupted cells were then subjected to enzymatic digestion in buffer at pH 7.42 (EDTA 0.001 M; Tris, HCl 0.002 N; NaCl 1%) at 37 °C:

1. by DNase (1% solution) for 1 hour. After centrifugation, the supernatant was discarded.
2. The sediment submitted to digestion by RNase under essentially the same conditions as specified for DNase.
3. The sediment recovered from this digestion was submitted to the action of Pronase (2% solution) for 90 hours [7].

After centrifugation the sediment was repeatedly washed with distilled water and recentrifuged until nucleic acids were no longer detectable in the supernatant (as verified by UV spectrophotometry). The sediment, resuspended in saline, was designated "Partly purified cell walls" (CW). The batch of corynebacteria from which cell walls were prepared is specified by the corresponding letter put in front of CW (for instance: DCW = cell walls from batch D).

b) Purified Cell Walls (CWZ)

Purification was performed by zonal centrifugation. Sucrose gradient centrifugation of CW was initially carried out in a B 60 zonal centrifuge (IEC) equipped with a transparent rotor Z 15. The value of $S\omega^2\, dt = 3{,}740 \times 10^5$ was determined by means of a "digital speed integrator" (IEC). These preliminary studies enabled specification of conditions suitable for centrifugation with two other zonal centrifuges, model B 20 and PR 6 (IEC). As previously described by [24], conditions with rotor Z 15 were; speed: 5.10^3 rev/min; duration: 30 min.

Electron microscope examination of the preparations obtained according to the process described under a) revealed a fairly large amount of undisrupted cells besides disrupted cells, cell walls, and cytoplasmic debris.

After two centrifugations in sucrose gradient as specified above, cell walls were isolated which contained only a small amount of undisrupted bacteria.

c) Cell Walls Obtained by Phenol Treatment

These were prepared essentially according to the general method described by [31] for the preparation of lipopolysaccharides. Briefly, the procedure was carried out as follows:

10 g bacteria (dry weight) were suspended in 350 ml distilled water and the suspension was kept in a water-bath at 65—68 °C. While stirring, 350 ml 90% phenol were added and the mixture was left for 30 min at 68 °C. The mixture was then cooled at 5 °C in crushed ice and centrifuged at 4,000 rev/min for 10 min. The sediment was taken up in 350 ml distilled water and the same treatment was repeated a second time. The sediment obtained at the end of these operations was washed three times with distilled water and resuspended in saline. The product was designated PWCW. The batch of origin is indicated as previously described.

Biological Tests

The carbon clearance test was performed according to the method of [11] and of [10]. Substances to be tested were injected i.v. at a dose of 400 μg. Clearance test was carried out 5 days later.

The clearance constant was calculated according to [11]

$$K = \frac{\log C - \log C'}{t' - t}$$

C and C' are the carbon concentrations at time t and t' in minutes following the injection of carbon.

A similar determination was made on 3 control mice and a clearance constant Ko was accordingly calculated for non-stimulated animals.

The results are reported in terms of the ratio K/Ko.

Hemagglutinins were measured in mice after i.v. injection of sheep red blood cells (SRBC) according to the technique used by [5], as modified by us, after we had stated that the minimum dose of SRBC to be administered was 5×10^6 cells per mouse [25].

The substances under investigation were injected i.v. 4 or 7 days before the antigen.

The effect on the production of antitetanus antibodies was investigated by estimating the 50% protective dose (PD_{50}) of tetanus toxoid in mice.

The immunostimulating effect is evidenced by the decrease of the amount of toxoid corresponding to 1 PD_{50}. The conditions of the determination were as follows:

— To determine the value PD_{50} of the preparation of toxoid used, groups of 10 Swiss mice, 20 g body weight, were injected s.c. with decreasing amounts of the toxoid adsorbed onto calcium phosphate after dilution with 0.9% saline. The thus immunized animals were challenged at the 28th day by an i.m. injection of 100 LD_{50} of pure toxin. The value PD_{50} was calculated according to the log. probit method of [26]. The conditions were those tentatively recommended by the Commission of the European Pharmacopoeae;

— the action of the stimulating substances was researched by s.c. administration of 0.2 ml of the mixture obtained by emulsion of the toxoid in incomplete Freund's adjuvant supplemented with the substances under test. The doses of tetanus toxoid were chosen to correspond to 0.5, 1.0 and 2.0 PD_{50}.

Induction of delayed hypersensitivity to ABA-TYR was achieved by injection into the four footpads of Hartley guinea pigs of a total of 100 μg ABA-TYR mixed with an equal volume of incomplete Freund's adjuvant (Difco) supplemented with the stimulating substances.

The incomplete Freund's adjuvant was supplemented with increasing amounts of corynebacteria or with fractions isolated from the latter.

The delayed hypersensitivity reaction eventually induced was obtained by injecting intradermally 0.1 ml of a solution in saline of the corresponding azo derivative with guinea pig serum albumin (ABA-GpSA) at a concentration of 20 μg/ml. The intensity of the reaction was estimated after 24 hours by measuring the diameter of erythema that had appeared and by noting the presence of infiltration. The characters of the lesions correspond to those of a cutaneous delayed-hypersensitivity reaction [15, 19].

L 1210 leukemia in mice was induced by injection of determined amounts of a cell suspension obtained by peritoneal puncture of leukemic mice. (We are indebted to Prof. MATHÉ for the strain of leukemic cells, which is maintained in DBA/2 mice, Orleans, CNRS.) The peritoneal fluid obtained was injected s.c. into hybrid mice (C 57 BL/6 × DBA/2) F_1 in dosages corresponding to 10^2 to 10^5 cells (cf. Results). Whole cells or fractions of corynebacteria were injected i.v. from the 4th day following the i.p. or i.v. injection of leukemic cells. Depending on the cases, the injection of the stimulating substances was repeated every four days up to 5 times as is indicated in the various tables. Results are expressed according to [13], as percentage Increase in Life Span (% ILS).

The effect of the stimulating substances was also investigated in DBA/2 mice inoculated with Friend leukemia virus. The inoculum consisted of a spleen homogenate from leukemic mice (1 g spleen per ml) diluted 1 : 100 and 1 : 1000. The inoculum that contained about 200 or 20 Spleen Doses 50 (SD_{50}) [28] was administered i.p. Under these conditions, non-stimulated animals usually died within approximately 45 days. In stimulated animals, survival time was often increased up to 100 days. 20 mice were used as control; 10 of these were sacrificed three weeks later to determine the increase of spleen weight. A mean weight of 2.5 g was found with the first dilution of virus, and 1.5 g for the second dilution.

The effect of the stimulating substances on the numbers of cells which form hemolytic plaques was studied in BALB/C mice injected i.v. with 5×10^6 SRBC. Spleens were excised after 4 days and the number of plaques of hemolysis corresponding to each spleen was determined according to the method of [8] in liquid medium. The numbers determined for mice stimulated 7 days before the injection of SRBC were compared with those obtained for mice which had received only the antigen.

Results

The results are presented in figures and tables.

The immunostimulating activity, as determined in the carbon clearance test for the various preparations used in this study is given in Table 1.

Table 1. K/Ko values of the various preparations of Corynebacteria used and of fractions isolated from them

Substances			K/Ko
C. granulosum S. 5196			
		A	3.54
		D	3.76
	Batches	F	3.26
		H	2.90
		I	3.70
Partly purified cell walls			
obtained from	Batch A (ACW)		3.78
	Batch D (DCW)		4.10
Purified cell walls obtained from batch D (DCWZ)			5.40
Phenol-water cell walls obtained from batch D (DPWCW)			3.30
Solubilized fraction in saline (SFS)			1.45
Autoclaved BCG	Strain Pasteur Institute		1.58

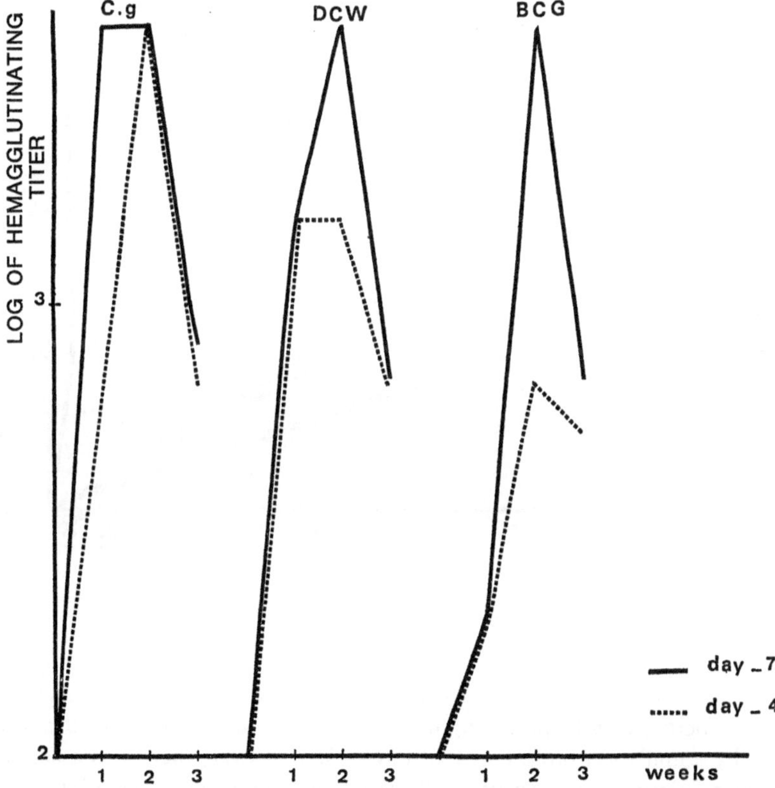

Fig 1. Determination of optimum time of stimulation for hemagglutinin formation. Cg = *Corynebacterium granulosum* S 5196; DCW = partially purified cell walls; sheep red blood cells (SRBC) = 5×10^7 cells/ml and 0.1 ml/mouse (i. v.). Stimulation with 1 mg substance per Swiss mouse (i.v.) on day — 7 (solid line) and on day — 4 (broken line)

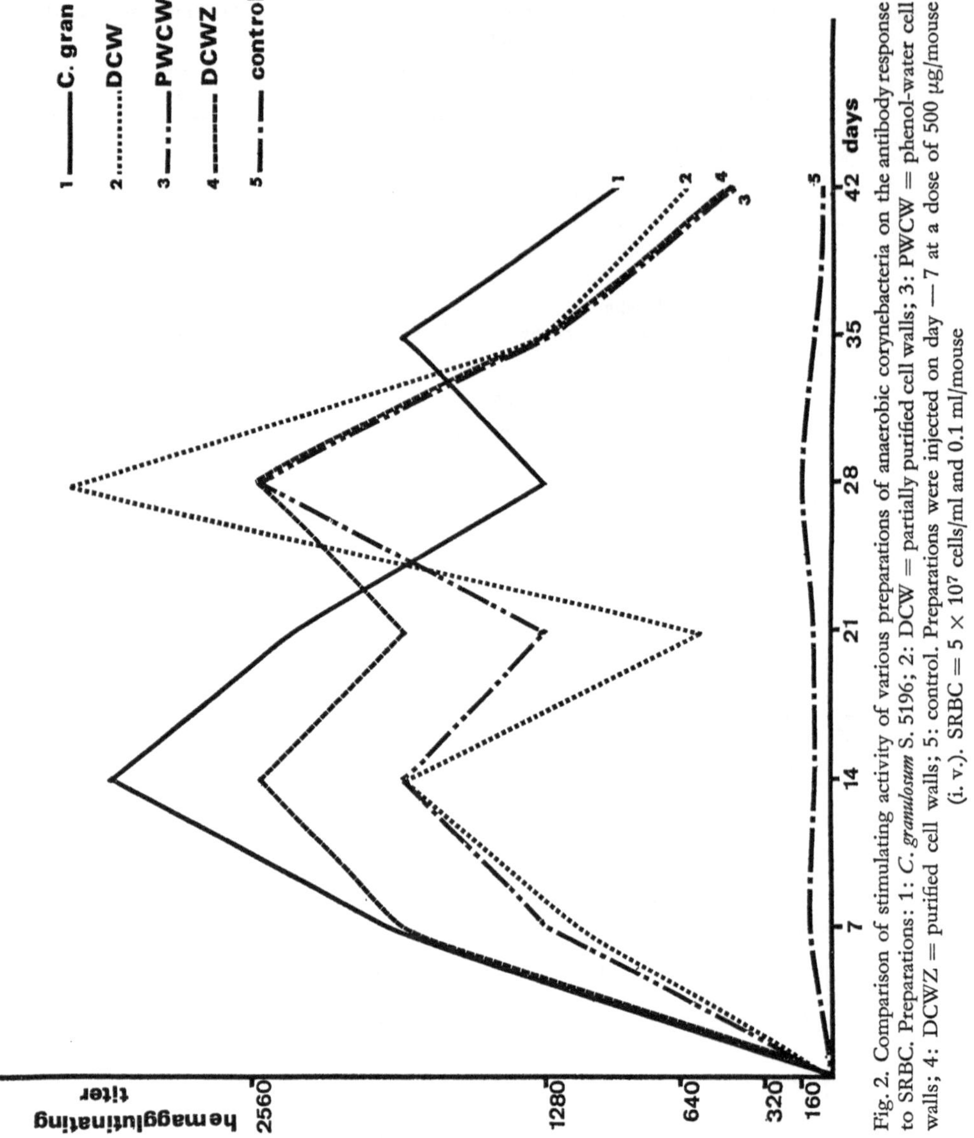

Fig. 2. Comparison of stimulating activity of various preparations of anaerobic corynebacteria on the antibody response to SRBC. Preparations: 1: *C. granulosum* S. 5196; 2: DCW = partially purified cell walls; 3: PWCW = phenol-water cell walls; 4: DCWZ = purified cell walls; 5: control. Preparations were injected on day —7 at a dose of 500 μg/mouse (i. v.). SRBC = 5×10^7 cells/ml and 0.1 ml/mouse

Fig. 1 summarizes the results of experiments on stimulation of hemagglutinin formation. There seems to be no significant difference in the amount of antibody produced by stimulation on day —4 or day —7. However, there was a slight advantage with prestimulation on day —7, particularly with the preparation of BCG used.

Figs. 2, 3, and 4 show the effect on hemagglutinin formation of the injection of different doses of corynebacteria and of the fractions obtained.

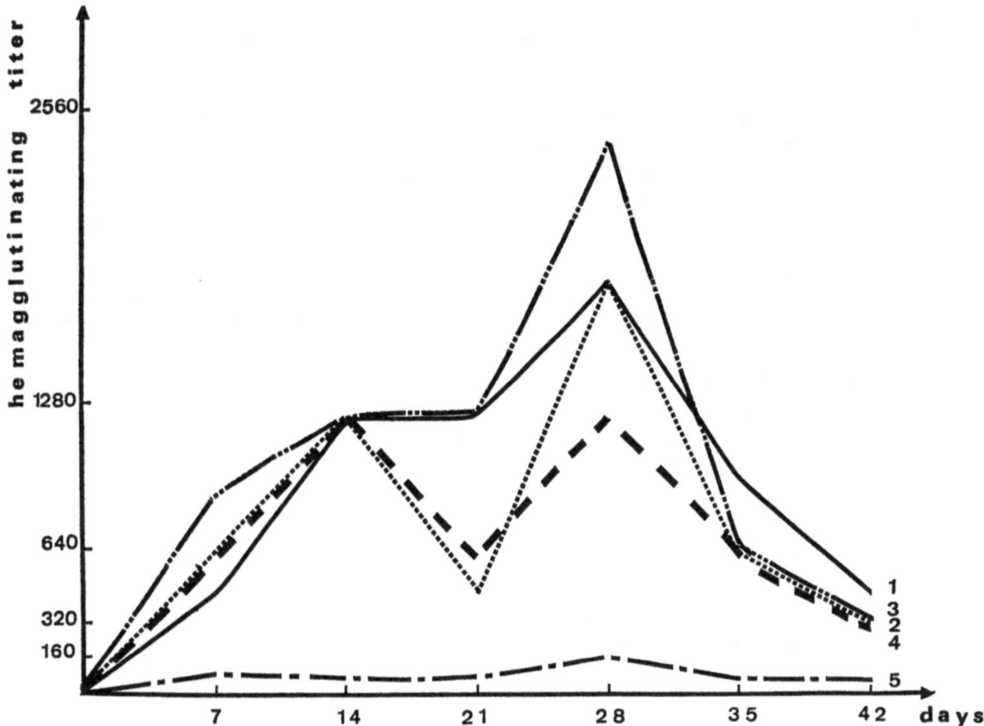

Fig. 3. Comparison of stimulating activity of various preparations of anaerobic corynebacteria on the antibody response to SRBC. Preparations: 1: *C. granulosum* S. 5196; 2: DCW = partially purified cell walls; 3: PWCW = phenol-water cell walls; 4: DCWZ = purified cell walls; 5: control. Preparations were injected on day —7 at a dose of 100 μg/mouse (i. v.). SRBC = 5 × 10^7 cells/ml and 0.1 ml/mouse

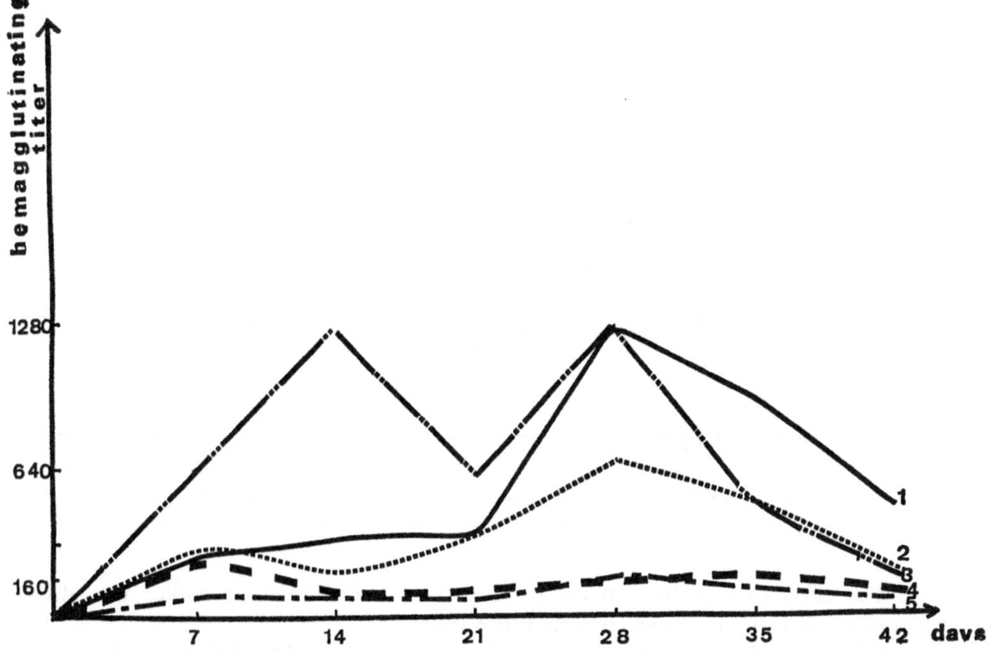

Fig. 4. Comparison of stimulating activity of various preparations of anaerobic corynebacteria on the antibody response to SRBC. Preparations: 1: *C. granulosum* S. 5196; 2: DCW = partially purified cell walls; 3: PWCW = phenol-water cell walls; 4: DCWZ = purified cell walls; 5: control. Preparations were injected on day — 7 at a dose of 10 μg/mouse (i. v.). SRBC = 5 × 10^7 cells/ml and 0.1 ml/mouse

Table 2. Enhanced protection of mice immunized against tetanus by injection of tetanus toxoid in oil combined with corynebacteria or fractions derived from them

Substances injected under 0.2 ml	Number of mice surviving in each group of 10 immunized with various doses of tetanus toxoid		
	0.05 Lf	0.10 Lf	0.20 Lf
Toxoid alone	0	5	9
Toxoid + incomplete Freund's adjuvant	3	7	10
Toxoid + incomplete Freund's adjuvant enriched with 2.5 mg/ml BCG	10	9	9
Toxoid + incomplete Freund's adjuvant enriched with 2.5 mg/ml *C. granulosum*, batch D	6	10	10
Toxoid + incomplete Freund's adjuvant enriched with 2.5 mg/ml DCW	10	10	10
Toxoid + incomplete Freund's adjuvant enriched with 2.5 mg/ml DPWCW	5	9	7

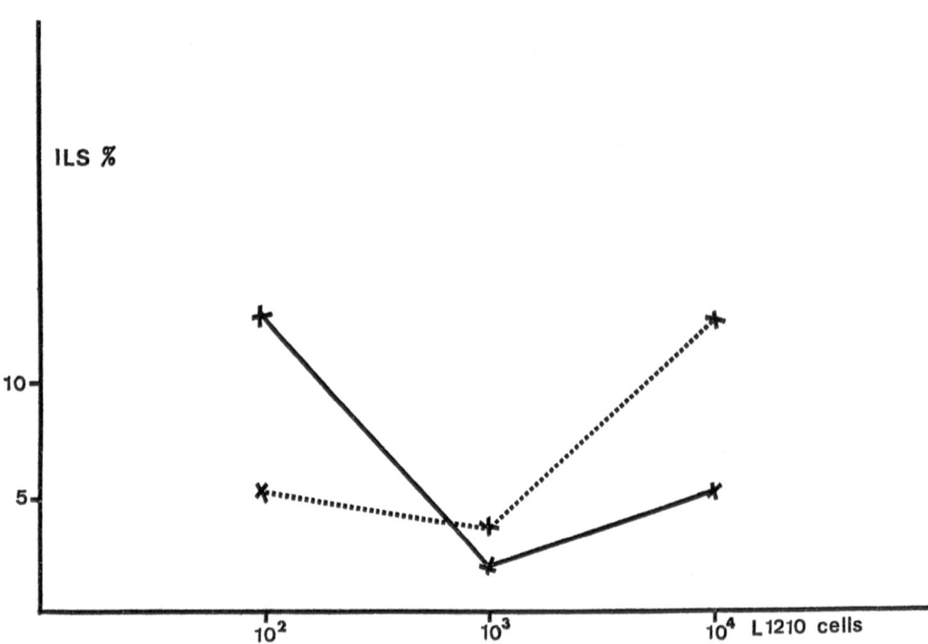

Fig. 5. Effect of route of inoculation of *C. granulosum* on L 1210 leukemia in mice: solid line = i. p., broken line = i. v. — *C. granulosum* given 4 days after grafting of the tumor

The effect of adjuvant on the production of antitetanus antibodies was also examined and the results are reported in Table 2.

Induction of a delayed-hypersensitivity reaction by ABA-TYR injected in incomplete Freund's adjuvant supplemented with whole corynebacteria or cell walls is clearly demonstrated in Table 3.

Table 3. Delayed hypersensitivity reaction in guinea pigs. Antigen = Azobenzenearsonate-N-acetyl-tyrosine 100 µg in incomplete adjuvant supplemented by various substances

Immunization on day 0 Substance added		Delayed hypersensitivity on day 15		
		Animals exhibiting a positive reaction after exposure to ABA-BSA [a]		Mean diameter of the cutaneous erythema
BCG	0.5 mg	18/20	90 p. 100	16 mm
	0.1 mg	1/17	5.9 p. 100	12 mm
C. granulosum	0.5 mg	17/28	60.7 p. 100	13 mm
	1 mg	52/56	93 p. 100	15 mm
	0.1 mg	1/16	6.2 p. 100	10 mm
DCW	0.5 mg	6/12	50 p. 100	14 mm
	1 mg	13/14	93 p. 100	14 mm

[a] The results are expressed according to the method of cumulative values of Reed and Muench.

Hartley guinea pigs, weight 350g were injected in each of their four footpads with 0.1ml of the supplemented adjuvant containing a total dose of azobenzene-arsonate-N-acetyl-tyrosine equal to 100 μg.

The figure in the first column corresponds to the total dose of substance administered.

Reactions to injection of 0.1 ml of a solution of a complex of azobenzene-arsonate and guinea pig serum albumin were studied.

The action of these stimulating substances was also investigated in L 1210 leukemia in mice. Firstly, the importance of the route of inoculation of the corynebacteria was determined. The choice of route had a definite effect on the results (Fig. 5), which were also influenced by the number of L 1210 cells inoculated.

Table 4 shows the differences between the various batches of corynebacteria in respect of their capacity to inhibit tumor development.

The results of similar experiments conducted with cell wall preparations of corynebacteria are summarized in Table 5.

The effect of the solubilized fraction in saline and the corresponding washed bacterial bodies is shown in Table 6.

Corynebacteria and fractions derived from the latter were assayed against Friend virus leukemia in animals stimulated 4 days before inoculation with the virus. Table 7 shows the results recorded after injection of 200 SD_{50} of virus. Table 8 shows the effect of the same substances with one tenth the dose of virus. Table 9 shows the effect of stimulation 7 days before immunization (11 days before excision of spleen) on the number of plaque-forming cells from mouse spleen.

Discussion

As Table 1 indicates, whole cells of heat-killed anaerobic corynebacteria exhibit a greater stimulating activity, as estimated by the carbon clearance test, than killed

Table 4. Effect of various batches of *Corynebacterium granulosum* S. 5196 on leukemia L 1210

ILS%: Increase in life span: $100 \times \frac{\text{life span of treated animals} - \text{life span of untreated animals}}{\text{life span of untreated animals}}$ MST = Median survival time in days.

No. of cells	Route of inoculation	Stimulating product	Route of inoculation	Dose µg	Days of inoculation	ILS %	MST	Range of death
10^5	s. c.	Corynebacteria "D"	i. v.	100	4, 8, 11	1.06	9.5	8—11
10^5	s. c.	Corynebacteria "F"	i. v.	100	4, 8, 11, 14	20.21	11.3	8—22
10^5	s. c.	Corynebacteria "H"	i. v.	100	4, 8, 11	—	9.4	8—12
10^5	s. c.	Corynebacteria "I"	i. v.	100	4, 8, 11	3.19	9.7	9—12
10^5	s. c.	BCG	i. v.	100	4, 8, 11	—	8.9	8—11
10^5	s. c.	none	—	—	0	—	9.4	8—10
10^4	s. c.	Corynebacteria "D"	i. v.	100	4, 8, 11, 14	12.06	13	12—16
10^4	s. c.	Corynebacteria "F"	i. v.	100	4, 8, 11, 14	25.86	14.6	12—21
10^4	s. c.	Corynebacteria "H"	i. v.	100	4, 8, 11, 14			
10^4	s. c.	Corynebacteria "I"	i. v.	100	4, 8, 11, 14	13.4	15.51	12—16
10^4	s. c.	BCG	i. v.	100	4, 8, 11, 14	12.2	5.17	11—15
10^4	s. c.	none	—	—	0		11.6	
10^3	s. c.	Corynebacteria "D"	i. v.	100	4, 8, 11, 14	22.72	16.2	14—22
10^3	s. c.	Corynebacteria "F"	i. v.	100	4, 8, 11, 14			
10^3	s. c.	Corynebacteria "H"	i. v.	100	4, 8, 11, 14	15.15	15.2	14—19
10^3	s. c.	Corynebacteria "I"	i. v.	100	4, 8, 11, 14			
10^3	s. c.	BCG	i. v.	100	4, 8, 11, 14	7.57	14.2	13—16
10^3	s. c.	none	—	—	0	—	13.2	12—15

Table 5. Effect of various preparations of cell walls on leukemia L 1210.

ILS%: Increase in life span: $100 \times \frac{\text{life span of treated animals} - \text{life span of untreated animals}}{\text{life span of untreated animals}}$ MST = Median survival time in days.

No. of cells	Route of inoculation	Stimulating product	Route of inoculation	Dose µg	Days of inoculation	ILS %	MST	Range of death
$5 \cdot 10^3$	s. c.	0	—	—	—		12.4	12—17
$5 \cdot 10^3$	s. c.	DCWZ	i. v.	100	3, 7, 11, 14	16.93	14.5	11—16
$5 \cdot 10^3$	s. c.	DPWCW	i. v.	100	3, 7, 11, 14	1.12	12.54	11—16
$5 \cdot 10^2$	s. c.	0					14.3	11—16
$5 \cdot 10^2$	s. c.	DCWZ	i. v.	100	3, 7, 11, 14	5.5	15.1	11—18
$5 \cdot 10^2$	s. c.	DPWCW	i. v.	100	3, 7, 11, 14	3.7	14.83	13—20

Table 6. Effect of the solubilized fraction in saline (SFS) compared with that of residual bacteria on leukemia L 1210.

ILS%: Increase in life span: $100 \times \frac{\text{life span of treated animals} - \text{life span of untreated animals}}{\text{life span of untreated animals}}$ MST = Median survival time in days.

No. of cells	Route of inoculation	Stimulating product	Route of inoculation	Dose µg	Days of inoculation	ILS %	MST (day)	Range of death
10^4	s. c.	0					11.5	11—13
10^4	s. c.	C. granulosum	i. v.	100	3, 7, 10	11.30	12.8	11—14
10^4	s. c.	SFS	i. v.	1000	3, 7, 10	5.2	12.1	11—15
10^4	s. c.	SFS	i. p.	1000	3, 7, 10	2.6	11.8	11—13
10^3	s. c.	—					13.5	11—15
10^3	s. c.	C. granulosum	i. v.	100	3, 7, 10, 15	3.7	14.0	13—16
10^3	s. c.	SFS	i. v.	1000	3, 7, 10	0	13.5	12—15
10^2	s. c.	—					13.2	12—14
10^2	s. c.	C. granulosum	i. v.	100	3, 7, 10, 15	5.3	13.9	13—18
10^2	s. c.	SFS	i. v.	1000	3, 7, 10	3.0	13.6	13—15
10^2	s. c.	SFS	i. p.	1000	3, 7, 10	3.0	13.6	13—15

Table 7. Effect of *C. granulosum* and its fractions on Friend leukemia.

$$\text{ILS\%}: \text{Increase in life span}: 100 \times \frac{\text{life span of treated animals} - \text{life span of untreated animals}}{\text{life span of untreated animals}}$$

MST = Median survival time in days

Stimulating substance [a]	Dose mg	ILS %	MST	Range of death	Number of survival after 100 days
C. granulosum	1.0	51.4	45.27	39—73	1
C. granulosum	0.1	62.2	48.7	32—77	0
C. granulosum	0.01	35.4	40.5	28—57	0
DCW	1.0	18.72	35.5	25—45	0
DCW	0.1	34.1	40.1	23—58	0
DCW	0.01	21.7	36.4	21—76	0
0 [b]			29.9	17—52	0
DPWCW	1.0	32.7	41.75	21—58	2
DPWCW	0.1	42.7	44.88	21—65	0
DPWCW	0.01	34.63	42.33	20—97	1
DCWZ	1.0	25.22	39.37	27—50	2
DCWZ	0.1	9.88	34.55	22—55	1
DCWZ	0.01	3.88	32.66	20—50	1
0 [b]			31.44	16—48	1

[a] Injected i.v. to mice on day — 4.
[b] Friend virus 200 (spleen dose 50) SD_{50} injected on day 0.

Table 8. Effect of *C. granulosum* and its fractions on Friend leukemia.

$$\text{ILS\%}: \text{Increase in life span}: 100 \times \frac{\text{life span of treated animals} - \text{life span of untreated animals}}{\text{life span of untreated animals}}$$

MST = Median survival time in days

Stimulating substance [a]	Dose mg	ILS %	MST	Range of death	Number of survival after 100 days
C. granulosum	1.0	21.96	50.25	23—69	2
C. granulosum	0.1	17.18	48.28	38—53	2
C. granulosum	0.01	6.8	43.75	27—56	2
DCW	1.0	32.40	54.55	32—98	1
DCW	0.1	—	39.44	29—57	1
DCW	0.01	—	39.44	35—56	1
0 [b]			41.2	31—52	0
DPWCW	1.0	6.86	47.66	13—90	1
DPWCW	0.1	10.4	49.25	33—67	2
DPWCW	0.01	30.04	58.0	26—97	1
DCWZ	1.0	1.21	45.14	36—60	2
DCWZ	0.1	—	39.66	9—50	3
DCWZ	0.01	11.81	49.87	44—55	2
0 [b]			44.6	34—62	0

[a] Injected i.v. to mice on day — 4.
[b] Friend virus 20 SD_{50} injected i.p. on day 0.

Table 9. Effect of injection of *C granulosum* on number of plaque-forming spleen cells (data from two separate experiments; each value is the mean obtained with two mice)

On day —7 *C. granulosum* dose (μg)	On day 0 SRBC dose	On day 4 Spleen weight (g)	PFC/10^6 cells	PFC/spleen
0	5 × 10^6 cells	0.125	186	25,550
500	0	0.510	3.3	1,531
500	5 × 10^6 cells	0.495	187	76,879
0	5 × 10^6 cells	0.110	324	54,621
1000	0	0.675	3.5	1,381
1000	5 × 10^6 cells	0.675	346	148,217

cells of BCG. There was no essential difference in the activity of the various batches of corynebacteria in this test. Cell wall preparations gave a slightly more pronounced effect, increasing with the degree of purity of the preparations. The soluble fraction isolated from corynebacteria by repeated washing with saline had a low activity, similar to that of autoclaved BCG.

A similar stimulating effect was seen in the enhanced antibody response to two antigens: SRBC and tetanus toxoid. Although the amount of antibodies produced in response to SRBC injection was not significantly modified by time of stimulation (day —4 or day —7), BCG cells effected a stronger stimulation, when injected on day —7 (Fig. 1). Therefore, we chose day —7 as the standard stimulation time.

Before we discuss the results presented in Figs. 2, 3 and 4, which compare the activity of various preparations of corynebacteria and their fractions at various doses, some introductory remarks should be made:

1. All preparations tested enhanced antibody formation.

2. The antibody produced by most preparations of *C. granulosum* exhibited maxima on day 14 and day 28 with a third maximum on day 35. This pattern of response emphasizes the need to continue such experiments for a sufficiently long time. With high doses the activity maximum is recorded on day 14 and with low doses on day 28.

3. The patterns of response differ with different preparations but depend on the dose administered. Of all the preparations tested, cell walls obtained by phenol treatment displayed the most marked activity in this test, the effect being as large with small doses as with large doses.

These results prompted us to study stimulation by corynebacteria at cell level. As shown in Fig. 6, an increase was recorded with all preparations tested in the number of plaque-forming cells per spleen, whereas the number per 10^6 spleen cells was not modified (Table 9). These experiments were carried out in collaboration with J.-C. Mazie and A. Bussard and the results will be published separately. The enhanced antibody formation is likely to result not from a specific augmentation of antibody-producing cells but from the increase in the total population of spleen cells. This conclusion is of limited relevance since we have up to now studied only IgM PFC.

A similar enhancement of antibody response was noted when tetanus toxoid was used as the antigen. In this instance, the effect is more like that of a true adjuvant, as the stimulating substances were injected in emulsion in incomplete Freund's adjuvant. Partially purified cell walls of corynebacteria had the most pronounced effect, but the activity of corynebacteria and BCG was about the same.

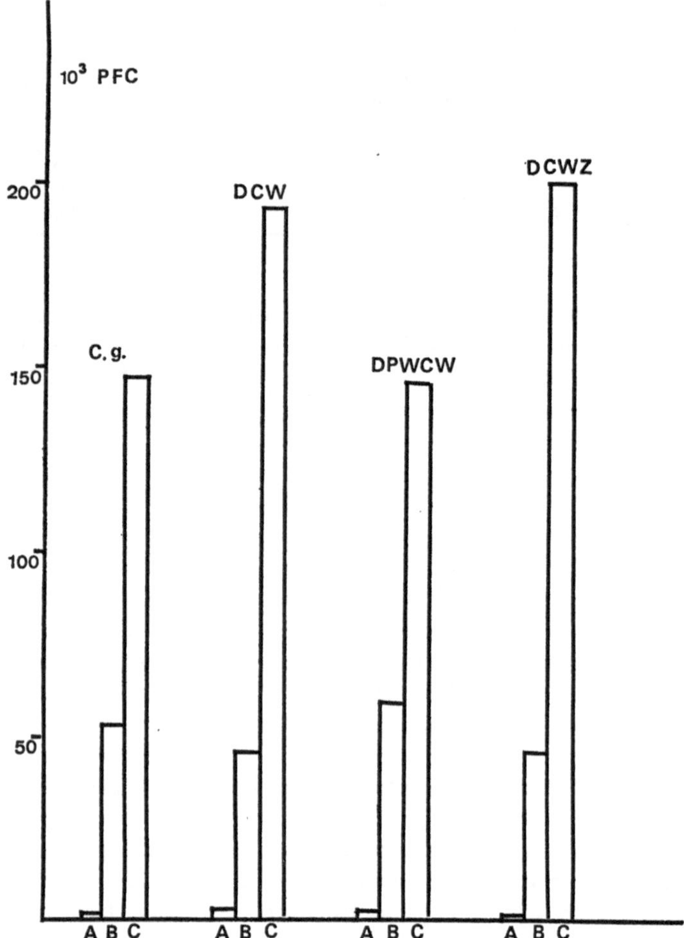

Fig. 6. Comparison of the effect of corynebacteria and various preparations obtained from the latter on the number of plaque-forming cells from spleen. Ordinate: number PFC/spleen. Abscissa: Control mice A stimulating substance, 1 mg/mouse on day — 7 alone; B SRBC, 5×10^6 cells/mouse on day 0 alone, C stimulating substance, 1 mg/mouse on day — 7 followed by SRBC, 5×10^6 cells/mouse on day 0. Each column represents the mean value calculated from two mice

Both corynebacteria and mycobacteria can induce a delayed-hypersensitivity reaction, provided they are injected in emulsion with incomplete Freund's adjuvant.

Preliminary experiments have shown that corynebacteria, or fractions isolated from them, exerted some protective effect against Friend leukemia virus when the experimental animals were stimulated on day —4 with the substance under test (Tables 7 and 8). In mice, protection sometimes lasted more than 100 days. As noted above (cf. hemagglutinin experiments) phenol-treated cell walls were more effective in low than in high doses. The mechanism that underlies such an effect has still to be elucidated. One may postulate the existence of more than one stimulating substance or of an antagonist inside the bacterial cell. Furthermore, the immunological reactions might differ (cellular or humoral) depending on the dose.

A comparative experiment was undertaken on L 1210 leukemia to determine the protection conferred by stimulation given 4 days after the tumor was grafted. Fig. 5

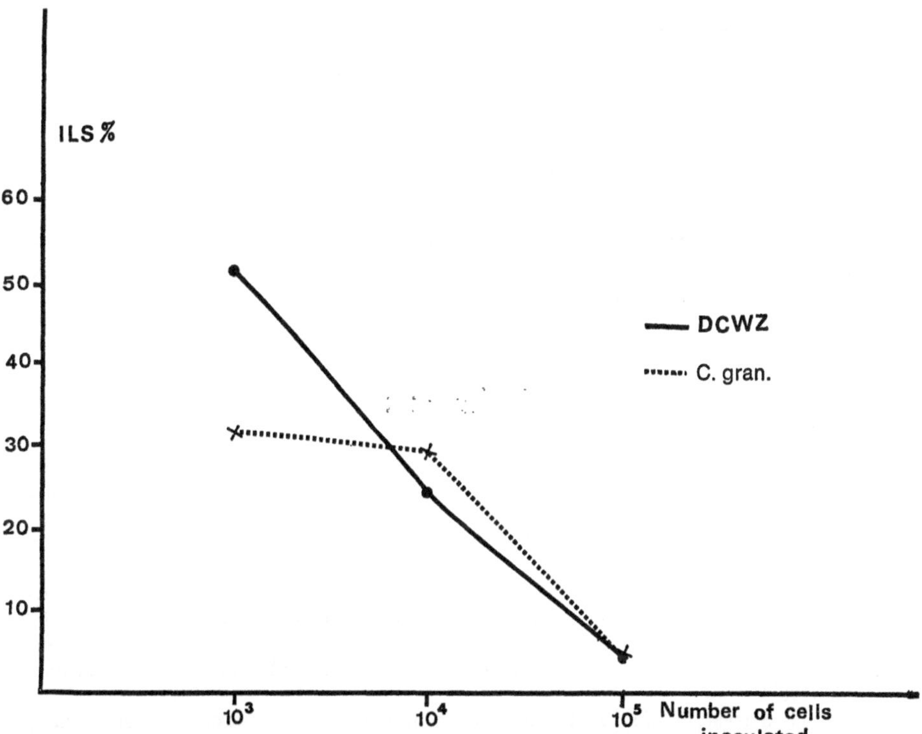

Fig. 7. Comparison of the effect of *C. granulosum* and purified cell walls on L 1210 leukemia in mice: solid line = purified CW; broken line = *C. granulosum*

shows the importance of the route of administration of the stimulating preparation. A given preparation was less effective when used intraperitoneally. This fact could account for the negative results reported by [17] and by [16]. However, when mice were given small doses of cells, only the i.p. route was effective. In contrast, corynebacteria administered intravenously invariably gave significant protection. Consequently, all experiments were conducted with i.v. administration. With small doses of leukemic cells, a marked difference was recorded in the activity of whole cells as against purified cell walls; this difference diminished as the number of L 1210 cells inoculated was increased (Fig. 7).

The results presented in Table 5 suggest that better protection is given by purified cell walls than by phenol-treated cell walls.

It is concluded from the L 1210 leukemia experiments that the substances tested could be used in combination with chemotherapy for the treatment of leukemia.

To sum up: the nonspecific immunostimulating effect of corynebacteria and their fractions is characterized by:

1. increased vascular clearance of colloidal carbon;
2. enhanced production of circulating antibodies;
3. induction of delayed-hypersensitivity to a chemically defined antigen (ABA-TYR);
4. protection against Friend virus leukemia and L 1210 leukemia.

In some cases cell walls have shown greater activity than whole cells.

Acknowledgements

We wish to thank Mr. L. Muller for having carried out the cultures in fermentor. We are pleased to acknowledge the excellent technical assistance of Misses A. Carlin, M. Pissavy and of Mr. F. Garcia-Pons.

References

1. Adlam, C., Broughton, E. S., Scott, M. T.: Enhanced resistance of mice to infection with bacteria following pretreatment with *Corynebacterium parvum*. Nature, New Biology **235**, 219 (1972).
2. Amiel, J. L., Litwin, J., Berardet, M.: Essai d'immunothérapie non spécifique par *Corynebacterium parvum* formolé. Rev. franç. Étud. clin. biol. **14**, 909 (1969).
3. Biozzi, G., Stiffel, C., Halpern, B. N., Mouton, D.: Recherches sur le mécanisme de l'immunité non spécifique produite par les Mycobactéries. Rev. franç. Étud. clin. biol. **5**, 876 (1960).
4. Biozzi, C., Howard, J. G., Mouton, D., Stiffel, C.: Modifications of graft-versus-host reaction induced by pretreatment of the host with *M. tuberculosis* and *C. parvum*. Transplantation **3**, 170 (1965).
5. Biozzi, G., Stiffel, C., Mouton, D., Liacopoulos-Briot, M., Decreusefond, C., Bouthillier, Y.: Etude du phénomène de l'immunocyto-adhérence au cours de l'immunisation. Ann. Inst. Pasteur **110** (Suppl. au N° 3), 7 (1966).
6. Biozzi, G., Stiffel, C., Mouton, D., Bouthillier, Y., Decreusefond, C.: A kinetic study of antibody producing cells in the spleen of mice immunized intravenously with sheep erythrocytes. Immunology **14**, 7 (1968).
7. Chermann, J.-C., Raynaud, M., Digeon, M.: Etudes des divers antigènes élaborés par *Salmonella typhi* R_2. II. Séparation et propriétés. Ann. Inst. Pasteur **113**, 375 (1967).
8. Cunningham, A. D.: A method of increased sensitivity for detecting single antibody-forming cells. Nature (Lond.) **207**, 1106 (1965).
9. Fauve, R. M., Hevin, M. B.: Pouvoir bactéricide des macrophages spléniques et hépatiques de souris envers *Listeria monocytogenes*. Ann. Inst. Pasteur **120**, 399 (1971).
10. Halpern, B. N., Biozzi, G., Mene, G., Benacerraf, B.: Etude quantitative de l'activité granulopexique du système réticuloendothélial par l'injection intraveineuse d'encre de Chine chez diverses espèces animales. I. Méthode d'étude quantitative de l'activité granulopexique du système réticuloendothélial par l'injection intraveineuse de particules de carbone de dimensions connues. Ann. Inst. Pasteur **80**, 582 (1951).
11. Halpern, B. N., Prevot, A.-R., Biozzi, G., Stiffel, C., Mouton, D., Morard, J.-C., Bouthillier, Y., Decreusefond, C.: Stimulation de l'activité phagocytaire du système réticuloendothélial provoquée par *Corynebacterium parvum*. J. reticuloendoth. Soc. **1**, 77 (1964).

12. Halpern, B. N., Biozzi, G., Stiffel, C., Mouton, D.: Inhibition of tumour growth by administration of killed *Corynebacterium parvum*. Nature (Lond.) **212**, 853 (1966).
13. Kessel, D.: Some determinants of camptothecin responsiveness in leukemia L 1210 cells. Cancer Res. **31**, 1883 (1971).
14. Lamensans, A., Stiffel, C., Mollier, M. F., Laurent, M., Mouton, D., Biozzi, G.: Effet protecteur de *Corynebacterium parvum* contre la leucémie greffée AKR. Relations avec l'activité catalasique hépatique et la fonction phagocytaire du système réticuloendothélial. Rev. franç. Étud. clin. biol. **13**, 773 (1968).
15. Leskowitz, S., Jones, V. E., Zak, S. J.: Immunochemical study of antigenic specificity in delayed hypersensitivity. V. Immunization with monovalent low molecular weight conjugates. J. exp. Med. **123**, 229 (1966).
16. Mathé, G.: Immunothérapie active de la leucémie L 1210 appliquée après la greffe tumorale. Rev. franç. Étud. clin. biol. **13**, 881 (1968).
17. Mathé, G., Pouillart, P., Lapeyraque, F.: Active immunotherapy of L 1210 leukemia applied after the graft of tumour cells. Brit. J. Cancer **23**, 814 (1969).
18. Mathé, G.: Active immunotherapy. Adv. Cancer Res. **14**, 1 (1971).
19. Nauciel, C., Raynaud, M.: Delayed hypersensitivity to azobenzenearsonate-N-acetyl-l-tyrosine. *In vivo* and *in vitro* study. Europ. J. Immunol. **I**, 257 (1971).
20. Pinckard, R. N., Weir, D. M., McBride, W. H.: Factors influencing the immune response. I. Effects of the physical state of the antigen and of lymphoreticular cell proliferation on the response to intravenous injection of bovine serum albumin in rabbits. Clin. exp. Immunol. **2**, 331 (1967).
21. Pinckard, R. N., Weir, D. M., McBride, W. H.: Factors influencing the immune response. II. Effects of the physical state of the antigen and of lymphoreticular cell proliferation on the response to intraperitoneal injection of bovine serum albumin in rabbits. Clin. exp. Immunol. **2**, 343 (1967).
22. Pinckard, R. N., Halonen, M.: The enhancement of rabbit anti-BSA IgE, homocytotropic antibody production by *Corynebacterium parvum* strain 10387. J. Immunol. **106**, 1602 (1971).
23. Prevot, A.-R., Halpern, B. N., Biozzi, G., Stiffel, C., Mouton, D., Morard, J.-C., Bouthillier, Y., Decreusefond, C.: Stimulation du système réticuloendothélial (S.R.E.) par les corps microbiens tués de *Corynebacterium parvum*. C. R. Acad. Sci. (Paris) **257**, (Série D), 13 (1963).
24. Prevot, A.-R., Raynaud, M., Bizzini, B., Chermann, J.-C., Kouznetzova, B., Sinoussi, F.: Activité réticulostimulante des parois de Corynébactéries anaérobies. C. R. Acad. Sci. (Paris) **274** (Série D), 2256 (1972).
25. Raynaud, M., Kouznetzova, B., Bizzini, B., Chermann, J.-C.: Étude de l'effet immunostimulant de diverses espèces de Corynébactéries anaérobies et de leurs fractions. Ann. Inst. Pasteur **122**, 695 (1972).
26. Reed, L. F., Muench, H.: Estimating fifty per cent end points. Amer. J. Hyg. **27**, 493 (1938).
27. Ribi, E., Hoyer, B. H.: Purification of Q fever Rickettsiae by density-gradient sedimentation. J. Immunol. **85**, 314 (1960).
28. Rowe, W. P., Brodsky, L.: A graded response assay for the Friend leukemia virus. J. nat. Cancer Inst. **213**, 1239 (1959).
29. Smith, L. H., Woodruff, M. F. A.: Comparative effect of two strains of *C. parvum* on phagocytic activity and tumour growth. Nature (Lond.) **219**, 197 (1968).
30. Turpin, A., Prevot, A.-R., Caille, B., Cruveiller, J.: Contribution à l'étude des antigènes des Corynébactéries aéro-anaérobies et à l'étude de leur pouvoir allergisant chez l'homme. Sem. Hôp. (Paris) **35**, 1774/P. 260 (1959).
31. Westphal, O., Lüderitz, O., Bister, F.: Über die Extraktion von Bakterien mit Phenol/Wasser. Z. Naturforsch. **7b**, 148 (1952).
32. Woodruff, M. F. A., Boak, J. L.: Inhibitory effect of injection of *Corynebacterium parvum* on the growth of tumour transplants in isogenic hosts. Brit. J. Cancer **20**, 345 (1966).

Nonspecific Stimulation by Inactivated or Ultrasonicated Brucella Abortus*

CH. PILET [1], Y. LE GARREC [1], L. TOUJAS [2], D. SABOLOVIC [3], J. C. MONTEIL, F. ROTHIER [1], U. MISHRA [1], B. GHEBREHIWET [1], J. GUELFI [2]

Laboratoire de Microbiologie — Immunologie — Pathologie Générale
Ecole Nationale Vétérinaire, Alfort [1],
Centre Eugène Marquis, Hôpital Pontchaillou, Rennes[2], and
Unité de Cancérologie de l'I.N.S.E.R.M. (U 95), Vandoeuvre-les-Nancy [3]

Brucella belongs to the large class of gram-negative bacteria, many members of which have long been known to produce a transient increase in the resistance of an organism to infection by both gram-negative and gram-positive bacteria. In their pathogenicity and ability to produce delayed hypersensitivity, Brucella have some resemblance to the Mycobacteria. Reports are available on the experimental and clinical results obtained by the use of BCG against tumors [3, 9, 10].

We report our findings on the activity of heat-inactivated or sonicated *Brucella abortus* against bacterial and viral infections and experimental tumors, including a hypothesis on its mechanism of action.

The adjuvant activity of Brucella in the production of antibody against tetanus and staphylococcal toxoid was demonstrated by RAMON *et al.* [15], and RICHOU *et al.* [16].

The antibacterial effect of inactivated Brucella was tested on the acute infection of the mouse by *Klebsiella pneumoniae* [13]. Other methods used to study its antiviral activity were *in ovo* infection with Newcastle disease virus (NDV) and mouse infections by foot-and-mouth disease virus (FMD), and influenza virus [14]. After preliminary results showing the inhibition of the growth of the Ehrlich ascites tumor [12] and L 1210 leukemia, we investigated the activity of Brucella on AKR spontaneous viral leukemia and on methylcholanthrene-induced sarcoma. Tests were carried out to determine the effect on the reticulo-endothelial system (RES), the macrophages, and the serum components, and changes in specific responses to an antigen.

Materials and Methods

1. Immunostimulant preparations were made from strains of B 19, B 19R and 45/20, heat-inactivated for 1 hr at 65 °C at a concentration of 5000 μg (dry weight).

* This work was carried out with financial help from the Institut National de la Santé et de la Recherche Médicale (no. 72.4.008), the World Health Organisation and the Institut National de la Recherche Agronomique.

The same concentration of B 19 S strain was sonicated (BUS) at 20 kHz in an MSE apparatus for 20 min, after which merthiolate was added to a final concentration of 1/10,000 to inactivate any non-disintegrated bacteria.

2. To demonstrate activity against bacterial infection, immunostimulation was carried out on CD1 mice by intraperitoneal injection of BUS, 3 days before various LD_{50}'s of *Klebsiella pneumoniae* in 2.5% mucin suspension were injected by the same route.

3. To test antiviral activity *in ovo*, various preparations were administered in the allantoic cavity of 10-day-old embryonated eggs; 10 infective doses of NDV were injected intro-allantoically at different times after stimulation. The results are expressed as hemagglutination titers of the allantoic fluid, 30 h after infection. The activity against FMD (C type) was analyzed in the newborn mouse by the intraperitoneal route, 3 days prior to intraperitoneal injection of 5 and 10 LD_{50} of virus. Heat-inactivated B 19 S was tested for antitumor activity at a single dose of 500 μg per mouse.

4. AKR female mice were divided into two groups. In the treated group, the mice received Brucella at the age of 1, 3.5 and 6.5 months, first intravenously and then intraperitoneally.

5. To test activity against chemically induced tumors, 0.1 mg methylcholanthrene (MCA) was injected subcutaneously into 5—6 week old mice of five strains: C57 BL6, DBA2, (C57BL6 × D DBD2) F_1, CBA and C_3H. Eight days later, one half of the mice in each group were injected intravenously with 500 μg of inactivated Brucella.

General Activity

Changes in the RES were measured by colloidal carbon clearance according to Stiffel [17].

Measurements of the acid phosphatase activity in the spleen were made at different times after intravenous injection of Brucella, according to Gianetto [5].

Serum parameters were analyzed; evaluation of the level of globulins by the electrophoretic method, assay of lysozyme by the Osserman method [11], and of complement by the Goto method [6].

Counts of plaque-forming cells (PFC) and rosette-forming cells (RFC) after immunization with sheep red blood cells (SRBC) were determined according to Jerne and Nordin [4] and Biozzi [2], respectively. Immunization with SRBC was preceded by a single dose of inactivated B 19 S.

Results

The mortality of mice after Klebsiella infection was significantly modified by administration of 1000 μg of BUS (Fig. 1); B 19 S and B 19 R were compared in inactivated form. No difference was observed between the two.

The antiviral activity is summarized in the Table. Multiplication of NDV *in ovo* is seriously impaired when BUS is injected 3 h, or 24 h, or 48 h before the injection of virus. No difference was observed when B 19 S was replaced by the rough strain 45/20. Activity on FMD and influenza disease of the mouse is also obvious from the percentage of mortality observed.

Survival time of mice was slightly increased by the treatment while studying evolution of AKR leukemia (Fig. 2).

Time of appearance of tumors as well as the percentage of tumor-bearing mice after MCA administration varied according to strain. (The result of nonspecific immunostimulation by heat-inactivated B19S also depended on the strain of mice.)

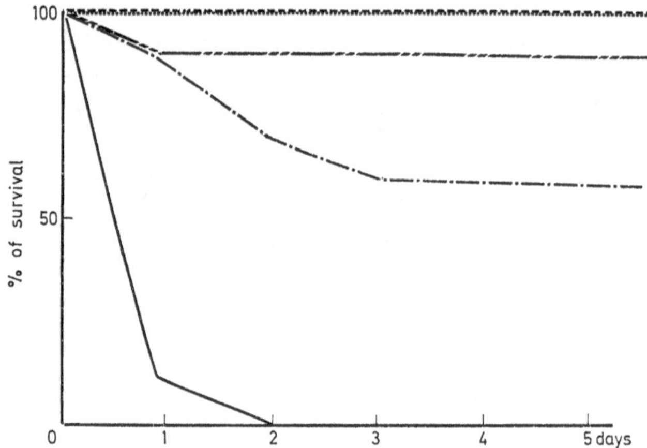

Fig. 1. Comparison of S and R strains of Brucella injected 3 days before injection of mice with *Klebsiella pneumoniae* at 26 LD_{50}. BUS R. 1000 μg, BUS S. 1000 μg, BUS R. 500 μg, BUS S. 500 μg, untreated

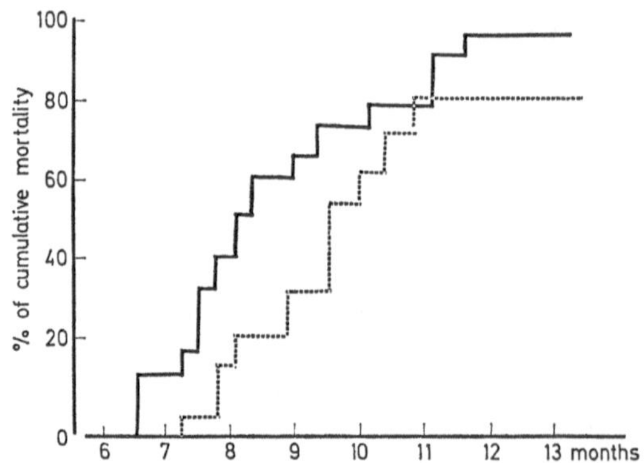

Fig. 2. Cumulative mortality of AKR mice untreated and treated with Brucella. —— Control, ------ treated

A tumor enhancement was observed in CBA and C57BL6 mice. The effect seemed inhibitory in DBA2 mice and a slight reduction was noted in C_3H and F_1 the hybrid (Fig. 3).

The speed of colloidal carbon clearance was found to reach its maximum after intraperitoneal injection of BUS between days 7 and 14 (Fig. 4). The acid phosphatase of the spleen increased to its maximum on 20 day and remained at a high level till day 40.

Table. Antiviral activity *in ovo* and in the mouse of ultrasonicated Brucella (BUS). Hemagglutination titer reveals the rate of multiplication of NDV. Results with FMD virus, and influenza virus are expressed as percentage of mortality

	NDV			FMD		Influenza	
	Hemagglutination titer			Percentage of mortality		Percentage of mortality	
	— 48 h	— 24 h	— 3 h	5 LD_{50}	10 LD_{50}	5 LD_{50}	10 LD_{50}
Control	1/3000	1/3000	1/3000	75	100	100	100
BUS	1/789	1/743	1/1067	0	0	0	0

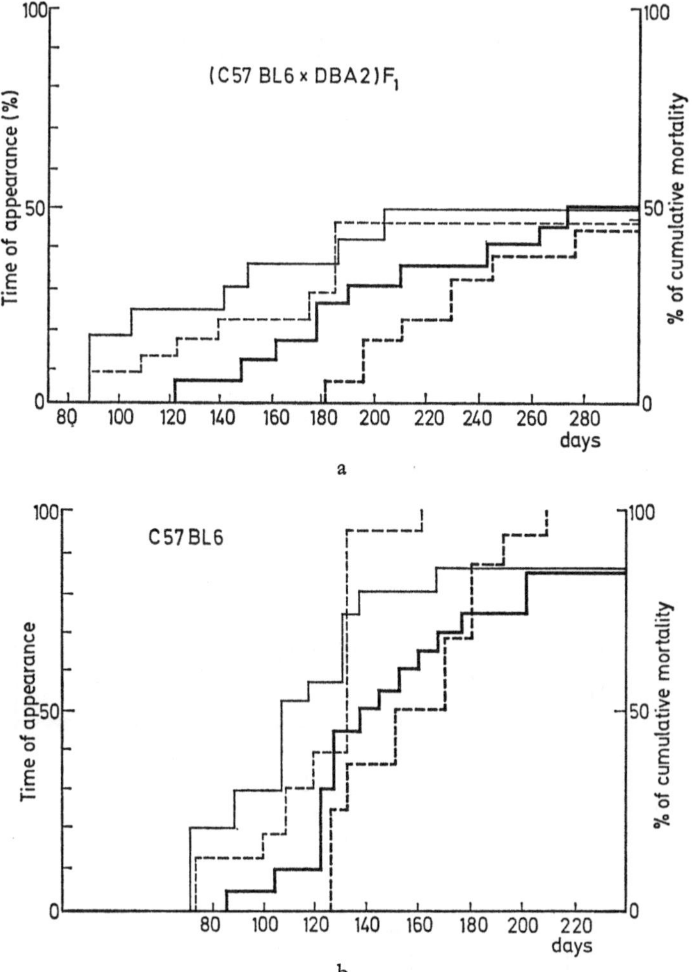

Fig. 3a-e. Time of tumor appearance and cumulative mortality in various strains of mice with tumors induced by methylcholanthrene and treated by heat-inactivated Brucella. Untreated: —— Time of appearance; ------ Cumulative mortality; treated by heat-inactivated Brucella: —— Time of appearance, —— Cumulative mortality

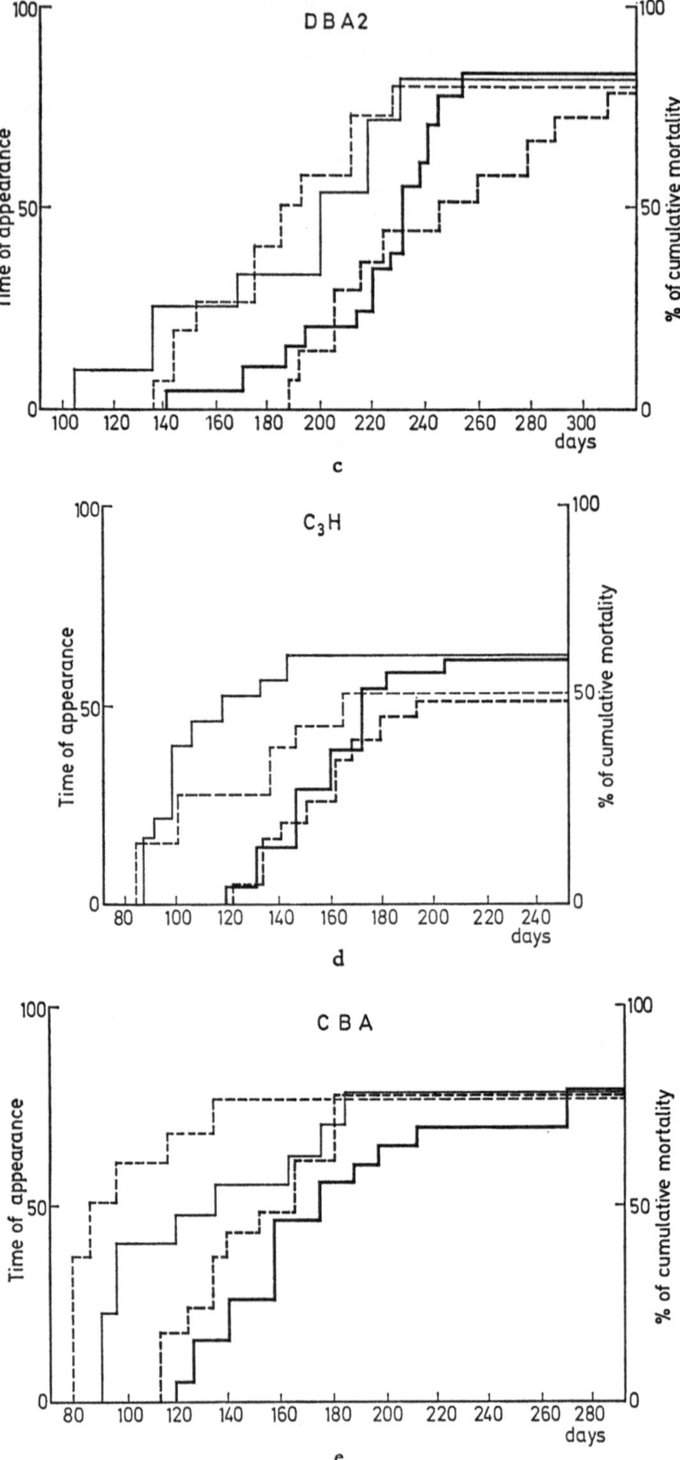
D B A 2
Time of appearance
% of cumulative mortality
100
50
0
100 120 140 160 180 200 220 240 260 280 300
days
C₃H
80 100 120 140 160 180 200 220 240
C B A
80 100 120 140 160 180 200 220 240 260 280

c

d

e

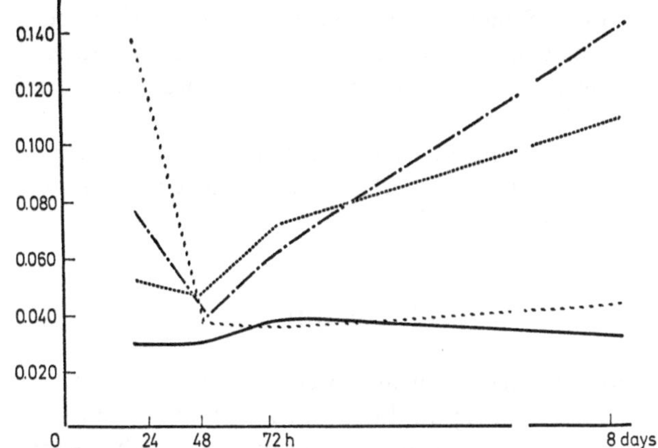

Fig. 4. Carbon clearance after intravenous, intraperitoneal and subcutaneous injection of BUS. 500 g i.p., 200 g i.v., 500 g s.c., i.v., Solvent s.c., i.p.

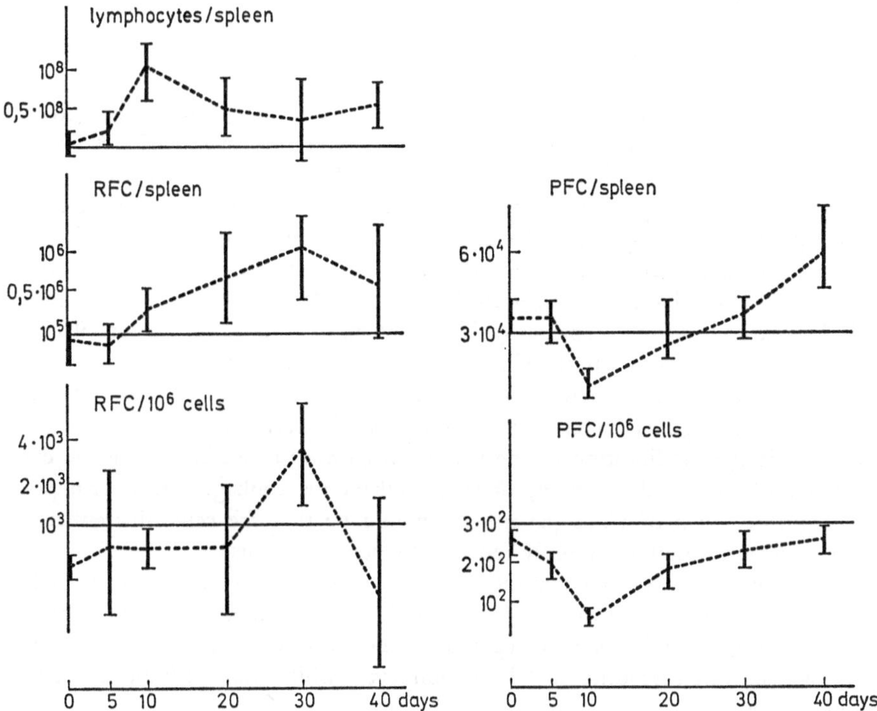

Fig. 5. Comparison of modification of the response to SRBC, expressed by plaque-forming cells (PFC) or rosette-forming cells (RFC) either per spleen, or per 10^6 cells, on different days after intravenous stimulation

After injection of B19 and BUS an early increase of globulins was noted.

Regarding complement and lysozyme, their maximum levels appeared approximately between days 9 and 12.

The stimulation of 19 S humoral antibodies against SRBC as measured by the number of PFC was slow and preceded by a phase of immunodepression around day 10. The change in response of the spleen in RFC was slightly different from that of PFC (Fig. 5).

Due to the great increase in the cellularity of the spleen, the curves expressing the number of PFC and RFC by 10^6 cells are very different from those expressing the number of PFC and RFC per spleen.

Discussion

Our observations of the activity against bacterial infection of inactivated Brucella confirm those of BERGER *et al.* [1]. In this case, somatic antigen does not seem to be required for the protective effect. At present, we cannot say what is the basis of this activity. However, the above results provide convincing evidence of the properties of Brucella against viral infection, probably unrelated to somatic antigen. Our current investigation suggests that interferon induction alone is not responsible for this antiviral resistance.

The activity of the filtered BUS and its fractions have been analyzed and the results will be reported in detail elsewhere [14].

The repeated treatment of AKR mice with heat-inactivated Brucella has given results comparable to those of LAMENSANS with *Corynebacterium parvum* [7]. A single dose of Brucella given several days after methylcholanthrene inoculation has given results which vary according to strain of mouse. A trial has been conducted on the association of specific and nonspecific stimulation and will be reported elsewhere [8].

The tests for nonspecific changes at both the cellular and the humoral level show that inactivated Brucella is a potent immunostimulant. The great increase in phagocytic index and in lysosomal enzymes (acid phosphatase) in the spelnic macrophages could explain the observed activity. Changes in lysozyme and complement occur too late to explain resistance to bacterial infection. One can speculate that macrophages play the main role against bacterial and, perhaps, viral infection.

As regards the modification of the specific response to SRBC, it could be explained by the accelerated processing of the stimulated macrophages. Another hypothesis, suggested in a previous paper [18], would be that the cells differentiated towards antigenic stimuli are rapidly replaced by new stem cells.

However, it is quite possible that the mechanisms of action of inactivated Brucella against these three type of disease (bacterial, viral and tumoral) are different. In each case, the situation must be analyzed separately. Therefore, we aim to investigate the activity of inactivated Brucella on "T" lymphocytes which play an important role in cellular defence.

Conclusion

The results obtained in bacterial and viral infections and in tumoral diseases lead to the conclusion that both inactivated and ultrasonicated Brucella are potent immunostimulants. An approach toward explaining the mechanism is reported in this article.

References

1. Berger, F. M., Fukui, G. M., Ludwig, B. J., Rosselet, J.: Increased host resistance to infection elicited by lipopolysaccharides from Brucella. Proc. Soc. exp. Biol. (N.Y.) **131**, 1376 (1969).
2. Biozzi, G., Stiffel, C., Mouton, D., Liacopoulos, Briot, M., Deucresefoud, C., Bouthillier, Y.: Etude du phénomène d'immuno-cyto-adhérence au cours de l'immunisation. Ann. Inst. Pasteur **110**, 7 (1966).
3. Halpern, B. N., Biozzi, G., Stiffel, C., Mouton, D.: Effet de la stimulation du système réticulo-endothélial par l'inoculation du BCG sur le développement de l'épithélioma atypique G 8 de Guerin chez le rat. C. R. Soc. Biol. (Paris) **153**, 919 (1959).
4. Jerne, N. K., Nordin, A. A.: Plaque formation in agar by a single antibody producing cell population. Science **140**, 405 (1963).
5. Gianetto, R., de Duve, C.: Tissue fractionation studies. IV. Comparative study of the binding of acid phosphatase, B glucuronidase and cathepsin by rat liver particles. Biochem. J. **59**, 433 (1955).
6. Goto, S., Fujii, G., Ishibashi, Y.: Studies on mouse serum. Jap. J. exp. Med. **41**, 311 (1971).
7. Lamensans, A., Stiffel, C., Mollier, M. F., Laurent, M., Mouton, D., Biozzi, G.: Effet protecteur de *Corynebacterium parvum* contre la leucémie greffée A.K.R. Relations avec l'activité catalasique hépatique et la fonction phagocytaire du SRE. Rev. franc. Étud. clin. biol. **13**, 773 (1968).
8. Le Garrec, Y., Sabolovic, D., Toujas, L., Dazord, L., Guelfi, J., Pilet, Ch.: Immunoprevention of murine tumours by inactivated Brucella and association to specific immunostimulation. Biomedicine (in press).
9. Mathe, G., Amiel, J. L., Schwarzenberg, L., Schneider, M., Cattan, A., Schlumberger, J. R., Hayat, M., de Vassal, F.: Active immunotherapy for acute lymphoblastic leukemia. Lancet **1969 I**, 697.
10. Old, L. J., Clarke, D. A., Benacerraf, B.: Effect of BCG injection on transplanted tumours in the mouse. Nature (Lond.) **184**, 291 (1959).
11. Osserman, E. F., Lawlor, D. P.: Serum and urinary lysozyme (muramidase) in monocytic and monomyelocytic leukemia. J. exp. Med. **124**, 921 (1966).
12. Pilet, Ch., Sabolovic, D.: Brucella abortus et immunothérapie active non spécifique de la tumeur d'Ehrlich. Bull. Ass. franc. Vét. Microbiol. Immunol. **7**, 43 (1970).
13. Pilet, Ch., le Garrec, Y.: Nonspecific immunostimulation by Brucella: protection of mice against Klebsiella infection. (In preparation.)
14. Pilet, Ch., Monteil, J.C., Mishra, U.: Nonspecific antiviral properties of inactivated *Brucella abortus*. (in preparation).
15. Ramon, G., Richou, R., Thiery, J. P., Gerbeaux, C.: De l'influence comparée de diverses substances stimulantes sur l'accroissement de l'immunité. C. R. Acad. Sci. (Paris) **229**, 278 (1949).
16. Richou, R., Gerbeaux, C., Schlaepfer, J.: De l'influence des suspensions de *Bacillus abortus* sur l'accroissement de l'immunité engendrée par l'anatoxine staphylococcique. C. R. Acad. Sci. (Paris) **229**, 858 (1949).
17. Stiffel, C.: Etude de la fonction phagocytaire du S.R.E. J. Physiol. (Paris) **50**, 911 (1958).
18. Toujas, L., Sabolovic, D., Dazord, L., le Garrec, Y., Toujas, J. P., Guelfi, J., Pilet, Ch.: The mechanism of immunostimulation induced by inactivated *Brucella abortus*. Rev. Europ. Étud. clin. biol. **17**, 267 (1972).

Increase of Brucella-Induced Immunostimulation by Administration in Combination with a Specific Antiserum

L. Toujas, L. Dazord, and J. Guelfi

Centre Régional Anticancéreux, Rennes

The immunostimulation induced by heat-killed *Brucella abortus* organisms strain B 19, as tested by the increase in plaque-forming cells (PFC) produced in response to challenge by sheep red blood cells (SRBC), is not detected until 40 days after the intravenous injection of the bacteria [6].

We have shown that when a hyperimmune brucella antiserum is added to this experimental system, the adjuvant properties could be detected soon after the injection of the Brucella [8].

The present paper deals with 1. the demonstration of the antiserum effect; 2. the optimal conditions for producing this effect; 3. the alterations in the humoral and cellular responses to SRBC and *Brucella* antigens provoked by the antiserum.

Materials and Methods

The isologous hyperimmune antiserum to *B. abortus* smooth strain B 19 (ASB 19) was prepared in (C57 Bl 6 × DBA 2) F_1 hybrid mice by s.c. injection (3 times a week, for 3 weeks) of 500 μg dry wt., of heat-killed B 19 organisms (kindly provided by C. Pilet). 7 different preparations of ASB 19 have been tested.

Inactivated B 19 was prepared as described previously [6] and injected into hybrid mice at a dose of 500 μg dry wt. per mouse. ASB 19 was usually given i.p. in different doses and at specified times relative to B 19 inoculation.

PFC response to SRBC challenge was determined by the direct technique of [3]. The spleens were tested 4 days after i.v. injection of 250×10^6 SRBC. The results were expressed as the number of PFC in the whole spleen.

The cellular response to SRBC was assessed as described previously [6]; the method consists in labeling with ^{3}H-thymidine the cells which divide after s.c. injection of 250×10^6 SRBC. The radioactivity is measured at the site of the challenge injection in one ear pinna. The results are expressed as the percentage increase in radioactivity in the challenged ear as against the control ear in the same animal (ear technique). This reaction was found to be greatly diminished in thymectomized, congenitally athymic, and antilymphocyte serum-treated mice [4]. The increase in radioactivity recorded in the challenged ear of animals which had not been previously immunized constituted a kind of baseline. B 19 was given i.v. in a dose of 500 μg administered at different times before SRBC.

For the determination of the cellular response to B19, an adaptation of the foregoing technique was devised: 6 or 10 days after s.c. injection of 500 µg B19 1,5 µCi ^{3}H-thymidine was given i.p. 2 days later, the mice were challenged with 5 µl of a 5000 µg per ml B19 suspension.

Results

In the experiments reported above, the day of injection of B19 was taken as day 0. Each table summarizes the particular experimental protocol. When not otherwise specified, the dose of ASB19 was 0.1 ml.

Evidence for the Adjuvant Properties of the Combination ASB19-B19

Of the protocols tested in the experiments reported in Table 1, only the combination ASB19-B19 increased the PFC response to SRBC. Replacement of ASB19 by a control serum or separate administration of B19 or ASB19 were ineffective.

Table 1. The different experimental protocols tested show that the number of PFC cannot be increased significantly by the addition of B 19 to SRBC or by the prior injection of control serum. Only the combination ASB 19 and B 19 is effective

	Experimental protocol		Number of PFC per spleen ± SE
Experiment no. 1	(Control group)	SRBC (day 0)	53,150 ± 4,865
		B 19 + SRBC (day 0)	55,550 ± 2,600
	Control serum (day — 1)	B 19 + SRBC (day 0)	61,800 ± 11,250
	ASB 19 (day — 1)	B 19 + SRBC (day 0)	164,300 ± 11,350
Experiment no. 2	(Control group)	SRBC (day 0)	16,250 ± 2,725
	ASB 19 (day — 1)	SRBC (day 0)	11,900 ± 1,500
	ASB 19 (day —1)	B 19 + SRBC (day 0)	44,750 ± 4,725

Requirements for the Optimal Effectiveness of the Combination (ASB19-B19)

a) Effect of dose ASB19.

The adjuvant effect was related to the dose of ASB19 given on day —1 (Fig. 1). The optimum dose was 0.1 ml for the antiserum investigated. Its agglutinating titer was 1/2560.

b) Effect of time of injection of ASB19.

The time of injection of ASB19 relative to that of B19 is very important: the antiserum is effective only when injected before the adjuvant (Table 2). It can be injected several weeks before B19 without significant loss of enhancing properties (Table 3).

c) Effect of time of injection of SRBC.

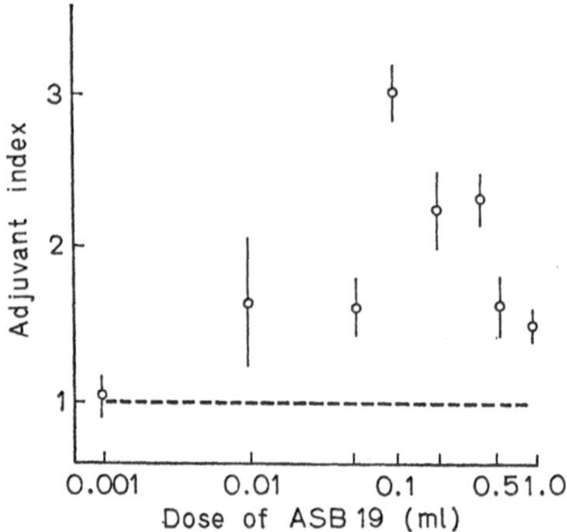

Fig. 1. ASB 19 dose-dependent increase in PFC response to SRBC. ASB 19 injected on day — 1. (The numbers on the ordinate refer to the number of PFC in treated mice divided by the corresponding control value.)

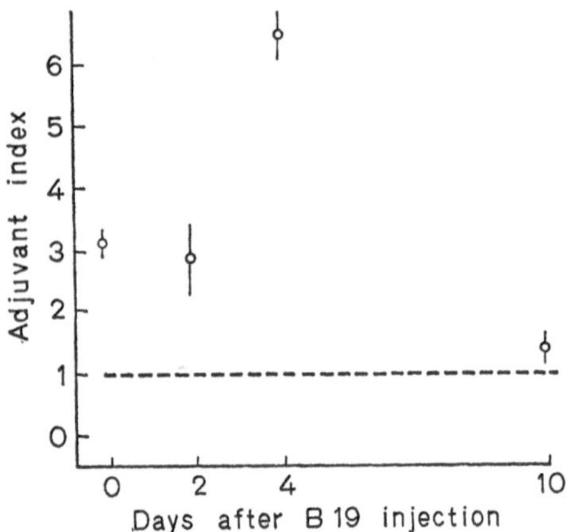

Fig. 2. Influence of the time of SRBC injection after ASB 19-B 19 administration on immunological stimulation. (The numbers on the ordinate refer to the number of PFC in treated mice divided by the corresponding control value.)

Table 2. Effect of time of injection of ASB 19 relative to that of Brucella B 19 administration ASB 19 must be given before B 19 to be effective in increasing the PFC response

Experimental protocol		Number of PFC per spleen ± SE
(Control group)	SRBC (day 2)	15,900 ± 2,625
ASB 19 (day — 1) B 19 (day 0)	SRBC (day 2)	44,150 ± 8,150
ASB 19 2 hours before B 19 (day 0)	SRBC (day 2)	43,500 ± 1,875
ASB 19 i.v. with B 19 (day 0)	SRBC (day 2)	33,200 ± 4,300
B 19 (day 0) ASB 19 (day 1)	SRBC (day 2)	23,600 ± 4,525

The immunostimulation reaches its peak value when SRBC are injected 4 days after B19 (Fig. 2). The adjuvant effect is no longer seen on day 10.

d) Use of an homologous ASB19.

The experiments with homologous ASB19 were carried out in Swiss mice. This strain has been demonstrated to be responsive to its own isologous antiserum. ASB 19 prepared in (C57 Bl 6 × DBA2) hybrids was active in Swiss mice (Table 4).

Table 3. ASB 19 injection at different times before B 19. A slight immunostimulation is still detected when ASB 19 is given 50 days prior to administration of B 19

Day of injection of ASB 19	PFC in ASB 19 + B 19 treated mice	PFC in corresponding control mice	Relative increase treated/control
— 1	43,500	15,900	× 2.7
— 3	33,400	16,250	× 2.1
— 7	55,100	16,250	× 3.4
— 14	49,350	12,150	× 4.1
— 30	46,875	25,000	× 1.9
— 50	45,625	31,250	× 1.5

Table 4. Stimulation of PFC response of Swiss mice by means of ASB 19 obtained from (C 57 Bl 6 × DBA 2) F_1 and combined with B 19

Experimental protocol		Number of PFC per spleen ± SE
(Control group)	SRBC (day 0)	27,150 ± 5,900
Homologous ASB 19 (day — 1)	SRBC (day 0)	43,150 ± 11,875
Homologous ASB 19 (day — 1)	B 19 + SRBC (day 0)	87,500 ± 11,950

ASB19-Induced Alterations of the Immune Response to B19 and SRBC

ASB19 given one day before B19 dit not prevent the increase in spleen weight which usually follows administration of *Brucella* organisms [7]. However, the increase in agglutinating antibodies to B19 was delayed by the use of the antiserum (Table 5). By contrast, the cellular response to B19, as assessed by the ear technique, seemed to be increased in the presence of antiserum (Fig. 3).

The cellular response to SRBC has been shown to be depressed by the systemic injection of different bacterial adjuvants: *Brucella*, *Corynabacterium granulosum*, BCG (to be published). Fig. 4 shows that B19 lowered the cellular response to SRBC to near the baseline level. The combination ASB19-B19 also depressed the response to the antigen, but to a significantly smaller extent (the difference between columns C and D in Fig. 4 was significant: $p < 0.01$).

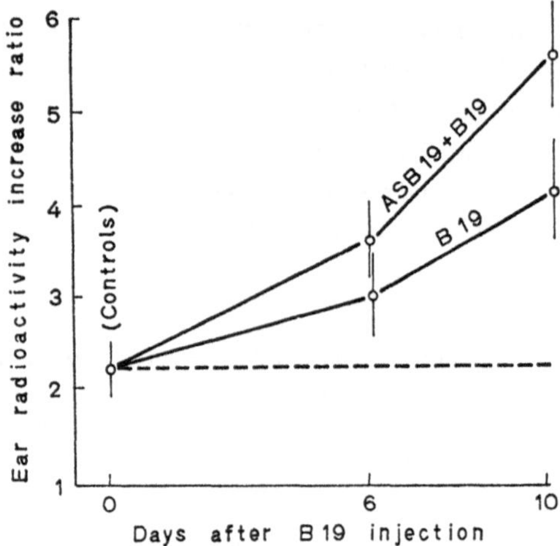

Fig. 3. Cellular response appreciated by the ear technique (see text) in mice, pretreated or notwith ASB 19, injected with B 19 on day 0

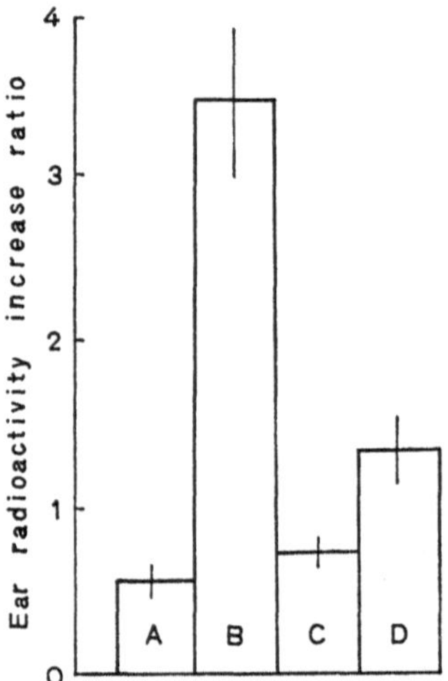

Fig. 4. Cellular response to SRBC in different experimental conditions. ASB 19 prevents the depression of cellular immunity induced by B 19 A: No SRBC immunization (background) B: SRBC immunization C: B 19 treatment + SRBC immunization D: ASB 19 B 19 treatment + SRBC immunization

Table 5. Spleen weight and agglutinating titer of sera sampled 8 and 13 days after B 19 with or without prior ASB 19. ASB 19 delays the rise of anti-Brucella antibodies

Experimental protocol	Spleen	Weight (mg)	Colog$_2$	Agglutinating titer
	day 8	day 13	day 8	day 13
No treatment	82	90	0[a]	0
B 19 (day 0)	672	369	5.8	7.1
ASB 19 (day — 1) B 19 (day 0)	656	235	0	4.9

[a] 0 = no agglutination.

Discussion

Combined treatment with brucella antiserum (ASB 19) and heat-killed Brucella B 19 induced immunological stimulation in experimental conditions where B 19 injected alone would be ineffective.

It is important for the activity of the antiserum that it is injected before the brucella. It may be given up to 7 weeks before. As the half-life of mouse immunoglobulins is up to 2 days, it seems unlikely that the main role of the antiserum is to block Brucella antigens at a peripheral level. Besides, the immunological enhancement is diminished when B 19 and ASB 19 are mixted together before injection. Thus ASB 19 probably acts at a central cellular level.

It has been suggested that antigenic competition may take place between SRBC and B 19 antigens. This phenomenon which is known to be thymus-dependent [1], would be weakened by the presence of brucella antiserum. Such a view is supported by the finding that the antiserum acts on a thymus dependent response to SRBC as indicated by its attenuation of the B 19-induced depression of the cellular response to SRBC.

An increase in the immunostimulating properties of an adjuvant correlated with a reduction in its antigenicity has been reported in other experimental systems in which the adjuvant material was chemically modified [2, 5]. The use of an anti-immunostimulant serum would represent a more generally applicable method, but it is not yet known to what extent it can be applied to other systemic adjuvants.

References

1. Gershon, R. K., Kondo, L.: Antigenic competition between heterologous erythrocytes: I. Thymic dependency. J. Immunol. **108**, 1524 (1971).
2. Hiu, I. J., Amiel, J. L.: Adjuvanticity and delayed type hypersensitivity by Bacillus Calmette-Guérin (B.C.G.). Experientia (Basel) **28**, 953 (1972).
3. Jerne, N. K., Nordin, A. A.: Plaque formation in agar by single antibody-producing cells. Science **140**, 405 (1963).
4. Sabolovic, D., Beugnot, M. C., Dumont, F., Bujadoux, M.: A new method to measure the specific cellular component of a delayed-hypersensitivity response in the ear of the mouse. Europ. J. Immunol. **2**, 604 (1972).
5. Tanaka, K., Tanaka, A., Suguyama, S.: Immunological adjuvants. I. Adjuvant activity and immunogenicity of acetylated wax D and its subfraction. Int. Arch. Allergy **34**, 495 (1968).
6. Toujas, L., Sabolovic, D., Dazord, L., Legarrec, Y., Toujas, J. P., Guelfi, J., Pilet, C.: The mechanism of immunostimulation induced by inactivated *Brucella abortus*. Rev. Europ. Etud. clin. Biol. **17**, 267 (1972a).
7. Toujas, L., Dazord, L., le Garrec, Y., Sabolovic, D.: Modification du nombre d'unités formatrices de colonies spléniques par des bactéries induisant l'immunostimulation non spécifique. Experientia (Basel) **28**, 1223 (1972b).
8. Toujas, L., Dazord, L., Guelfi, J.: Augmentation des propriétés immunostimulantes de *Brucella abortus* B_{19} inactivée par l'utilisation conjuguée d'un antisérum spécifique. C. R. Acad. Sci. (Paris) **276**, 433 (1973).

Alterations in Immune Response to Experimental Murine Tumor-Associated Antigens Following Administration of BCG or Polysaccharide from Proteus vulgaris*

M. DONNER and D. VAILLIER

Research Unit of Experimental Cancerology and Radiobiology, INSERM, Vandoeuvre-les-Nancy

Introduction

It is now well established that most experimental tumors have associated antigens which are able to evoke immune reactions in syngeneic hosts [8, 18, 20]. Much experimental evidence has been accumulated indicating that the resulting antitumor immunity is weak [6, 13]. This led investigators to test adjuvant substances as nonspecific stimulators of the immune response to tumor-associated antigens. Various trials were made with numerous bacterial adjuvants and their effects on the development of transplanted tumors were studied.

It was found that treatment with BCG [2, 3, 14], or *Corynebacterium parvum* [1], or a lipopolysaccharide from *Proteus vulgaris* [16] significantly inhibited the development of leukemia and ascites tumors.

In the case of transplanted solid tumors, results were contradictory: some workers reported that the growth of nonspecific solid tumors was inhibited by BCG [10] or *C. parvum* [11]. It was also demonstrated that *C. parvum* delayed the development of isogeneic transplants of mammary carcinoma and chemically induced sarcomas [22, 29].

In contrast, other investigators have shown that BCG could in some cases increase the growth rate of tumors [17, 19, 24]. This paradoxical effect has been also reported with fractions of tubercle bacillus [27], *Bordetella pertussis* [7], and *C. parvum* [15].

There is no satisfactory explanation as yet for these contrasting results. It is possible that the experimental parameters, such as route of administration, dose, timing of adjuvant administration might be of crucial importance. We consider this last possibility here. We chose for this investigation the experimental models involving chemically induced solid tumors and two bacterial adjuvants: BCG, and a polysaccharide extracted from *P. vulgaris*.

* This work was supported by a grant from INSERM.

The experiments described below were designed to study the effects of the timing of adjuvant administration on the immune response to challenge by tumor cells in hosts previously sensitized to tumor-associated antigens.

In addition, we wondered whether humoral enhancement might not be responsible for the increased tumor growth sometimes recorded following treatment with immunological adjuvants. Therefore, we investigated, whether serum from mice treated with bacterial adjuvants could be shown to have a neutralizing effect on tumor cells.

Lymphoid cells obtained from animals immunized with cellular antigens are known to release lymphotoxins when exposed to sensitizing antigens *in vitro*. It is not known whether similar events occur *in vivo*. To obtain some precise data on the conditions of lymphotoxin production, we undertook studies to determine whether adjuvants can induce modifications in the release of lymphotoxins by spleen cells of mice immunized with tumor antigens.

Materials and Methods

Animals and Tumors

Inbred C_3H/He mice, 3—5 months old and weighing 20—22 g each, were used throughout the experiments. The mice were housed in air-conditioned quarters and given water and commercial pellets of complete mouse diet *ad libitum*.

Rhabdomyosarcomas, originally induced in a female C_3H mouse by i.m. injection of a chemical carcinogen were maintained by serial transplantation in syngeneic female recipients. The sarcoma CB1 was induced by methylcholanthrene and the experiments performed from passage 75 to passage 85. The sarcoma TCH1 was induced by benzpyrene and used before the 15th passage.

In some experiments, dissociated tumor-cell suspensions were used as target cells. They were obtained from a methylcholanthrene-induced sarcoma (RV2) in a male C_3H mouse.

Tumor Immunization

Syngeneic mice were immunized against transplanted sarcomas according to the method described in [21]. They received two heavily irradiated (8000 rad) tumor grafts at 2 weeks intervals. Fragments of uniform size (1 mm^3) were implanted s.c. into the back with a trocar.

Adjuvants

Two weeks after the last tumor immunization, one half of the mice were injected i.p. twice with either BCG or polysaccharide from *P. vulgaris*. For the former, mice received 0.6 mg of living BCG (Institut Pasteur, Paris); for the latter, each animal received 0.1 mg of polysaccharide in physiological saline. Polysaccharide was prepared as described in [25] in a modification of WESTPHAL's method [28]. The endoxin obtained by the water-phenol method at 3—5 °C consisted of lipopolysaccharide and proteinaceous material. The protein-free lipopolysaccharide was isolated by means of a further 50% aqueous phenol extraction at 65 °C.

The species-specific polysaccharide was obtained from lipopolysaccharide by gentle hydrolysis with 0.1 N CH_3COOH. The dose of either BCG or polysaccharide from *P. vulgaris* which was used throughout these experiments did not itself produce any toxic symptoms. Immunized mice treated with i.p. injections of physiological saline served as controls.

Assays

At various times (1—46 days) after the last injection of adjuvant, mice were used for determinations of a) *in vivo* level of antitumor immunity, b) enhancing properties of serum, or c) release of lymphotoxins by spleen cells.

In vivo Measurement of Antitumor Immunity

Antitumor immunity was assessed by s.c. inoculation of single viable tumor cells into the back. Within each experiment, two groups of control mice (immunized and unimmunized) were grafted in the same way but not injected with adjuvants. Single tumor cell suspensions were prepared as described in [5], with some minor modifications. Briefly, a tumor-bearing animal was killed and the tumor excised. All necrotic tissue was discarded and the tumor mass cut into small pieces with a pair of fine scissors. The pieces of tumor were placed in Hank's medium with trypsin and transferred to a plastic tube. The ends of the tube were connected to a peristaltic pump. The movement of the pump induced a circular displacement of the fluid inside the tube and ensured a progressive dispersal of tumor cells. Cell suspensions obtained in this way were then cooled to 4 °C, filtered through several layers of sterile gauze to remove tissue debris, centrifuged twice and resuspended in Hank's medium. The cells were then counted, tested for viability with the trypan-blue exclusion procedure and injected without delay. Mice were inspected twice weekly for tumor incidence and survival time.

For comparison of tumor incidence, the χ^2 test was used to evaluate the significance of differences in number of tumor as between experimental and control groups.

Assay for Tumor Growth-Enhancing Capacity of Serum

Sera of experimental and control groups were tested for tumor-enhancing capacity by a neutralization method. Mice were exsanguinated and the blood was pooled and allowed to clot at room temperature for 1 h then left at 4 °C overnight. The serum was collected by two centrifugations at 1200 g for 30 min. The general design of the experiment consisted of incubating a known number of single viable tumor cells in 2 ml of serum. These suspensions were well mixed and incubated at 37 °C for 30 min with occasional gentle shaking. Following this, aliquots of each preparation were injected s.c. into normal C_3H recipients.

Measurement of Release of Lymphotoxins

Secretion of lymphotoxins by tumor-activated immune lymphoid cells was assayed as described in [12]. Briefly, tests were carried out in two compartment diffusion chambers. Millipore filters, effective pore size 0.1 μ, were cemented on two plastic rings with filling cacheters, thus forming two closed compartments (A and B) separated by the filter. The porosity of the filter prevented the passage of cells but allowed that of fluids.

Spleen cells harvested from mice immunized against sarcomas were used as the source of lymphotoxins. Spleens were removed aseptically and sliced into small pieces in Medium 199 supplemented with penicillin (100 U/ml) and streptomycin (100 µg/ml). The cells were gently dispersed from the tissue fragments with a loosely fitting Potter homogenizer. The cell suspension was then filtered through 4 layers of sterile gauze and diluted to the appropriate concentration. One volume of spleen-cell suspension at a concentration of 100×10^6 nucleated cells/ml was added to the same volume of tumor-cell suspension at a concentration of 2×10^6 cells/ml and 0.15 ml of this mixture was dispensed into compartment A of the diffusion chambers. Each series of experiments included control diffusion chambers containing only immune spleen cells in compartment A.

In all groups, compartment B of the diffusion chambers was filled with 0.15 ml of the target cell suspension at a concentration of 2×10^6 cells/ml. Target cells consisted of a single tumor cell suspension obtained from a solid rhabdomyosarcoma (RV2) unrelated to the sensitizing sarcomas TCH1 and CB1.

The filled chambers were inserted s.c. into the back of C_3H recipients and the wound was closed by metal clips. After 5 days, the chambers were withdrawn and the trypan blue-excluding target cells counted after dissecting out the occasional clumps with a gauze 23 needle. Each experimental and control group included 5 or 6 diffusion chambers and the mean number of harvested target cells was calculated in each group.

The level of lymphotoxin release was expressed by a cytotoxic index (CI) which was determined as follows:

$$\text{Cytotoxic index in } \% = 100 \times \left(1 - \frac{\begin{array}{c}\text{mean number of target cells in chambers}\\ \text{with immune spleen cells + tumor cells in}\\ \text{compartment A}\end{array}}{\begin{array}{c}\text{mean number of target cells in chambers with}\\ \text{only immune cells in compartment A}\end{array}} \right)$$

Results

1. Modifications of the Level of *in-vivo* Anittumor Immunity after Treatment with BCG or Polysaccharide from *Proteus Vulgaris*

In a first series of experiments, mice were sensitized with s.c. implants of heavily irradiated pieces of sarcoma TCH1 as described above. Immunizations were performed on days —28 and —14. Half the mice were then injected with 0.6 mg of living BCG on days —4 and 0 and divided into groups A, B and C.

The level of antitumor immunity in these various groups was then tested with a single s.c. challenge of suspended viable tumor cells. Group A was given a living tumor challenge on day +1, group B on day +2 and group C on day +30 after the last injection of BCG. Each group had controls of sensitized and normal mice which had received physiological saline and were challenged in the same way. The level of antitumor immunity is known to be subject to variations with time [23] and only groups immunized and challenged at exactly the same time can be compared. Each animal was given 10^5 living tumor cells.

Fig. 1 A shows the results, expressed as the percentage of mice resistant to this challenge in the experimental and control groups.

Only 5% of normal mice failed to develop tumors. As expected the sensitization procedure induced a significant immune resistance to challenge implantation of viable tumor cells, and about 40% of mice survived the challenge. Inoculation of BCG into sensitized recipients led to important modifications of the level of antitumor immunity. The immune response was markedly depressed when the tumor challenge was given one day after the last injection of BCG and only 11% of the mice failed to develop tumors.

Statistical evaluation of the results shows that the difference in tumor incidence in the groups which received BCG or physiological saline was highly significant ($\chi^2 = 11.07, p < 0.001$). However, immune resistance was only supressed for a short time, since it returned to its normal level if the tumor challenge was given 10 days after BCG. The tumor incidence was analogous to that observed in sensitized mice which received no adjuvant. Fig. 1 A also shows that resistance was enhanced when the period between BCG and living tumor challenge was extended to 30 days. About 70% of mice failed to develop tumors. The differences in tumor "takes" between sensitized mice which received BCG or saline were significant ($\chi^2 = 7.24, p < 0.01$).

In a second series of experiments, a similar experimental design was used with tumor CB1 and polysaccharide from *Proteus vulgaris*. Sensitized mice received 0.1 mg of polysaccharide on days —4 and 0. They were challenged with 8×10^4 living cells of sarcoma CB1 at various time intervals after the last injection of polysaccharide.

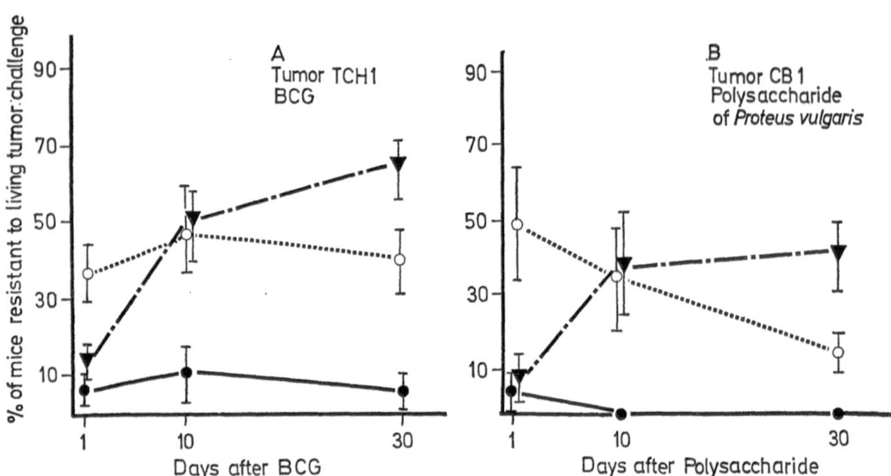

Fig. 1. Effect of BCG (A) and polysaccharide of *Proteus vulgaris* (B) on *in vivo* antitumor immunity in mice immunized specifically against syngeneic solid rhabdomyosarcomas. Mice were sensitized against tumor on days — 28 and — 14. One half of the mice received BCG or polysaccharide on days — 4 and 0. Antitumor immunity was assessed by a living tumor challenge at various intervals after the last dose of adjuvant. ○------○ Mice immunized and *not treated* with adjuvant, ▼—-—▼ Mice immunized and *treated* with adjuvant, ●——● Controls. Vertical bars represent 95% confidence limits

The results shown in Fig. 1B were identical to these described for the tumor TCH1-BCG experimental model. The level of antitumor immunity was related to the time interval between the treatment with polysaccharide and the living tumor challenge. A depression of antitumor immunity was seen in the early days after the last inoculation of adjuvant. The differences between the tumor incidence in sensitized mice which received either polysaccharide or saline were significant ($\chi^2 = 10.46, p < 0.005$). The level of antitumor immunity returned to normal values on day 10 and was significantly increased 30 days after treatment with adjuvant ($\chi^2 = 4.37, p < 0.05$).

2. Changes in Properties of Serum Following BCG or Polysaccharide from *P. Vulgaris*

The observation that antitumor immunity was depressed in the early days after inoculation of both adjuvant substances suggested that enhancing antibodies may have been responsible. This possibility was tested by means of a neutralization method, as described in materials and methods.

Identical procedure were used for tumors TCH1 and CB1. Mice sensitized against sarcomas were bled at 7 or 22 days after the last injection of adjuvants. Sensitized mice which had received no BCG and normal mice were exsanguinated simultaneously, and 3×10^3 living tumor cells were mixed with 2 ml of each serum. After incubating at 37 °C for 30 min, the same aliquot of each preparation was inoculated subcutaneously into normal recipients. Tumor incidence in each group was the criterion of the effect of serum on tumor cells.

The results are illustrated in Fig. 2. For the tumor TCH1, about 70% of mice displayed tumors when tumor cells were mixed with normal serum. It was also

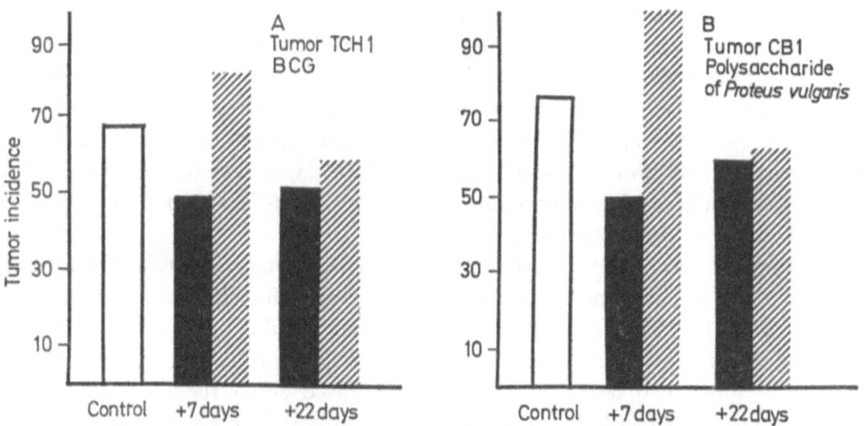

Fig. 2. Effect of BCG or polysaccharide of *Proteus vulgaris* on the properties of serum in mice sensitized against syngeneic solid tumors. Mice were immunized against tumor on days —28 and —14. One half of the mice received BCG or polysaccharide. In each of these groups, the serum was collected 7 or 22 days after the last dose of adjuvant. The properties of serum were assessed by a neutralization test: normal mice were grafted with living tumor cells which had been previously incubated with serum. Closed columns: serum from mice immunized against tumor and *not treated* with adjuvant. Hatched columns: serum from mice immunized against tumor and *treated* with adjuvant. Open column: serum from normal mice served as control

apparent that tumor incidence was slightly inhibited in recipients which were given tumor cells incubated with immune serum. In marked contrast, the action of serum is strongly modified after administration of BCG. When blood was collected 7 days after BCG, tumor growth was enhanced as compared with the control group given normal serum. This effect of serum decreased when mice were bled 22 days after the last injection of BCG. Statistical evaluation of the results shows that the difference was not significant.

As Fig. 2B shows, quite similar results were obtained with mice sensitized against sarcoma CB1 and treated with polysaccharide from *P. vulgaris*. When mice were bled 7 days after the last injection of polysaccharide, sera were found to cause a considerable enhancement of tumor growth. As with BCG, the effect of polysaccharide was of short duration. The enhancing capacity of serum was greatly reduced when sera were collected 22 days after treatment with polysaccharide.

3. Effect of BCG and Polysaccharide from *P. Vulgaris* on the Release of Lymphotoxins by Spleen Cells Sensitized Against Syngeneic Tumors

The results observed with serum demonstrated that administration of BCG or polysaccharide from *P. vulgaris* presumably alters the humoral immune response. However, adjuvants can also change a cell-mediated immune response.

In order to test whether this was the case in our experimental system, the spleen cells of sensitized mice which had been treated with adjuvants were examined for their capacity to release lymphotoxins over a period of time ranging from 4 to 46 days after the last injection of adjuvant. Indeed, results show that lymphotoxins were released when lymphoid cells from mice immunized against a syngeneic tumor were cultured with the sensitizing tumor [26].

Tests were conducted in two-compartment diffusion chambers, as described in Materials and Methods. At different times after the last injection of adjuvants, spleen cells were harvested from mice treated with BCG or polysaccharide from *P. vulgaris*; 10×10^6 spleen cells were cultured with or without 2×10^5 living tumor cells in one compartment of diffusion chambers, and 2×10^5 target cells in the second compartment. Production of lymphotoxins was quantitatively assessed by a cytotoxic index, calculated as described previously.

In a parallel series of control experiments, spleen cells harvested from immunized mice which had received no adjuvant were also tested for their ability to release lymphotoxins. The results are summarized in Tables 1 and 2.

In all control experiments, it may be seen that spleen cells harvested from sensitized mice which had received no adjuvant released about the same amount of cytotoxic factor when cultured with sensitizing tumor. For the tumor CB1, the cytotoxic index was near 30%; in the case of tumor TCH1, it was about 35%. Following administration of BCG or polysachcharide, release of lymphotoxins was markedly modified. When the spleens were harvested a few days after the last injection of adjuvant. the production of non-specific cytotoxic factors was very weak. In some cases, a negative value of cytotoxic index was found indicating that, when reexposed to antigen, sensitized spleen cells released soluble products which stimulated the growth of target cells. This result was somewhat surprising. However, it

Table 1. Effect of BCG on the release of lymphotoxins from spleen cells sensitized to tumor TCH 1-associated antigens

Time interval in days [a]	Number of viable target cells ($\times 10^6$/ml) harvested in compartment B of diffusion chambers when compartment A [b] was filled with					
	Control [c] spleen cells alone	Control spleen cells and tumor cells	Cototoxic index in %	Experimental [d] spleen cells alone	Experimental spleen cells and tumor cells	Cytotoxic index in % [e]
4	3.17 ± 0.32 [f]	2.06 ± 0.33	35.0	3.14 ± 0.32	3.17 ± 0.42	— 0.9
9	3.93 ± 0.29	2.38 ± 0.25	39.4	4.27 ± 0.28	4.27 ± 0.28	3.2
12	2.35 ± 0.17	1.47 ± 0.12	37.4	2.40 ± 0.23	2.92 ± 0.21	— 21.6
19	3.23 ± 0.27	2.07 ± 0.22	35.9	3.31 ± 0.44	2.05 ± 0.45	38.0
26	2.32 ± 0.17	1.51 ± 0.34	34.9	2.10 ± 0.22	1.65 ± 0.87	21.4
28	3.75 ± 0.41	2.52 ± 0.55	32.8	3.62 ± 0.18	2.40 ± 0.18	33.7
32	2.16 ± 0.16	1.57 ± 0.22	27.3	2.25 ± 0.52	1.08 ± 0.21	52.0
43	4.46 ± 0.38	2.88 ± 0.26	35.4	4.60 ± 0.45	3.15 ± 0.51	31.5
46	2.56 ± 0.24	1.72 ± 0.32	33.6	2.13 ± 0.12	1.07 ± 0.23	49.3

[a] Mice were sensitized to tumor on days — 28 and — 14. One half of the mice received BCG on days — 4 and 0. Spleen cells in each of these two groups were harvested at various intervals after the last dose of BCG.

[b] The experiments were performed in two compartment diffusion chambers.

[c] Control groups consisted of spleen cells from mice sensitized to tumor TCH 1 and *not treated* with BCG.

[d] Experimental groups consisted of spleen cells from mice sensitized to tumor TCH 1 and *treated* with BCG.

[e] Calculated as described in Materials and Methods.

[f] Each figure represents the mean number of viable target cells ($\times 10^6$/ml) harvested on day + 5 in 5 diffusion chambers ± standard error.

Table 2. Effect of polysaccharide of *Proteus vulgaris* on the quantitative production of lymphotoxins released by spleen cells sensitized to tumor CB 1-associated antigens

Time interval in days [a]	Number of viable target cells ($\times 10^6$/ml) harvested in compartment B of diffusion chambers when compartment A [b] was filled with					
	Control [c] spleen cells alone	Control spleen cells and tumor cells	Cytotoxic index in %	Experimental [d] spleen cells alone	Experimental spleen cells and tumor cells	Cytotoxic index in % [e]
6	1.73 ± 0.10 [f]	1.24 ± 0.09	28.3	1.80 ± 0.51	1.80 ± 0.16	0.0
9	2.73 ± 0.33	1.83 ± 0.45	32.9	2.75 ± 0.54	2.73 ± 0.93	0.7
14	2.27 ± 0.29	1.63 ± 0.29	28.2	2.60 ± 0.16	2.44 ± 0.26	6.1
15	4.05 ± 0.47	3.05 ± 0.39	24.7	4.02 ± 0.21	4.39 ± 0.47	— 9.2
25	3.90 ± 0.10	2.92 ± 0.22	25.1	3.92 ± 0.22	3.15 ± 0.33	19.6
32	2.21 ± 0.66	1.47 ± 0.40	33.4	2.90 ± 0.56	1.10 ± 0.12	62.1
39	2.49 ± 0.12	1.61 ± 0.21	35.3	2.63 ± 0.32	1.18 ± 0.11	55.2

[a] Mice were sensitized to tumor on days — 28 and — 14. One half of the mice received polysaccharide on days — 4 and 0. Spleen cells in each of these two groups were harvested at various intervals after the last dose of polysaccharide.

[b] The experiments were performed in two-compartment diffusion chambers.

[c] Control groups consisted of spleen cells from mice sensitized to tumor CB 1 and *not treated* with polysaccharide.

[d] Experimental groups consisted of spleen cells from mice sensitized to tumor CB 1 and *treated* with polysaccharide.

[e] Calculated as described in Materials and Methods.

[f] Each figure represents the mean number of viable target cells ($\times 10^6$/ml) harvested on day + 5 in 5 diffusion chamber ± standard error.

has been suggested that small amounts of lymphotoxins could stimulate protein biosynthesis [9].

In contrast to these findings, spleen cells harvested from mice treated about two weeks earlier with BCG or polysaccharide released a normal amount of lymphotoxins upon stimulation with tumor antigen.

Finally, it was also apparent from Tables 1 and 2 that spleen cells produced more non-specific cytotoxic factors when they were harvested one month after administration of adjuvant.

Discussion

The main object of our work was to collect information on the action of adjuvant substances on the immune response to murine solid tumor-associated antigens. The results demonstrate that BCG and a polysaccharide extracted from *Proteus vulgaris* induce similar modifications of this immune response. The effect of both adjuvants on the level of *in vivo* antitumor immunity can be divided into three phases: antitumor immunity is strongly depressed in the early days after two injections of either BCG or polysaccharide; in the second phase, immunity returns to a normal level; the third phase is characterized by a significant increase in the immune response of mice to tumor-associated antigens.

We have also shown that the decline in antitumor immunity is associated with a marked change in the properties of serum. In the early days following adjuvant administration, humoral substances are able to stimulate the growth of tumors.

Finally, the present study has also demonstrated that adjuvants influence the release of lymphotoxins from spleen cells sensitized to tumor antigens.

These results require some comments. First, the present studies confirm that the depression of antitumor immunity is due to a classical phenomenon of enhancement, particularly in the case of experiments utilizing sera for neutralization of tumor cells. Indeed, tests indicate that humoral substances are able to promote tumor growth. It may be that injections of adjuvants result in an increased production of circulating antibodies. It is conceivable that tumor cells become coated with these antibodies, which prevents the access of lymphocytes and allows the growth of tumors. It is interesting to note that the production of these antibodies appears to decline rapidly. Further experimentation will obviously be needed to clarify this particular point.

Second, both adjuvants cause important modifications in lymphotoxin release by sensitized cells; this is more difficult to explain. Some workers suggest that the quantitative production of soluble mediators may be regarded as a reflection of cell-mediated immune response [4]. If this is correct, our findings show that administration of adjuvants is followed by a depression of the cell-mediated immune response. It is not yet known whether enhancing antibodies produce this effect by acting at the central level of cellular response, or whether the production of such antibodies and the depression of the cell-mediated response are unrelated. In a later phase after administration of adjuvants, the quantitative estimation of lymphotoxin release indicates that the cell-mediated immune response is increased. In this case, no humoral factor seems to play an important role. These results are somewhat surprising since the production of lymphotoxins is a specific phenomenon. Further studies on the action of adjuvants on the effector molecules of cellular immunity might provide some information on the mechanism of action of adjuvants.

In the present state of knowledge, these results cannot be directly extrapolated to other systems. It seems prudent to perform complementary investigations with other adjuvants, and other experimental tumors.

Acknowledgements

The skilful technical assistance of Mrs. Michéle Batoz and Suzanne Droesch is gratefully acknowledged.

References

1. Amiel, J. L., Litwin, J., Berardet, M.: Essai d'immunothérapie active non spécifique par le *Corynebacterium parvum* formolé. Rev. franç. Étud. clin. biol. **14**, 909 (1969).
2. Amiel, J. L., Berardet, M.: Effects of active specific and non-specific immunotherapy on E ♂ G 2 leukemia according to the route of administration and combination of immunological adjuvants. Europ. J. Cancer **7**, 419 (1971).
3. Biozzi, G., Stiffel, C., Halpern, B. N., Mouton, D.: Effet de l'inoculation du Bacille de Calmette-Guérin sur le développement de la tumeur ascitique d'Ehrlich chez la souris. C. R. Soc. Biol. (Paris) **153**, 987 (1959).
4. Bloom, B. R.: *In vitro* methods in cell-mediated immunity (Bloom, B. R., Glade, P. R., Eds.), p. 3. New York, London: Academic Press 1971.
5. Boyse, E. A.: A method for the production of cell suspensions from solid tumors. Transplant. Bull. **7**, 100 (1960).
6. Donner, M., Oth, D., Vaillier, D., Burg, C.: Analyse quantitative *in vivo* des réactions immunitaires dirigées contre les antigènes associés à des tumeurs murines solides. Int. J. Cancer **9**, 30 (1972).
7. Floersheim, G. L.: Facilitation of tumor growth by *Bacillus pertussis*. Nature (Lond.) **216**, 1235 (1967).
8. Foley, E. J.: Antigenic properties of methylcholanthrene-induced tumors in mice of the strain origin. Cancer Res. **13**, 835 (1953).
9. Granger, G. A.: In: Mediators of cellular immunity (Sherwood, H., Lawrence, M., Landy, Eds.), p. 321. New York, London: Academic Press 1969.
10. Halpern, B. N., Biozzi, G., Stiffel, C.: Action de l'extrait microbien Wxb 3148 sur l'évolution des tumeurs expérimentales. In: Colloque Int. du CNRS (Halpern, B. N., Ed.), p. 221, 1963.
11. Halpern, B. N., Biozzi, G., Stiffel, C., Mouton, D.: Inhibition of tumor growth by administration of killed *Corynebacterium parvum*. Nature (Lond.) **212**, 853 (1966).
12. Hottier, D., Donner, M., Burg, C.: Release of non specific cytotoxic factors by splenic cells immunized against allogeneic tumour cells. Rev. europ. Étud. clin. biol. **16**, 240 (1971).
13. Klein, G., Sjögren, H. O., Klein, E., Hellström, K. E.: Demonstration of resistance against methylcholanthrene-induced sarcoma in the primary autochtonous host. Cancer Res. **20**, 1561 (1960).
14. Mathé, G., Pouillart, P., Lapeyraque, F.: Active immunotherapy of L 1210 leukemia applied after the graft of tumour cells. Brit. J. Cancer **23**, 814 (1969).
15. Mathé, G.: Application de l'immunotherapie active au traitement des tumeurs solides. Etude expérimentale et humaine. Compte rendu contrat D.G.R.S.T. n° 70-7-2361, 1 (1971).
16. Mizuno, D., Yoshioka, O., Akamatu, M., Kataoka, T.: Antitumor effect of intracutaneous injection of bacterial polysaccharide. Cancer Res. **28**, 1531 (1968).
17. Old, L. J., Benacerraf, B., Clarke, D. A., Carswell, E. A., Stockert, E.: The role of the reticuloendothelial system in the host reaction to neoplasia. Cancer Res. **21**, 1281 (1961).

18. OLD, L. J., BOYSE, E. A., CLARKE, D. A., CARSWELL, E. A.: Antigenic properties of chemically-induced tumors. Ann. N.Y. Acad. Sci. **101**, 80 (1962).
19. PIESSENS, W. F., LACHAPELLE, F. L., LEGROS, N., HEUSON, J. C.: Facilitation of rat mammary tumour growth by B.C.G. Nature **228**, 1210 (1970).
20. PREHN, R. T., MAIN, J. M.: Immunity to methylcholanthrene-induced sarcomas. J. nat. Cancer Inst. **18**, 769 (1957).
21. REVESZ, L.: Detection of antigenic differences in isologous host-tumor systems by pretreatment with heavily irradiated tumor cells. Cancer Res. **20**, 443 (1960).
22. SMITH, L. H., WOODRUFF, M. F. A.: Comparative effect of two strains of *Corynebacterium parvum* on phagocytic activity and tumor growth. Nature (Lond.) **219**, 197 (1968).
23. SNELL, G. D., WINN, H. J., KANDUTSCH, A. A.: A quantitative study of cellular immunity. J. Immunol. **87**, 1 (1961).
24. STJERNSWÄRD, J.: Immune status of the primary host towards its own Methylcholanthrene-induced sarcomas. J. nat. Cancer Inst. **40**, 13 (1968).
25. TOUPLICHEVA, A. P., IVANOV, K. K., SILINOVA, N. G.: Influence of antigens and their degradation products on the resistance of animals to irradiation (in Russian). Radiobiologiia **5**, 243 (1965).
26. VAILLIER, D., DONNER, M., VAILLIER, J., BURG, C.: Release of lymphotoxins by spleen cells sensitized against mouse tumor associated antigens. Cell. Immunol. **6**, 466 (1973).
27. WEISS, D. W., BONHAG, R. S., LESLE, P.: Studies on the heterologous immunogenicity of a methanol-insoluble fraction of attenuated tubercle bacilli. II. Protection against tumor isografts. J. exp. Med. **124**, 1039 (1966).
28. WESTPHAL, O., LÜDERITZ, O., BISTER, F.: Über die Extraktion von Bakterien mit Phenol/Wasser. Z. Naturforsch. **7**b, 148 (1952).
29. WOODRUFF, M. F. A., BOAK, J. L.: Inhibitory effect of injection of *Corynebacterium parvum* on the growth of tumor transplants in isogeneic hosts. Brit. J. Cancer **20**, 345 (1966).

Cell-Mediated Immunity in AKR Mice Treated with Lentinan, a Fungal Polysaccharide*

M. M. Bortin [1], A. A. Rimm [1], E. C. Saltzstein [1], M. R. Shalaby [1], and G. E. Rodey [2]

May and Sigmund Winter Research Laboratory, Mount Sinai Medical Center [1] and Milwaukee Blood Center [2], Medical College of Wisconsin, Milwaukee, Wisc.

A number of recent reports from the National Cancer Center Research Institute in Tokyo have indicated that a polysaccharide extracted from *Lentinus edodes* possesses marked antitumor activity against sarcoma 180 [1, 2, 3, 4]. In the doses tested, the purified extract from this edible mushroom was not toxic [2]. It was not cytocidal in tumor-cell cultures [2] but exhibited marked antitumor activity *in vivo* when administered in 10 daily doses of 1 mg/kg [2, 3, 4]. The antitumor effect occurred whether the series of lentinan injections was completed prior to tumor inoculation or started on the day after tumor inoculation. Its antitumor effect was largely abolished when tested in neonatally thymectomized hosts [3] or when lentinan was administered in conjunction with antilymphocyte serum [4]. Chihara, Maeda and their colleagues in Japan have proposed that lentinan is a potent nonspecific stimulant of cell-mediated immunity.

This preliminary report describes some effects of lentinan as measured a) *in vivo* in young AKR mice bearing a long-passage lymphocytic leukemia, and b) *in vitro* by culturing spleen cells from lentinan-treated mice with PHA or mitomycin-treated allogeneic cells.

Materials and Methods

Inbred 8—10 week old AKR/J and C57 BL/6J female mice obtained from the Jackson Laboratory, Bar Harbor, Maine were used. A long-passage lymphocytic leukemia (BW 5147) was the source of leukemia cells. BW 5147 leukemia originated spontaneously in an AKR mouse at the Jackson Laboratories in 1954 [6]. It has been paasaged there as a solid tumor through more than 800 transplant generations. It had been maintained as a lymphocytic leukemia by serial i.v. passage in our laboratory through more than 100 transplant generations when these experiments were initiated. Donor mice bearing BW 5147 leukemia for 7 days were sacrificed,

* Research supported by American Cancer Society grant ET-55, the Board of Trustees, Mount Sinai Medical Center, HE 13-629 Grant from the National Heart and Lung Institute (U.S.A.) and the Milwaukee Blood Center Research Fund.

their spleens removed, and the cells flushed from the spleens with Hanks' solution. Spleen cells were counted in a hemocytometer, the percentage of "blast" (large) cells was noted, and viability verified by the dye-exclusion test. The concentration of blast cells in the spleen cell suspensions ranged from 49% to 65%, and viability was 90% or higher. All mice that died were autopsied and examined grossly for evidence of leukemia.

The radiation conditions [7], technique for spleen bioassay [8], *in vitro* methods for mouse spleen PHA response [9], and mouse one-way mixed leukocyte culture (MLC) tests [10] have been described.

Results

The model used to test the cytocidal and cytostatic properties of lentinan against BW 5147 leukemia cells is shown in Fig. 1. On day zero, young AKR mice were

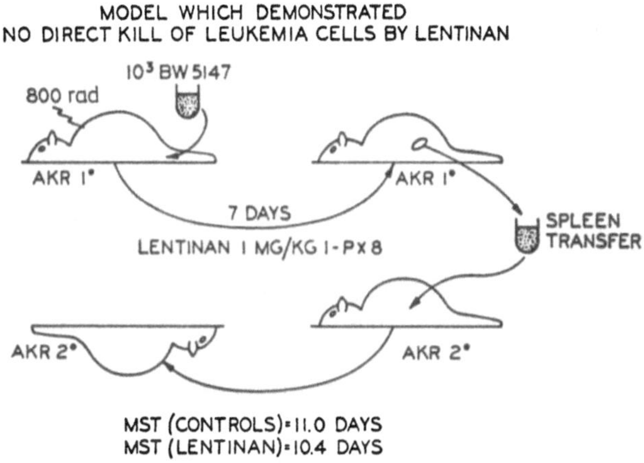

MODEL WHICH DEMONSTRATED
NO DIRECT KILL OF LEUKEMIA CELLS BY LENTINAN
10^3 BW 5147
800 rad
AKR 1°
AKR 1°
7 DAYS
LENTINAN 1 MG/KG I-P x 8
SPLEEN TRANSFER
AKR 2°
AKR 2°
MST (CONTROLS) = 11.0 DAYS
MST (LENTINAN) = 10.4 DAYS

Fig. 1. Experimental model to test the cytocidal and/or cytostatic effects of lentinan. On day zero, immunosuppressed AKR mice were given leukemia cells and daily injections of lentinan were started. Spleens from individual mice were bioassayed in individual syngeneic secondary recipients on day 7. Spleen cells from lentinan-treated and control mice produced leukemia in all (59/59) secondary recipients with no significant difference in their median survival times

exposed to 800 rad whole-body X-irradiation ($LD_{100/15}$) to impair or eliminate the immunological reaction of the host to the leukemia. Within 4 hours following radiation the AKR primary hosts were given 10^3 BW 5147 leukemia blast cells; 30 min later they were given the first of 8 daily i.p. inoculations of lentinan (generously provided by Dr. G. CHIHARA) in a dose of 1 mg/kg/day. On day 7, the primary hosts were sacrificed and spleen cell suspensions from individual mice were inoculated i.p. into individual normal young AKR secondary recipients. The secondary recipients were observed for survival. The median survival time (MST) of 10.4 days for secondary recipients that received spleen cells from lentinan-treated mice was not significantly different from the MST of 11.0 days for controls. Control mice were treated similarly in all respects except that injections of the suspending vehicle (double-distilled sterile water) were given instead of lentinan. All lentinan-treated (39/39) and control (20/20) bioassay secondary recipients died of leukemia. Lentinan exhibited no detectable cytocidal or cytostatic effect on a dose of 10^3 long-passage leukemia cells in immunosuppressed AKR host mice.

Groups of normal young AKR mice were given i.v. injections of 10^3 BW 5147 leukemia blast cells and treated with 3 different dose schedules of lentinan. The dose schedules and results are shown in the Table. There were no significant differences

Table. Effect of lentinan on survival of young AKR mice given 10^3 long-passage leukemia cells

Number of mice	Schedule for i.p. lentinan (1 mg/kg) [a]	Median survival time (days) [a]
54	None(controls)	11.6
30	Days —11 to —1	10.9
30	Days —4 to +5	11.2
30	Day —11 only	12.0

[a] 10^3 BW 5147 blast cells were given i.v. on day zero.

between the MST of the treated and control mice. None of the control or treated mice survived, and all died with the characteristic gross anatomic findings of AKR long-passage leukemia (massive splenomegaly and either thymic enlargement and/or lymphadenopathy). The dose schedule for lentinan (1 mg/kg/day from days —11 to —1) which had been so effective in Swiss mice bearing a long-passage sarcoma [2, 3, 4], was ineffective in the AKR long-passage leukemia.

Spleen cells from normal young AKR mice were cultured for 2 days with lentinan. No mitogenic effect was apparent when a suspension of 7.5 μg of lentinan was added to 2 ml cultures of 4×10^6 AKR spleen cells (Fig. 2).

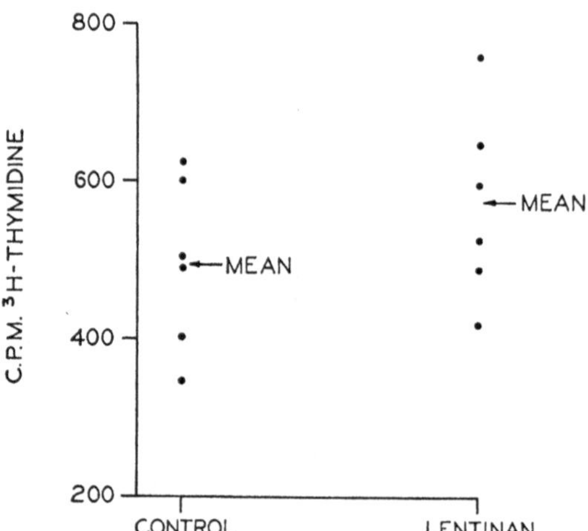

Fig. 2. Effect of 7.5 μg lentinan per 2 ml culture on ^{3}H-thymidine uptake by spleen cells from normal 8—10 week old AKR mice. Each point represents the mean value of triplicate cultures computed from individual experiments

Normal young AKR mice were given 1 mg/kg lentinan i.p. on day —11 only or daily on days —11 to —1. On day zero, their spleen cells were placed in culture. Incorporation of ^{3}H-thymidine was measured 2 days later. Spleen cells from mice treated with 10 injections of lentinan exhibited a small but significant increase ($p < 0.01$) in DNA synthetic activity over that observed in spleen cells obtained from mice that received no lentinan or one injection of lentinan (Fig. 3).

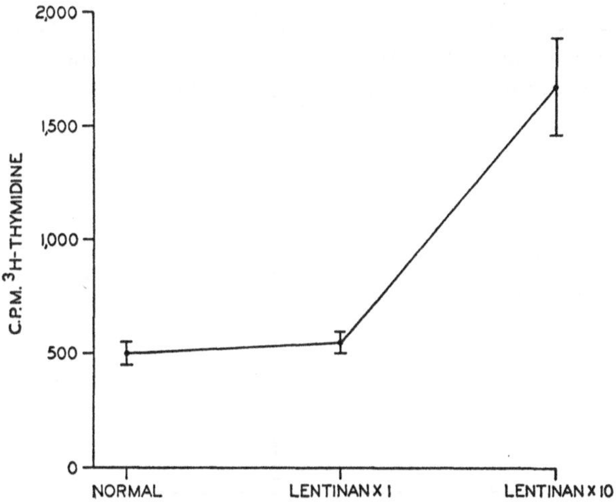

Fig. 3. Relationship between lentinan dose *in vivo* and ^{3}H-thymidine uptake *in vitro*. Each point represents the mean value of triplicate cultures computed from 6 individual experiments, ± the standard error of the mean

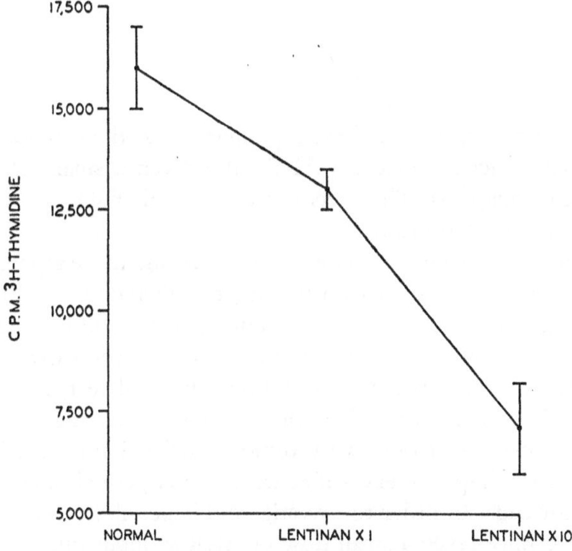

Fig. 4. Relationship between lentinan dose *in vivo* and response to PHA *in vitro*. Each point represents the mean value of triplicate cultures computed from 6 individual experiments, ± the standard error of the mean

Incubation of spleen cells from lentinan-treated AKR mice with PHA showed marked diminution from normal in their uptake of ^{3}H-thymidine (Fig. 4). When cultured with PHA, spleen cells from mice that received one injection of lentinan on day —11 incorporated less ^{3}H-thymidine than controls ($p < 0.01$); and spleen cells from mice that received 10 injections of lentinan incorporated less ^{3}H-thymidine than cells from mice that received one dose of lentinan ($p < 0.01$).

Spleen cells from C57BL/6 mice were treated with mitomycin-C [11] and served as the stimulating cells in one-way MLC tests. Responding cells were obtained from the spleens of normal and lentinan-treated AKR mice. No significant differences were detected in ^{3}H-thymidine uptake by the 3 responding cell populations in 4-day cultures (Fig. 5).

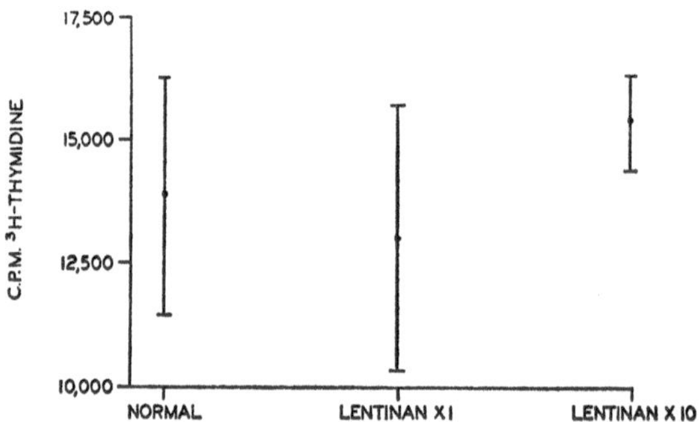

Fig. 5. Response of spleen cells from lentinan-treated AKR mice to C 57 BL/6 spleen cells in one-way MLC tests. Each point represents the mean value of triplicate cultures computed from 6 individual experiments, $\pm$ the standard error of the mean

Discussion

The most significant finding in these experiments was the absence of a detectable antileukemic effect in lentinan-treated AKR mice given a small cell dose of long-passage AKR leukemia cells. The precise cause for this failure is not known, but several possibilities merit mention.

We believe that the differences between our results and those reported for sarcoma 180 [2, 3, 4] may be explained, at least in part, by differences in antigenicity in the two tumor systems. It is well known that long-passage experimental tumors often "lose" tumor-associated antigens and, with time, become progressively less antigenic. In studies on BW 5147 leukemia, we have been unable to detect an immune response of AKR mice against the tumor [12] (in press). This finding suggests that BW 5147 leukemia cells possess no, or only weak tumor-associated antigens. Of course, one would not expect a therapeutic effect if *no* antigenic target existed for the immunocompetent effector cells. In order to investigate this possibility, studies have begun in lentinan-treated mice given a small dose of AKR spontaneous (first-passage) leukemia-lymphoma cells known to carry tumor-associated antigens [13]. Preliminary results indicate that an antileukemic effect does occur in the presence of this antigenic tumor and details of these experiments will be published. Although sarcoma 180 is a long-passage tumor, it is likely that it is antigenic, since it is carried in outbred Swiss mice. It is probable that sarcoma 180 carries histocompatibility antigens from the donor (in addition to possible tumor-associated antigens) which are foreign to outbred Swiss hosts. Thus, it is probable that the long-passage sarcoma 180 is more antigenic than the long-passage leukemia, which is carried in highly inbred AKR mice. Also, in contrast to long-passage AKR leukemia, sarcoma 180 has previously been shown to be vulnerable to nonspecific immunotherapy [14, 15].

The possibility exists that tumors associated with the Gross virus are refractory to nonspecific immunotherapy. MATHÉ *et al.* [16] reported that BCG was ineffective as a nonspecific immunostimulant in another leukemia associated with the Gross virus. However, with this same tumor they found that specific immunotherapy (leukemia cells treated with formalin) was quite effective.

Other differences between the long-passage leukemia and sarcoma, or differences in lentinan dose requirements for AKR and Swiss mice, may have been responsible for the discrepancy in results. It is possible that the observations reported here imply that lentinan may be active as an immunostimulant only in certain strains of mice, or that the failure of lentinan was due to an inherent defect in cell-mediated immune capability, which has been reported (by some) to occur in AKR mice [17].

The *in vitro* studies of cell-mediated immune function were of interest. Since lentinan was not mitogenic in cell culture (Fig. 2) and because the mouse spleen is primarily a lymphoid organ, the observed small increase in ^{3}H-thymidine uptake by spleen cells from mice given repeated injections of lentinan (Fig. 3) may have reflected immunostimulation. The inverse relationship between lentinan dose and PHA response (Fig. 4) was striking. It was not known whether lentinan administration blocked the mitogenic effect of PHA on T lymphocytes, or whether it promoted the emigration of T lymphocytes from the spleen to the peripheral lymphoid tissues. Additional experiments are planned to test the latter possibility. In the MLC tests (Fig. 5), spleen cells from untreated AKR control mice may already have been maximally stimulated by C57BL/6 cells so that additional uptake of ^{3}H-thymidine could not occur.

From the results reported here, and from the preliminary results indicating that lentinan may be effective against the slower growing, more antigenic first-passage AKR leukemia-lymphoma, it is apparent that additional studies are needed in order to evaluate the potential role of lentinan as a drug for immunotherapy.

Acknowledgement

Skilled technical assistance was provided by EVANGELINE R. REYNOLDS, ANITA LAPP, MARCIA R. HILGER, J. SPRADER and R. GILLER.

References

1. CHIHARA, G., MAEDA, Y., HAMURO, J., SASAKI, T., FUKUOKA, F.: Inhibition of mouse sarcoma 180 by polysaccharides from *Lentinus edodes* (Berk.) Sing. Nature (Lond.) **222**, 687 (1969).
2. CHIHARA, G., HAMURO, J., MAEDA, Y. Y., ARAI, Y., FUKUOKA, F.: Fractionation and purification of the polysaccharides with marked antitumor activity, especially lentinan, from *Lentinus edodes* (Berk.) Sing. (an edible mushroom). Cancer Res. **30**, 2776 (1970).

3. Maeda, Y. Y., Chihara, G.: Lentinan, a new immunoaccelerator of cell-mediated responses. Nature (Lond.) **229**, 634 (1971).
4. Maeda, Y. Y., Hamuro, J., Chihara, G.: The mechanisms of action of anti-tumor polysaccharides. I. The effects of antilymphocyte serum on the anti-tumor activity of lentinan. Int. J. Cancer **8**, 41 (1971).
5. Tokuzen, R.: Comparison of local cellular reaction to tumor grafts in mice treated with some plant polysaccharides. Cancer Res. **31**, 1590 (1971).
6. Fekete, E., Kent, E.: Transplantable mouse tumors. Transplantation Bull. **2**, 61 (1955).
7. Bortin, M. M., Saltzstein, E. C.: Graft versus host inhibition: fetal liver and thymus cells to minimize secondary disease. Science **164**, 316 (1969).
8. Saltzstein, E. C., Glasspiegel, J. S., Rimm, A. A., Giller, R. H., Bortin, M. M.: Graft versus leukemia for "cell cure" of long-passage AKR leukemia after chemoradiotherapy. Cancer Res. **32**, 1658 (1972).
9. Rodey, G. E., Good, R. A.: The *in vitro* response to phytohemagglutinin of lymphoid cells from normal and neonatally thymectomized adult mice. Int. Arch. Allergy **36**, 399 (1969).
10. Rodey, G. E., Good, R. A., Yunis, E.: Progressive loss in vitro of cellular immunity with ageing in strains of mice susceptible to autoimmune disease. Clin. exp. Immunol. **9**, 305 (1971).
11. Bach, F. H., Voynow, N. K.: One-way stimulation in mixed leukocyte cultures. Science **153**, 545 (1966).
12. Bortin, M. M., Rimm, A. A., Saltzstein, E. C., Rodey, G. E.: Graft versus leukemia. III. Apparent independent antihost and antileukemic activity of transplanted immunocompetent cells. Transplantation (in press).
13. Wahren, B.: Demonstration of a tumor-specific antigen in spontaneously developing AKR lymphomas. Int. J. Cancer **1**, 41 (1966).
14. Bradner, W. T., Clarke, D. A., Stock, C. C.: Stimulation of defense against experimental cancer. I. Zymosan and sarcoma 180 in mice. Cancer Res. **18**, 347 (1958).
15. Bradner, W. T., Clarke, D. A.: Stimulation of host defense against experimental cancer. II. Temporal and reversal studies of the zymosan effect. Cancer Res. **19**, 673 (1959).
16. Mathé, G., Pouillart, P., Lapeyraque, F.: Active immunotherapy of mouse RC 19 and E ♀ Kl leukemias applied after the intravenous transplantation of the tumor cells. Experientia (Basel) **27**, 446 (1971).
17. Friedman, H , Ceglowski, W. S.: Defect in cellular immunity of leukemia virus-infected mice assessed by a macrophage migration-inhibition assay. Proc. Soc. exp. Biol. (N.Y.) **136**, 154 (1971).

The Antitumor Effects of Interferon

I. Gresser

Institut de Recherches Scientifiques sur le Cancer, C.N.R.S., Villejuif

Interferon exerts a marked antitumor activity in experimental animals. Thus, interferon treatment of mice, hamsters, rabbits and chickens inoculated with oncogenic viruses has resulted in a delay in tumorigenesis and an increase in animal survival. Interferon treatment of mice inhibits the appearance and the progression of the spontaneously appearing lymphoid leukemia of AKR mice, and the development of mammary tumors in R III mice. Interferon inhibits the growth of transplantable tumors (syngeneic or allogeneic; of viral or nonviral origin) in different strains of mice (Table 1).

Table 1. Antitumor effect of interferon

Virus-induced neoplasms	Spontaneous virus-associated	Radiation-induced	Transplantable tumors
RNA: Leukemia-sarcoma DNA: Polynoma	Leukemia (Gross) Mammary carcinoma (Bittner)		Viral or nonviral origin Syngeneic or allogeneic Ascitic or solid

Table 2. Reprinted from Gresser *et al.* [J. nat. Cancer Inst. **45**, 365 (1970)]
Effect of interferon on BALB/c mice inoculated with Ehrlich ascites cells

No. of cells inoculated	Treatment	Total no. mice surviving > 60 days	Mean survival (days)
10^6	none	0/11	11
	interferon	2/11	29
10^5	none	0/11	16
	inteferon	4/11	59
10^4	none	0/11	18
	interferon	9/11	—

In each of the above examples interferon was of therapeutic value. In several instances treatment was initiated at a time when splenomegaly, or a palpable tumor, had already developed in the test animals. Table 2 illustrates the marked effect of interferon on the survival of BALB/c mice inoculated with Ehrlich ascites cells. For example, the mean survival time of untreated mice inoculated with 10^4 Ehrlich ascites cells (equivalent to approximately 5,000 LD_{50}) was 18 days, and all mice were dead by the 60th day. In the group treated with interferon (treatment beginning 24 h *after* tumor inoculation and continued daily for 1 month) all mice were alive by the 30th day and 90% survived beyond the 6th month. These mice can be considered cured.

Lewis lung carcinoma transplanted s.c. in mice metastasizes to the lung, and these metastatic foci can be counted macroscopically. This tumor has been adopted by the National Cancer Institute as a model for the assay of potential anticancer chemotherapeutic substances. In general, it is unresponsive to antimetabolites; although somewhat affected by alkylating agents and natural products, it is rather unresponsive to present antitumor agents. Table 3 shows the inhibitory effect of daily interferon

Table 3. Reprinted from Gresser and Bourali [Nature **236**, 78 (1969)]
Inhibition of the primary 3LL tumor and pulmonary metastases by interferon

Treatment	No. of mice	Primary tumor (weight)	Mean number of pulmonary metastases
none	19	4.7 g	30
interferon day + 1 to 20	20	2.6 g	7.7
interferon day + 6 to 20	20	2.9 g	6.1

treatment on the growth of the primary 3 LL tumor and on the development of pulmonary metastases in C 57 B1/6 mice. Note that an inhibitory effect was observed even when treatment was initiated 6 days *after* tumor inoculation.

In contrast to endotoxin, BCG, and similar substances; interferon does not seem to have a significant antitumor effect when administered *prior* to inoculation of tumor cells. It is effective only when it is administered repeatedly during the test period. It is therefore active *therapeutically* rather than prophylactically.

What is the mechanism of its antitumor activity? There are three apparent possibilities:

1. interferon inhibits the multiplication of tumor cells *in vivo*;
2. interferon enhances the capacity of the host to reject the tumor;
3. both mechanisms are operative.

Our results to date do not permit a definitive answer. Some recent data do suggest that both mechanisms may be operative.

Interferon can inhibit the multiplication of tumor cells *in vitro* (Fig. 1). Interferon can also enhance the specific cytotoxicity of sensitized lymphocytes for target tumor cells (Fig. 2). If a similar phenomenon occurred *in vivo*, it might suggest a mechanism whereby interferon induced a host-mediated response.

Interferon acts therapeutically: it appears to be non-toxic, the host does not develop tolerance to interferon, nor are antibodies to interferon detected even after prolonged administration. Interferon should certainly be tried in the treatment of neoplasia in man.

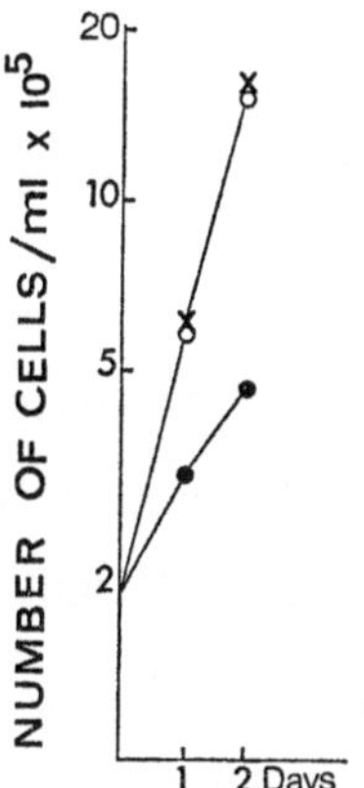

Fig. 1. Effect of interferon on the multiplication of L 1210 cells. × No treatment; ○ treatment with control preparation; ● treatment with interferon. Reprinted from GRESSER *et al.* [Nature New Biol. **231**, 20 (1971)]

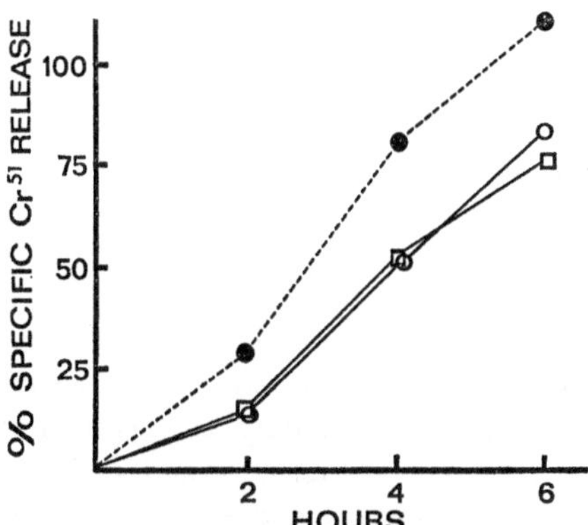

Fig. 2. Effect of interferon on the cytotoxic action of C 57 BL/6 mouse lymphocytes on L 1210 target cells expressed as % specific ^{51}Cr-release. □ Sensitized lymphocytes pretreated with medium; ○ sensitized lymphocytes pretreated with control preparation; ● sensitized lymphocytes pretreated with semipurified C 57 BL/6 brain interferon. Reprinted from LINDAHL *et al.* [Proc. nat. Acad. Sci. (Wash.) **69**, 721 (1972)]

Use of Double-Stranded Synthetic Polynucleotides in Amplifying Immunologically Induced Lymphocyte Proliferation

M. R. MARDINEY, Jr., L. CHESS, C. LEVY, M. SCHMUKLER, and K. SMITH

Section of Immunology and Cell Biology, National Institutes of Health, National Cancer Institute, Baltimore Cancer Research Center, Baltimore, Md.

We have been interested in models of adjuvant immune activation which would be capable of amplifying responsiveness both *in vivo* and *in vitro*, and we have spent some time studying the ability of the synthetic polyribonucleotides, namely polyadenylic-polyuridylic acids, in amplifying the specific immune responsiveness of lymphocytes *in vitro*. We have found that the synthetic double-stranded polyribonucleotide polyadenylic-polyuridylic acid (poly AU) will enhance both the response of sensitized leukocytes to suboptimal concentrations of strong soluble antigens and the response of nonsensitized leukocytes to suboptimal concentrations of allogeneic leukocytes. Furthermore, our experience with the measles virus a poor stimulus in leukocyte cultures, indicates that poly AU may be useful in *in vitro* studies designed to detect cellular immune reaction to this type of antigen preparation.

Poly AU complexes have been shown to stimulate macrophage activity and increase phagocytosis, to amplify T-cell activity as measured by graft-versus-host disease, delayed hypersensitivity and graft rejection and, in addition, to enhance B-cell activity as reflected in increased primary and secondary responsiveness [3, 6, 9]. Particularly interesting is that these agents are capable of restoring normal antibody formation in aged mice [1] and can restore normal graft rejection in neonatally thymectomized mice [7]. Our own work extends the original observation of Friedman and Johnson, that poly AU could amplify the immune responsiveness in short-term leukocyte cultures [4].

Our data indicate that poly AU enhances responsiveness of sensitized leukocytes to suboptimal concentrations of strong cellular and soluble antigenic stimuli while depressing responses to PHA. In addition, poly AU consistently enhances responsiveness to measles virus, a preparation which has elicited varied responsiveness in lymphocyte cultures.

Materials and Methods

Preparation of Synthetic Double-Stranded Complexes of Poly AU

Polyadenylic acid (poly AU) potassium salt (Lot no. 68) and polyuridylic acid (poly U) ammonium salt (Lot no. 81) were purchased from Miles Laboratories,

Elkhart, Indiana. Each polymer was reconstituted with RPMI 1640 media to a concentration of 3 mg/ml and stored at —20 °C. Prior to use, double stranded complexes of poly AU were formed by mixing equimolar amounts of each polymer at room temperature for 5—10 min. The poly AU complexes were then diluted to the final concentrations in RPMI 1640 media prior to use in lymphocyte cultures. 100 μg of poly AU indicates the complex resulting from 50 μg of poly A and 50 μg of poly U.

Culture Conditions and Cell Preparations

Our methods of cell culture, evaluation of thymidine incorporation and statistical evaluation have been described [2, 8]. In brief, 3×10^6 leukocytes obtained from sedimented heparinized whole blood were cultured in a final volume of 1.5 ml of RPMI 1640 media containing 15—20% autologous plasma, 50 units/ml penicillin, 50 μg/ml streptomycin, 300 μg/ml of glutamine, in addition to antigens and synthetic polynucleotides. All cultures were maintained at an angle of 5 ° from the horizontal in a 95% air, 5% CO_2 humid atmosphere at 37 °C. At appropriate times after initiating cultures, 0.5 ml of RPMI 1640 media containing 2 μCi of tritiated thymidine (specific activity 1.9 Ci/mmole, Schwartz Bio Research, Inc.) was added to each tube. Triplicate tubes were incubated subsequently for 4 h, washed with chilled saline, and later analyzed for tritiated thymidine incorporation into DNA by methods previously described [2, 8]. All data are presented as disintegrations per min (DPM) $\pm$ the standard error of triplicate cultures. Any two means greater than three standard errors apart are significantly different at greater than the 95% confidence level.

Preparation of Antigens and PHA

The preparation of PHA-M [Difco], and purified protein derivative (PPD) [Parke Davis Company, Detroit, Michigan] are as previously described [2, 8]. Measles complement-fixation antigen was obtained from Microbiological Associates, Bethesda, Md. (Cat. no. 30—850), and inactivated with betapropiolactone (Betaprone; Testagar Company, Oakpark, Michigan) at a final concentration of 1 : 4000. All antigens were diluted to appropriate concentrations in RPMI 1640 medium and added directly to leukocyte cultures.

Results

The responsiveness of an individual sensitive to PPD and an individual insensitive to PPD in the presence of various concentrations of this antigen with and without poly AU was assessed by ^{3}H-thymidine incorporation on day 7. No response to PPD is observed in the non-sensitive individual at any of the concentrations used (Fig. 1). In contrast, peak responsiveness to PPD occurred at the 2 μg level. This concentration of PPD has generally elicited maximal responsiveness in most individuals sensitive to this antigen in our laboratory. Analysis of the data obtained from cultures containing both PPD and poly AU indicate that, in the sensitive individual, poly AU significantly augmented lymphocyte responsiveness at the suboptimal antigen concentrations. The PPD-negative individual did not respond to PPD at any of these concentrations and no amplification of response was effected by the addition of poly AU.

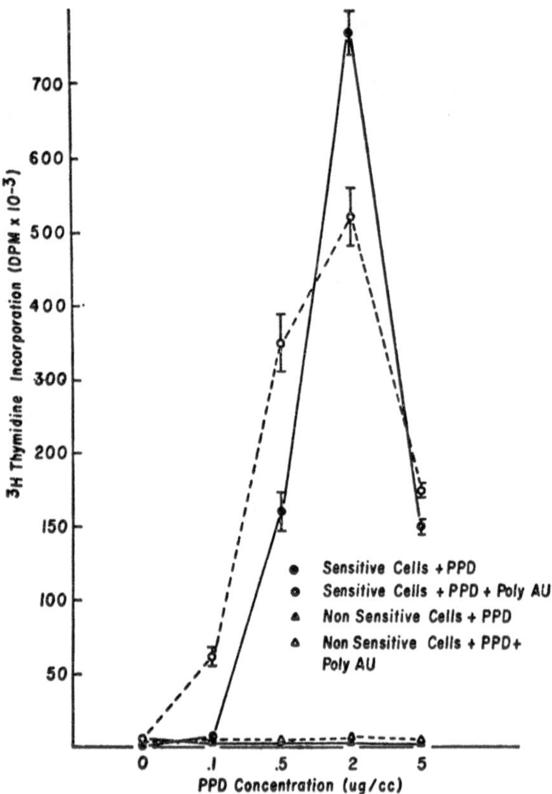

Fig. 1. Effect of 100 μg of poly AU on ^{3}H-thymidine incorporation (measured on day 7) induced by varying concentrations of PPD in sensitized and nonsensitized leukocytes

Table. Poly AU-induced amplification of ^{3}H-thymidine incorporation (DPM ± SE) by sensitized leukocytes in response to PPD. All cultures contained 3.0×10^6 leukocytes in a final volume of 1.5 ml. The poly AU concentration utilized was 100 μg/ml. The concentration of PPD was 0.25 μg per culture. ^{3}H-thymidine incorporation was measured on day 7 of culture

Expt.	Cells alone	Cells + Poly AU	Cells + PPD	Cells + PPD + Poly AU
1	1515 ± 260	4,131 ± 910	160,730 ± 27,055	349,514 ± 40,353
2	3537 ± 757	2,264 ± 188	2,249 ± 140	439,925 ± 10,799
3	5143 ± 592	6,450 ± 1244	9,347 ± 1250	38,729 ± 3,038
4	4851 ± 829	5,230 ± 1350	7,188 ± 1075	38,422 ± 6,270
5	2922 ± 721	11,764 ± 2652	10,478 ± 2316	17,119 ± 3,905

The amplification of tritiated thymidine incorporation effected by poly AU in the lymphocytes of five additional PPD-sensitive donors stimulated by the suboptimal PPD dose of 0.25 μg is shown in the Table. We should first note that amplification of response to antigen was seen in all cultures. In addition, it is important to emphasize that poly AU had a variable effect on cells cultured without antigen; it stimulated some cultures and inhibited others. This response was variable but was in no way connected with the amplification effect to specific antigen. For example, although reactivity of control cells in Experiment 2 was somewhat inhibited by poly AU, the response to specific antigen was markedly enhanced.

The effects of poly AU on the kinetics of lymphocyte responsiveness to specific antigen are presented in Fig. 2. Cells from an individual sensitive to PPD were cultured alone, in the presence of poly AU, in the presence of PPD, and in the presence of PPD and poly AU. Tritiated thymidine incorporation was measured at 4-h intervals on each day subsequent to culture for a total of 8 days. The kinetics of

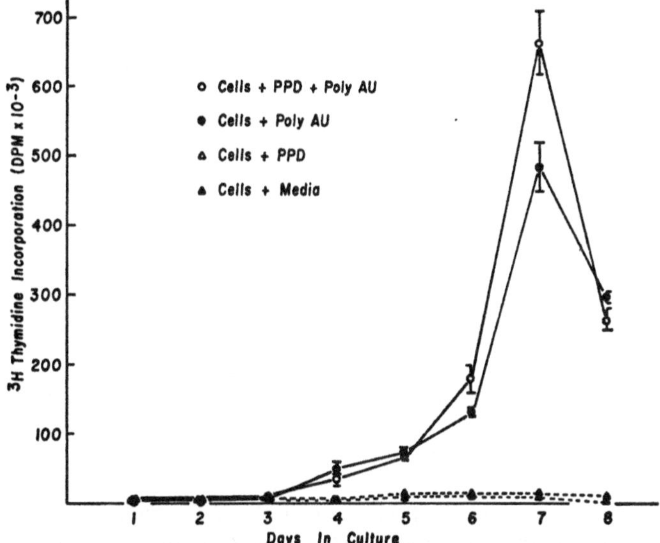

Fig. 2. Effect of 100 μg of poly AU on PPD-induced ^{3}H-thymidine incorporation in sensitized cells, measured daily for 8 days (PPD was 0.25 μg per culture)

responsiveness to PPD were unaffected by the presence of poly AU. Amplification of response was first noted on day 6 and was most marked on day 7. This finding is in accord with the work of Jaroslow [5] who demonstrated that the poly AU-induced amplification of plaque-forming cell responses to SRBC did not depend on changes in the rate of proliferation of reactive cells; poly AU-induced amplification may be secondary to more cells being initially activated by antigen or perhaps recruited.

The data in Figs. 3 and 4 represent our experience with the measles-virus antigen as a stimulus of specifically sensitized cells *in vitro*. This antigen preparation has had a variable effect in culture with sensitized cells stimulating some, inhibiting others, and apparently having no effect on others. The measles preparation utilized in this experiment was a complement fixation antigen preparation prepared by Microbiological Associates, Bethesda, Maryland and treated with β-propiolactone. The cells used for the experiment of which the results are shown in Fig. 3 were taken from an individual having a positive history of clinical measles approximately 15 years prior to testing. The antigen was not stimulatory over a wide range of concentrations

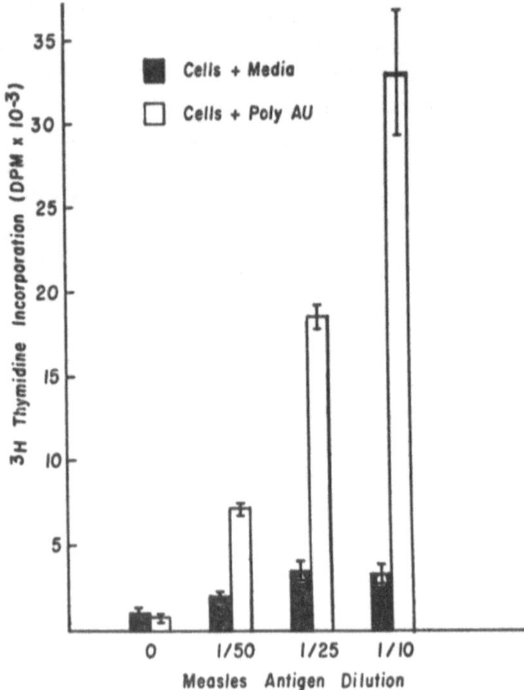

Fig. 3. Amplification of measles antigen-induced ^{3}H-thymidine incorporation by 100 μg of poly AU, measured on day 7. Per culture: 0.5 ml of each dilution of measles antigen shown on the abscissa

in the absence of poly AU. In the presence of poly AU, significant amplification of tritiated thymidine incorporation measured on day 7 of culture was observed.

Our experience with measles as a stimulus of lymphocytes response *in vitro* in the absence of poly AU, like that of others, has been variable: minimal stimulation was observed in some cases and lack of response or absolute depression in others. It appears that the factors present in the measles preparation responsible for the depression or inhibition of lymphocyte responsiveness can be overridden by the stimulus to immune reactivity aided by poly AU. This can be seen in Fig. 4. Measles antigen alone not only did not stimulate but also suppressed thymidine incorporation as compared to control cultures. In contrast, poly AU markedly enhanced responsiveness, overriding this inhibition.

The effect of poly AU on the immunological response to cellular antigens was studied in mixed leukocyte cultures: 1.5×10^6 responding cells were reacted with varying concentrations of allogeneic irradiated (1000 rad) leukocytes in the presence or absence of 100 μg of poly AU. As Fig. 5 shows, the results are analogous to our data with strong soluble antigenic stimuli. Amplification of response is most apparent at suboptimal stimulatory cell concentrations.

In contrast to our results with specific antigens and allogeneic cells, poly AU depressed responses to PHA (Fig. 6). At no concentration did poly AU augment responses to PHA, and depression was observed at high concentrations. These results are in accord with those previously reported by [4].

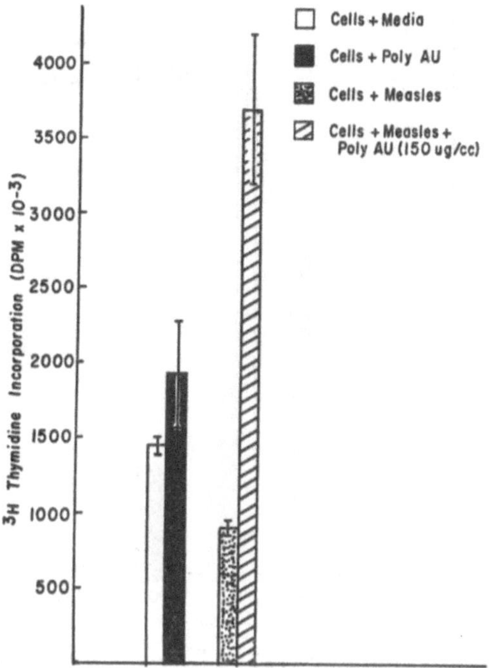

Fig. 4. Amplification of measles antigen-induced ^{3}H-thymidine incorporation by poly AU, measured on day 7. Per culture: 0.5 ml of poly AU (150 μg/ml) and 0.5 ml of measles antigen (1/50)

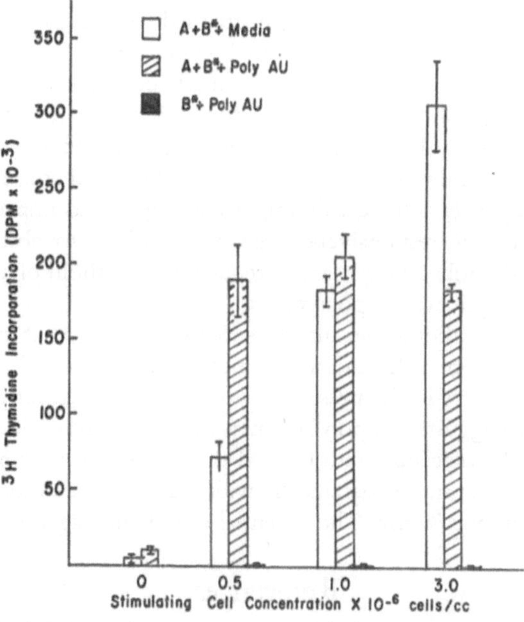

Fig. 5. Effect of poly AU (100 μg) on one-way mixed leukocyte reaction. The concentration of responding cells was 1.5×10^{6} per culture, 0.5 ml of irradiated allogeneic cells was added at each concentration shown on the abscissa. ^{3}H-thymidine incorporation was measured on day 7 of culture

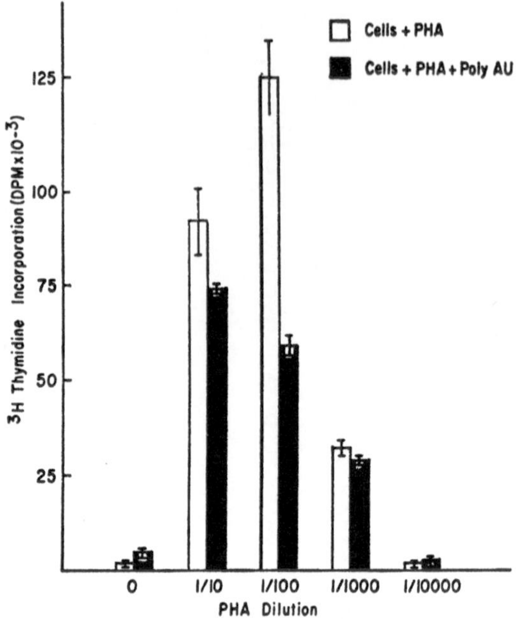

Fig. 6. Depressive effect of poly AU (100 μg) on PHA-induced ³H-thymidine incorporation, measured on day 4 of culture

Discussion

The present study indicates that double-stranded complexes of poly AU enhance tritiated thymidine incorporation by cultured leukocytes in response to both weak and strong antigenic stimuli. Thus, strong stimuli such as PPD, tetanus toxoid, or allogeneic cells, when diluted to concentrations which are minimally stimulatory, will significantly augment the incorporation of tritiated thymidine in the presence of poly AU. Poly AU appears to lower the threshold of antigen concentration essential for lymphocyte response, and, equally important, appears to impart responsiveness in situations where such responsiveness has been difficult to observe (i.e. measles virus). Thus, overall, poly AU appears to reduce the threshold of antigenic stimulation essential for lymphocyte responsiveness.

Past work in other laboratories indicates that poly AU acts at many levels of the immune response system. The molecular mechanisms responsible for augmented reactivity of lymphocytes in the presence of poly AU are currently being explored. The work of Braun suggests that poly AU may activate adenyl cyclase and secondarily increase cyclic AMP associated with the cell membrane [1]. Our own laboratory is now involved in evaluating the parameters which may be useful for monitoring host responsiveness to tumor *in vitro*. The potential use of such agents *in vivo* is obvious.

References

1. BRAUN, W., NAKANO, L., JARASKOVA, Y., YASIMA, Y., JIMENEZ, L.: Stimulation of antibody formation by nucleic acids and their derivatives. In: Nucleic Acids in Immunology (PLESCIA, O. J., BRAUN, W., Eds.), p. 379. Berlin-Heidelberg-New York: Springer 1968.

2. Bredt, A. B., Mardiney, M. R., jr.: Effects of amantadine on the reactivity of human lymphocytes stimulated by allogeneic lymphocytes and phytohemagglutinin. Transplantation **8**, 763 (1969).
3. Cone, R. E., Johnson, A. G.: Regulation of the immune system by synthetic polynucleotides. III. Action of antigen reactive cells by thymic origin. J. exp. Med. **133**, 665 (1971).
4. Friedman, H. M., Johnson, A. G., Pan, P.: Stimulatory effect of polynucleotides on short-term leukocyte cultures. Proc. Soc. exp. Biol. (N.Y.) **132**, 916 (1969).
5. Jaroslow, B. N., Ortiz-Ortiz, L.: Influence of Poly A-Poly U on early events in the immune response in vitro. Cell. Immunol. **3**, 123 (1972).
6. Johnson, A. G., Cone, R. E., Friedman, H. M., Han, I. H., Johnson, H. G., Schmidtke, J. R., Stout, R. D.: Stimulation of the immune system by homopolyribonucleotides. In: Biological Effects of Polynucleotides (Beers, R., Braun, W., Eds.). Berlin-Heidelberg-New York: Springer 1971.
7. Johnson, H. G., Johnson, A. G.: Regulation of the immune system by synthetic polynucleotides. II. Action on peritoneal exudate cells. J. exp. Med. **133**, 649 (1970).
8. Mangi, R. J., Mardiney, M. R., jr.: The *in vitro* transformation of frozen-stored lymphocytes in the mixed lymphocyte reaction and in culture with phytohemagglutinin and specific antigens. J. exp. Med. **132**, 401 (1970).
9. Schmidtke, J. R., Johnson, A. G.: Regulation of the immune system by synthetic polynucleotides. I. Characteristics of adjuvant action on antibody synthesis. J. Immunol. **106**, 1191 (1971).

Immunoenhancing and Antitumor Effects of Agents that Elevate Endogenous Cyclic AMP Levels*

W. BRAUN and C. SHIOZAWA

Institute of Microbiology, Rutgers University, New Brunswick, N. J.

Among the various immunoenhancing agents that can produce some antitumor effects are the double-stranded synthetic polynucleotides, such as poly I : C (poly I. poly C) and poly A : U (poly A. poly U) [1, 4, 8, 9, 14, 15, 16, 19, 22]. These agents have received increasing attention in recent years because they are chemically well-defined, easy to reproduce and, at least in the case of poly A:U, devoid of toxicity and pyrogenicity in experimental animals [7]. It is this lack of undesirable side-effects that motivated us to study the effects of poly A:U on both immune responses and tumor growth; another reason for our preference for poly A : U was its poor interferon-inducing activity; this permitted the exclusion of antiviral effects in studies of virus-induced tumors.

Two apparently significant developments in our recent studies with poly A:U furnish the basis for our remarks. First, we were able to obtain evidence that immunoenhancing effects of poly A:U and poly I : C, as well as those of interferon preparations and endotoxin, are associated with an alteration of the level of regulatory cAMP in immunocompetent cells [5, 6, 12, 15]. Secondly, we were able to show that a significant portion of the antitumor activity of polynucleotides, and of other agents that modify endogeneous cAMP levels, is not exerted via familiar immune responses, but seems to involve more direct effects on the tumor cells [22]. The latter finding prompted us to explore relationships between endogeneous cAMP levels and control of proliferation of neoplastic cells, and we have found that intracellular cAMP levels are indeed significantly altered following contact of virus-transformed tumor cells with normal syngeneic spleen cells.

I would like to start by sketching the steps in cAMP formation and degradation, a process now known to regulate various cellular functions including those involved in immune responses. As indicated in Fig. 1, the interaction between a variety of exogenous agents and appropriate receptor sites on the surface of relevant cells will activate a membrane-bound enzyme, adenyl cyclase, which converts intracellular ATP into cAMP. Cyclic AMP in turn activates kinases that influence transcription, translation, the activity of preformed enzymes, and apparently DNA replication itself [18, 20]. Once formed, cAMP is fairly rapidly degraded with the help of phospho-

* These studies were supported by grants from the NIH, NSF and the N.Y. Cancer Research Institute.

diesterases into inactive AMP. Methylxanthines, such as theophylline and caffeine, have been recognized as phophodiesterase inhibitors that can prevent or retard degradation of cAMP and thus enhance its effects. Catecholamines, including epinephrine, norepinephrine and isoproterenol, are well-known adenyl cyclase stimulators; we have demonstrated that poly A:U and poly I:C also are also potent enhancers of adenyl cyclase activity [6, 18].

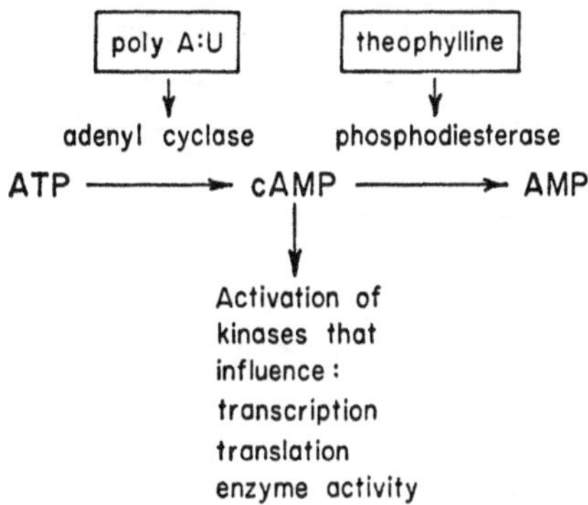

Fig. 1. Steps in cAMP formation and degradation, outlining the sites of influence of polynucleotides and methylxanthines

In hormone-dependent cells, cAMP is known to act as a "second messenger", mediating and regulating the triggering actions of hormones [6]. In cells involved in the immune response, a some what more complex situation appears to exist: while changes in intracellular cAMP levels following the interaction of antigen and cell receptor are not ruled out, a principal contribution of cAMP-mediated events appears to be due to a separate second chain of events involving the activation of a cAMP-dependent regulatory system. This system can, depending on the strength of the second signal and the state of differentiation of the cell, magnify or reduce the events triggered by the specific antigenic signal [3].

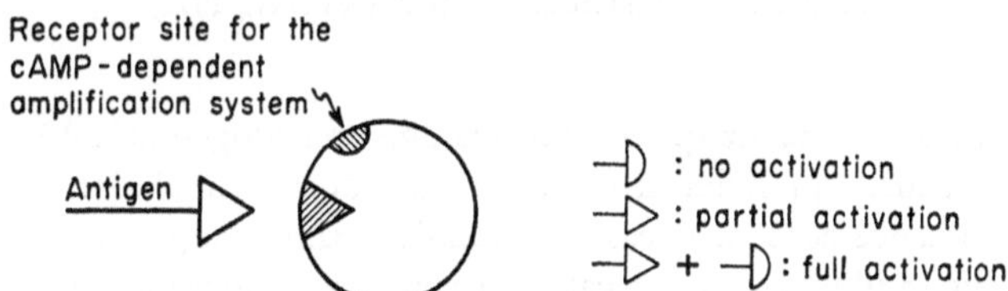

Fig. 2. Diagram of presumed receptors on B lymphocytes

Fig. 2 shows our current concept of signals required for the detectable activation of functions of antibody-forming B lymphocytes. In the case of most but not all immunogens, neither an antigenic signal alone, nor a signal to the cAMP-dependent amplification system will suffice to produce a full activation of the cells, leading to detectable antibody secretion, whereas a combination of both signals will do so. Similarly, the activity of T lymphocytes (involved in cell-mediated immunity) is enhanced by the presence of stimulators of cAMP formation or by stabilizers of cAMP levels during exposure to antigen [7, 13]; in addition, changes in intracellular cAMP levels have been shown to occur following contact of T lymphocytes with mitogens [21]. Macrophage activity is stimulated by cAMP itself and by modifiers of endogenous cAMP levels [7]; furthermore, it has been demonstrated that alterations in cAMP levels occur during phagocytosis [17].

The magnitude of immune responses seems to be regulated, both normally and in the presence of many adjuvants, by cAMP-dependent events. Experimental documentation for this conclusion has been published by several groups, including my own, during the past two years [2, 5, 6, 11, 12, 17, 21] and will not be reviewed here.

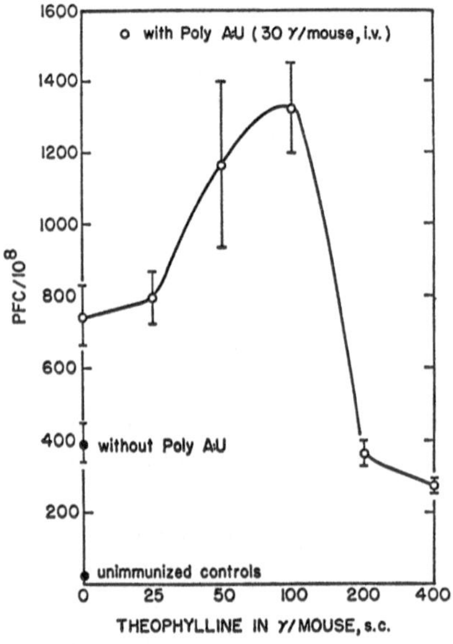

Fig. 3. Influence of different concentrations of [theophylline]$_2$ · ethylenediamine, given s. c., on antibody formation to SRBC in CFW mice in the absence or presence of poly A:U. All assays were made 48 h after immunization. (Ishizuka *et al.*, 1971)

During activation of immunocompetent cells, changes in endogenous cAMP levels can lead either to enhanced or reduced responses: a modest stimulation of the cAMP system causes enhancement, whereas an excessive stimulation reduces or inhibits responses [5]. Fig. 3 illustrates a typical biphasic dose-response curve depicting the influence of increasing levels of theophylline in the presence of a constant low level of poly A:U on the activation of mouse spleen cells that form antibodies to SRBC.

In contrast to this biphasic response in the course of activation of immature or resting cells, *already activated* immunocompetent cells tend to be inhibited in their functions when exposed to antigen in the presence of stimulators of cAMP production. Studies by Lichtenstein and associates and by Park's and Austen's groups have provided a good deal of information on this phenomenon [2, 11, 17, 21].

A suppression of functions of already activated cells by agents that elevate endogenous cAMP levels also seems to occur in the case of tumor-cell populations. We became aware of this during our work with chemically or virus-induced mouse tumors implanted into syngeneic hosts [22]. As illustrated in Fig. 4, which shows results obtained with Rauscher leukemia virus-induced tumor cells implanted i.d. into syngeneic BALB/c mice, we confirmed that the rate of growth of many tumor cell lines can be retarded by i.p. injection of poly I : C. We also showed that a similar but somewhat less pronounced retardation can be produced by treatment with poly A:U. Next, we found that theophylline administered at the time of injection with poly A:U increased the anti-tumor effect of the polynucleotides, and that even

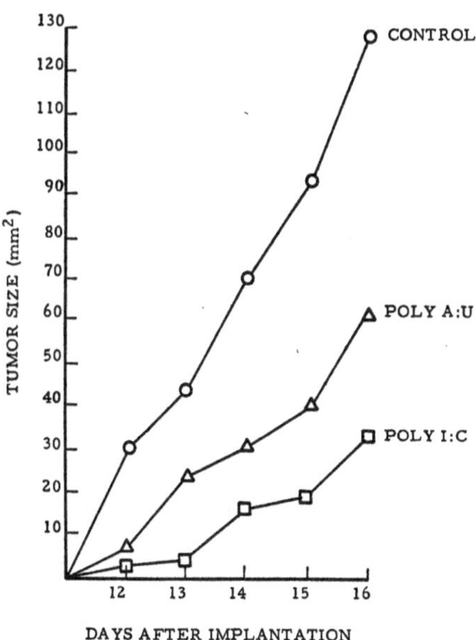

Fig. 4. Influence of poly A:U and poly I:C on the growth of Rauscher leukemia virus-induced tumor ascites cells, implanted i. d. into syngeneic BALB/c mice. Tumor inoculum size, 10^4 cells. Treatment with i. p. poly A:U (300 γ per injection) or poly I:C (300 γ per injection) was on days 0 and 1. The ordinate indicates tumor size (mm^2)

theophylline alone retarded the growth of a number of tumor-cell lines (Fig. 5). Other modifiers of endogenous cAMP levels, such as isoproterenol and cAMP itself, produced comparable effects which we, like other investigators, believed to be due to an alteration of appropriate host immune responses. We then discovered that essentially identical effects were produced when the mice were irradiated just prior to tumor implantation, using an X-ray dose that should have sufficed to impair immune mechanisms (Table). Subsequent tests showed that *in vitro* exposure of tumor cells to poly A:U or theophylline prior to the cells' implantation into untreated hosts was sufficient to retard tumor growth.

We thus recognized that agents influencing intracellular cAMP levels can have an inhibitory effect on tumor cells that is independent of any stimulation of the conventional host immune responses. In agreement with the results of others with BCG and fractions of tubercle bacilli [24], we also found that direct injection of poly A:U,

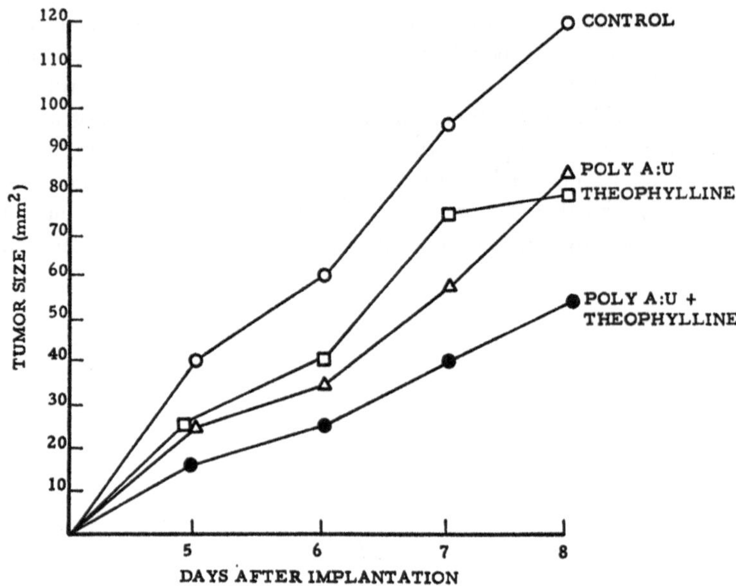

Fig. 5. Influence of poly A:U and theophylline on the growth of Rauscher leukemia virus tumors in BALB/c mice. Tumor inoculum size, 10^6 cells. Treatment on days 0 and 1 with i. p. poly A:U (450 γ per injection) or theophylline, or both (200 γ per injection)

Table. Effects of poly I:C and poly A:U (450 γ i.p. on days 0 and + 1) on the growth of Rauscher leukemia virus-induced tumor cell populations in irradiated and non-irradiated, syngeneic, BALB/c mice. Five animals/group

Group	Average tumor size (mm^2) ± S.E. on day 7
Poly I:C non-irradiated	32 ± 7.8
Poly I:C irradiated	35 ± 2.0
Poly A:U non-irradiated	58 ± 13.5
Poly A:U irradiated	54 ± 11.1
Controls non-irradiated	95 ± 6.2
Controls irradiated	82 ± 8.0

theophylline, isoproterenol, or cAMP itself into a growing tumor produced better antitumor effects than systemic treatment. In fact, with a number of virus-induced tumor cell lines that failed to respond to systemic treatment, fair therapeutic effects were obtained by the direct injection of the agents into the growing tumor 6—8 days after the i.d. implantation of 10^6 tumor cells.

Finally, we have measured cAMP levels directly in Rauscher leukemia virus-induced tumor cell suspensions exposed to poly A:U or theophylline *in vitro*. No changes were observed. However, when we added normal, syngeneic spleen cells to the tumor-cell suspension, a rapid and significant temporary increase in endogenous cAMP levels was detected in both tumor and spleen cells (Fig. 6) and this increase was further elevated by the addition of poly A:U. Klein and associates previously noted phenomena resembling mixed-lymphocyte reactions following interactions of normal cells with autochthonous tumor cells [23]. It is now tempting to speculate whether a modest alteration of endogenous cAMP levels following contact of transformed cells with neighboring normal cells might contribute to the triggering of proliferative events (for which changes in cAMP levels appear to be required), whereas any additional elevation of such intracellular cAMP levels might result in inhibition of cell functions.

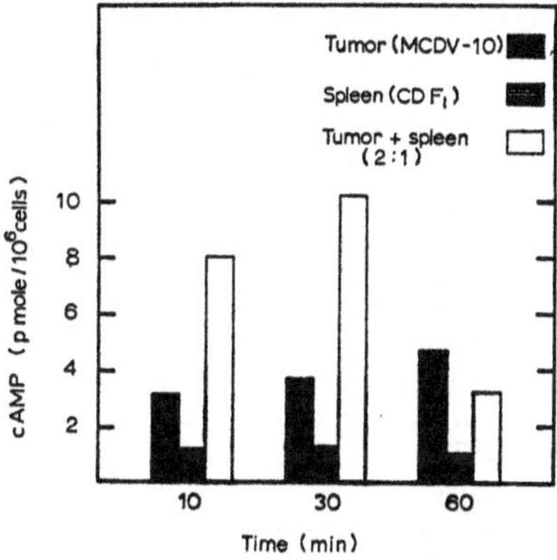

Fig. 6. Cyclic AMP levels measured by the Gilman method in Rauscher leukemia virus-induced tumor ascites cells suspended in Eagle's medium *in vitro*, and in normal, dissociated spleen cells of syngeneic CDF_1 mice or in (2:1) mixtures of such cell suspensions

In cooperation with H. Levy, we recently demonstrated that interferon preparations also stimulate endogenous cAMP formation (and immune responses) and one wonders whether this also may explain the antitumor effects of interferon reported by others [10]. The long-recognized antitumor activity of bacterial endotoxin and the more recently recognized antitumor effects of localized hypersensitivity reactions may have a similar mode of action, causing an inhibitory elevation of cAMP levels in tumor cells. Unfortunately, there seem to be significant differences among different tumor cell lines in regard to their susceptibility to modifiers of endogenous cAMP regard to their susceptibility to modifiers of endogenous cAMP levels, and this difference, possibly attributable to inherent differences in basal cAMP levels and the dynamics of their alteration, may preclude immediate clinical utilization of these recent experimental findings.

In summary, many immunoenhancing agents, including double-stranded synthetic polynucleotides, seem to exert their effects by altering endogenous cAMP levels which regulate the magnitude of immune responses. Alterations in cAMP levels also occur after direct exposure of tumor cells to such agents or to cells that influence the cAMP system of the neoplastic cells. In the presence of appropriate alterations of intracellular cAMP levels, inhibition of cell proliferation will occur.

References

1. Bart, R. S., Kopf, A. W.: Inhibition of the growth of murine malignant melanoma with synthetic double-stranded ribonucleic acid. Nature (Lond.) **224**, 372 (1969).
2. Bourne, H. R., Melmon, K. L., Lichtenstein, L. M.: Histamine augments leukocyte adenosine 3',5'-monophosphate and blocks antigenic histamine release. Science **173**, 743 (1971).
3. Braun, W.: Ann. N.Y. Acad. Sci. (in press).
4. Braun, W.: New approaches to immunology as potential adjuncts to chemotherapy. In: Progress in antimicrobial and anticancer chemotherapy, vol. I, p. 17. Tokyo: University of Tokyo Press 1970.
5. Braun, W., Ishizuka, M.: Antibody formation: Reduced responses after administration of excessive amounts of nonspecific stimulators. Proc. nat. Acad. Sci. (Wash.) **68**, 1114 (1971a).
6. Braun, W., Ishizuka, M.: Cyclic AMP and immune responses. II. Phosphodiesterase inhibitors as potentiators of polynucleotide effects on antibody formation. J. Immunol. **107**, 1036 (1971b).
7. Braun, W., Ishizuka, M., Yajima, Y., Webb, D., Winchurch, R.: Spectrum and mode of action of Poly A:U in the stimulation of immune responses. Biological effects of polynucleotides. p. 139 (Beers, R., Braun, W., Eds.). New York: Springer 1971c.
8. Braun, W., Plescia, O J., Raskova, J., Webb, D.: Basic proteins and synthetic polynucleotides as modifiers of immunogenicity of syngeneic tumor cells. Israel J. med. Sci. **7**, 72 (1971d).
9. Gelboin, H. V., Levy, H. B.: Polyinosinic-polycytidylic acid inhibits chemically induced tumorigenesis in mouse skin. Science **167**, 205 (1970).
10. Gresser, I., Bourali, C., Levy, J. P., Fontaine-Brouty-Boye, D., Thomas, M. T.: Increased survival in mice inoculated with tumour cells and treated with interferon preparations. Proc. nat. Acad. Sci. (Wash.) **63**, 51 (1969).
11. Henney, C. S., Lichtenstein, L. M.: The role of cyclic AMP in the cytolytic activity of lymphocytes. J. Immunol. **107**, 610 (1971).
12. Ishizuka, M., Braun, W., Matsumoto, T.: Cyclic AMP and immune responses. I. Influence of poly A:U and cAMP on antibody formation *in vitro*. J. Immunol. **107**, 1027 (1971).
13. Johnson, A. G., Cone, R. E., Friedman, H. M., Han, I. H., Johnson, H. G., Schmidke, J. R., Stout, R. D.: Stimulation of the immune system by homopolyribonucleotides. Biological effects of polynucleotides, p. 157 (Beers, R., Braun, W., Eds.). New York: Springer 1971.
14. Lacour, F., Spira, A., Lacour, J., Prade, M.: Polyadenylic-polyuridylic acid, an adjunct to surgery in the treatment of spontaneous mammary tumors in C 3 H-He mice and transplantable melanoma in the hamster. Cancer Res. **32**, 648 (1972).
15. Larson, V. M., Clark, W. R., Hilleman, M. R.: Influence of synthetic (Poly I:C) and viral double-stranded ribonuleic acids on adenovirus 12 oncogenesis in hamsters. Proc. Soc. exp. Biol. (N.Y.) **131**, 1002 (1969).
16. Levy, H. B., Law, L. W., Rabson, A. S.: Inhibition of tumor growth by polyinosinic-polycytidylic acid. Proc. nat. Acad. Sci. (Wash.) **62**, 357 (1969).
17. Park, B. H., Good, R. A., Beck, N. P., Davis, B. B.: Concentration of cyclic adenosine 3',5'-monophosphate in human leukocytes during phagocytosis. Nature (Lond.) New Biol. **229**, 27 (1971).
18. Robison, G. A., Butcher, R. W., Sutherland, E. W.: Cyclic AMP. New York: Academic Press 1971.
19. Sarma, P. S., Shiu, G., Neubauer, R. H., Baron, S., Huebner, R. J.: Virus-induced sarcoma of mice: Inhibition by a synthetic polyribonucleotide complex. Proc. nat. Acad. Sci. (Wash.) **62**, 1046 (1969).
20. Sheppard, J. R.: Difference in the cyclic adenosine. 3',5'-monophosphate levels in normal and transformed cells. Nature (Lond.) New Biol. **236**, 14 (1972).
21. Smith, J. W., Steiner, A. L., Parker, C. W.: Human lymphocyte metabolism: Effects of cyclic and noncyclic nucleotides on stimulation by phytohemagglutinin. J. clin. Invest. **50**, 442 (1971).
22. Webb, D., Braun, W., Plescia, O. J.: Antitumour effects of polynucleotides and theophylline. Cancer Res. **32**, 1814 (1972).
23. Vanky, F., Stjernsward, J., Klein, G., Nilssone, U.: Serum-mediated inhibition of lymphocyte stimulation by autochthonous human tumors. J. nat. Cancer Inst. **47**, 95 (1971).
24. Zbar, B., Rapp, H. J., Ribi, E. E.: Tumor suppression by cell walls of *Mycobacterium bovis* attached to oil droplets. J. nat. Cancer Inst. **48**, 831 (1972).

BCG Immunotherapy of Pulmonary Deposits from Experimental Rat Tumors of Defined Immunogenicity*

R. W. BALDWIN and M. V. PIMM

Cancer Research Campaign Laboratories, University of Nottingham

Introduction

Studies with several chemically-induced animal tumors have demonstrated that implantation of tumor cells in admixture with viable Bacillus Calmette-Guérin (BCG) prevents their growth in genetically compatible hosts [1, 3, 5]. Deliberate infection of established local tumors may also lead to their suppression [1, 7] and the inhibition of metastases [7]. The mechanism of this tumor inhibition is not yet understood, although factors other than immunostimulation are involved, since intimate contact between BCG organisms and tumor cells is necessary [1, 5] and may contribute to this effect.

The objective of the present experiments was to evaluate immunotherapeutic methods for the treatment of pulmonary deposits of 3-methylcholanthrene(Mc)-induced rat sarcomas which have substantial immunogenicity. In comparison, the methods were used to treat pulmonary deposits of other rat tumors varying in immunogenic potential, including one which lacked detectable tumor-associated rejection antigens.

Materials and Methods

Tumors induced with chemical carcinogens or arising without deliberate inducement in rats of an inbred Wistar strain were maintained by s.c. transplantation.

Sarcomas Mc 7, Mc 40 A and Mc 52 A. Induced by s.c. injection of 3-methylcholanthrene were highly immunogenic; rats treated by excision of s.c. tumors rejected a subsequent challenge with trocar grafts.

Sarcoma Sp 24. Arose spontaneously and was weakly immunogenic. Graft-immunized rats rejected a maximum of 10^3 viable tumor cells.

Mammary carcinoma AAF 57. Induced by feeding N-hydroxy-2-acetylaminofluorene lacked significant antigenicity; graft-immunized rats failed to reject a challenge inoculum of 2×10^3 viable tumor cells.

Epithelioma Sp 1. A spontaneously arising tumor, was weakly immunogenic; immunized rats rejected a maximum of 5×10^4 viable tumor cells.

* Supported by a grant from the Cancer Research Campaign.

Assessment of Pulmonary Tumor Growth

Pulmonary growth of intravenously transferred tumor cells was demonstrated by perfusion of lungs with diluted Indian ink [4].

BCG

Freeze-dried BCG vaccine Percutaneous (supplied by Glaxo Laboratories Ltd., Greenford, Middlessex, England) was used at a concentration of 10 mg wet weight of organisms per ml.

Results

Immunotherapy of Pulmonary Deposits of 3-Methylcholanthrene-Induced Sarcomas

Active immunotherapy. Rat sarcoma cells were injected i.v. and their pulmonary growth treated by active immunotherapy. This was given by s.c. injection of viable cells of the same sarcoma in admixture with viable BCG (Table 1). This local inoculum did not develop and consistent with previous studies on immunotherapy of local tumors showed marked inhibition of pulmonary tumor growth [1]. Control rats had to be killed within 14 to 21 days, all but two having multiple (more than 200) discrete pulmonary tumor nodules. In comparison, 9/13 rats receiving immunotherapy had no macroscopic tumor in their lungs when experiments were terminated. Moreover, in the case of sarcoma Mc 52 A, growth was suppressed in a proportion of rats even when treatment was delayed for 10 days following i.v. injection of tumor cells.

Adjuvant immunotherapy. Previous studies showed that direct contact between BCG organisms and Mc sarcoma cells was necessary to inhibit local tumor growth

Table 1. Active immunotherapy of i. v. transferred rat sarcomas

Expt.	Sarcoma	No. cells injected	Treatment Day [a]	Treatment Inoculum [b]	Expt. terminated (day [a])	No. rats with lung tumors	No. nodules/lung
1	Mc 40 A	5×10^6	0	1.5 mg BCG + 5×10^6 Mc 40 A cells	14	1/5	1 × 200 +
		5×10^6	—	—	14	5/5	5 × 200 +
2	Mc 40 A	5×10^5	0	1.0 mg BCG + 3×10^6 Mc 40 A cells	19	1/4	1 × 70
		5×10^5	—	—	19	4/5	4 × 200 +
3	Mc 52 A	1×10^6	0	1.0 mg BCG + 1×10^6 Mc 52 A cells	21	2/4	48,200 +
		1×10^6	10	1.0 mg BCG + 1×10^6 Mc 52 A cells	21	2/4	75,200 +
		1×10^6	—	—	21	4/4	3,3 × 200 +

[a] With respect to tumor cell injection.

[b] Viable sarcoma cells in admixture with BCG injected s. c.

Table 2. BCG-adjuvant treatment of i. v. transferred rat sarcomas

Expt.	Sarcoma	No. cells injected	BCG [b] treatment (day [a])	Expt. terminated (day [a])	No. rats with lung nodules	No. nodules/lung
1	Mc 40 A	5×10^6	—	14	5/5	5 × 200 +
			0	14	0/5	—
2	Mc 40 A	5×10^5	—	19	4/5	4 × 200 +
			0	19	0/5	—
			5	19	0/5	—
3	Mc 40 A	5×10^5	—	21	5/5	40, 140, 3 × 200 +
			0	21	0/5	—
			6	21	0/5	—
4	Mc 7	2×10^6	—	14	4/4	40, 140, 2 × 200 +
			0	14	0/4	—
			7	14	0/4	—
5	Mc 52 A	1×10^6	—	21	4/4	3, 3 × 200 +
			0	21	0/4	—
			6	21	0/5	—

[a] With respect to tumor cell injection.
[b] BCG (1 mg wet weight) injected i. v.

and evoke concomitant tumor-specific immunity [1]. Tests were therefore carried out to evaluate whether pulmonary growth of i.v. transferred sarcoma cells could be inhibited by systemic infection with BCG, also administered i.v. (Table 2). Almost all (21/23) control rats receiving tumor cells alone developed multiple pulmonary nodules so that experiments had to be terminated after 14 to 21 days. In contrast,

Table 3. BCG-adjuvant treatment of i. v. transferred rat tumors

Expt.	Tumor	No. cells injected	Dose of BCG [a] (mg wet weight)	Expt. terminated (day)	No. rats with lung nodules	No. nodules/lung
1	Mammary					
	carcinoma	1×10^5	—	17	3/3	23, 37, 47
	AAF 57	1×10^5	1.0	17	3/3	3 × 200 +
2	Mammary					
	carcinoma	1×10^5	—	40	4/4	0 [b], 0 [b], 1, 2
	AAF 57	1×10^5	0.5	40	5/5	11, 11, 12, 12, 23
3	Carcinoma	2×10^5	—	35	2/3	0, 5, 7
	Sp 1	2×10^5	1.0	35	4/4	4, 11, 24, 43
4	Carcinoma	1×10^5	—	35	4/4	1, 1, 2, 17
	Sp 1	1×10^5	1.0	35	5/5	2, 5, 5, 8, 10
5	Fibrosarcoma	5×10^4	—	19	5/5	44, 67, 70, 74, 85 (68 ± 7)
	Sp 24	5×10^4	1.0	19	5/5	72, 87, 88, 113, 124 (97 ± 9)

[a] BCG injected i. v. in admixture with tumor cells.
[b] Rats had large thoracic tumor masses.

none of the BCG-treated rats developed detectable pulmonary tumors during this time. It should be noted that suppression of tumor growth was obtained even when BCG treatment was given 5 to 7 days after tumor-cell injection.

Adjuvant Immunotherapy of Pulmonary Deposits of Other Rat Tumors

In view of the inhibitory effect of systemically administered BCG on the growth of i.v. transferred cells of highly antigenic sarcomas, the effectiveness of this treatment was evaluated using a range of tumors (AAF57, Sp 1, Sp 24) of low immunogenicity. In these tests (Table 3), tumor cells were injected i.v. in admixture with BCG, but in no case did this treatment prevent pulmonary tumor growth. Moreover, in experiments with carcinoma AAF57 and the spontaneously arising fibrosarcoma Sp 24, growth in the lung was enhanced rather than restricted.

Discussion

These studies establish that BCG immunotherapy can inhibit the development of artificial pulmonary metastases, although this depends upon the antigenicity of the target tumor. Where the tumor has substantial immunogenicity, as in the case of the 3-methylcholanthrene-induced sarcomas described in this paper, active immunotherapy with viable sarcoma cells in admixture with BCG, or systemic treatment with BCG alone will inhibit or completely suppress growth of pulmonary tumor deposits. On the other hand, tests with several rat tumors lacking immunogenicity (Table 3) indicate that i.v. injection of BCG does not inhibit and may even enhance tumor growth in the lungs. These observations are relevant to the application of BCG to treatment of spontaneous metastases. Thus, with the weakly immunogenic epithelioma Sp1, which spontaneously metastasizes from subcutaneous growths, repeated i.v. injection of BCG following surgical removal of tumor grafts only partially suppresses pulmonary tumor growth, the major response being an increase in survival and a decrease in the number of pulmonary metastases [2].

Intimate contact of tumor cells with BCG organisms is essential for inhibition of local tumor growth [1, 5]. It is therefore likely that the inhibition of pulmonary tumor deposits following i.v. injection of BCG reflects direct contact between BCG organisms and tumor cells in the lungs. It is clear, however, that viable BCG organisms are not ideal for this purpose, particularly in a clinical situation, and one advantage of the experimental rat sarcomas described in this communication is that they provide a reproducible system for screening the tumor-inhibitory properties of other mycobacterial preparations such as cell-wall fractions [6] and defined soluble extracts.

References

1. BALDWIN, R. W., PIMM, M. V.: Influence of BCG infection on growth of 3-methylcholanthrene-induced rat sarcomas. Rev. Europ. Étud. clin. biol. **16**, 875 (1971).
2. BALDWIN, R. W., PIMM, M. V.: BCG immunotherapy of local subcutaneous growths and post-surgical pulmonary metastases of a transplanted rat epithelioma of spontaneous origin. Int. J. Cancer **12**, 420 (1973).

3. Barlett, G. L., Zbar, B., Rapp, H. J.: Suppression of murine tumor growth by immune reaction to the bacillus Calmette-Guérin strain of *Mycobacterium bovis*. J. nat. Cancer Inst. **48**, 245 (1972).
4. Wexler, H.: Accurate identification of experimental pulmonary metastases. J. nat. Cancer Inst. **36**, 641 (1966).
5. Zbar, B., Bernstein, I. D., Rapp, H. J.: Suppression of tumor growth at the site of infection with living bacillus Calmette-Guérin. J. nat. Cancer Inst. **46**, 831 (1971).
6. Zbar, B., Rapp, H. J., Ribi, E. E.: Tumor suppression by cell walls of *Mycobacterium bovis* attached to oil droplets. J. nat. Cancer Inst. **48**, 831 (1972).
7. Zbar, B., Tanaka, T.: Immunotherapy of cancer: Regression of tumors after intralesional injection of living *Mycobacterium bovis*. Science **172**, 271 (1971).

Specific and Nonspecific Immunotherapy: Use of BCG

B. Zbar

Biology Branch, National Cancer Institute, Bethesda, Md.

We have reported that tumor growth is suppressed at the site of infection with living BCG [7]. This observation has been confirmed [1, 3]. Guinea pigs that suppressed tumor growth at sites of BCG infection developed strong specific systemic tumor immunity [7, 8]. These observations prompted us to examine the basis of BCG-mediated tumor killing and the conditions required for optimal development of tumor immunity.

The central factor underlying BCG-mediated tumor regression is the ability of the host to develop and express an inflammatory reaction of the delayed hypersensitivity type at the tumor site. Manipulations that impair either the ability of the host or the ability of bacterial antigen(s) to generate delayed-hypersensitivity reactions decrease tumor killing. For example, treatment of guinea pigs with antilymphocyte serum, or large i.v. doses of BCG prevented the development of tuberculin sensitivity and BCG-mediated tumor killing [4, 7]. Treatment of adult mice with thymectomy and sublethal whole-body X-irradiation prevented the development of tuberculin sensitivity and BCG-mediated tumor regression [3].

Nonliving mycobacterial antigen preparations that did not produce tuberculin sensitivity did not lead to suppression of tumor growth. A chronic inflammatory reaction of the delayed-hypersensitivity type is essential for tumor suppression. This chronic inflammatory reaction is characterized histologically by the presence of granulomas [5].

The current view of the basis of BCG-mediated tumor regression is as follows: following BCG infection, the host produces lymphocytes capable of recognizing distinctive antigens of BCG; these lymphocytes come into contact with BCG in tissues and release soluble mediators of cellular immunity. Some of these molecules may directly kill tumor cells; other molecules induce accumulation of "activated" macrophages that may kill tumor cells. These "activated" macrophages process tumor antigens; this leads to development of specific tumor immunity.

Specific tumor immunity does not invariably develop following tumor regression at sites of BCG infection. This has been well documented with murine tumors [3]. The conditions required for enhancement of immunogenicity of weakly antigenic murine tumors remain to be defined. It is noteworthy that production of experimental allergic encephalomyelitis in mice required particular ratios of antigen and mycobacteria [6]. We have examined the conditions required for effective adjuvant activity of mycobacteria in a guinea-pig tumor system. In this system, guinea pigs receive simultaneous contralateral i.d. injections of vaccine (BCG and tumor cells) and challenge (tumor cells). The growth of the tumor cells is a sensitive and quantitative test of the immunogenicity of the BCG-tumor cell vaccine. The results of the investigation were clearcut: 1. more than 10^6 BCG cells were required for optimal development of specific tumor immunity; 2. water-in-oil emulsions containing mycobacteria and tumor cells were ineffective in producing systemic tumor immunity; 3. BCG cell walls attached to oil droplets (oil-in-water emulsion) mixed with tumor cells produced potent systemic immunity (75 μg was optimal; 300 μg was less effective); 4. living tumor cells in the vaccine were occasionally tumorigenic; X-irradiated tumor cells were not tumorigenic and retained immunogenicity; 5. no benefit was gained from multiple injections of vaccine or from increasing numbers of tumor cells in vaccine (standard dose equals 1.5×10^6 cells); 6. host response under these conditions can cope with 10^6 tumor cells, but not with 10^7 tumor cells [2, 9].

The molecular and cellular basis for this adjuvant effect remains unknown. We do not know whether 1. the host needs to be able to respond immunologically to BCG antigens; 2. tumor cells and BCG must be at the same site; and 3. whether "activated" macrophages indeed play a crucial role in development of specific tumor immunity. Answers to these questions may lead to effective use of BCG as an adjuvant in human tumor immunology.

References

1. Baldwin, R. W., Pimm, M. V.: Influence of BCG infection on growth of 3-methylcholanthrene-induced rat sarcomas. Europ. J. clin. biol. Res. **16**, 875 (1971).
2. Bartlett, G. L., Zbar, B.: Tumor specific vaccines containing *Mycobacterium bovis* and tumor cells: Safety and efficacy. J. nat. Cancer Inst. **48**, 1709 (1972).
3. Bartlett, G. L., Zbar, B., Rapp, H. J.: Suppression of murine tumor growth by immune reaction to the bacillus Calmette-Guérin strain of *Mycobacterium bovis*. J. nat. Cancer Inst. **48**, 245 (1972).
4. Hanna, M. G., jr., Snodgrass, M. J., Zbar, B., Rapp, H. J.: Histopathology of tumor regression after intralesional injection of *Mycobacterium bovis*. IV. The development of antitumor and anti-BCG immunity. J. nat. Cancer Inst. (submitted for publication 1973).
5. Hanna, M. G., jr., Zbar, B., Rapp, H. J.: Histopathology of tumor regression mediated by *Mycobacterium bovis* (BCG). I. Effect on tumor growth and metastases. J. nat. Cancer Inst. **48**, 1441 (1972).
6. Lee, J. M., Schneider, H. A.: Critical relationships between constituents of the antigen-adjuvant emulsion affecting experimental allergic encephalomyelitis in a completely susceptible mouse genotype J. exp Med. **115**, 157 (1961).
7 Zbar, B., Bernstein, I. D., Rapp, H. J.: Suppression of tumor growth at the site of infection with living bacillus Calmette-Guérin. J. nat. Cancer Inst. **46**, 831 (1971).
8. Zbar, B., Bernstein, I. D., Tanaka, Rapp, H. J.: Tumor immunity produced by the intradermal inoculation of living tumor cells and living *Mycobacterium bovis* (strain BCG). Science **170**, 1217 (1970).
9. Zbar, B., Rapp, H. J., Ribi, E. A.: Tumor suppression by cell walls of *Mycobacterium bovis* (BCG) attached to oil droplets. J. nat. Cancer Inst. **48**, 831 (1972).

Poly A. Poly U as an Adjunct to Surgery in the Treatment of Spontaneous Murine Mammary Adenocarcinoma*

F. Lacour, J. Lacour, and A. Spira

Institut Gustave-Roussy, Villejuif

Introduction

Certain complexes of multistranded synthetic polynucleotides possess two biological activities, induction of interferon (discovered by [4]), and stimulation of immunological reactions (demonstrated by [1]). There have consequently been numerous attemps to determine whether such polynucleotides have any effect on neoplasia. Two double-stranded complexes of synthetic polynucleotides have been used: poly I. poly C and poly A. poly U Poly I. poly C was initially employed because of its efficiency in inducing interferon. Poly A. poly U is a poor inducer of interferon but has been utilized as a nonspecific stimulator of the immune system. Repeated injections of poly I. poly C have protected animals from virus-induced and chemical-induced transplantable syngeneic tumors [9], and can prevent induction of leukemia or tumors by viruses [11, 12, 14].

It has been clearly established, however, that the antitumor effect is not correlated with poly I. poly C-induced circulating interferon [5, 13] but can be related in part to an enhancement of cell-mediated immunity. In addition to protective effects, such deleterious characteristics as pyrogenicity in rabbits [10] and toxicity in other species have been described [8].

Nonspecific stimulators of the immune response (generally bacterial products) can enhance host resistance to transplantable or autochthonous tumors. In occasional experiments however, these substances have increased tumor growth rather than resistance.

We decided to test the effect on host resistance to malignant tumors of poly A. poly U since this is a well-defined substance, easily accessible to study by the methods of molecular biology. Moreover, we hoped that this complex would not induce any of the noxious effects associated with some other nonspecific stimulators of the immune system. In contrast to poly I. poly C, poly A. poly U has no toxic or pyrogenic effects.

Materials and Methods

We chose for our experiments a spontaneous mammary carcinoma in the mouse since it can be correlated with a human cancer; C3H/He mice inbred at the Institut

* This work was supported by the Ligue Nationale Française contre le Cancer and by the Annie Dalsace grant.

Gustave-Roussy were used. We decided to administer the homopolyribonucleotide complex at a time when the tumor load confronting the host had been reduced by surgery.

The appearance of tumors (beginning at 3 months of age) was monitored weekly by manual palpation. In the first experiment, mice bearing tumors 5 to 10 mm in diameter were divided into 3 groups: Group I — controls; Group II — treated by surgery; Group III — subjected to both surgery and poly A. poly U. The animals were anaesthetized with ether and a simple mastectomy was performed under aseptic conditions one week to one month after detection of the tumor.

The homopolymers poly A and poly U were purchased from Miles Laboratories and further purified in our laboratory before preparation of the double-stranded complex [6].

An intravenous injection of 150 μg of poly A. poly U was given to the mice weekly for 6 weeks.

Animals remained in the study until their death, when autopsy and histological examination of tumor, lungs and spleen were performed.

Results

We assessed results on the number of lung metastases found and the survival period following the onset of the tumor (Table 1).

Table 1. Effect of surgery and surgery complemented with Poly A. Poly U on spontaneous mammary tumors of mice

	Number of mice	Metastases		Mean survival time after the onset of the tumor (days)
		No.	%	
I Controls	50	18	36	69
II Surgery	23	5	22	100 [a]
III Surgery + Poly A. poly U	23	5	22	120 [b]

[a] Surgery vs. controls $P < 0{,}001$ (calculated by Student's b.f.test).
[b] Surgery + Poly A. Poly U vs. surgery: $P = 0.10$.

Survival was significantly higher in the two groups treated by surgery than in the controls. In the group treated by surgery in conjunction with poly A. poly U, survival was longer than in the group treated by surgery alone, though the difference was on the borderline of statistical significance. The incidence of metastases was lower in the surgical groups than in the controls.

The distribution of survival periods among the 3 groups was plotted (Fig. 1). It should be noted that, in contrast to Groups I and II, Group III (surgery + poly A. poly U) had no deaths prior to day 50. From this analysis and a comparison of the body weight of mice in the three groups at autopsy we concluded that multiple injections of poly A. poly U (150 μg) had no toxic effects [7].

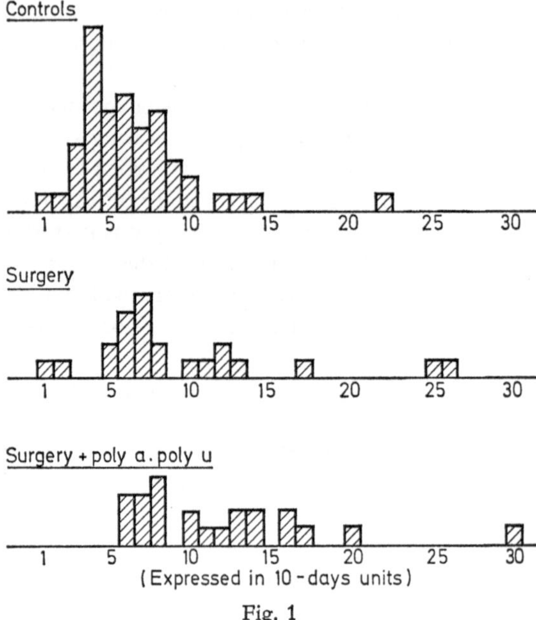

Fig. 1

The second experiment was designed to determine whether the results could be improved by increasing the dose of poly A. poly U and whether this double-stranded complex would influence the development of spontaneous mammary tumors in the absence of surgery.

To permit more accurate statistical analysis of the results, the animals were randomized into four groups: Group I — controls; Group II — poly A. poly U; Group III — surgery; and Group IV — surgery + poly A. poly U.

Material and methods were similar to those of the first experiment, except that poly A. poly U was injected in a dose of 250 μg instead of 150 μg. The results are summarized in Table 2.

Table 2. Effect of Poly A. Poly U on survival of mice bearing spontaneous mammary tumors and mice in which the tumor was surgically removed

	Number of mice	Metastases		Mean survival time after the onset of the tumor (days)
		No.	%	
I Controls	41	13	32	78
II Poly A. Poly U	33	14	42	83
III Surgery	25	8	32	102 [a]
IV Surgery + Poly A. poly U	23	5	22	132 [b]

[a] Surgery vs. controls: $P < 0.02$.
[b] Surgery + Poly A. poly U vs. surgery: $P < 0.02$ (calculated by Student's b.f.test).

1. The mean survival time of animals treated with poly A. poly U alone is not appreciably different from that of the controls.

2. Survival is significantly ($p < 0.01$) increased (31%) by surgery alone (Group III).

3. Survival is better in Group IV (surgery + poly A. poly U) than in Group III (surgery alone); the difference is statistically significant ($p < 0.02$). The mean survival time in this group was strikingly longer (69%) than that of the controls, and 29% longer than that of Group III.

4. The incidence of metastases was lowest in Group IV.

A similar observation was made in the first experiment.

There was no evidence of hematological or systemic toxicity of poly A. poly U, even at high doses. Histological observation of the spleen showed hyperplasia of lymphocytes and megakaryocytes.

Discussion and Conclusion

Our results indicate that the polyribonucleotide complex poly A. poly U is non-toxic and has a definite inhibitory effect on tumor growth. This effect may be due to stimulation of cell-mediated immunity. No effect was noted in the absence of surgical treatment, probably because of the presence of a large number of tumor cells, or a lack of immunologically reactive tissue available for stimulation of host resistance, or both. The conspicuous delay in the recurrence of virus-induced mammary tumors in mice after surgical treatment is not yet understood. It is unlikely to be due to some virus-mediated mechanism triggered by poly A. poly U, since a similar effect was obtained with a transplantable hamster tumor which, so far as is known, does not contain any infectious oncogenic virus [6].

[2] working with the same synthetic polynucleotide complex, observed decreased recurrence of a transplantable syngeneic tumor, removed by surgery before treatment.

Poly A. poly U is a poor inducer of interferon and the benefit obtained from surgery complemented by this complex may be due to the reduction of tumor cells, i.e. lowered antigen levels and amplified activity of antigen-reactive cells. [3] reported that poly A. poly U can much enhance the capacity of neonatally thymectomized mice to respond to skin homografts. However, a direct action of this complex on the tumor cells cannot be excluded.

These studies demonstrate that clinically significant improvement can be achieved in a spontaneous breast cancer when surgery is combined with administration of the double-stranded synthetic polynucleotide complex poly A. poly U.

References

1. Braun, W., Nakano, M.: Antibody formation: Stimulation by polyadenylic and polycytidylic acids. Science **157**, 819 (1967).
2. Braun, W., Plescia, O. J., Raskowa, J., Webb, D.: Basic proteins and synthetic polynucleotides as modifiers of immunogenicity of syngeneic tumor cells. Israel J. med. Sci. **7**, 72 (1971).
3. Cone, E. R., Johnson, A. G.: Regulation of the immune system by synthetic polynucleotides. III. Action on antigen reactive cells of thymic origin. J. exp. Med. **133**, 665 (1971).
4. Field, A. K., Tytell, A. A., Lampson, G. P., Hilleman, M. R.: Inducers of interferon and host resistance. II. Multistranded synthetic polynucleotide complexes. Proc. Nat. Acad. Sci. (Wash.) **58**, 1008 (1967).

5. GAZDAR, A. F., WEINSTEIN, A. J., SIMS, H. L., STEINBERG, A. D.: Enhancement and suppression of murine sarcoma virus-induced tumors by polyriboinosinic-polyribocytidylic acid. Proc. Soc. Exp. Biol. (N.Y.) **139**, 279 (1969).
6. LACOUR, F., SPIRA, A., LACOUR, J., PRADE, M.: Poly A. poly U: a potent adjunct to surgery in the treatment of spontaneous mammary tumors in C 3 H/He mice and transplantable melanoma in hamster. Cancer Res. **32**, 648 (1972).
7. LACOUR, J., LACOUR, F., FLAMANT, R.: Essai thérapeutique sur le cancer mammaire spontané: chirurgie et ARN synthétique (Poly A. poly U). Mém. Acad. Chir. **99**, 364 (1970).
8. LEONARD, B. J., ECCLESTON, E., JONES, D.: Toxicity of interferon inducers of double-stranded RNA type. Nature (Lond.) **224**, 1023 (1969).
9. LEVY, H. B., LAW, L. W., RABSON, A. S.: Inhibition of tumor growth by polyinosinic-polycytidylic acid. Proc. Nat. Acad. Sci. (Wash.) **62**, 357 (1969).
10. LINDSAY, H. L., TROWN, P. W., BRANDT, J., FORBES, M.: Pyrogenicity of poly I. poly C in rabbits. Nature (Lond.) **223**, 717 (1969).
11. SARMA, P. S., SHIU, G., NEUBAUER, R. H., BARON, S., HUEBNER, R. Y.: Virus-induced sarcoma of mice. Inhibition by a synthetic polyribonucleotide complex. Proc. Nat. Acad. Sci. (Wash.) **62**, 1046 (1969).
12. VANDEPUTTE, M., DATTA, S. V., BILLIAU, A., DE SOMMER, P.: Inhibition of polyoma virus oncogenesis in rats by polyriboinosinic-ribocytidylic acid. Europ. J. Cancer **6**, 323 (1970).
13. WEINSTEIN, A. J., GAZDAR, A. F., SIMS, H. L., LEVY, H. B.: Lack of correlation between interferon induction and antitumour effect of poly I. poly C. Nature (Lond.) **231**, 53 (1971).
14. YOUN, J. K., BARSKI, G., HUPPERT, J.: Inhibition de leucémigenèse virale chez la souris par traitement aux polynucléotides synthétiques. C. R. Acad. Sci. (Paris) **267**, 816 (1968).

Combined Chemotherapy and Immunotherapy of Transplantable and Spontaneous Murine Leukemia in DBA/2 and AKR Mice*

J. G. Bekesi and J. F. Holland

Department of Neoplastic Diseases, Mt. Sinai School of Medicine New York, N. Y.

Introduction

Glycoprotein is an integral part of the surface structure of normal and neoplastic cells. Glycoprotein components play a significant role in such substances as blood-group antigens [12] and histocompatibility antigens [14], and may act as receptors in mitogenic interaction of phytohemagglutinin with lymphocytes. Membrane glyco-

Sialic acid
- **N-Acetylneuraminic acid**
- **N-Glycolylneuraminic acid**
- **N-Acetyl-4-O-acetyneuraminic acid**
- **Methoxy neuraminic acid**
- **N-Acetoglycolyl-4-methyl-4,9-dideoxy-neuraminic acid**

In Leukemia L-1210 as well as other experimental tumors

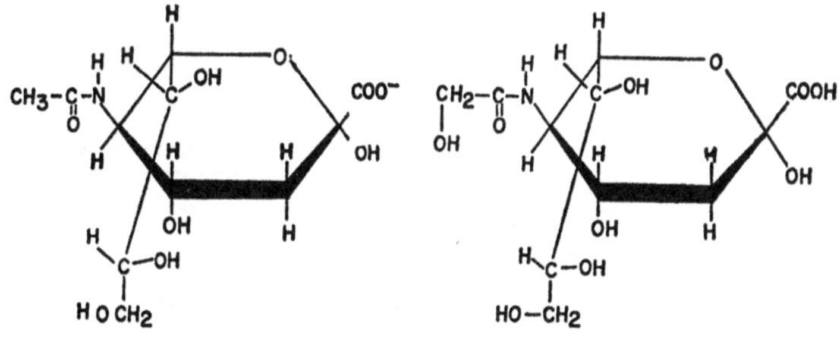

N-Acetylneuraminic acid **N-Glycolylneuraminic acid**

Fig. 1. Chemical structure of N-acetylneuraminic acid and N-glycolylneuraminic acid

* This investigation was supported by NIH 72-2014 from the National Cancer Institute.

proteins also probably play a role in self-recognition. It is therefore an attractive hypothesis that glycoprotein components of cell membranes may have a significant influence on metastasis and invasion of neoplastic cells [10, 15].

Most experimental tumors carry tumor-specific transplantation antigens (TSTA) and histocompatibility antigens (H_2) which they may not share with the recipient host [9]. That the host does not reject these antigenically different tumors implies tolerance. This tolerance has been attributed to a) antigens on the neoplastic cells being concealed by a terminal sugar residue, N-acetylneuraminic acid, on the surface glycoproteins (Fig. 1) [1—3], or b) antigenic sites of the tumor cells being coated with nonspecific glycoproteins [2, 8, 17]. Either circumstance might prevent antigen detection by the host's immunosurveillance system. Sialo-glycoproteins (glycoproteins rich in sialic acid) are generally very poor immunogens. However, a significant increase of immunogenicity of glycoproteins has been demonstrated after removal of the terminal N-acetylneuraminic acid (NANA) residue with neuraminidase (Fig. 2), indicating that the terminal NANA may directly influence the antigenic expression of the parent molecule [1, 16, 19]. Recently, considerable efforts have been made to elucidate the biological role of sialic acid in normal and neoplastic tissue. [13] demonstrated that i.v. injection of desialated glycoproteins (orosomucoid, fetuin, ceruloplasmin, heptoglobin, and α_2 macroglobulin) into rats resulted in their prompt

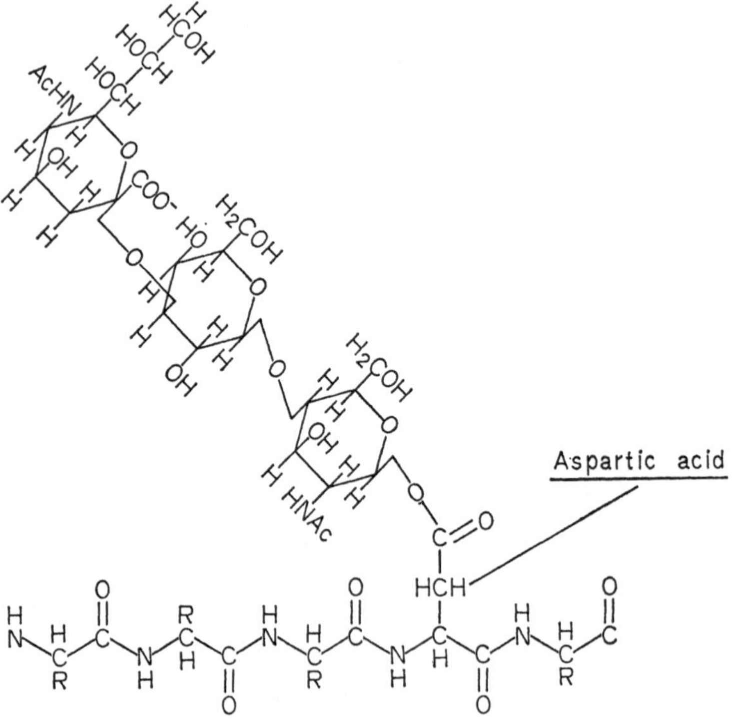

Fig. 2. Diagrammatic segment of the carbohydrate portion of glycoprotein

removal from the circulation and accumulation within the parenchymal cells of the liver.

The function of sialic acid on the surface membrane of neoplastic cells has been intensively investigated since [4, 5, 6, 11, 18] almost simultaneously reported that *Vibrio cholerae* neuraminidase treatment of tumor cells led to increased immunogenicity.

The present work deals with several problems related to the enzymatic release of neuraminic acid and the subsequent change of immunogenicity of leukemia L 1210 cells in DBA/2 mice and of spontaneous leukemic thymocytes and leukemic spleen cells in AKR mice. The influence of chemotherapy on the immunological response to tumors is also discussed.

Methods and Materials

Leukemia L 1210 cells, maintained by weekly intraperitoneal passage in DBA/2 mice, were harvested 6 days after transplantation and were freed from contaminating red blood cells (RBC) by a 5 second osmotic shock treatment. They were washed 3 times with physiological saline, then incubated in acetate buffer (0.05 M sodium acetate, 0.154 M NaCl, and 0.005 M $CaCl_2$; pH 5.6) or in Hanks' balanced salt solution at pH 7.0 in the presence of *Vibrio cholerae* neuraminidase at 37 °C. Final enzyme concentration was 30—50 units per 2.5×10^7 cells per ml incubation medium. A unit of activity is defined as the amount of enzyme which will release 1 μg of NANA from neuraminolactose or orosomucoid in 15 min at 37 °C. At predetermined times, reaction flasks were removed, cooled rapidly, and the cells washed once with 40 volumes of saline-EDTA, then twice with physiological saline. Supernatants and washings were combined and kept for quantitation of N-acetylneuraminic acid.

Leukemia L 1210 cells treated with neuraminidase were suspended in physiological saline to give a final concentration of 2×10^7 tumor cells per ml. For immunization, 10^5, 10^6 or 10^7 treated cells were injected i.p. into each DBA/2 recipient mouse. Animals remaining tumor-free at the end of 30 days were challenged with 10 to 10^7 freshly harvested viable L 1210 cells (i.p., i.v., or s.c.).

Experiments to determine the efficacy of chemotherapy and chemotherapy followed by immunization with neuraminidase-treated tumor cells were conducted as follows: DBA/2 mice (2—3 months of age) were inoculated i.p. on day 0 with 10^7 viable L 1210 cells. The tumor-bearing mice were then treated on day 1 or 3 or 5 with Cytoxan, BCNU or methyl CCNU. A group of 20 mice received no treatment and served as the untreated control. Animals were randomized after chemotherapy: a) chemotherapy alone, b) chemotherapy followed by immunotherapy. A single immunization was performed with 10^7 neuraminidase-treated L 1210 cells i.p. on days 1, 4, 7, 10, 13 or 16 after chemotherapy. In both experimental groups, challenge of surviving mice with untreated L 1210 tumor cells was carried out 30 days after the initial tumor transplant.

The studies of effectiveness of chemotherapy plus immunotherapy in AKR mice with spontaneous lymphoma were carried out after positive confirmation of the disease (palpation and WBC count) by treating the diagnosed AKR mice with a combination of vincristine and dexamethasone. 2 to 3 days after drug therapy, animals were randomized into two groups, a) chemotherapy alone; b) chemotherapy followed by immunization with 10^7 neuraminidase-treated leukemic thymocytes or spleen cells at the times indicated in the figures.

Results

Effect of Neuraminidase Treatment on the Immunogenicity of Leukemia L1210 Tumor Cells in DBA/2 Mice

The total NANA content of leukemia L 1210 is 1.09 μmole per 10^9 cells. Results presented in Fig. 3 show the release of N-acetylneuraminic acid from L 1210 tumor cells by *Vibrio cholerae* neuraminidase under various incubation conditions. When incubation was performed at pH 5.6 in the presence of Ca^{++}, sialic acid was rapidly hydrolyzed from the neoplastic cells, reaching a plateau after 60 min of incubation. At this point, about 70% of the total cellular NANA had been cleaved from 10^9 L 1210 cells. At the same time, neuraminidase treatment resulted in a loss of oncogenic potential of L 1210 cells, since 10^7 tumor cells treated in this manner failed to produce tumor when inoculated i.p. into DBA/2 mice. Loss of oncogenic potential of L 1210 cells was not apparent, however, when the incubation with neuraminidase was performed at pH 7.0, or in sodium acetate buffer alone at pH 5.6, or when the Ca^{++} was omitted from the neuraminidase-containing sodium acetate buffer.

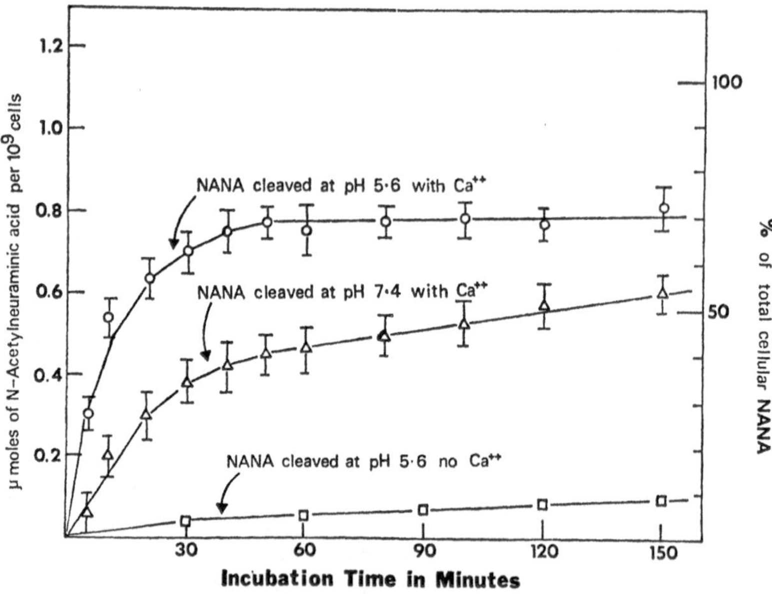

Fig. 3. Release of N-acetylneuraminic acid from leukemia L 1210 cells during incubation with *Vibrio cholerae* neuraminidase. Supernatants obtained after neuraminidase treatment at pH 5.6 and 7.0 were directly applied to a Dowex-2x 8 acetate form resin column and NANA was eluted with 1.0 M sodium acetate buffer (pH 5.6). Qualification of NANA was done by Warren's TBA method. N-acetylneuraminic acid released at pH 5.6 with Ca^{++} △—△—△; at pH 7.0 with Ca^{++} □—□—□; at pH 5.6 with no Ca^{++} ○—○—○

The immunity induced by single or multiple immunization with neuraminidase-treated L 1210 cells in DBA/2 mice was tested by challenge with untreated leukemia L 1210 cells 30 days after the last immunization. The data presented in Fig. 4 leave little doubt that neuraminidase treatment resulted in a significant increase in the immunogenicity of L 1210 tumor cells, since all mice immunized by single or multiple

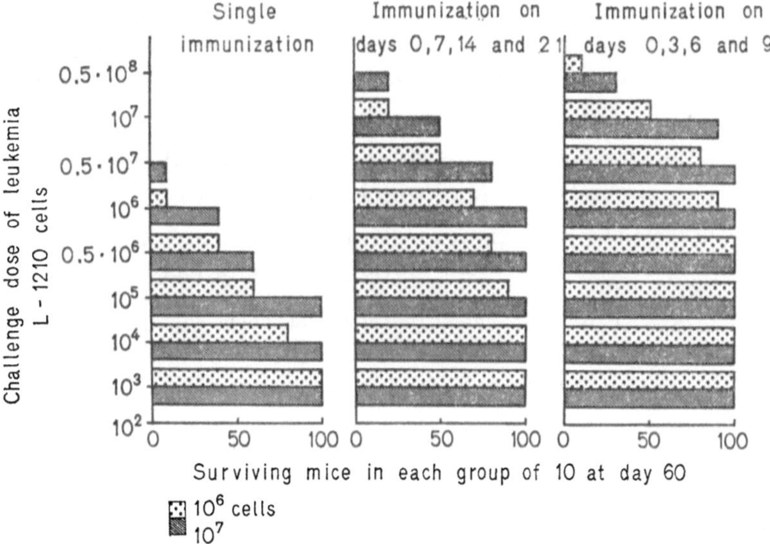

Fig. 4. Refractoriness of DBA/2 mice after a single or multiple immunization with neuraminidase-treated leukemia L 1210 tumor cells. DBA/2 mice were immunized with 10^6 or 10^7 neuraminidase-treated L 1210 cells i. p. and 30 days later challenged i. p. with 10—10^7 untreated leukemia L 1210 cells Results are expressed as percent of challenged DBA/2 mice free of tumor on day 60

Table 1. Specificity of immunity in DBA/2 Ha mice to *V. cholerae* neuraminidase-treated L 1210 tumor cells

	Tumor grafts	Challenge with 10^5 tumor cells TF/T[a]	Mean survival time ± S.D. (days)
Control	L 1210	0/15	8.1 ± 0.6
DBA/2 Ha mice	Sarcoma 180	0/15	20.6 ± 3.1
	Ehrlich carcinoma	0/15	16.2 ± 1.6
	Krebs-2	0/15	17.6 ± 2.3
	Mammary tumor[b]	0/10	49.8 ± 6.1
Immunized	L 1210	14/15	
DBA/2 Ha mice[c]	Sarcoma 180	0/15	19.7 ± 1.9
	Ehrlich carcinoma	0/15	17.1 ± 1.8
	Krebs-2	0/15	16.8 ± 2.8
	Mammary tumor[b]	0/10	51.6 ± 4.8

[a] Number of animals free of tumor at day 60/number of immunized mice challenged.

[b] Spontaneous mammary carcinoma was obtained from a 10-months-old DBA/2 mouse.

[c] DBA/2 mice were immunized with a single injection of 10^7 neuraminidase treated L 1210 tumor cells. Mice were challenged 30 days after immunization.

immunization with 10^7 treated cells were refractory to 10^5 or 5×10^6 virulent L 1210 tumor cells, respectively. Progressive booster challenges with untreated L 1210 tumor cells produced refractoriness to 3 to 5×10^8 virulent L 1210 cells.

The specificity of anti-tumor immunity induced by neuraminidase-treated leukemia L 1210 cells was examined (see Table 1). All control animals died after injection of 10^5 untreated tumor cells. Mice immunized with neuraminidase-treated L 1210 cells resisted a challenge of 10^5 virulent L 1210 cells but died at the same rate as the controls when the challenge tumor graft was other than L 1210. This indicates that the neuraminidase-treated L 1210 cells did not induce nonspecific immunity in the DBA/2 mice.

Effectiveness of Chemotherapy and Immunotherapy in DBA/2 Mice with Leukemia L1210

In view of these observations, we investigated whether a combination of chemotherapy with immunotherapy could provide a better therapeutic approach than

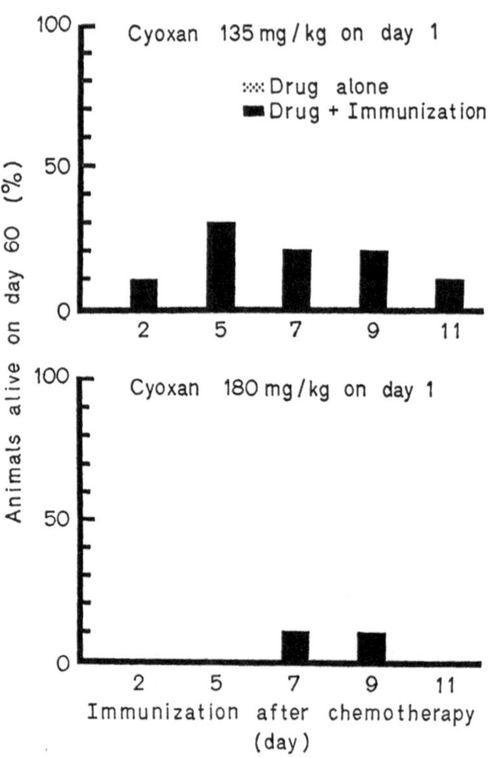

Fig. 5. Effect of cyclophosphamide (Cytoxan) alone and in combination with immunization in DBA/2 mice with L 1210 leukemia. On day 0 DBA/2 mice were inoculated with 10^7 untreated L 1210 tumor cells i.p. and on day 1 with cyclophosphamide at dose level indicated (for details see "Materials and Methods")

chemotherapy alone. We realized at the beginning of this study that a) the dosage of the chemotherapeutic agents had to be adjusted so that host immunocompetence was not irreversibly depressed, yet the tumor load was sufficiently reduced; b) the timing of immunization after chemotherapy was a highly critical factor. It is evident from Fig. 5 that tumor-bearing DBA/2 mice receiving more than 135 mg/kg cyclophosphamide (Cytoxan) did not benefit from the combination of chemo- and immunotherapy. On the other hand, treatment with 135 mg/kg cyclophosphamide followed by immunization with neuraminidase-treated L 1210 tumor cells resulted in 20—30% of animals free of tumor. No animals which received cyclophosphamide alone survived free of tumor. The data presented in Fig. 6 demonstrate that the combination of BCNU treatment followed by immunization with neuraminidase-treated leukemia L 1210 cells proved better than treatment with cyclophosphamide. Under these experimental conditions, about 10% of the animals which received BCNU on day 1 or 3 survived free of disease. On the other hand, 40—60% of DBA/2 mice with leukemia L 1210 treated with BCNU followed by immunization were cured. Methyl CCNU treatment appeared to be highly effective against leukemia L 1210 in

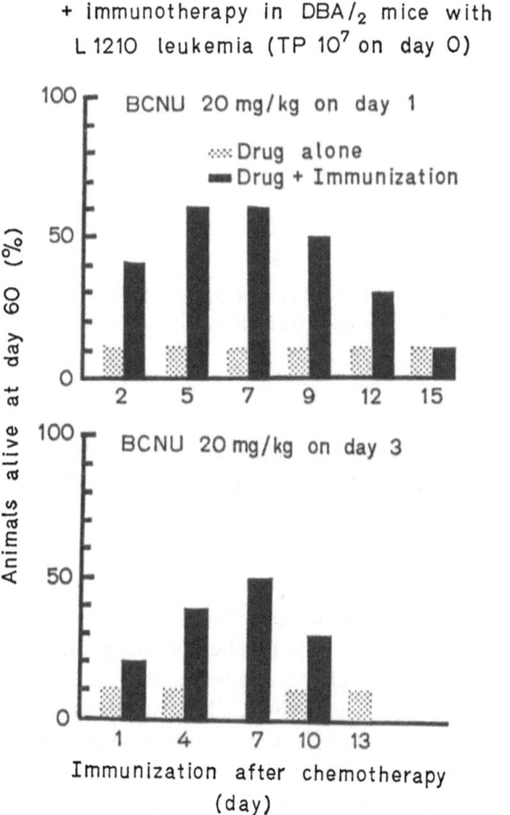

Fig. 6. Efficacy of BCNU and BCNU plus immunotherapy in DBA/2 mice with leukemia L 1210 (for details see "Materials and Methods")

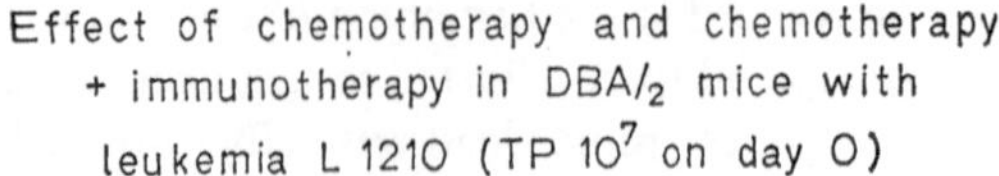

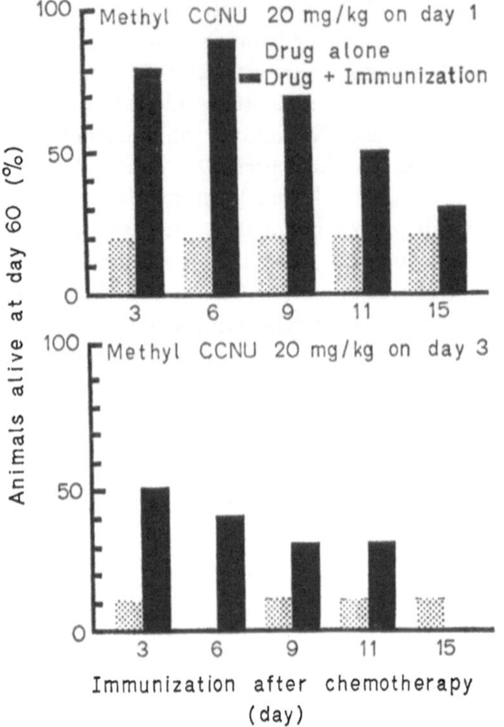

Fig. 7. Effect of chemotherapy (methyl CCNU) and combined with immunotherapy in DBA/2 mice with transplanted leukemia L 1210 tumor cells (for further information see "Materials and Methods")

DBA/2 mice; it reduced the tumor load without significantly altering the immunocompetence of the treated animals. Data presented in Fig. 7 indicate that the combination of this therapeutic agent with immunotherapy resulted in the highest percentage of mice cured (50—80%) of leukemia L 1210.

In order to investigate whether cure was associated with different degrees of immunological response, we examined the resistance of the surviving DBA/2 mice which had received chemotherapy alone or chemotherapy plus immunotherapy to untreated leukemia L 1210 cells. Table 2 summarizes these experiments. Mice surviving free of tumor after BCNU or methyl CCNU treatment alone rejected L 1210 tumor cell inocula of less than 1,000 cells. On the other hand, animals surviving after combination chemotherapy and immunotherapy were refractory to 10^6 untreated L 1210 tumor cells, irrespective of site of injection of the challenge dose (s.c., i.p., i.v. or i.cr.). This indicates the presence of a powerful immunity in mice immunized with neuraminidase-treated L 1210 cells after chemotherapy.

Table 2. Immunocompetence of DBA/2 mice following BCNU or MCCNU therapy or BCNU or MCCNU + immunization with neuraminidase-treated L 1210 tumor cells

Source of animals	Challenge dose	TF/T [a]
Control DBA/2 mice	10^3	0/10
Chemotherapy [a]	10^3	5/6
	10^4	2/6
	10^5	1/7
Chemo-immunotherapy [a]	10^3	10/10
	10^4	10/10
	10^5	17/17
	10^6	9/10
	10^7	5/10

[a] Number of animals free of tumor at day 30/number of animals challenged with untreated tumor cells (s.c., i.p., i.v., or i.cr.).

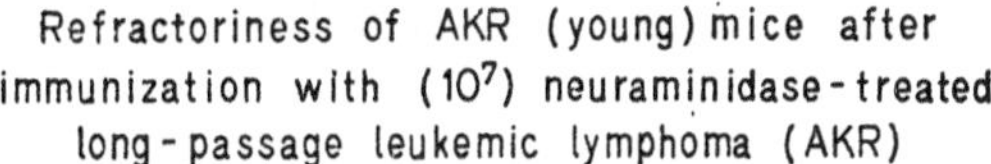

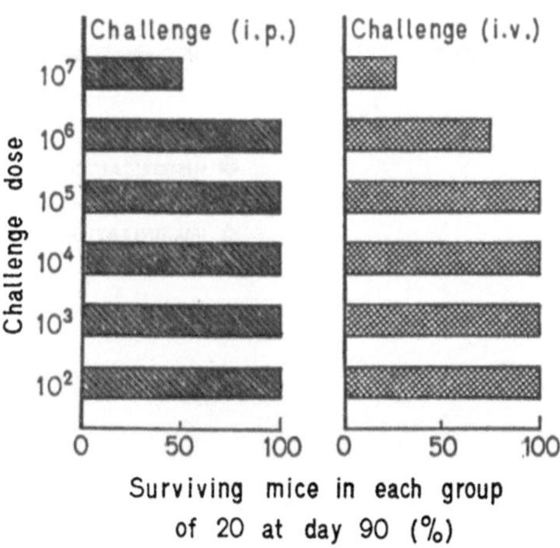

Fig. 8. Refractoriness of AKR mice after immunization with neuraminidase-treated long-passage leukemic lymphoma. Female 2—4 months old AKR mice were immunized with 10^7 neuraminidase-treated long-passage (46th) leukemic lymphoma cells i.p. 30 days after immunization, animals were randomized into 2 groups: Group 1 were challenged i.p., and Group 2 challenged i.v. with 10 to 10^7 untreated long-passage leukemic lymphoma cells. The LD_{50} of this tumor line is < 10 cells

Immunogenicity of Long-Line Passage Leukemia (AKR) After Neuraminidase Treatment in Young AKR Mice

Until recently it has been generally accepted, albeit without incontrovertible evidence, that AKR mice are tolerant to leukemia induced by Gross virus. Dore, Ajuria and Mathé [7], however, successfully immunized young AKR mice with

BCG K_{36} cells (leukemia induced by Gross virus) against K_{36} tumor. They demonstrated the presence of a cytotoxic antibody against K_{36} leukemia in the serum of immunized, mice thus throwing doubt on the validity of the above hypothesis. Our results in Fig. 8 substantiate and extend the work of Dore *et al.* We have shown strong refractoriness in AKR mice after immunization with neuraminidase-treated long-passage leukemic cell against the challenge of untreated leukemic cells. This immunity was found to be specific and can be transferred in non-immunized young AKR mice.

Immunization of Leukemic (Spontaneous) AKR Mice After Chemotherapy with Neuraminidase-Treated Leukemic (AKR) Thymocytes

AKR mice acquire Gross virus prior to their birth but the virus remains dormant until they reach the age of 6 months, when spontaneous leukemia develops. About 90—95% of the AKR mice die from leukemia before 12 months of age. We undertook the study of various carcinostatic agents, with and without neuraminidase-modified syngeneic tumor cells in this animal model system, because of the similarity of the disease to human acute lymphocytic leukemia. Spontaneously leukemic AKR mice were selected from the colony of 4,500 retired female breeders. The clinical diagnosis of leukemia was made with 94% accuracy by splenic and lymph node palpation

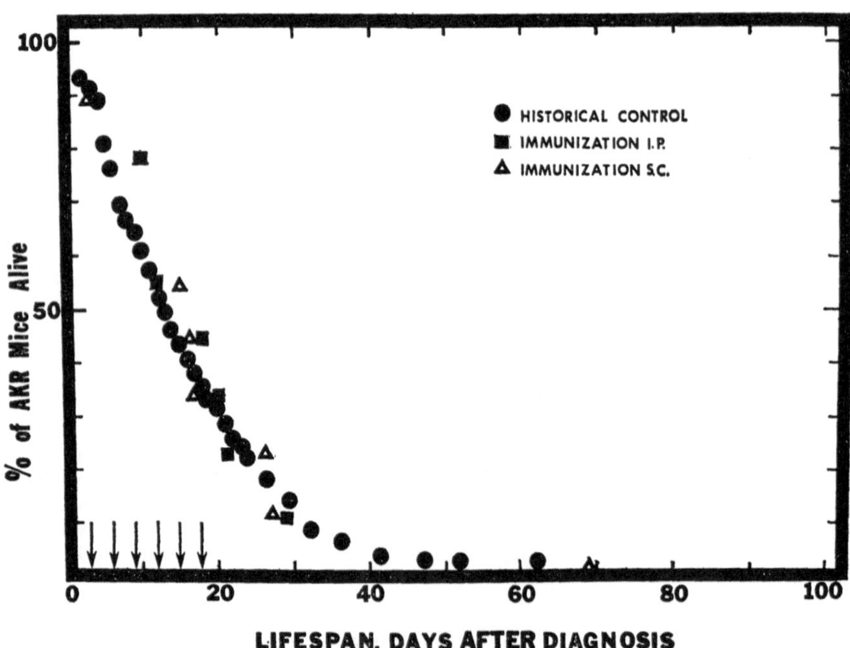

Fig. 9. Immunization of leukemic AKR mice with neuraminidase-treated leukemic thymocytes without chemotherapy. AKR mice with spontaneous lymphoma were randomized into three groups: Group 1 untreated control; Group 2 immunized with 10^7 neuraminidase-treated leukemic (spontaneous) thymocytes i.p.; Group 3 immunized s.c. The number of immunizations is indicated by arrows on the abscissa

followed by leukocyte count (see the historical control curves in Fig. 9, 10, 11 and 12 which represent 320 AKR mice obtained from 25 different experiments). At the time of diagnosis, the average splenic weight was 410 mg, the thymus 650 mg, and the leukocyte count 23,400/mm^3. It is not surprising that, with such a tumor load, immunization with neuraminidase-treated leukemic thymocytes injected either i.p. or s.c. did not change the survival pattern of the tumor-bearing animals (see Fig. 9).

Treatment with a combination of vincristine and dexamethasone for 4 days resulted in a reduction of organ weights and leukocyte count (spleen to approximately 70 mg, thymus to approximately 50 mg, and WBC to approximately 8,000/mm^3). Animals treated with drugs alone had a 92% increase in life-span but none survived 100 days (see drug survival curves in Figs. 10, 11 and 12).

Immunization of vincristine plus dexamethasone-treated AKR mice with X-irradiated spontaneous AKR leukemic cells (see Fig. 10) or immunization with neuraminidase-treated leukemia L 1210 cells (see Fig. 11) resulted in an essentially similar survival pattern to the drug-treated control groups.

The combination of drug therapy and immunization with neuraminidase-treated AKR leukemic thymocytes s.c. caused 30% of animals to survive 100 days without evidence of the disease (Fig. 12). For those mice which died, the increase in life-span was 160%.

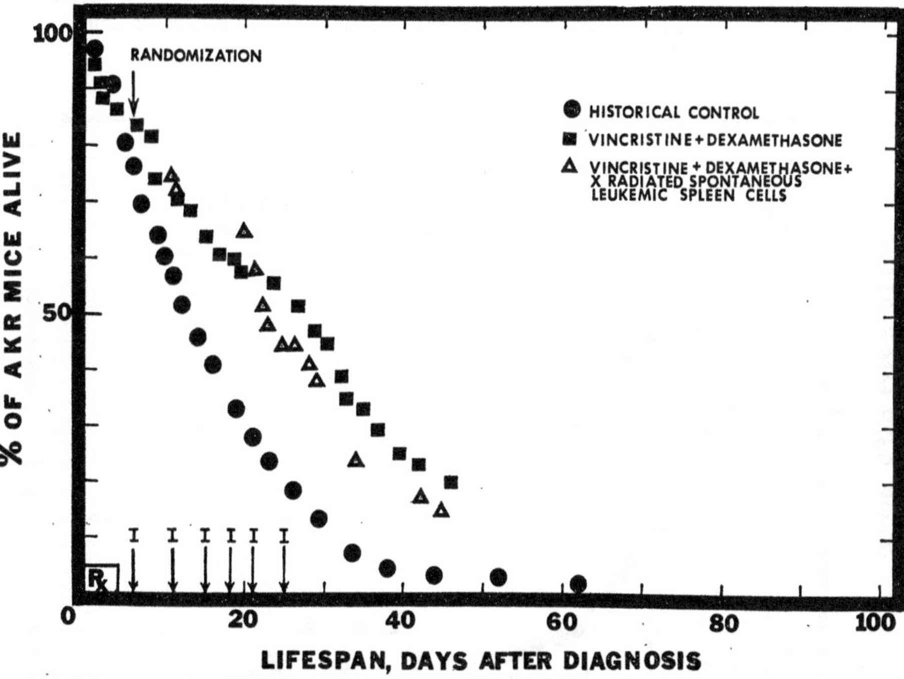

Fig. 10. Immunization of leukemic AKR mice with X-irradiated spontaneous AKR lymphoma spleen cells after vincristine and dexamethasone treatment. AKR mice with spontaneous leukemia were treated on day 1 with 0.75 mg/kg vincristine and on days 1, 2, 3 and 4 with 4.5 mg/kg dexamethasone i.p. Animals were randomized into two groups: Group 1 drug controls and Group 2 immunized s.c. as indicated by arrows on abscissa with 10^7 X-irradiated spontaneous lymphoma cells

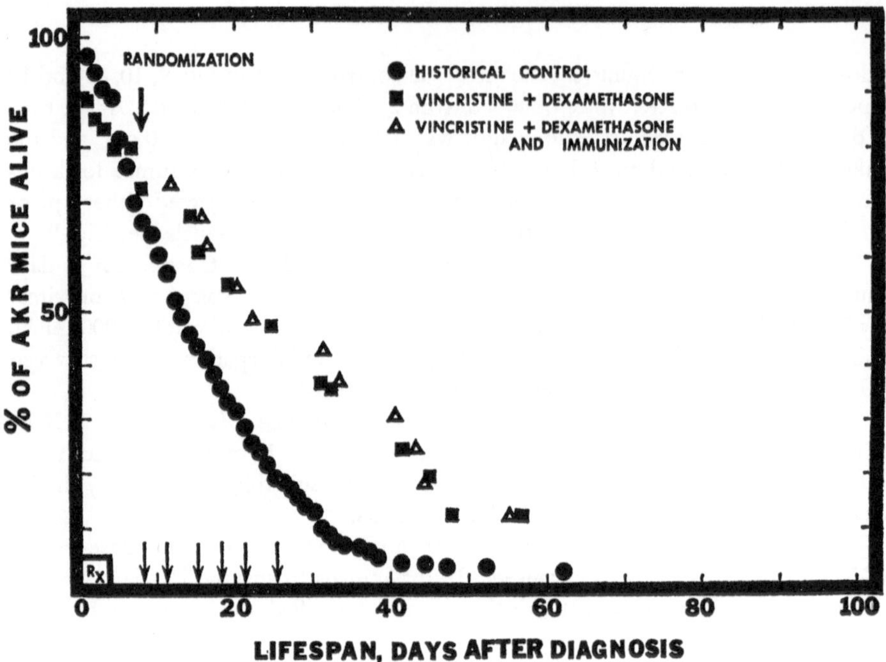

Fig. 11. Immunization of leukemic AKR mice after chemotherapy with neuraminidase-treated leukemia L 1210 cells. Treatment of mice with chemotherapeutic agents was as described under Fig. 10. Immunizations with 10^7 neuraminidase-treated L 1210 cells were performed as indicated by arrows on abscissa

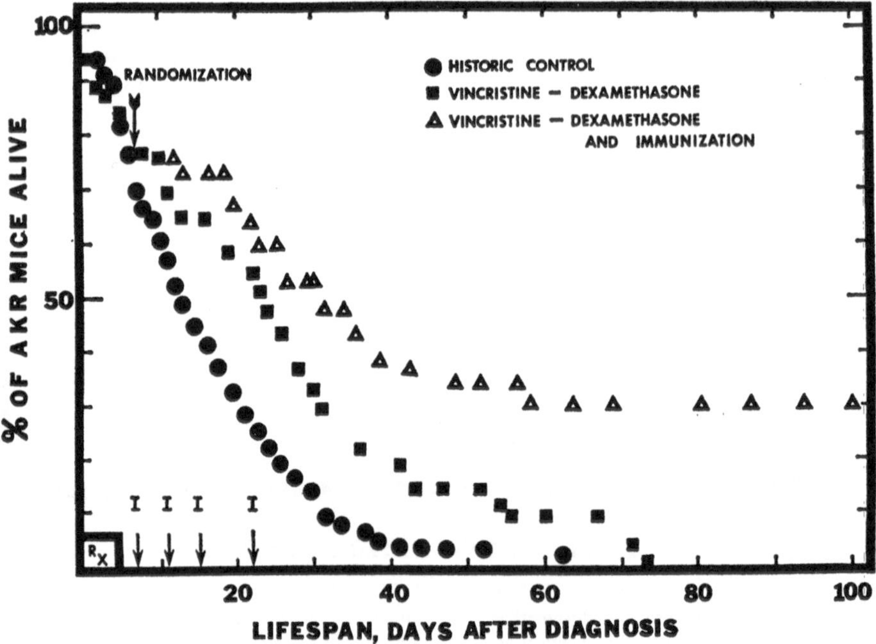

Fig. 12. Effectiveness of immunization in leukemic AKR mice after chemotherapy with neuraminidase-treated leukemic thymocytes (for details see "Materials and Methods")

References

1. APFELL, C. A., PETERS, J. H.: Tumors and serum glycoprotein "The Symbodies". Progr. exp. Tumor Res. (Basel) **12**, 1 (1969).
2. APFELL, C. A., PETERS, J. H.: Regulation of antigenic expression. J. theor. Biol. **26**, 47 (1970).
3. BAGSHAWE, K. D., CURRIE, G. A.: Immunogenicity of L 1210 murine leukemia cells after treatment with neuraminidase. Nature (Lond.) **218**, 1254 (1968).
4. CURRIE, G. A., BAGSHAWE, K. D.: The effect of neuraminidase on the immunogenicity of the Landschutz ascites tumor: site and mode of action. Brit. J. Cancer **22**, 588 (1968).
5. CURRIE, G. A., BAGSHAWE, K. D.: The role of sialic acid in antigenic expression: further studies of the Landschutz ascites tumor. Brit. J. Cancer **22**, 843 (1968).
6. CURRIE, G. A., BAGSHAWE, K. D.: Tumor-specific immunogenicity of methylcholanthrene-induced sarcoma cells after incubation in neuraminidase. Brit. J. Cancer **23**, 141 (1969).
7. DORE, J. F., AJURIA, E., MATHÉ, G.: Non-leukemic AKR mice are not tolerant to cells of leukemia induced by Gross virus. Rev. Europ. Étud. clin. biol. **15**, 81 (1970).
8. GASIC, G., GASIC, T.: Removal and regeneration of the cell coating in tumor cells. Nature (Lond.) **196**, 170 (1962).
9. KLEIN, G.: Experimental studies in tumor immunology. Fed. Proc. **28**, 1739 (1969).
10. KOJIMA, K., SAKAI, I.: On the role of stickiness of tumor cells in the formation of metastasis. Cancer Res. **24**, 1887 (1964).
11. LINDENMAN, J., KLEIN, P. A.: Immunological aspects of viral oncolysis, p. 63—66. Berlin-Heidelberg-New York: Springer 1967.
12. LLOYD, K. O., KABAT, E. A.: Immunochemical studies on blood groups. XLI. Proposed structures for the carbohydrate portion of blood groups A, B, H, Lewis ^{a} and Lewis ^{b} substances. Proc. nat. Acad. Sci. (Wash.) **61**, 1470 (1968).
13. MORELL, A. G., GREGORIADIS, G., SCHEINBERG, H. I., HICKMAN, J., ASHWELL, G.: The role of sialic acid in determining the survival of glycoproteins in the circulation. J. biol. Chem. **246**, 1461 (1971).
14. NATHENSON, S. G., SHIMADA, A., YAMANE, K., MURAMATSU, T., CULLEN, S., MANN, D. L., FAHEY, J. L., GRAFF, R.: Biochemical properties of papain solubilized murine and human histocompatibility alloantigens. Fed. Proc. **29**, 2026 (1970).
15. NOSSAL, G. J. V.: Self recognition. Ann. N.Y. Acad. Sci. **124**, 37 (1965).
16. PETERS, J. H.: Immunogenic basis of nephritis. Biochem. Clin. **2**, 137 (1963).
17. SANFORD, B. H.: An alteration in tumor histocompatibility induced by neuraminidase. Transplantation **5**, 1273 (1967).
18. SANFORD, B. H., CODINGTON, J. F.: Further studies on the effect of neuraminidase on tumor cell transplantability. Tissue Antigens **1**, 153 (1971).
19. SCHULTZE, H. E.: Influence of bound sialic acid on electrophoretic mobility of human serum proteins. Arch. Biochem. Biophys. **1** (Suppl.), 290 (1962).

Modification of Immunogenicity in Experimental Immunotherapy and Prophylaxis*

R. L. SIMMONS ** and A. RIOS

Mayo Memorial Building University of Minnesota, Minneapolis, Minn.

Sialic acid residues are the principal constituents on the surface of plasma membranes [5] and make the chief contribution to the negative charge of the cell surface [1]. A number of functional alterations of the cell can be induced by removal of the sialic acid from the surface membrane by neuraminidase [7, 8, 10, 23]. These include enhanced phagocytosis [15, 31], inhibition of viral [4] or mycoplasma [11] induced hemagglutination, inhibition of cell aggregation [14], increased cell deformability [30], alterations in the patterns of cellular migration [32] and interference with amino acid transport across treated cell membranes [6]. CURRIE and BAGSHAWE [8] postulated that, because of their negative charges, the sialomucins on cells interfered with detection of cellular immunogens by lymphocytes. APFFEL and PETERS [2] have broadened this concept by suggesting that masking of antigens is one of the normal natural biological roles of glycoproteins, and that sialoglycoprotein on the cell surface may be a distinct system of immunoregulation. These hypotheses are supported by the finding of SANFORD [23] that TA-3 tumor, which has lost strain specificity, would not kill recipient mice if the cells were treated *in vitro* with neuraminidase before i.p. inoculation. Independently, CURRIE and BAGSHAWE [8] showed that neuraminidase-treated Landschutz ascites tumor cells, L 1210 leukemia cells [3], and methylcholanthrene-induced sarcoma cells [9] grew less well in normally susceptible mice. Recipients were subsequently shown to be immune to the tumor. Ehrlich's ascites tumor was found [16] to be rendered more immunogenic when treated with neuraminidase before inoculation, and CURRIE *et al.* [10] also claimed that mouse trophoblast could be made to express histocompatibility antigens by treatment with neuraminidase. They suggested that these changes in immunogenicity were more likely to be attributable to an "unmasking" of antigens on cell surfaces than to changes in surface charge.

Our experiments were all designed to determine whether neuraminidase could be used prophylactically in immunization against future inoculations of tumor, or therapeutically to induce the regression of well-established tumors in syngeneic

* This work was supported from Grant no. CA 11605 from the United States Public Health Service and Grant no. IC-9 from the American Cancer Society, Inc.

** R. L. SIMMONS is a Professor of Surgery and Microbiology. He is also a John and Mary Markle Foundation Scholar in Academic Medicine.

animals. In the process, we were able to induce immunospecific regression of spontaneous mammary carcinomas utilizing immunotherapeutic techniques.

Materials and Methods

Two different fibrosarcomas (MC-42, MC-43) were induced with 3-methylcholanthrene in C3H/HeJ female mice [12]. The tumors have been serially transplanted in syngeneic female mice without evidence of loss of antigen. In unimmunized mice, an inoculum of 120 MC-42 cells or 1280 MC-43 cells will kill 50% of the recipients. Spontaneous regression does not occur. The tumors are specific for the strain in which they arose and do not grow in allogeneic mice. These tumors are weakly immunogenic; that is, inoculation of the tumor followed by excision leads to tumor-specific resistance against subsequent inoculation. The MC-42 tumor, however, does not immunize against MC-43 or vice versa [12].

Suspensions of sterile tumor cells were prepared by pressing the tumor through stainless steel screens (mesh 45) in medium 199 (M 199). No trypsin was utilized at any time. Counted viable cells were injected s. c. into the lateral posterior flank of recipient mice. The mice were inspected daily to determine the day of appearance of the tumor, the largest diameter of a growing tumor was measured with calipers at bi-weekly intervals, and the day of death was recorded. The tumors had usually reached palpable size by day 8 and measured 0.5 to 1.0 cm by day 15 when challenge with *Vibrio cholerae* neuraminidase (VCN) (obtained from General Biochemicals, Chagrin Falls, Ohio) was started. Suspended tumor cells for the immunotherapy step were incubated for one hour with 25 units of VCN/ml/10^6 cells plus mitomycin C (25 μg/ml) to prevent the growth of the tumor challenge. The cells were then washed three times, mixed with M 199, and inoculated at sites distant from the growing tumor.

Experiment I. Prevention of MC-42 Tumor Growth by Post-Inoculation Challenge with VCN-Treated Tumor Cells

20,000 untreated MC-42 tumor cells were injected into C3H/HeJ mice. At intervals up to 20 days following inoculation, 20,000 living MC-42 cells, which had been incubated with VCN or heat-inactivated VCN, were injected s. c. into the opposite flank. Secondary challenges of cells treated with heat-inactivated VCN had no effect on the growth of the initial inoculum; 30/30 animals supported tumor growth and died. In contrast, VCN-treated MC-42 cells strongly inhibited the growth of the initial inoculum. Only 4/30 of these animals manifested tumor growth from the initial inoculum [27].

Experiment II. Regression of MC-42 Tumors by Secondary Challenge with Neuraminidase-Treated MC-42 Cells

Fig. 1 illustrates the tumor growth of s. c. inoculations of 20,000 normal MC-42 fibrosarcoma cells in C3H/HeJ mice. At various intervals following inoculation, 10^6 living MC-42 cells were injected s. c. into the opposite flank. Treatment of the

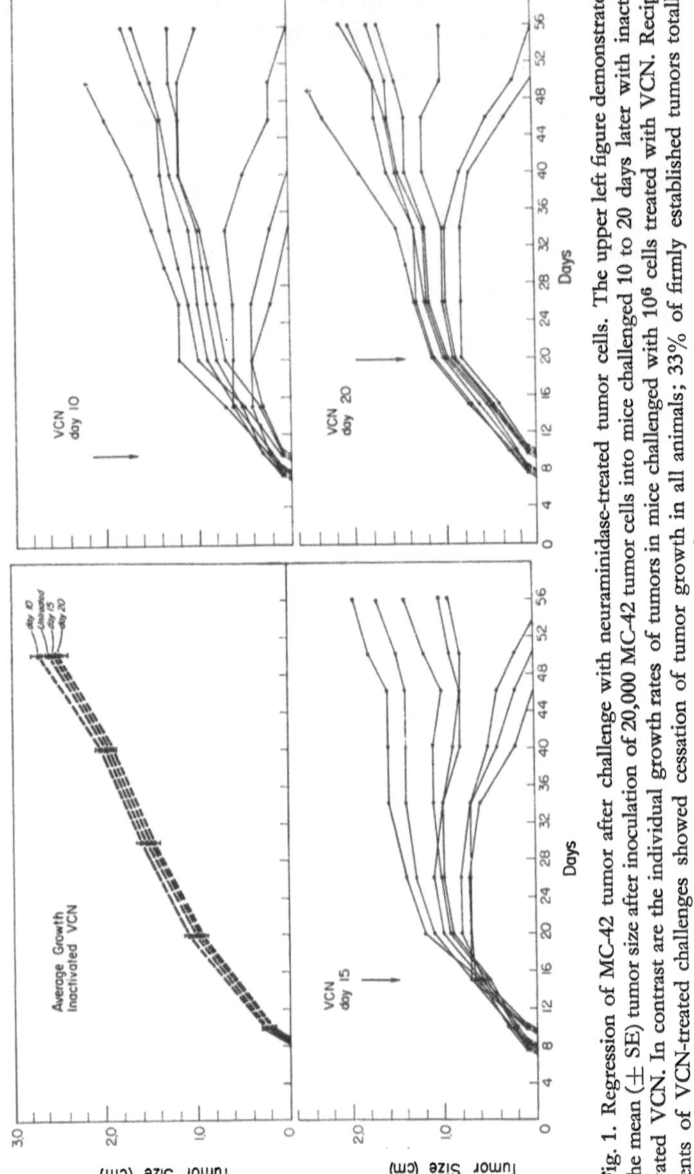

Fig. 1. Regression of MC-42 tumor after challenge with neuraminidase-treated tumor cells. The upper left figure demonstrates the mean (± SE) tumor size after inoculation of 20,000 MC-42 tumor cells into mice challenged 10 to 20 days later with inactivated VCN. In contrast are the individual growth rates of tumors in mice challenged with 10^6 cells treated with VCN. Recipients of VCN-treated challenges showed cessation of tumor growth in all animals; 33% of firmly established tumors totally regressed

tumor challenge with heat-inactivated VCN had no effect on the growth of the initial inoculum. In contrast, VCN-treated MC-42 cells strongly inhibited the growth of the tumor, which was already firmly established and growing rapidly. All the tumors showed temporary cessation of growth and many tumors regressed and disappeared. All animals whose tumors regressed survived for an indefinite period [18, 25].

Experiment III. Immunospecificity of Tumor Regression Induced by VCN Treatment of MC-42 Tumor Cells

C3H/HeJ mice were inoculated s. c. with 20,000 untreated MC-42 tumor cells in the left flank and 20,000 untreated MC-43 tumor cells in the right flank. All tumors became established. 13 days later these animals were challenged s. c. with 10^6 MC-42 or 10^6 MC-43 tumor cells which had been treated with either VCN or heat-inactivated VCN. Regression of firmly established MC-42 tumors took place only in animals challenged with VCN-treated MC-42 tumors. MC-42 tumors did not regress when challenged with MC-42 cells exposed to inactivated VCN, nor did the MC-42 tumor regress when treated with MC-43 cells exposed to VCN. Conversely, MC-43 tumors regressed only if challenged with MC-43 cells which had been treated with VCN. MC-43 tumors did not regress if challenged with MC-43 cells exposed to inactivated VCN or to MC-42 cells in any form [27].

Experiment IV. Combined Effect of BCG and VCN-Treated Tumor Cells on MCA Tumors

The previous experiments were repeated by challenging tumor-bearing C3H/HeJ mice with 10^6 VCN-treated tumor cells plus 1 mg BCG (obtained from Research Foundation, Chicago, Illinois). BCG was either mixed with the tumor cells (1:1) or injected alone into the tumor nodule itself, or at another site. A single injection of BCG, or MC-42 cells exposed to heat-inactivated VCN, plus mitomycin C, or any combination of these treatments did not produce total regression in any of the firmly established MC-42 tumors. In contrast, a single injection of MC-42 tumor cells exposed to VCN plus mitomycin induced the regression of 2 out of 7 tumors. When the VCN-treated tumor cells were injected in combination with BCG, 16 out of 56 tumors totally regressed. When BCG was injected directly into the tumor mass and the VCN-treated tumor vaccine was injected elsewhere, only 1 out of 14 tumors regressed. However, if the BCG was injected at a separate location from the injection of VCN tumor vaccine, or mixed with VCN tumor, 15 out of 42 tumors totally regressed and the animals survived.

This experiment was repeated with the use of a total of six injections of BCG or 10^6 tumor cells, or both, on alternate days beginning 15 days after the inoculation of 20,000 normal MC-42 tumor cells. Regression of a well-established tumor was never induced in animals that received no treatment, or that received tumor cells previously incubated with heat-inactivated VCN, even if the injections were given simultaneously with or at the same site as BCG inoculations. The BCG by itself induced the regression of only 1 out of 21 tumors. In contrast, six injections of VCN-treated tumor cells induced total regression of 6 out of 17 tumors; when combined with BCG injections, 24 out of 42 tumors totally regressed. In this experiment, it appeared that combining BCG with VCN-treated tumor cells at the same injection site was slightly more effective than giving them simultaneously at different sites [25].

Experiment V. Effect of Intralesional Injections of VCN on the Growth of MCA Fibrosarcomas

Further experiments were carried out to determine the effect of direct injections of VCN into the sites of growing fibrosarcomas: 50 units of VCN or heat-inactivated

VCN were injected into tumor masses growing simultaneously in the opposite flanks of the same C3H/HeJ mice; MC-42 tumors were inoculated on the left and MC-43 tumors on the right. When MC-42 tumors were injected with VCN, there was definite inhibition of the growth of the injected tumor; 4/12 MC-42 tumors totally regressed. The MC-43 tumor on the opposite side continued to grow and did not differ significantly in size from MC-43 tumors growing in recipients of heat-inactivated VCN or M 199. Such animals died in approximately the same time as animals bearing MC-42 tumors injected with heat-inactivated VCN of M 199. The converse was also true. When animals bearing MC-42 tumors on the left and MC-43 tumors on the right were injected with VCN into the right-sided tumor, there was a definite inhibition of the injected MC-43 tumor, but not of the MC-42 tumor. 4/8 injected MC-43 tumors totally regressed while their MC-42 counterparts on the opposite side continued to grow unabated and the animals died [26].

Experiment VI. The effect of Intralesional Injections of VCN and BCG on the Growth of Spontaneous Mammary Carcinomas

C3H/HeJ female mice, aged 9 to 15 months, were observed for the development of mammary tumors. The tumor masses (0.7 to 1.0 cm) were injected with 50 units VCN and/or 1 mg BCG twice weekly. Fig. 2 illustrates the mean diameter of tumors

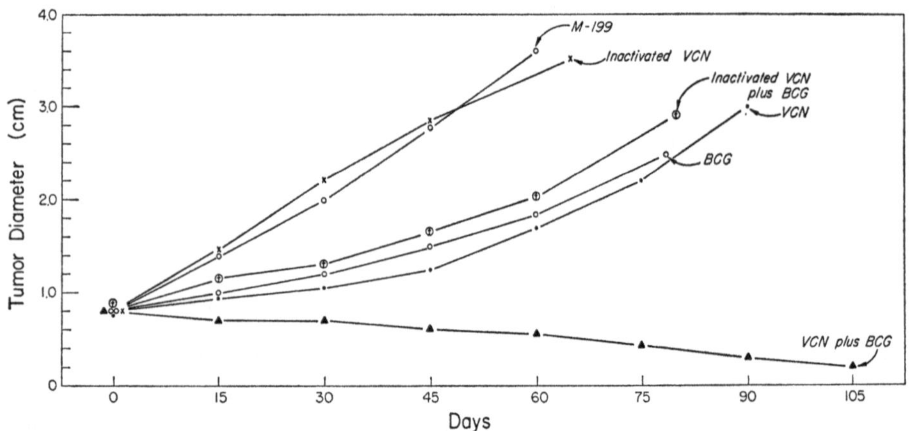

Fig. 2. Mean tumor diameter of spontaneous mammary carcinomas in C 3 H/HeJ female mice. The tumors were injected with 0.1 ml of the substances indicated every 4 days from the time of discovery (day 0). The tumor sizes are significantly different ($p \leqq 0.05$) from each other (M 199, inactivated VCN vs. BCG, VCN, inactivated VCN plus BCG vs. VCN plus BCG) after day 45

treated with the various substances. Neither M 199 nor heat-inactivated VCN injected directly into the spontaneous mammary adenocarcinomas had any effect on the progressive tumor growth and early death of the mice. Metastases were found in the livers and lungs of such mice only 60 days following treatment. The intra-tumor injection of 1 mg viable BCG organisms or 50 units VCN significantly slowed tumor growth and prolonged survival. The combination of VCN plus BCG, however, led to tumor regression: 4/13 tumors totally disappeared in recipients of intratumor injections of 50 units of VCN plus 1 mg BCG every 4 days. Survival in these animals was significantly prolonged when compared with the intratumor injections of VCN or BCG alone.

Table. Development of secondary mammary adenocarcinomas in treated mice

Intratumor treatment	Mean day of death	Secondary tumors	Days to secondary tumor
M 199	66.5	0/11	—
IVCN	60.8	0/11	—
VCN	88.4	4/10	28, 35, 47, 51
BCG	79.5	1/10 [a]	32
IVCN + BCG	83.1	2/10 [a]	24, 118
VCN + BCG	107.0	9/13 [a]	27, 28, 50, 52, 54, 57, 62, 83

[a] Three mice developed 3rd and in one case 4th tumors.

The Table demonstrates that second mammary adenocarcinomas frequently developed in mice treated with VCN and/or BCG. Secondary tumors developed only in animals who demonstrated some slowing of growth of the first tumor. The more effective the treatment, the more often did secondary tumors arise. Three animals developed a third tumor, and one even a fourth. Regression was induced in 2/9 tumors by the same treatment as used for treatment of the primary tumor, and the growth of most was inhibited by the local injection of the substance which had induced regression of the primary tumor.

Discussion

A number of observations have previously suggested that VCN increases the immunogenicity of cells exposed to it *in vitro*.

a) Fetal tissue incubated in VCN and injected into allogeneic recipients results in a greater degree of sensitization of those recipients than animals injected with fetal tissue exposed to heat-inactivated VCN [24].

b) When small nonimmunogenic doses of lymphoid cells were injected into allogeneic recipients, donor skin grafts were rejected significantly more rapidly [28].

c) Cyclophosphamide pre-treated mice do not become tolerant of VCN-treated bone marrow cells.

d) Human lymphocytes treated with VCN and mitomycin are several times more stimulating to allogeneic lymphocytes in one-way mixed lymphocyte culture than are lymphocytes treated with mitomycin alone [17, 18].

e) TA-3 tumor [23], Landschütz ascites tumor [8], L 1210 leukemia [3], methylcholanthrene-induced fibrosarcoma [7, 27, 29], and Ehrlich's ascites tumor [16] grow less well in normally susceptible recipients if the tumor cells have been incubated in VCN. Recipients who survive the primary tumor inoculum are rendered immune to subsequent inocula of untreated cells [9, 16, 29]. This paper has briefly summarized the experiments which showed that immunospecific total regression of well-established methylcholanthrene fibrosarcomas can be induced by challenging the tumor-bearing animals with syngeneic tumor cells treated *in vitro* with VCN. The effect was clearly due to the enzymatic action of VCN on the sialic acid residues of the tumor cell surfaces, since heat-inactivation of the VCN, or incubation of VCN and tumor cells with an excess of sialic acid (specific feedback inhibitor of VCN) destroyed the ability of such cells to induce tumor regression [27]. VCN itself was nontoxic to normal or tumor cells in any concentration utilized [3, 8, 9, 21, 23, 27, 32].

Subsequent experiments demonstrated that immunospecific regression of tumors can be induced by injecting VCN directly into the tumor mass even after it has become firmly established and is growing actively [21]. With injections of VCN beginning on day 15 when the tumors were small (0.6—0.9 cm), complete disappearance of the tumor could be achieved in a number of treated animals. The treatment was totally immunospecific and regression of untreated tumor nodules could be induced by injecting VCN into immunologically identical tumors on the opposite side. Tumors which were not identical to the treated tumor, however, continued to grow and killed the animal [26].

BCG by itself will induce the regression of syngeneic hepatomas in guinea pigs [33] and a few melanomas in man [19], and if used repeatedly will induce the regression of a few methylcholanthrene-induced fibrosarcomas in mice [22]. However, BCG is relatively ineffective on its own.

The present experiments demonstrate not only that transplantable MCA tumors will regress, but also that spontaneous tumors can be induced to regress by the combined intratumor injection of VCN and BCG. Lesser degrees of tumor inhibition were induced by either agent alone. This is the first demonstration that immunotherapeutic techniques will induce the regression of spontaneous syngeneic tumors in animals. One cannot, however, rule out the possibility that BCG and/or VCN induced nonspecific changes leading to tumor regression which have nothing to do with immunotherapy. By analogy with the experimental transplanted tumor, however, it is likely that the effect is immunological.

Surprisingly, animals who demonstrated best immunoregressive response to intratumor injections of VCN and/or BCG developed new tumors of identical histological types in other mammary glands. Some of these tumors also regressed in the face of intratumor injections of VCN and/or BCG. If the treatment of the primary tumor had induced immunity to the MTV-associated cellular antigen, the secondary tumors could not have developed. Several investigators have demonstrated that mice infected with MTV are completely tolerant to the common MTV-related antigen on mammary adenocarcinoma cells induced by this virus [13, 20]. However, these mice were not tolerant to a second type of antigen, unrelated to the MTV. Such antigens are individually unique for each mammary carcinoma and usually are much weaker than the common MTV-related tumor antigen [20]. Since MTV-infected mice are completely tolerant to the stronger common antigen, the major defense against mammary carcinogenesis is probably their immune response to the weaker group of tumor-specific antigens. These events are perfectly consistent with our findings that immunotherapy of firmly established spontaneous mammary adenocarcinomas can be induced, but this does not prevent the appearance of other mammary adenocarcinomas. Thus, immunity to the primary tumor is probably directed against the weaker specific antigen on the treated tumor and not against the MTV antigen.

References

1. AMBROSE, E. J.: Electrophoretic behavior of cells. Progr. Biophys. molec. Biol. **16**, 241 (1966).
2. APFFEL, C. A., PETERS, J. H.: Regulation of antigenic expression. J. theor. Biol. **26**, 47 (1970).
3. BAGSHAWE, K. D., CURRIE, G. A.: Immunogenicity of L 1210 murine leukemia cells after treatment with neuraminidase. Nature (Lond.) **218**, 1254 (1967).
4. BAYLOR, M. E.: The reaction of receptor glycoprotein with influenza virus and neuraminidase: An electron microscopic study. Trans N.Y. Acad. Sci. **26**, 1103 (1964).
5. BENEDETTI, E. L., EMMELOT, P.: Studies on plasma membranes. IV. The ultrastructural localization and content of sialic acid in plasma membranes isolated from rat liver and hepatoma. J. Cell Sci. **2**, 499 (1967).
6. BROWN, D. M., MICHAEL, A. F.: Effect of neuraminidase on the accumulation of alpha-aminoisobutyric acid in HeLa cells. Proc. Soc. exp. Biol. (N.Y.) **131**, 568 (1969).
7. CURRIE, G. A., BAGSHAWE, K. D.: The masking of antigens on trophoblast and cancer cells. Lancet **1967 I**, 708.
8. CURRIE, G. A., BAGSHAWE, K. D.: The role of sialic acid in antigenic expression: Further studies of the Landschutz ascites tumour. Brit. J. Cancer **22**, 843 (1968).
9. CURRIE, G. A., BAGSHAWE, K. D.: Tumor specific immunogenicity of methylcholanthrene-induced sarcoma cells after incubation in neuraminidase. Brit. J. Cancer **23**, 141 (1969).
10. CURRIE, G. A., VAN DOORNICK, W., BAGSHAWE, K. D.: Effect of neuraminidase on the immunogenicity of early mouse trophoblast. Nature (Lond.) **219**, 191 (1968).
11. GESNER, B., THOMAS, L.: Sialic acid binding sites: Role in hemagglutination by *Mycoplasma gallisepticum*. Science **151**, 590 (1966).
12. HAYWOOD, G., MCKHANN, C. F.: Antigenic specificities on murine sarcoma cells: Reciprocal relationship between normal transplantation antigens (H-2) and tumor specific immunogenicity. J. exp. Med. **133**, 1171 (1971).
13. HEPPNER, G. H.: Studies on serum-mediated inhibition of cellular immunity to spontaneous mouse mammary tumors. Int. J. Cancer **4**, 608 (1969).
14. KEMP, R. B.: Effect of the removal of cell surface sialic acids on cell aggregation *in vitro*. Nature (Lond.) **218**, 1255 (1968).
15. LEE, A.: Effect of neuraminidase on the phagocytosis of heterologous red cells by mouse peripheral macrophages. Proc. Soc. exp. Biol. (N.Y.) **128**, 891 (1968).
16. LINDENMANN, J., KLEIN, P. A.: Immunologic aspects of viral oncolysis. Recent Results in Cancer Research, Vol. 9. Berlin-Heidelberg-New York: Springer 1967.
17. LUNDGREN, G., JEITZ, L., LUNDIN, L., SIMMONS, R. L.: Increased stimulation by neuraminidase treated cells in mixed lymphocyte cultures. Fed. Proc. **30**, 395 (1971 a).
18. LUNDGREN, G., SIMMONS, R. L.: Effect of neuraminidase on the stimulatory capacity of cells in human mixed lymphocyte cultures. Clin. exp. Immunol. **9**, 915 (1971 b).
19. MORTON, D. L., EILBER, F. R., JOSEPH, W. L., WOOD, W. C., TRAHAN, E., KETCHAM, A. S.: Immunological factors in human sarcomas and melanomas: A rational basis for immunotherapy. Ann. Surg. **172**, 740 (1970).
20. MORTON, D. L., GOLDMAN, L., WOOD, D. A.: Acquired immunological tolerance and carcinogenesis by the mammary tumor virus. II. Immune responses influencing growth of spontaneous mammary adenocarcinomas. J. nat. Cancer Inst. **42**, 321 (1969).
21. RAY, P. K., SIMMONS, R. L.: Failure of neuraminidase to unmask allogeneic antigens on cell surfaces. Proc. Soc. exp. Biol. (N.Y.) **138**, 600 (1971).
22. RIOS, A., SIMMONS, R. L.: Comparative effect of BCG and neuraminidase treated tumor cells on the growth of established methylcholanthrene fibrosarcomas in syngeneic mice. Cancer Res. **32**, 16 (1972).
23. SANFORD, B. H.: An alteration in tumor histocompatibility induced by neuraminidase. Transplantation **4**, 1273 (1967).

24. Simmons, R. L., Lipschultz, M. L., Rios, A., Ray, P. K.: Neuraminidase does not unmask histocompatibility antigens on trophoblast. Nature (Lond.) **231**, 111 (1971a).
25. Simmons, R. L., Rios, A.: Immunotherapy of cancer: Immunospecific rejection of tumors in recipients of neuraminidase-treated tumor cells plus BCG. Science **174**, 591 (1971b).
26. Simmons, R. L., Rios, A.: Immunospecific regression of methylcholanthrene fibrosarcoma using neuraminidase. II. Intratumor injections of neuraminidase. Surgery **71**, 556 (1972).
27. Simmons, R. L., Rios, A., Lundgren, G., Ray, P. K., McKhann, C. F., Haywood, G. R.: Immunospecific regression of methylcholanthrene fibrosarcoma with the use of neuraminidase. Surgery **70**, 38 (1971c).
28. Simmons, R. L., Rios, A., Ray, P .K.: Immunogenicity and antigenicity of lymphoid cells treated with neuraminidase. Nature (Lond.) **231**, 179 (1971).
29. Simmons, R. L., Rios, A., Ray, P. K., Lundgren, G.: Effect of neuraminidase on the growth of methylcholanthrene fibrosarcoma in normal and immunosuppressed syngeneic mice. J. nat. Cancer Inst. **47**, 1087 (1971e).
30. Weiss, L.: Studies on cell deformability. I. Effect of surface charge. J. Cell Biol. **26**, 735 (1965).
31. Weiss, L., Mayhew, E., Ulrich, K.: The effect of neuraminidase on the phagocytic process in human monocytes. Lab. Invest. **15**, 1304 (1966).
32. Woodruff, J. J. Gesner, B. M.: The effect of neuraminidase on the fate of transfused lymphocytes. J. exp. Med. **129**, 551 (1969).
33. Zbar, B., Tanaka, T.: Immunotherapy of cancer: Regression of tumors after intralesional injection of living *Mycobacterium bovis*. Science **172**, 271 (1971).

Aspects of the Immunology of the Tumor-Host Relationship and Responsiveness to Modified Lymphoma Cells

M. D. Prager, R. J. Ribble, and J. M. Mehta

Department of Surgery and Biochemistry,
University of Texas Southwestern Medical School, Dallas, Texas

There are various approaches to cancer immunotherapy currently under investigation by many groups. We are studying use of modified cells from the tumor to be treated. Immunization with modified cells may be useful in two situations: 1. When an immune response occurs as part of the natural reaction of the host to tumor, the strength of the response may be increased; 2. in the absence of a host response, the possibility exists that an altered tumor cell preparation could be used to break the unresponsive state.

Modified cells for immunization of the host have been used in a number of studies with mouse lymphomas and leukemias. Vaccination of C 57 BL/6 mice with iodoacetate-modified EL-4 cells [2] and vaccination of C 3 H mice with 6 C 3 HED and EPF-1 lymphomas [10, 11] modified by the sulfhydryl reagents iodoacetate, iodoacetamide, or N-ethylmaleimide protected the host against challenge with the viable, unaltered tumor cells. Iodoacetamide modification of Rauscher virus-induced leukemia cells was only moderately successful in producing a vaccine in (DBA/2 × CBA) F_1 mice [5]. After X-irradiation, L 5178 Y [1], I_b [8], and 6 C 3 HED [10] cells protected DBA/2, C 58, and C 3 H mice respectively; partial protection of DBA/2 and AKR mice was achieved following irradiation of L 1210 [4, 14] and AKR [7] leukemia cells. WL 3, WL 4, SL 1, and LNSA leukemias [14] and P 1798 lymphoma [10] were not protective in their respective hosts following irradiation of the cells. Formaldehyde treatment of I_b cells gave a protective vaccine in C 58 mice [8], but similar treatment of L 1210 [4] gave a preparation which only partially protected DBA/2 mice against this tumor. Recent work with neuraminidase from *Vibro cholerae* indicates that this could be a useful reagent for modifying leukemic cells. L 1210 cells [4] treated with this enzyme were immunogenic and protective in DBA/2 mice. Furthermore, injection of neuraminidase-treated AKR leukemic cells delayed the appearance of the spontaneous disease in this high-incidence leukemic strain of mice [6].

The approach in this laboratory has been to examine a variety of tumor cell modifications for development of a vaccine which protects the syngeneic host against a lethal inoculum of tumor cells and then to use the vaccine for developing a therapeutic regimen for treatment of the tumor-bearing host. Successful vaccines have been prepared for two C 3 H mouse lymphomas: 6 C 3 HED, an old transplant line, and EPF-1, an early-generation transplanted tumor [10, 11]. With failure to achieve successful vaccination of BALB/c mice against the P 1798 lymphoma (also an old transplant line) [10], attention was directed to the immunological relationship between tumor and host in the hope of elucidating features of the interaction which might control success or failure [13]. These studies form the subject of this report.

Materials and Methods

Three lymphomas in ascites form were studied in the mouse strain of origin. These include 6 C 3 HED and EPF-1 in C 3 H mice and P 1798 in BALB/c mice. Techniques for modifying the lymphoma cells, vaccinating the mice, and presenting them with an intraperitoneal challenge of viable tumor cells have been described [10, 11]. The quantity of modifying reagent per ml of tumor cells is given in Table 1. More recently, the immunology of the tumor-host system has been examined for 6 C 3 HED in C 3 H mice and P 1798 in BALB/c mice. In order to permit adequate time for an immune response prior to death of the animal from tumor growth, there were implanted intraperitoneally 10^4 lymphoma cells, a dose requiring 2.5 to 3.0 weeks to kill the host. At various times after implantation, cells were withdrawn and examined for antibody coating by means of a rabbit fluorescein isothiocyanate conjugated anti-mouse globulin (Sylvana Co.). The technique for performing immunofluorescent studies was essentially that of [3]. Cells were washed with ACD saline, and then 0.1 ml (10^6 cells) was incubated with 0.1 ml antiglobulin reagent (diluted 1:4 with phosphate-buffered saline (PBS), pH 7.4) for 15 min at 37°C. Cells were washed 3 times with ACD saline, resuspended in 0.5 ml of a 1:1 glycerol-PBS solution and wet-mounted for viewing. In parallel studies mice were examined for antibody to the tumor cells. These serum samples (0.1 ml) were incubated with 10^6 cells collected at various times after implantation and then immunofluorescent studies were performed as described.

Results

Three vaccinating doses of modified cells were given at weekly intervals followed by challenge one week later with 10^6 6 C 3 HED or EPF-1 cells and either 10^4 or 10^6 P 1798 cells. In the majority of experiments the equivalent of 10^8 cells was given per vaccinating dose. A rather extensive series of alterations of 6 C 3 HED have been examined and the results are summarized in Table 1. Of the various physical treatments used to alter the cells only X-irradiation (5400 r) gave an effective vaccine. Sulfhydryl blocking reagents in the range of 10—40 μmoles/ml 6 C 3 HED cells yielded preparations effective for vaccination purposes. Release of carbohydrate by either β-glucosidase or β-glucuronidase from iodoacetamide-modified cells had no adverse effect on their ability to immunize the host. The one ineffective sulfhydryl blocking agent was p-hydroxymercuribenzoate. It was suggested that this reagent might be ineffective because it introduces the benzoate group, which is a strong antigenic determinant, onto the cell surface, and this could result in antigenic

Table 1. Summary of results of vaccination of C3H mice with modified 6C3HED lymphoma cells

Modifying agent or process	Treatment of 6C3HED cells Quantity/ml cells	Survivors/total
Physical treatment		
X-ray	5400 rad	5/5
Freeze-thaw	—	0/8
Lyophilization	—	0/10
Heat, 56 °C	—	0/10
Sulfhydryl-blocking agents		
Iodoacetamide	10—40 μmoles	16/16
Iodoacetate	10—40 μmoles	10/10
N-ethylmaleimide	10—40 μmoles	16/16
p-hydroxymercuribenzoate	10 μmoles	0/6
Iodoacetamide + β-glucosidase	80 μmoles + 60 I.U. [a]	6/6
Iodoacetamide + β-glucuronidase	80 μmoles + 0.04 I.U.	6/6
Carbohydrate reagents		
Concanavalin A	7.5 mg	9/12
Sodium periodate ($NaIO_4$)	3 mmoles	0/6
β-Glucosidase	60 I.U. [a]	0/4
Other treatments		
pH 3.1, Earle's solution	—	10/12
Diazotized p-aminobenzoic acid	2.4 mmoles	0/6
Fluorodinitrobenzene	3—300 μmoles	0/18
Polypropyleneimine	10 mg	1/6

[a] From supplier's assay at pH 5.25; incubation was at pH 7.2.

competition thus causing the immune response to be directed away from the weaker tumor-specific antigen. With reagents that affect carbohydrate, concanavalin-A treatment of the cells resulted in successful vaccination. The loss of effectiveness of 6 C 3 HED cells after $NaIO_4$ treatment leads us to consider tentatively that, if cleavage of monosaccharide units by this reagent reduces the immunogenicity of the altered cells, then carbohydrate may be an important part of the antigen to which the host is capable of responding. Neither diazotized p-aminobenzoic acid nor fluorodinitrobenzene were effective reagents for production of protective vaccines. The polycation polypropyleneimine was used as a reagent, which might reduce the negative charge on the tumor cells and possibly render them more immunogenic, as has been observed for neuraminidase. However, only 1 of 6 mice vaccinated with cells modified by this reagent survived challenge with 10^6 6 C 3 HED cells. Exposure of 6 C 3 HED to Earle's solution at pH 3.1 (bicarbonate was not added to attain physiological pH) was an effective procedure for producing a vaccine which protected 10 of 12 mice.

Since most of these experiments were performed with vaccinating doses of 10^8 modified cells, an experiment was undertaken to determine the number of cells required to achieve immunization. When 10^5 N-ethylmaleimide-modified cells were used, only 40% of the mice were protected. The number rose to 100% as the cell number increased to 10^8 (Table 2). Although most of the mice receiving 10^6 or

10^7 modified cells survived, those which succumbed to the lethal effects of the tumor inoculum showed only minimally prolonged survival.

As indicated by uptake of trypan blue, cells used for immunization after treatment with sulfhydryl reagents constitute a killed-cell vaccine. Of considerable concern is the length of time a killed-cell vaccine may render the host immune. A study was therefore undertaken to determine the effect of the time interval between the third immunizing dose and the challenge dose. The results summarized in Table 3 indicate

Table 2. Effect of vaccine size on resistance of C3H mice to 6C3HED lymphoma

No. of N-ethylmaleimide-modified 6C3HED cells	Survivors/total	Mean survival (days) of dead mice ± S.E.
10^5	6/15	17.3 ± 0.75
10^6	14/17	16.7 ± 1.76
10^7	9/11	18.5 ± 1.50
10^8	12/12	—
Control	0/12	14.3 ± 0.33

Table 3. Effect of time lag between vaccination with Iodoacetamide-modified 6C3HED and challenge

Time lag (weeks)	Survivors/total	Time lag (weeks)	Survivors/total
1	(100%)	8	5/6
2	6/6	12	2/4
3	3/6	Unvaccinated	0/18
6	4/6		

that the animals were fully protected when challenged after 1 or 2 weeks, but at later times only partial protection was observed. However, half the animals challenged 3 months after vaccination were still protected. This problem may be eliminated by challenging mice 1 to 2 weeks after the immunizing doses when they are capable of rejecting the live cells. C 3 H mice re-challenged 9—10 months later were still resistant to 6 C 3 HED. This time interval represents a significant portion of the life span of the animal.

It was previously reported [11] that iodoacetamide modification of EPF-1 cells produced a protective vaccine, but a cell homogenate was toxic and did not protect C 3 H mice against the tumor.

The P 1798 lymphoma of BALB/c mice was selected as an additional tumor for study because of indications in the literature that it might be difficult to immunize against it. The approach was similar to that used for 6 C 3 HED except that the challenging dose of viable tumor cells was 10^4 in the majority of trials. Cells altered by treatment with the following agents have been studied: X-irradiation, iodoacetamide, N-ethylmaleimide, concanavalin A, phytohemagglutinin, sodium periodate, iodoacetamide with either β-glucosidase or β-glucuronidase, and polypropyleneimine. None of these preparations have yielded protective vaccination.

In view of the grossly different results obtained with 6 C 3 HED and P 1798, an investigation of the immunology of the tumor-host relationship was undertaken. At various times after implanting 10^4 ascites tumor cells in the syngeneic host, mice were bled and serum was collected to determine the presence of antibody. At the same time live cells from the peritoneum were examined for antibody coating using a fluorescent antiglobulin reagent, and the percentage demonstrating positive membrane fluorescence was recorded. Cells which fluoresced throughout the cytoplasm were not counted as they were considered nonviable. This study indicated a remarkable difference in the response of the host mice to the two tumors (Fig. 1).

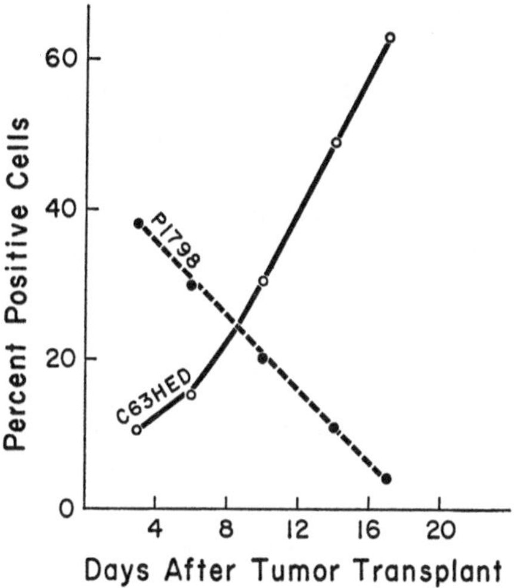

Fig. 1. Fraction of ascites cells giving positive membrane fluorescence with fluorescent rabbit anti-mouse globulin. The ascites cells were collected at various times after tumor implantation. Data points are mean values for 2—5 experiments

C 3 H mice bearing 6 C 3 HED gave a small percentage of positively staining cells at day 3, and the fraction of positive cells increased continuously to 63% just before the death of the animals. With BALB/c mice bearing P 1798, the converse was observed; whereas the day-3 cell preparation gave 38% positive staining cells, this fraction decreased continuously to 4% at the time of death. However, between day 3 and day 14 the absolute number of positively staining cells obtained by washing the peritoneal cavity of BALB/c mice increased about 50-fold. Although significant, this number is small compared to the 1000-fold increase in positive cells recovered from the C 3 H mice. In an additional experiment, serum collected from mice during the period of tumor growth was incubated with cells collected from the peritoneum of tumor-bearing mice prior to addition of the antiglobulin reagent. C 3 H mouse serum collected on day 6 or later markedly increased the percentage of positive cells collected on day 3 and day 6, as would be expected if antibody were present (Fig. 2). However, the percentage of positive cells reached a pleteau at 60—70%, suggesting that even in the late phases of tumor growth about one third of the cells were either not tumor cells or were incapable of reacting with the fluorescent antiglobulin antibody. None of the serum samples collected from tumor-bearing BALB/c mice increased the percentage of stained cells collected on any given day after tumor implantation (Fig. 2). This result suggested that there was no free antibody to P 1798 in the serum of the tumor-bearing mice.

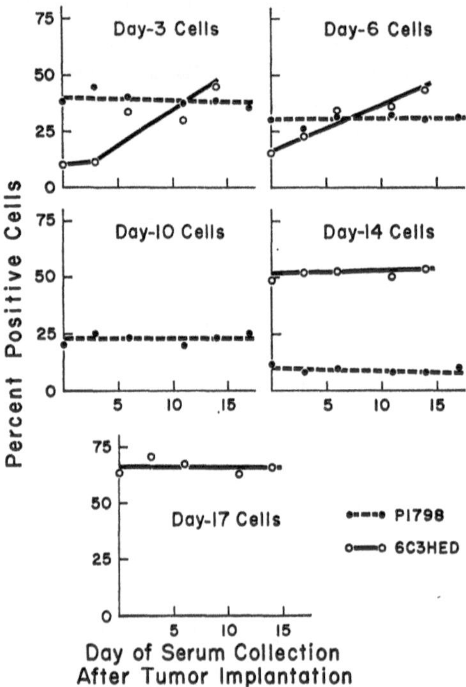

Fig. 2. Fraction of ascites cells giving positive membrane fluorescence with fluorescent rabbit anti-mouse globulin after incubation of the cells with serum of tumor-bearing mice. The control value without added serum is plotted as the intercept on the vertical axis. Serum as well as cells were collected at various times after tumor implantation

Discussion

The studies recorded in this report extend earlier work on the use of modified cells to prepare vaccines against the specific tumor from which the cells were obtained. Vaccination with 6 C 3 HED cells altered by treatment with N-ethylmaleimide showed that three doses of 10^5 cells protected only 40% of mice subsequently challenged with 10^6 viable tumor cells. With individual vaccinating doses of 10^6 and 10^7 cells most of the animals were protected, and an inoculum of 10^8 modified cells protected all mice. The problem of using a killed cell vaccine has been considered, and animals challenged one to two weeks after the immunization schedule were resistant to 10^6 6 C 3 HED cells. Mice challenged after an interval of 3 weeks or more were only partially protected. It is particularly pertinent in this regard that mice which once rejected the viable tumor cell challenge were still resistant when rechallenged up to 10 months later. A similar result was noted after

L-asparaginase treatment of the tumor-bearing host [12]. The use of the early challenge may then completely obviate the problem of a killed-cell vaccine.

The lack of success in finding a modifikation ofP 1798 cells to provide protective vaccination for BALB/c mice stands in sharp contrast to the results with 6 C 3 HED. The difference may lie in the pattern of immunologic responsiveness of the host to the tumor. Data presented here support this contention. In C 3 H mice antibody to 6 C 3 HED is produced throughout the period of tumor growth. Evidence for this comes from 1. the increasing fraction of cells staining positively with fluorescent anti-mouse globulin as the tumor progressively grows, and 2. the increased fluorescence of day-3 or day-6 cells after reaction with serum from tumor-bearing mice. A very different picture was presented by the antiglobulin staining pattern for cells collected from the peritoneum of BALB/c mice after implanting P 1798. Although the day-3 cells demonstrated a higher fraction of positive cells than was observed for 6 C 3 HED, this fraction decreased throughout the period of tumor growth. None of the serum samples collected up to day 17 after tumor implantation increased the antiglobulin-staining reaction of cells collected on any given day. Although identification of the cells which gave the positive reaction is the object of continuing investigation, several possibilities may be considered. If there is an immune response to the tumor, it would seem to be short-lived because of either 1. an adverse effect of progressive growth of P 1798 on the immune system or 2. antigenic modulation [9, 15]. The latter might result from antigen release from the tumor cell, rearrangement of membrane components so as to leave antigen unavailable, or suppression of antigen synthesis. Alternatively, since no antibody was demonstrable in the serum of tumor-bearing BALB/c mice, it seems more likely that there is no immune response to P 1798 and that the positive cells were normal peritoneal cells with immunoglobulin receptors. If it is assumed that there is indeed no immunologic response as part of the natural history of this tumor-host relationship, than, rather than attempting to strengthen an already present response as was the case with 6 C 3 HED, future experimental work should be directed toward attempting to break the state of tolerance.

Acknowledgements

This work was supported by Public Health Service Research Grant No. CA 12089 from the National Cancer Institute. The aid of Corinne Merrill with a portion of these studies is gratefully acknowledged.

References

1. Alexander, P., Connell, D. I., Mikulska, Z. B.: Treatment of a murine leukemia with spleen cells or sera from allogeneic mice immunized against the tumor. Cancer Res. **26**, 1508 (1966).
2. Apffel, C. A., Arnason, B. G., Peters, J. H.: Induction of tumour immunity with tumour cells treated with iodoacetate. Nature (Lond.) **209**, 694 (1966).
3. Baldwin, R. W., Barker, C. R.: Demonstration of tumour-specific humoral antibody against aminoazo dye-induced rat hepatoma. Brit. J. Cancer **21**, 793 (1967).
4. Bekesi, J. G., St-Arneault, G., Holland, J. F.: Increase of leukemia L 1210 immunogenicity by *Vibrio cholerae* neuraminidase treatment. Cancer Res. **31**, 2130 (1971).

5. JASMIN, C., PITON, C., ROSENFELD, C.: Effets de l'iodoacetamide sur les cellules de leucémie virale de rauscher. Int. J. Cancer **3**, 254 (1968).
6. HOLLAND, J. F.: *E Pluribus Unum*: Presidential address. Cancer Res. **31**, 1319 (1971).
7. LATARJET, R.: Action inhibitrice d'Extraits leucémiques isologues irradiés sur la leucémogenèse spontanée de la souris AkR. Ann. Inst. Pasteur **107**, 1 (1964).
8. LIN, J. S. L., HUBER, N., MURPHY, W. H.: Immunization of C 58 mice to line I_b leukemia. Cancer Res. **29**, 2157 (1969).
9. OLD, L. J., STOCKERT, E., BOYSE, E. A., KIM, J. H.: Antigenic modulation. Loss of TL antigen from cells exposed to TL antibody. Study of the phenomenon *in vitro*. J. exp. Med. **127**, 523 (1968).
10. PRAGER, M. D.: Vaccination and immunotherapy with chemically modified cancer cells. Bibl. Haemat. **39**, 706 (1973).
11. PRAGER, M. D., DERR, I., SWANN, A., COTROPIA, J.: Immunization with chemically modified lymphoma cells. Cancer Res. **31**, 1488 (1971).
12. PRAGER, M. D., ROBERTS, J., BACHYNSKY, N.: Immunity to the 6 C 3 HED ascites tumor following treatment of tumor-bearing mice with *Escherichia coli* L-Asparaginase. J. Immunol. **98**, 1045 (1967).
13. PRAGER, M. D., TICARIC, S., MERRILL, C. L.: Tumor-host relationship in immune response to modified lymphoma cells. Proc. Amer. Ass. Cancer Res. **13**, 103 (1972).
14. REVESZ, L.: Detection of antigenic differences in isologous host-tumor systems by pretreatment with heavily irradiated tumor cells. Cancer Res. **20**, 443 (1960).
15. TAKAHASHI, T., OLD, L. J., MCINTIRE, K. R., BOYSE, E. A.: Immunoglobulin and other surface antigens of cells of the immune system. J. exp. Med. **134**, 815 (1971).

Use of Enzyme-Treated Cells in Immunotherapy of Leukemia

J. F. DORÉ, M. J. HADJIYANNAKIS, A. COUDERT, C. GUIBOUT, L. MARHOLEV, and K. IMAI

Institut de Cancérologie et d'Immunogénétique, Hôpital Paul Brousse, Villejuif

The *in vitro* treatment of tumor cells with *Vibrio cholerae* neuraminidase (VCN) increases their immunogenicity [5, 6, 9]. VCN-treated tumor cells frequently fail to grow in animals, and the recipients are rendered immune to a subsequent challenge with untreated viable tumor cells. Moreover, inoculation of VCN-treated cells into animals grafted with cells from the same tumor is able to impair the growth of the initial tumor-cell inoculum [10, 11]. However, using a transplantable murine leukemia, we have observed that immunotherapy with VCN or papain-treated leukemia cells abolishes the expected effects of active specific immunotherapy.

Mice of the C 57 Bl/6 strain randomly assigned to 4 groups were grafted with 10^3 isogeneic E (AkR) leukemic cells [1], given i. p. on day 0. Mice in one group received no further treatment and served as controls. Mice in a second group received, on days 1, 5, 9, 13 and 17, five injections of 5×10^6 irradiated E (AkR) cells given s. c. [8]. Mice in a third and a fourth group received (on the same days) 5 injections of the same number of irradiated E (AkR) cells treated with either VCN (2 units of VCN per 5×10^6 cells, 20 min incubation at 37 °C) [7] or papain (0.1 mg/ml of crude Papaya extract per 10^7 cells, 10 min incubation at room temperature) [4]. Fig. 1 shows that a percentage of mice treated with irradiated E (AkR) cells survived

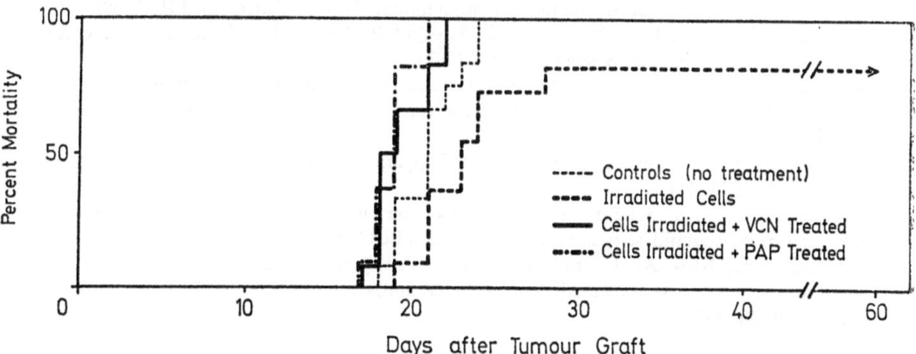

Fig. 1. Mortality of C 57 Bl/6 mice grafted with 10^3 E (AkR) leukemia cells and receiving on days 1, 5, 9, 13 and 17, 5×10^6 E (AkR) leukemia cells irradiated (12,000 rad) or both irradiated and enzyme-treated

the leukemia, as previously shown with a similar protocol [8]. On the other hand, no mice in the groups receiving enzyme-treated leukemia cells survived. Mice in these groups died earlier than in the previous group ($p = 0.001$) or in the control group ($p = 0.02$ for the group receiving papain-treated leukemia cells).

Quantitative estimation of the cytotoxic activity for E (AkR) cells of lymphoid cells from identically treated mice, based on a radiochromium-release assay [3], showed that lymph-node cells from mice receiving VCN-treated leukemia cells destroyed the target cells more efficiently than those from other groups. This is contrary to the clinical results. Preliminary studies, which are still in progress, tend to demonstrate the presence of humoral antitumor antibodies in mice receiving enzyme-treated leukemia cells. Therefore it is not unlikely that we may have produced an immunological enhancement of the tumor graft mediated by a blocking antibody in these animals.

We think that these data, which do not necessarily contradict previously reported positive results [10, 11], emphasize the need for exhaustive investigation of immunotherapy with enzyme treated-tumor cells on experimental animal models before applying it to man, paying particular attention to the possible effect of the enzyme dosage [2].

References

1. Amiel, J. L., Berardet, M.: Induction d'une leucémie isogénique virale de Gross chez des $C_{57}Bl/6$ adultes par des injections répétées de cellules leucémiques AkR. Rev. franç. Étud. clin. biol. **14**, 587 (1969).
2. Bekesi, J. G., St. Arneault, G., Walter, L., Holland, J. F.: Immunogenicity of leukemia L 1210 cells after neuraminidase treatment. J. nat. Cancer Inst. **49**, 107 (1972).
3. Brunner, K. T., Mauel, J., Cerottini, J. C., Chapuis, B.: Quantitative assay of the lytic action of immune lymphoid cells on ^{51}Cr-labelled allogeneic target cells *in vitro*; inhibition by isoantibody and by drugs. Immunology **14**, 181 (1968).
4. Coudert, A., Ajuria, E., Doré, J. F., Hadjiyannakis, M. J., Marholev, L.: Augmentation de l'antigénicité de cellules tumorales traitées par la papaïne. C. R. Acad. Sci. (Paris) **274**, 2833 (1972).
5. Currie, G. A., Bagshawe, K. D.: The role of sialic acid in antigenic expression: Further studies of the Landschütz ascites tumour. Brit. J. Cancer **22**, 843 (1968).
6. Currie, G. A., Bagshawe, K. D.: Tumour specific immunogenicity of methylcholanthrene-induced sarcoma cells after incubation in neuraminidase. Brit. J. Cancer **23**, 141 (1969).
7. Grothaus, E., Wayne Flye, M., Yunis, E., Amos, D. B.: Human lymphocyte antigen reactivity modified by neuraminidase. Science **173**, 542 (1971).
8. Mathé, G., Pouillart, P., Lapeyraque, F.: Active immunotherapy of mouse RC 19 and E ♀ K 1 leukaemias applied after the intravenous transplantation of the tumour cells. Experientia (Basel) **27**, 446 (1971).
9. Sanford, B. H.: An alteration in tumor histocompatibility induced by neuraminidase. Transplantation **5**, 1273 (1967).
10. Simmons, R. L., Rios, A.: Immunotherapy of cancer: immunospecific rejection of tumors in recipients of neuraminidase-treated tumor cells plus BCG. Science **174**, 591 (1971).
11. Simmons, R. L., Rios, A., Lundgren, G., Ray, P. K., McKhann, C. F., Haywood, G. R.: Immunospecific regression of methylcholanthrene fibrosarcoma with the use of neuraminidase. Surgery **70**, 38 (1971).

Active Immunotherapy of AKR Mouse Spontaneous Leukemia

G. MATHÉ, O. HALLE-PANNENKO, and C. BOURUT

Institut de Cancérologie et d'Immunogénétique*, Hôpital Paul-Brousse**

Active immunotherapy (AI), which is the immune stimulation applied after the establishment of the tumor, has been shown by our first experiments conducted on L 1210 grafted leukemia, to be able to eradicate the neoplastic cell population and to cure the animals. However, the leukemic cell population must not exceed 10^5 [7] and this is a limiting factor. These experiments also showed that the most active modality of immune stimulation for immunotherapy is the combination of irradiated tumor cells and of agents we have called "systemic adjuvants of immunity", because they potentiate the effect of the specific stimulation produced by these cells, even when applied at different sites and at different times [7, 12]. The most active of these agents is BCG, as shown by a systematic study with a battery of screening tests [11]. BCG given alone, though active in immunoprophylaxis, i.e. when administered before the establishment of the tumor, is usually inactive for therapy [12].

An experiment conducted with POUILLART on L 1210 leukemia has shown that a leukemic cell population in excess of 10^5 can be reduced by chemotherapy to the number that can be eradicated by immunotherapy [8].

Such was the principle of a trial conducted on acute lymphoid leukemia (ALL) in man, which has maintained remission for more than 5 years in 7 of 20 patients in the immunotherapy group, whereas 10 out of 10 relapsed in the randomized control group [10]. Further trials of AI conducted on more than 100 ALL patients have shown that the curve of the cumulative duration of first remission levels out to a plateau between 16 and 32 months; this is the statistical expression of "cure expectancy" for about 40% of all patients [14].

Using a similar protocol based on the combination of BCG and irradiated tumor cells, [6] have confirmed these results in acute myeloid leukemia [6].

There are still many operational problems to be studied before active immunotherapy can be used as a routine. They need to be studied on experimental models which are as close to human leukemias as possible. We have been able to confirm our L 1210 leukemia results on grafted leukemias, more recently induced leukemias and leukemias induced by viruses, namely the RC 19 (Rauscher virus) and the E♀K1 (Gross virus). Cells were inoculated i.v. in order to simulate human leukemias

* INSERM et Association Claude-Bernard

** 14-16, avenue Paul Vaillant Couturier, Villejuif, France

as closely as possible [13], but it is evident that no murine model can simulate human ALL better than spontaneous leukemia in AKR mice.

However, this model had always been considered an improper model for immunotherapy, because theoretically there should be immune tolerance in AKR mice due to the vertical transmission of Gross virus. [4] showed that this tolerance was a myth. The possible rejection of isogeneic leukemic cells by AKR mice pretreated with a systemic immunity adjuvant or allogeneic leukemic cells carrying the same tumor-associated antigen was demonstrated. We observed the presence of antibodies against G antigen. This was confirmed by [15] and by [1]. This suggests that AKR spontaneous leukemia can serve as model for experimental active immunotherapy trials.

[3] are presently conducting similar experiments. They treat the animals at the time leukemia is detectable after reduction of the disease by a moderate chemotherapy. Their preliminary results are very encouraging.

The object of the present work was to see whether active immunotherapy could be efficient when applied at the age of 6 months, when leukemia is starting. The aim was to find out (i) whether the results with a combination of BCG and allogeneic leukemia cells for the AI can be improved by *in vitro* treatment of the cells by neuraminidase, as suggested by [2], and (ii) whether a preceding intensive chemotherapy, which should be able to reduce the number of leukemic cells considerably [17], in fact improves the action of AI.

Materials and Methods

308 6-months-old AKR mice (obtained from CNEAL, Orleans) were randomized among 7 groups of 44 mice (18 males and 26 females).

44 mice were sacrificed and examined macroscopically and histologically.

Experimental Group 1 served as controls for studying spontaneous mortality.

Experimental Group 2 were treated by a chemotherapy protocol suggested by Skipper's results [17]: the animals received, as shown in Fig. 1, (a) cyclophosphamide (CPM), 150 mg/kg on days 0 and 12, and 100 mg on days 24 and 36; (b) cytosine arabinoside (ARAC), 7.5 mg/kg t.i.d. from day 3 to 9, then from day 15 to 21 and day 27 to 33.

The mice of Group 3 received intra-peritoneally on day 225 of their life, 1 mg of living Pasteur Institute BCG per mouse, and subcutaneously 10^7 cells of E♂G2 leukemia, a leukemia induced by Gross virus in C 57 Bl/6 mice and transferred for 2 years in this strain.

BCG was repeated every 7 days and the leukemic cells every 30 days.

The treatment of the mice in Group 4 was a combination of the chemotherapy given to Group 2, followed by AI as in Group 3.

The animals of Group 5 received AI as in Group 3, except the cells were treated *in vitro* with *Vibrio cholerae* neuraminidase (VCN) (Behringwerke AG., Marburg/Lahn) in a concentration of 500 units of enzyme/ml in the following manner: the washed E♂G2 cells were incubated for 20 min at 37 °C with 2 units of VCN/ml/5×10^6 cells; after incubation, the cells were washed 4 times in buffered saline

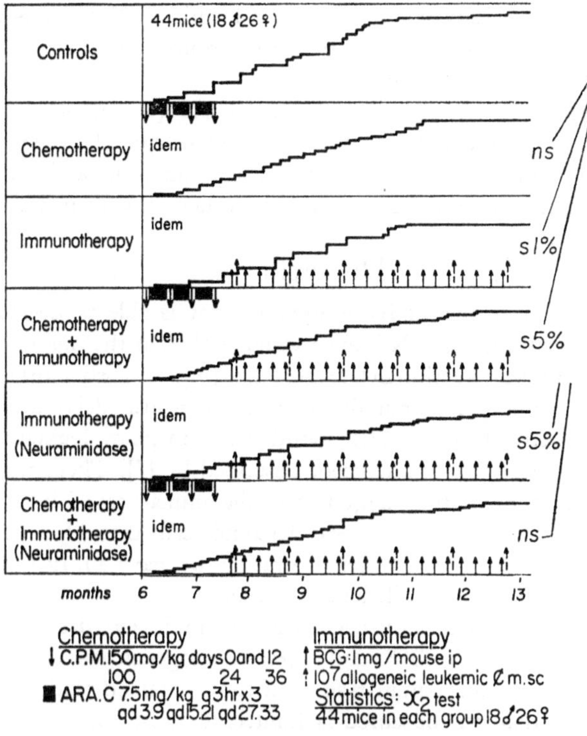

Fig. 1. Cumulative mortality of six groups of AKR mice given different treatment

(PBS) pH 7.6 and then resuspended at a concentration of 5×10^7 cells/ml for injection.

Group 6 received chemotherapy as in Group 2 followed by AI as in Group 5.

Results

The results (on animals taken at 6 months and representing a leukemia detectable in 40% of the population) are shown in Fig. 1.

Group 1. 92% of controls had died by 13 months. The curve of cumulative mortality shows that death is most frequent between the 6th and the 10th months, then becomes rare.

Group 2. Chemotherapy, though intensive, did not significantly decrease mortality, which is in accordance with the results published by [16].

Group 3. Active immunotherapy combining BCG and allogeneic leukemic cells untreated by neuraminidase did not delay mortality but reduced it; 30% of the animals were normal at month 11 and there were no deaths between this date and month 13. The difference between the mortality of the treated and the control group is significant ($p > 0.01$).

Group 5. Immunotherapy using cells treated with VCN did not improve the results. On the contrary, the difference between Group 5 mortality and that of the control group is only significant at $p > 0.05$.

Intensive chemotherapy, administered before AI (Group 4 and 6) did not improve the results; on the contrary, it made them worse. The difference between Group 4 (immunotherapy without neuraminidase) and controls is only $p > 0.05$, and the difference between the Group 6 (immunotherapy with neuraminidase) and controls is not significant.

Discussion

These results indicate that active immunotherapy is able to decrease mortality from spontaneous leukemia in AKR mice when applied at the onset of the disease. Contrary to a significant reduction in late mortality (Fig. 1), early mortality in Group 3 (immunotherapy without neuraminidase) is not significantly delayed. This suggests that animals that died before the 11th month had too many leukemic cells to be sensitive to AI according to the concept described by [7]. There were no deaths between months 11 and 13; this suggests that the animals saved by AI were those that at 6 months had only the number of leukemic cells that AI can eradicate.

This result again confirms the demonstration we gave in 1970 with [4] that AKR mice are not tolerant to AKR leukemic cells.

The fact that the treatment of the cells by neuraminidase *in vitro* does not improve the effect of the combination of BCG and untreated allogeneic leukemic cells suggests that the maximum immune stimulation is already obtained with the latter. The number of animals that can be cured is limited to those carrying not too many leukemic cells at 6 months. Any small decrease of the results of AI by neuraminidase-treated cells may be due to the fact that cells treated by this enzyme may stimulate humoral immunity, hence blocking antibodies, more than cell mediated-immunity as observed by [5].

One is tempted to explain the worsening of the AI effect by chemotherapy by the immunosuppressive effect of the intensive chemotherapy. [3] however, enhanced the effect of AI by administering mild chemotherapy. We are presently conducting an experiment in which the variable is the intensity of chemotherapy. This question is very important. We have treated more than 120 acute lymphoid leukemia patients with different protocols applying the same principle, i.e. cell-reducing chemotherapy followed by AI. In all protocols except one, chemotherapy was prolonged (about 5 months) and mild, and about 40% of the patients have not relapsed. In this one protocol, chemotherapy was short and very intensive (remission-induction chemotherapy with prednisone, vincristine and daunomycin, repeated 3 times); with this protocol alone, all patients relapsed very soon [9]. An immunotherapy trial conducted by "Acute Leukemia Group A" in which the patients were submitted to BCG immediately after intensive remission-induction chemotherapy also gave a negative result (personal communication).

References

1. Allison, A. C.: Potential of viral carcinogenesis by immunosuppression. Brit. med. J. **4**, 419 (1970).

2. Bagshawe, K. D., Currie, G. A.: Immunogenicity of L 1210 murine leukemia cells after treatment with neuraminidase. Nature (Lond.) **218**, 1254 (1968).

3. Bekesi, J. G., Holland, J. F.: Combined chemotherapy and immunotherapy of transplantable and spontaneous murine leukemia in DBA/2 and AkR mice. This volume.
4. Doré, J. F., Ajuria, E., Mathé, G.: Non leukaemic AkR mice are not tolerant to cells of leukaemia induced by Gross virus. Europ. J. clin. biol. Res. **15**, 81 (1970).
5. Doré, J. F., Hadjiyannakis, M. J., Coudert, A., Guibout, C., Marholev, L., Imai, K.: Use of enzyme-treated cells in immunotherapy of leukaemia. This volume.
6. Powles R., Kay, H. E. M., McElwain, T. J., Alexander, P., Crowther, D., Hamilton-Fairley, G., Pike, M.: Immunotherapy of acute myeloblastic leukemia in man. This volume.
7. Mathé, G.: Immunothérapie active de la leucémie L 1210 appliquée après la greffe tumorale. Rev. franç. Étud. clin. biol. **13**, 881 (1968).
8. Mathé, G.: Active immunotherapy. Advanc. Cancer Res. **14**, 1 (1971).
9. Mathé, G.: Results of active immunotherapy in acute lymphoid leukemia according to the preimmunotherapy chemotherapy. To be published, 1973.
10. Mathé, G., Amiel, J. L., Schwarzenberg, L., Schneider, M., Cattan, A., Schlumberger, J. R., Hayat, M., de Vassal, F.: Active immunotherapy for acute lymphoid leukaemia. Lancet **1969 I**, 697.
11. Mathé, G., Kamel, M., Dezfulian, M., Halle-Pannenko, O., Bourut, C.: An experimental screening for "systemic adjuvants of immunity" applicable in cancer immunotherapy. This volume.
12. Mathé, G., Pouillart, P., Lapeyraque, F.: Active immunotherapy of experimental leukaemias applied after the graft of leukaemia. Brit. J. Cancer **23**, 814 (1969).
13. Mathé, G., Pouillart, P., Lapeyraque, F.: Active immunotherapy of mouse RC 19 and E ♀ Kl leukaemias applied after the intravenous transplantation of the tumour cells. Experientia (Basel) **27**, 446 (1971).
14. Mathé, G., Pouillart, P., Schwarzenberg, L., Amiel, J. L., Schneider, M., Hayat, M., de Vassal, F., Jasmin, C., Rosenfeld, C., Weiner, R., Rappaport, H.: Attempts at immunotherapy of 100 acute lymphoid leukemia patients. Some factors influencing results. nat. Cancer Inst. **35**, 361 (1972).
15. Oldstone, M. B. A., Aoki, T., Dixon, F. J.: The antibody response of mice to murine leukemia virus in spontaneous infection: absence of classic immunologic tolerance. Proc. nat. Acad. Sci. (Wash.) **69**, 134 (1972).
16. Pollard, M., Sharon, N.: Prevention and treatment of spontaneous leukemia in germ free AkR mice. Proc. Soc. exp. Biol. (N.Y.) **137**, 1494 (1971).
17. Skipper, H. E., Schabel, F. M. jr., Trader, M. W., Russel Laster, W. jr.: Response to therapy of spontaneous first passage, and long passage lines of AkR leukemia. Cancer Chemother. Abstr. **53**, 345 (1969).

Augmented Immunogenicity of Tumor Cell Homogenates Infected with Influenza Virus

C. W. Boone

Cell Biology Section, Viral Biology Branch, National Cancer Institute, National Institutes of Health, Bethesda, Md.

We have studied the use of influenza virus to augment the immunogenicity of tumor-transplantation antigens (TTA) isolated from tumor homogenates [1, 2, 3, 4]. The data to be presented here refer to a transplantable SV 40-induced fibrosarcoma in BALB/c mice infected with the WSA strain of mouse-adapted influenza virus [1]. We have obtained similar results with methylcholanthrene-induced fibrosarcomas and a Moloney virus-induced lymphoma of mice. In addition, the Hong Kong strain of influenza virus appears to be as effective as the WSA strain after adaption to growth in mouse cells.

Table 1. Viability dependence of TTA of SV3T3-T4 fibrosarcoma cells [a]

Inoculated with	Number of tumors/number challenged
X-irradiated tumor cells (5×10^6)	0/20
Frozen-thawed tumor cells (5×10^7)	19/20
No treatment, control	20/20

[a] Inoculation: s. c. on days 0 and 3; challenge: 10^6 SV3T3-T4 cells s. c. on day 14; tumors scored 30 days after challenge.

Very early in our work we were confronted with the general phenomenon of the *viability dependence of TTA* illustrated in Table 1. Whereas a dose of 5×10^6 intact X-irradiated tumor cells was perfectly immunogenic, a frozen-thawed homogenate of 5×10^7 cells was not at all immunogenic. Some years ago Lindenmann [6] reported on a way to prevent this loss of TTA in tumor homogenates. Working with the allogeneic Ehrlich ascites tumor, he showed that homogenates of tumor cells that had been infected with influenza virus retained the capacity to immunize mice against tumor challenge, whereas homogenates of cells not infected by virus did not. We therefore infected the SV 40 fibrosarcoma cells with influenza virus and tested homogenates of these cells for TTA activity, with the good results shown in Table 2. Note the important specificity control: animals inoculated with homo-

Table 2. Augmented immunogenicity of tumor cell homogenates infected with influenza virus [a] (Table reproduced from reference [3])

Inoculated with	Number of tumors/number challenged	Mean tumor weight (g)
Homogenate of SV3T3-T4 cells previously infected with influenza virus	3/35	0.125
Homogenate of SV3T3-T4 cells not infected with influenza virus	20/26	0 642
Homogenate of 3T3 cells previously infected with influenza virus	15/17	0.370
No treatment, control	17/19	0.307

[a] Inoculation: 0.5 ml of a 10% homogenate s. c. on days 0 and 3; challenge: 10^6 SV3T3-T4 cells s. c. on day 14; recording: tumors scored 30 days after challenge.

genates of normal BALB/c cells that had been infected with influenza virus were not made resistant to tumor transplant challenge. Clearly, the virus must infect the tumor cells. Simply mixing egg-grown influenza virus with a tumor homogenate did not make the homogenate immunogenic.

In another experiment testing the specificity of the TTA-enhancing effect, animals were immunized with a virus-infected homogenate of one type of tumor and challenged with tumor cells of another type. The results are shown in Table 3. The M 3 T tumor in this table is a neoplastic variant of the BALB 3T3 line. These results definitely indicate that the TTA-enhancing effect of the virus is not due to a simple non-specific stimulation of the immune system in a manner analogous to the effect of BCG.

Live virus is not necessary for the TTA-enhancing effect. Formalin-inactivated virus-infected tumor homogenates are still immunogenic [2].

Having found a way to produce tumor homogenates with retained TTA activity approaching that of intact tumor cells, we are now in the process of isolating and

Table 3. Specificity of the TTA-enhancing effect produced by influenza virus (Table reproduced from reference [4])

Group	Cell type infected with influenza virus and used for immunizing inoculum	Result of challenge with E 4 cells		
		Tumor incidence [a]	Mean tumor weight (g)	S.D.
I	SV 40 tumor cells (E 4 cells)	5/20	0.79	0.47
II	M3T tumor cells	19/20	1.67	1.36
III	3T3 normal cells	15/20	1.28	0.96
IV	No treatment	18/20	1.74	0.99

[a] Number with tumors/number challenged.
Immunization: One s. c. dose of 0.5 ml of virus-infected tumor homogenates.
Challenge: 2×10^6 SV 40 tumor cells (E 4 cells) given s. c. 14 days after immunization.
Recording: Tumors tallied and weighed 30 days after challenge.

purifying the TTA. Since TTA on the surface of a tumor cell may exist in the form of a particular conformational pattern extending over a broader surface area than a single macromolecule, we refrained from using antigen isolation techniques involving solvent extraction (3 m KCl, non-ionic detergents, butanol, chloroform-methanol) or enzymatic hydrolysis (papain) for fear that they might overdegrade the TTA and produce a macromolecule having serological reactivity but no tumor-protective capacity. Instead, we isolated the membrane fractions of influenza virus-infected tumor cells on sucrose density gradients. Table 4 shows that the TTA

Table 4. TTA activity of membrane fractions from influenza virus-infected tumor cells. Two immunizing doses (Table reproduced from reference [4])

Group	Gradient fraction used for immunizing inoculum	Dose [a]	Tumor incidence [d]	Mean tumor weight (g)	S.D.
1	30% [b]	N.D. [c]	8/20	0.26	0.19
2	30/40%	0.75 mg	1/25	0.65	
3	40/45%	0.75 mg	2/24	0.29	0.15
4	No treatment	—	16/20	0.34	0.18

[a] Protein content (Lowry procedure).
[b] Mixture of small amounts of material at the 20/30% interface and air-liquid interface.
[c] Not determined. Estimated at 0.15 mg.
[d] Number with tumors/number challenged.
Immunization: Two s. c. doses in 0.2 ml spaced two days apart.
Challenge: 10^6 E 4 cells given s. c. 14 days after first inoculation.
Recording: Tumors tallied and weighed 30 days after challenge.

activity is retained in these fractions. The 33—40% fraction also contains influenza virus. During virus maturation in the cell, the influenza virus-coded hemagglutinin and neuraminidase antigenic proteins are inserted in high density into the entire plasma membrane, not just into the portion that becomes th evirus envelope [5]. Most of the augmented TTA in the 33—40% fraction may therefore exist in the form of plasma-membrane microvesicles containing both TTA and viral antigens. The virus itself may possibly contain TTA in its envelope. We feel that a stable suspension of virus and virus antigen-containing plasma-membrane microvesicles, where the virus is inactivated with ultraviolet irradiation, may form the most effective immunizing preparation for practical use.

In connection with TTA isolation, we needed a faster assay for TTA activity than tumor-graft rejection, which takes 40 days. We therefore developed the useful radioisotopic footpad assay for delayed hypersensitivity to tumor cells in the mouse (Table 5). At the same time as the eliciting dose of tumor cells is injected into the footpad of a tumor-immune mouse, radioiodine-labeled serum protein is inoculated i.p. The increased vascular permeability associated with delayed-hypersensitivity reaction in the footpad results in leakage of the labeled mouse serum protein from the vascular compartment into the interstitial fluids of the inflamed area. 24 hours later, both feet are cut off and counted in a gamma spectrometer. The ratio of counts in the test foot to counts in the contralateral control foot is taken as the measure of the intensity of the reaction. The delayed hypersensitivity reaction against the tumor cells is adoptively transferable with spleen cells but not with serum [7].

We have found that although a homogenate of SV 40-transformed tumor cells will not induce immunity to tumor transplant challenge, it will elicit a delayed-hypersensitivity reaction in animals made tumor-immune either by being given a tumor that is later excised, or by being inoculated with X-irradiated tumor cells. Intact X-irradiated tumor cells will immunize animals against tumor transplant

Table 5. Delayed hypersensitivity to tumor cells in BALB/c mice demonstrated by a radioisotopic footpad assay (table taken from reference [7])

Footpad inoculum	Status of recipient	Foot-count ratio [a]	Average
10^6 tumor cells	Immune to tumor challenge	4.08, 3.67, 3.30, 2.76, 2.58, 2.19	3.13
10^6 tumor cells	Normal	1.62, 1.53, 1.27, 1.24, 1.20, 1.02	1.31
10^6 syngeneic normal cells	Immune to tumor challenge	1.44, 1.34, 1.24, 1.18, 0.81	1.20
10^6 tumor cells	Immunized with complete Freund's adjuvant (CFA)	1.27, 1.26, 1.24, 1.09, 1.07	1.40
10 µg *Mycobacterium tuberculosis* extract	Immunized with CFA	3.63, 3.52, 3.45, 2.24, 2.18	3.00

[a] cpm test paw/cpm control paw: mice inoculated with ^{125}I-labeled mouse serum protein at the time of footpad inoculation.

challenge and also elicit a delayed hypersensitivity reaction in tumor-immune animals. Ten times the dose of tumor cells in the form of a homogenate will not immunize against tumor-transplant challenge; but a small dose of the same homogenate will elicit a delayed-hypersensitivity reaction in tumor-immune animals. Finally, homogenates of tumor cells infected with influenza virus will both induce tumor immunity and elicit delayed hypersensitivity. The simplest conclusion from these results is that the footpad assay is more sensitive than the tumor transplant rejection assay and will detect amounts of TTA insufficient to immunize against tumor challenge. We are careful at this stage to distinguish three empirically defined immunologic determinants on the tumor cells that may or may not be structurally the same: 1. a delayed hypersensitivity-eliciting determinant, 2. a delayed hypersensitivity-sensitizing antigen, or the molecular configuration that primes an animal to react to the eliciting determinant, and 3. the TTA, which makes the animal immune to tumor-transplant challenge.

We have also been investigating the mechanism of the enhancement of TTA activity mediated by influenza virus. The phenomenological situation is shown in Fig. 1. The possible mechanisms for the virus augmentation of TTA are: 1. simple adjuvant action; 2. chemical stabilization; 3. helper antigen; or 4. neuraminidase action.

1. The virus could act as a simple adjuvant, which would be like mixing the tumor homogenate with complete Freund's adjuvant. However, when we mixed the tumor homogenate with egg-grown influenza virus, the very slight degree of tumor protection that occurred was insufficient to account for the relatively marked immunogenicity of virus-infected tumor homogenates.

2. Infection with the virus could chemically stabilize the viability-dependent portion of the TTA (VD). This is the chemical stabilization hypothesis.

3. If the influenza-virus antigens and the viability-independent TTA (VI) together induce an immune response against the TTA alone, then a helper antigen action could be operating.

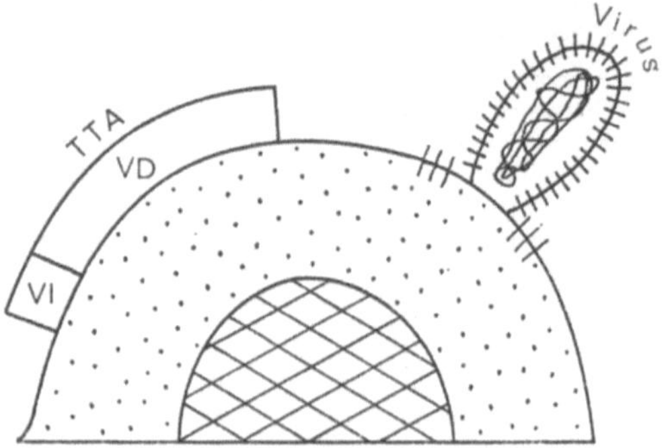

Fig. 1. Mechanism of enhancement of TTA activity mediated by influenza virus. VD viability-dependent portion of TTA (eliminated by homogenization); VI viability-independent portion of TTA

We have just finished an experiment which appears to distinguish between the chemical stabilization and the helper antigen hypothesis. We made animals tolerant to egg-grown influenza virus by means of Cytoxan, and then inoculated them with homogenates of virus-infected tumor cells. These animals did not become immune to challenge with tumor cells, whereas non-tolerant animals become immune as usual. We interpret this as strong evidence for the helper-antigen hypothesis: the virus-tolerant animals did not recognize the viral helper antigens and therefore could not be immunized. If the virus had worked through a chemical stabilizing mechanism, the homogenate of virus-infected cells would still have been immunogenic to the virus-tolerant animals.

4. Another possible mechanism of action related to the helper-antigen hypothesis is that the neuraminidase of the influenza virus could modify the host-cell membrane structure to produce a "non-self" transplantation antigen. We have recently found that infection of tumor cells with vesicular stomatitis virus (VSV) also enhances TTA activity to about the same extent as influenza virus (unpublished observations). Since VSV does not possess a neuraminidase, the mechanism of TTA enhancement must involve something other than the action of this enzyme.

Human tumors treated by surgery not infrequently recur at the operative site. Here is a situation in which some immunotherapeutic maneuver might be especially effective once the main tumor load has been removed. We therefore conducted a series of immunotherapy experiments in which homogenates of virus-infected tumor cells were used to treat animals left with a small amount of residual tumor after surgical excision of the main tumor mass. The protocol was as follows: Tumor cells were inoculated into the footpad on day 0. On day 14, when the tumor was approximately 1 cm in diameter, the tumors were amputated except for a small amount definitely visible to the naked eye. Immunization of these animals with homogenates of tumor cells infected with influenza virus was begun on day 7 (after inoculation of the tumor cells, and repeated on days 10, 14, 21, and 28. Control animals were inoculated according to the same schedule with tumor homogenate not infected with influenza virus. The results of the first experiment of this type are shown in Fig. 2. The survival time of the animals treated with virus-augmented

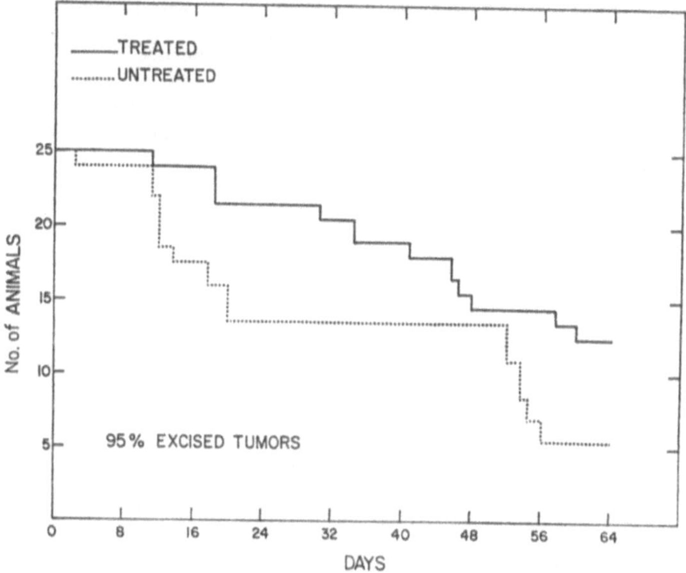

Fig. 2. Effect of immunotherapy with homogenates of virus-infected tumor cells following surgical excision of main tumor mass

TTA was definitely prolonged, and there were more survivors than in the control group. These highly encouraging results are being repeated and will form the subject of a subsequent report.

In summary, while seeking to isolate biologically effective tumor transplantation antigens from SV 40-induced mouse fibrosarcomas, we found that the immunogenicity of tumor homogenates was markedly augmented if the tumor cells were first infected with influenza virus. The plasma-membrane fraction of the virus-infected tumor cells appeared to contain most of the virus-augmented TTA. A fast footpad assay for TTA is speeding the isolation work considerably, and the mechanism of action of the influenza virus effect appears to be that of a "helper antigen". Initial immunotherapy experiments are encouraging in that animals left with a small amount of residual tumor after surgery exhibit prolonged survival after treatment with homogenates of influenza virus-infected tumor cells.

References

1. Boone, C. W., Blackman, K., Brandchaft, P.: Tumor immunity induced in mice with cell-free homogenates of influenza virus-infected tumor cells. Nature (Lond.) **231**, 265 (1971).
2. Boone, C. W., Blackman, K.: Augmented immunogenicity of tumor cell homogenates infected with influenza virus. Cancer Res. **32**, 1018 (1972).
3. Boone, C. W.: Augmented immunogenicity of tumor cell homogenates produced by infection with influenza virus. Nat. Cancer Inst. Monogr. **35**, 301 (1972).
4. Boone, C. W., Orme, T. W., Blackman, K., Gillette, R : Preparation of membrane fractions with augmented tumor transplantation antigen activity from tumor cells infected with influenza virus. J. nat. Cancer Inst. **51**, 1141 (1973).
5. Duc-Nguyen, H., Rose, H. M., Morgan, C.: An electron microscopic study of changes at the surface of influenza-infected cells as revealed by ferritin-conjugated antibodies. Virology **28**, 404 (1966).
6. Lindemann, J., Klein, P. A.: Viral oncolysis: increased immunogenicity of host cell antigen associated with influenza virus. J. exp. Med. **126**, 93 (1967).
7. Paranjpe, M. S., Boone, C. W.: Delayed hypersensitivity to SV 40 tumor cells in BALB/c mice demonstrated by a radioisotopic footpad assay. J. nat. Cancer Inst. **48**, 563 (1972).

Characterization and Purification of Rauscher Leukemia-Associated Transplantation Antigens

M.-C. Martyre, O. Halle-Pannenko, and P. Jolles

Institut de Cancérologie et d'Immunogénétique, Hôpital Paul Brousse, Villejuif and Laboratoire de Biochimie, Université de Paris VI

1. Introduction

The antigenic changes which have been found in virtually every experimental tumor system studied, as well as many tumors studied in man, can be divided into two main groups. The first are quantitative changes in the density of normal histocompatibility antigens on malignant cells [4, 11, 18]. These changes have been found by antibody absorption studies as well as by light and electron microscope studies using antibodies labeled with appropriate markers. The other major change in antigenicity has been qualitative, that is to say, antigenic determinants have been found on tumor cells which are not present on cells of the non-tumor bearing isogenic host and to which the host is, in most cases, capable of responding immunologically [5, 13, 16].

The relationship between the antigenic changes observed in both chemically and virally induced tumors and the malignant transformation is poorly understood and indeed is a central question in tumor immunology today [9]. The various reports which have dealt with the quantitative aspects of tumor-associated membrane antigens have generally agreed that they are poorly represented on the membrane surface as compared to the histocompatibility antigens on the same cell [4, 18]. They are, however, present and immunologically active in the isogeneic host. As we report in the succeeding communication, the transplantable ascitic murine leukemia (RC_{19}) induced in Balb/c mice by Rauscher virus carries an extractable and immunologically active cellular antigen. Pre-immunization with the soluble fraction obtained from the ascites tumor cells can inhibit the induction of the leukemia by cell-free virus and can facilitate the growth of the ascitic graft of leukemia cells. We have partially purified the antigenic fractions of the extract by isoelectric focusing as previously used to purify the soluble H-2 antigens of C_3H mice [7]. Moreover we have used isoelectric focusing to compare the isoelectric pH, charge, and mobility of the tumor-specific and normal transplantation antigens of our extract.

2. Material and Methods

Mice. Young adult male and female Balb/c mice were used.

Tumor. RC_{19} is a murine leukemia induced by the Rauscher virus in Balb/c mice and carried in ascites form in Balb/c mice.

Preparation of the membrane fraction. The method of preparing the membrane fraction has been described in detail [2, 8]. The ascites cells from RC_{19} bearing Balb/c mice were submitted to lysis by successively hypotonic solutions of NaCl (0.07 M; 0.035 M) and finally distilled water. After each 30 min incubation the material is centrifuged for 10 min at 800 g at room temperature and the supernatant is saved. The 3 supernatant fractions are pooled and centrifuged at 75,000 g for 90 min. The precipitate obtained represents the membrane fraction.

Solubilization of the membrane fraction. The tumor cell membrane fractions were solubilized by the autodigestion method previously described [3, 12]. The pellet obtained from the rapid centrifugation (75,000 g) of the cell lysate was suspended in a solution of 0.05 M Tris-HCl at pH 7.7 at 37 °C for 3 h. The suspension was then centrifuged for 1 h at 105,000 g and the supernatant was used as the soluble fraction.

Isoelectric focusing of the soluble fractions. The isoelectric focusing technique used was as described for the purification of the H-2 antigens of the C_3H mouse [7]. The carrier ampholyte was selected to give a gradient between pH 3 and pH 10. Isoelectric focusing was performed for 48 h at 10 °C with a potential of 600 V. Absorbance of each 2 ml fraction collected was determined at 280 mμ.

Determination of biologic activity. The biologic activity of the soluble extracts and the fractions obtained after electrofocusing was determined *in vitro* by inhibition of cytotoxic activity of reference sera. The activity was assayed by the ability to absorb the cytotoxic activity of an allogeneic antiserum directed against the FMR (Friend-Moloney-Rauscher) antigen as well as another allogeneic serum directed against the $H\text{-}2^d$ antigens.

The anti-FMR sera was prepared in C 57 Bl/6 ($H\text{-}2^b$) mice by injections of ascitic cells from RC_{19} tumor bearing Balb/c mice. The resulting serum was absorbed with normal Balb/c spleen cells until no cytotoxic activity against the normal cells could be found. The anti $H\text{-}2^d$ serum was prepared in C 57 Bl/6 mice by the injection of DBA/2 spleen cells.

3. Results

Purification by Isoelectric focusing of the Soluble Fractions of Cell Lysates

Purification of the soluble fraction of malignant cell lysates by the method of isoelectric focusing has been carried out on different samples. The results are reproducible. Fig. 1 is a representative elution profile of RC_{19} cell antigens obtained by isoelectric focusing (absorption at 280 mμ). The relationship between the total fraction eluted and the biologically active fraction indicates a 3 to 4-fold purification (see Fig. 1).

Biologic Activity

The biologic activity was determined as the absorptive capacity of each fraction after dialysis of each eluate against 0.9% NaCl buffered with Na_2HPO_3 to pH 7.8 at 4 °C for 48 h.

The isoelectric focusing of the cell extract yielded antigenic material absorbable by anti-FMR serum in only 2 or 3 fractions eluted between pH 6.3 and pH 7.4.

Moreover, when the eluates were tested for absorptive activity against the anti H-2^d serum, the activity was again found in the same fractions as the absorptive activity of the leukemia-associated antigens.

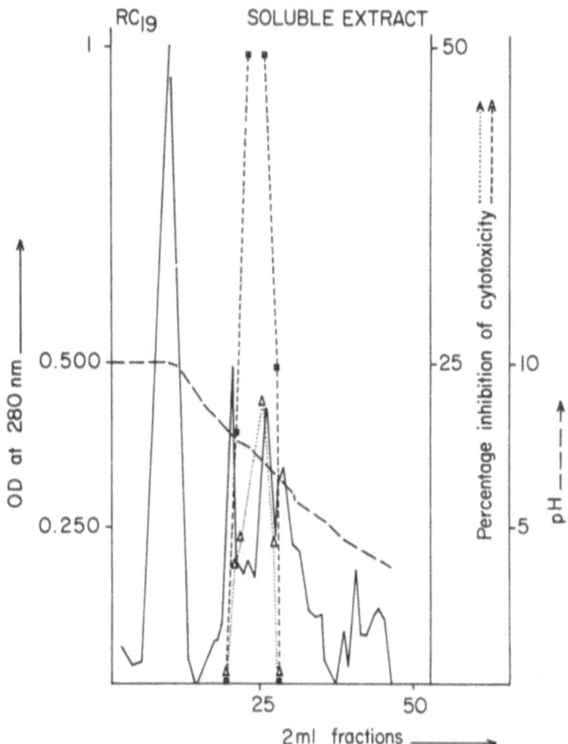

Fig. 1. Isoelectric focusing between pH 3 and pH 10 of the soluble fraction obtained by autodigestion from murine RC 19 (Balb/c) tumor cell membranes. —— absorbance at 280 nm ----- pH ■ · · · ■ inhibition of cytotoxicity of anti-FMR antiserum ▲ · · · ▲ inhibition of cytotoxicity of anti-H-2^d antiserum

4. Discussion

All the biological activity was eluted in a narrow pH range and yielded products purified 3 to 4-fold in terms of protein concentration. The extract retained its characteristic antigenic pattern as determined by absorption capacity after purification. The active fractions of tumor-cell extract absorbed the cytotoxic activity of both the anti-H-2 and the anti-FMR sera.

The attempts at solubilization, separation and purification of normal and tumor-associated antigens which have interested our laboratory and many others have been motivated by the possibility of specific immune manipulation by modifying antigenic determinants. While certain immunological effects have been demonstrated by the altered immunogenicity of intact cells, the mechanisms remain obscure [1, 6, 10, 17]. Modification of cell-free extracts [15] have likewise been shown to modulate host response, but again little knowledge has been gained of the criteria necessary for specific immunogenicity. By contrast, specific modification of a well-defined molecule has recently revealed some of the factors involved in the production of either immunity or tolerance in both the humoral and cell-mediated immune response [14].

The key term is "well-defined", and it is our objective to pursue the definition of antigenic determinants. In this way we may hope to approach systematically the manipulations of the immune response.

References

1. Blakeslee, J. R., jr.: The effect of various enzymes and chelating agents on the TSTA of SV 40 induced tumor cells. Proc. Amer. Ass. Cancer Res. **13**, (1972).
2. Davies, D. A. L.: Mouse histocompatibility isoantigens derived from normal and from tumour cells. Immunology **17**, 115 (1966).
3. Halle-Pannenko, O., Florentin, I., Kiger, N., Jolles, P.: Advances in transplantation proceedings of the 1st international congress of the transplantation society. Paris: June 1967.
4. Haywood, G. R., McKhann, C. F.: Antigenic specificities on murine sarcoma cells. J. exp. Med. **133**, 1171 (1971).
5. Hollinshead, A., Glew, D., Bunnag, B., Gold, P., Herberman, R.: Skin reactive soluble antigen from intestinal cancer cell membrane and relationship to carcinoembryonic antigens. Lancet **1970 I**, 1191.
6. Jasmin, C., Piton, C., Rosenfeld, C.: Effets de l'iodoacetamide sur les cellules de la leucémie virale de Rauscher. Int. J. Cancer **3**, 254 (1968).
7. Jolles, P., Schoentgen, F., Halle-Pannenko, O., Martyre, M. C.: Purification of soluble murine transplantation antigens by isoelectric focusing. FEBS Letters **8**, 167 (1970).
8. Kahan, B. D., Holms, E. C., Reisfeld, R. A., Morton, D. L.: Water soluble guinea pig transplantation antigen from carcinogen-induced sarcomas. J. Immunol. **102**, 28 (1969).
9. Klein, G.: Tumor specific transplantation antigens. Cancer Res. **28**, 625 (1968).
10. Martin, W. J., Wunderlich, J. R., Fletcher, F., Inman, J. K.: Enhanced immunogenicity of chemically coated syngeneic tumor cells. Proc. nat. Acad. Sci. (Wash.) **68**, 469 (1971).
11. Motta, R., Bruley, M.: Quantitative study of the histocompatibility antigens on the surface of normal and leukaemic cells in mice. Transplantation **15**, 22 (1973).
12. Nathenson, S., Davies, D. A. L.: Transplantation antigen: Study of the mouse model system, solubilisation and partial purification of H 2 isoantigen. Ann. N.Y. Acad. Sci. **129**, 6 (1966).
13. Old, L. J., Boyse, E. A.: Antigens of tumors and leukemias induced by viruses. Fed. Proc. **24**, 1009 (1965).
14. Parish, C. R.: Immune response to chemically modified flagellin. I. Inducting of antibody tolerance to flagellin by aceto acetylated derivatives of the protein. J. exp. Med. **134**, 1 (1971).
15. Prager, M. L., Ticaric, S., Merril, C. L.: Tumor-host relationship in immune response to modified lymphoma cells. Proc. Amer. Ass. Cancer Res. **13**, (1972).
16. Prehn, R. T.: Cancer antigens in tumors induced by chemicals. Fed. Proc. **24**, 1018 (1965).
17. Simmons, R. L., Rios, A., Lundgren, G., Ray, P. K., McKhann, C., Haywood, G.: Immunospecific regression of methylcholanthrene induced fibrosarcoma using neuraminidase. Surgery **70**, 38 (1971).
18. Watanabe, T., Yagi, Y., Pressman, D.: Antibody against neoplastic plasma cells. 1) Specific surface antigens on mouse myeloma cells. Immunology **106**, 1213 (1971).

The *in vivo* Activity of Soluble Extracts Obtained from RC 19 Leukemia: Effect of the Method of Extraction

M.-C. Martyre, R. Weiner, and O. Halle-Pannenko

Institut de Cancérologie et d'Immunogénétique, Hôpital Paul Brousse, Villejuif

Soluble antigens from tumor cells have been shown to be biologically active in animal systems [1] and in man [2]. Soluble antigens can be conveniently stored, purified and manipulated; they are thus much more useful as investigative tools than whole tumor cells. Their extraction and characterization have been subject of intense study. In the preceding communication, Martyre *et al.* have described some biochemical and antigenic properties of a soluble antigen obtained by the hypotonic lysis of murine RC 19 tumor cells [3]. We report here the *in vivo* activity of this extract when used to immunize Balb/c mice against an i. p. challenge of live autochthonous RC 19 tumor cells. The activity of the hypotonic extract was compared to the activity of an extract of the same tumor cells prepared in hypertonic potassium chloride.

Materials and Methods

Mice. Young adult (6—12 weeks old) male and female mice obtained from the C.N.R.S. Animal Center at Orleans, La Source (France) were vaccinated against variola at 4 weeks of age and maintained in the germ-free animal quarters of our Institute. The mice were used both to carry the RC 19 tumor in ascites form and for the *in vivo* experiments.

Tumor cells. RC 19 is a leukemia induced by the Rauscher virus in Balb/c mice. The tumor cells used for this study were maintained in the ascites of mice and harvested 11 days after the i.p. injection of 1.5×10^6 viable cells. The tumor has been maintained in ascites form for 3 years. Cell-free serum from tumor-bearing animals is capable of inducing the same tumor.

Hypotonic cell extracts. Cell extracts were made from hypotonic sodium chloride lysates as described in the preceding paper. After concentration by dialysis against dry Sephadex G-200, they were stored at — 20 °C and used within one month.

Hypertonic cell extracts. The membrane antigen extraction procedure using 3 M KCl was that reported by [4] with minor modifications.

Ascites tumor cells were incubated with 3 M KCl for 18—24 h at 4 °C with constant stirring. A ratio of 10^9 cells to 20 ml 3 M KCl was used. The lysed cells were then centrifuged in a "Superspeed 50" centrifuge (MSE) using the 10×10 ml head at 50,000 r.p.m. ($150{,}000 \times g$) for 3 h. The supernatant was then dialysed against 1 M KCl in phosphate-buffered saline (PBS) followed by PBS and distilled water. The final dialysate was cleared by centrifugation at 1500 × g, lyophilized, and stored at — 20 °C.

Results

Immunizations with the soluble membrane extracts were performed according to the schema in the Table. Series A and B with three injections prior to and three

Table. Immunization schedule. The first injection was given in complete Freund's adjuvant; subsequent injections were given in saline. All doses were given s. c. and divided among at least four different sites. Day 0 is the day of the i. p. graft of 1×10^3 tumor cells

Product and dose	Days — 6	— 4	— 2	0	+ 2	+ 4	+ 6
Series A							
HSA 3 mg (2 mg protein)	+	+	+		+	+	+
KSA 3 mg (1.8 mg protein)	+	+	+		+	+	+
Series B							
HSA 3 mg (2 mg protein)	+	+	+		+	+	+
KSA 1 mg (0.600 mg protein)	+	+	+		+	+	+
Series C							
HSA 3 mg (2 mg protein)	+	+	+				
KSA 3 mg (1.8 mg protein)	+	+	+				

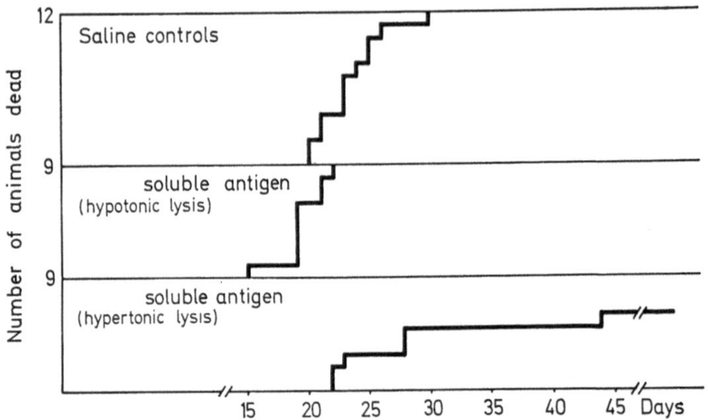

Fig. 1. Influence of soluble antigen on mortality from RC 19 leukemia. Cumulative survival curve of BALB/c mice treated in Series A (see the Table)

injections following the i.p. tumor graft gave the clearest differences in biological activity of the two extracts. While the hypotonic extract resulted in mild but significant ($p < 0.01$) shortening of survival, the hypertonic extract at both doses significantly ($p = 0.03$) prolonged survival (Fig. 1).

Neither extract was demonstrably active when given only prior to the tumor graft in a purely prophylactic system (series C).

Discussion

While the 3 M KCl-derived extract has not as yet been characterized to the same extent as that obtained by hypotonic lysis, the differences in biological activity obtained in our system are noteworthy. The extract obtained by hypotonic lysis shortens survival, either by a mechanism of tolerance induction, or, by an enhancing effect, possibly mediated by blocking antiserum, though we have been unable to demonstrate such humorally mediated activity (unpublished results).

The hypertonic KCl extract, however, clearly protected the animals when given in the same doses by dry weight and when given in one half the dose of the hypotonic extract. While we have not excluded an antigenic dose-related phenomenon as being a qualitative one related to the method of extraction, we are in the process of better defining our extracts antigenically as well as continuing our efforts to define them physicochemically.

These preliminary data confirm the potential response of the autochthonous host to the tumor antigens and reaffirm the dependence of response on the form of presentation of the antigen.

References

1. Baldwin, R. N., Embleton, H. J.: Detection and isolation of tumour specific antigen associated with a spontaneously arising rat mammary carcinoma. Int. J. Cancer **6**, 373 (1970).
2. Hollinshead, A., Glew, D., Bunnag, B., Gold, P., Herberman, R.: Skin reactive soluble antigen from intestinal cancer cell membranes and relationship to carcino-embryonic antigen. Lancet **1970 I**, 1191.
3. Martyre, M. C., Halle-Pannenko, O., Jolles, P.: Characterization and purification of Rauscher leukemia-associated transplantation antigens. This volume.
4. Reisfeld, R. A., Pellegrino, M. A., Kahan, B. D.: Salt extraction of soluble HLA antigens Science **172**, 1134 (1971).

The Preferential Induction of Cell-Mediated Immunity and Some Preliminary Observations on its Application to Tumor Immunotherapy*

E. Benjamini and R. T. Scibienski

Department of Medical Microbiology, School of Medicine,
University of California, Davis, Cal.

The role of the immune response in cancer has been under intense investigation in recent years in the hope of finding means both to enhance immunological rejection of tumor cells and to provide serological methods for early diagnosis of cancer. These studies have been the subject of recent reviews [6, 8, 9, 10]. A short description of major findings relevant to this communication is presented.

It has been conclusively demonstrated that most if not all neoplastic cells possess tumor-specific antigens. Much effort has been directed to elucidating the physico-chemical properties of these antigens, yet their exact nature is still obscure. Nevertheless, there is general agreement that tumor antigens are mainly associated with the cell membrane and are composed of proteins or lipoproteins.

Both circulating antibodies and cell-mediated immunity have been implicated in tumor growth and regression. Much experimental evidence indicates that circulating antibodies against tumor antigens play a role in prolonging tumor survival. Humoral antibodies may protect tumor cells from destruction by immune lymphoid cells by blocking receptor sites on target cells, which are the antigenic sites to which immune lymphocytes are directed [7]. Thus, in many instances immunization of experimental animals with tumor cells or tumor antigens to produce circulating antibodies enhances the growth of transplanted tumors. Clinically, there seems to be little correlation between the presence of tumor-specific circulating antibodies and tumor regression. Although cytotoxic antibodies to tumor cells have been demonstrated, it is now generally accepted that cellular immunity plays the major role in the rejection of cancer.

Cellular immunity has been postulated by Burnet to be a surveillance system against neoplastic mutations, which are continually arising in the body and are continually suppressed by lymphocytes [3]. Cell-mediated immunity appears to be implicated in tumor regression, as shown by numerous *in vivo* and *in vitro* experiments and clinical observations [6, 7, 8, 9, 10]. Moreover, even non-specific recruitment of lymphocytic cells to a tumor area, induced by inflammatory agents or non-specific enhancement of cell-mediated immunity have been shown to adversely

* Supported in part by Grant No. GB 30697 from the U.S. National Science Foundation.

affect tumor growth to various degrees [19]. Thus immunization with tumor-specific antigens to induce cell-mediated immunity without humoral antibodies would be expected to lead to an intensification of immunologically mediated tumor regression and/or rejection.

Until recently, attempts to induce cell-mediated immunity to a given protein antigen without the concomitant induction of humoral antibodies (by varying dosages of injected antigen, by incorporation with adjuvants, by manipulation of injection schedule, etc.) have been unsuccessful. Very recently, investigations in two laboratories have indicated that careful chemical modification of an antigen can create a situation in which the native and modified forms will exhibit cross-reactivity with respect to many immunological parameters but not with respect to humoral antibodies.

Parish [13] reported that certain degrees of acetoacetylation of flagellin resulted in modification of the protein to the extent where the native and modified forms showed very little or no serological cross-reactivity, but still exhibited cross-reactivity with respect to delayed hypersensitivity. Similarly, work in our laboratory [18] has shown that whereas the protein lysozyme and its reduced and carboxymethylated form (CM lysozyme) exhibited no serologic cross-reactivity, both forms cross-reacted with respect to delayed hypersensitivity (Table 1).

Table 1. Delayed skin reactions in guinea pigs, elicited by lysozyme and by CM-lysozyme [a]

Immunizing antigen	Test antigen	Skin reactions (24 h)
Lysozyme	Lysozyme	8/8 [b]
Lysozyme	CM lysozyme	7/8
CM lysozyme	CM lysozyme	15/20
CM lysozyme	lysozyme	15/20

[a] According to [18]. — [b] Number of animal reacting/number tested.

Investigations on the relationship between lysozyme and CM lysozyme with respect to several immunological parameters revealed that the two forms of the protein exhibited cross-reactivity in their ability to inhibit the migration of peritoneal exudate cells, an *in vitro* correlate of delayed hypersensitivity. Data in Table 2 demonstrate that lysozyme or CM lysozyme was capable of inhibiting the migration of peritoneal exudate cells obtained from guinea pigs immunized with either lysozyme or CM lysozyme.

The cross-reactivity between lysozyme and CM lysozyme is further demonstrated by the capacity of the native and modified antigens to stimulate splenic lymphocytes obtained from lysozyme- or from CM lysozyme-immunized guinea pigs (Table 3). To determine whether or not cross-reactivity would also be demonstrated with respect to both adult and neonatal tolerance, several groups of mice (BAB/14) were treated as follows: one group was injected with 1 mg lysozyme for 20 days from the first day of life. Another group was injected with 5 mg on the first day of life. A third group was injected with 5 mg on the 1st, 2nd, 3rd and 4th day of life. All the injections were given s.c. in saline. The animals were challenged at 6 weeks of age by

Table 2. The inhibition of migration of guinea pig peritoneal exudate cells by various antigens [a]

Immunizing antigen	Test antigen	Inhibition %
Lysozyme	Lysozyme	60
Lysozyme	CM lysozyme	44
Lysozyme	Bovine γ globulin	0
CM lysozyme	Lysozyme	69
CM lysozyme	CM lysozyme	73
CM lysozyme	Bovine γ globulin	0
TMVP [b]	Lysozyme	0
TMVP	CM lysozyme	0
TMVP	TMVP	75

[a] According to [18]. — [b] Tobacco Mosaic Virus Protein.

Table 3. *In vitro* stimulation of splenic cells obtained from guinea pigs immunized with lysozyme or with CM lysozyme [a]

Immunogen	Test antigen Lysozyme			CM lysozyme		
	0.25 [b]	2.5	25	0.25	2.5	25
Lysozyme	1.6	3.1	4.2	2.2	3.4	3.9
CM lysozyme	1.5	3.0	4.0	3.2	4.3	5.5

[a] According to [18]. — [b] Numbers in this row represent μg per ml culture.

Table 4. Cross-tolerance between lysozyme and CM lysozyme [a]

Induction procedure with lysozyme	Proportion of animals tolerant [b] Challenged with lysozyme	Challenged with CM lysozyme
Neonatal		
1 mg on days 1—20	9/18 [c]	13/13
5 mg on days 1—4	12/12	5/6
5 mg on days 1—2	11/13	6/6
5 mg on day 1	3/4 [b]	3/3
Control	0/20	0/20
Adult		
50 mg	0/12 [c]	3/5
Control	0/20	0/20

[a] According to [15].
[b] As determined by radioimmunoassay.
[c] Those animals which did respond had severely depressed titers.

footpad and i.p. injections of 0.2 ml containing 100 μg of either lysozyme or CM lysozyme incorporated in Freund's complete adjuvant. Booster injections consisting of 100 μg of the respective antigens in 0.1 ml saline were given 2 weeks later. The animals were bled 2 weeks after the booster injection (the time for peak titers as established in animals which had not been made tolerant). Results shown in Table 4 indicate that neonatal induction of tolerance by lysozyme rendered the animals tolerant to lysozyme as well as to CM lysozyme. Those animals which were not completely tolerant had severely depressed titers.

Table 4 indicates further that tolerance induced in adults (6—8 weeks old mice) by i.p. injection of 50 mg lysozyme in 1 ml saline also rendered the animals tolerant to both lysozyme and CM lysozyme when challenged 10 days later (100 μg antigen in Freund's complete adjuvant followed 2 weeks later by 100 μg antigen in saline, with bleeding 2 weeks after the last injection). These results support our earlier findings on the cross-reactivity of the two forms of the antigen with respect to cyclophosphamide-induced adult tolerance [18].

Thus, the two forms of antigen, although not cross-reacting on a serological level, show marked cross-reactivity with respect to all the other immunological parameters investigated (delayed hypersensitivity, release of migration inhibition factor, stimulation of splenic lymphocytes, neonatal tolerance and adult tolerance). The results demonstrate that it is possible to chemically modify a protein molecule and eliminate those antigenic determinants to which circulating antibodies are directed without drastically alterning other areas on the molecule which are recognized by other arms of the immune response.

In terms of current theories on the participation of bone marrow-derived cells (B cells) and thymus-derived cells (T cells) in the immune response, the data presented here may be interpreted to indicate that the native and the modified forms of the proteins exhibit cross-reactivity by virtue of common sites which interact with T cells but not with B cells.

Indeed, functionally diffrent areas on the same molecule may be recognized: some for carrier recognition and delayed hypersensitivity, and others to which circulating antibodies are directed [5, 12, 16, 17]. It has been proposed that lymphocyte stimulation, delayed skin reactions, and release of migration inhibition factor are carrier-specific (although not necessarily against the same areas) [1, 2, 4, 11]. Therefore, the cross-reactivity we observed may be due to common sequences serving as carrier for distinct determinants of lysozyme and of CM lysozyme to which specific circulating antibodies are directed.

Cross-reactivity with respect to delayed hypersensitivity but not with respect to humoral antibodies may be useful as a tool for studying the sequence of stages in the immune response, since it distinguishes at least two major steps, antigenic recognition and antibody production. The use of modified proteins as immunogens for induction of delayed hypersensitivity to the native antigen (without the concomitant production of circulating antibodies) has great potential for clinical applications when delayed hypersensitivity is preferred. This approach may be highly valuable in tumor immunotherapy where one would strive to minimize possible immunological enhancement by humoral antibodies and maximize delayed hypersensitivity to neoplasms.

However, since it is likely that the tumor-bearing individual possesses circulating antibodies to the tumor, which may be competing for tumor cells with cell-mediated immunity it seems advisable to reduce their titers. This may be achieved by conventional chemotherapeutic regimens, which results in various degrees of immunosuppresion at both the cellular and the humoral levels. It seems reasonable to suppose that discontinuation of chemotherapy to allow for the minimal restoration of immune competence (2—3 weeks, as determined by skin tests with common antigens) and institution of immunotherapy with modified tumor antigens would enhance the induction of cell-mediated immunity to the tumor while minimizing the production of circulating antibodies to the tumor. If the tumor mass has not been sufficiently reduced prior to immunotherapy, a recurrence of circulating antibodies and clinical relapse would be expected. In such cases it would seem advisable to reinstitute chemotherapy for the purpose of reducing the tumor mass and, more importantly, to again reduce the titers of humoral antibodies. At this stage chemotherapy should be stopped, following by a period of immune recovery and immunotherapy. Perhaps such an approach would eliminate the residual tumor or at any rate keep the residual tumor in stasis. This may be of particular importance for patients who cannot tolerate prolonged chemotherapy.

We have recently begun experiments to evaluate the potential of chemically modified extracts of tumor cells in the immunoprophylaxis and immunotherapy of cancer. The preliminary nature of the results merit only a short description.

One model system under investigation is methylcholanthrene-induced mammary carcinoma in BALB/c mice. One immunization of mice with preparations consisting of chemically modified (by acetoacetylation to various degrees) extracts of tumor cells conferred a high degree of immunity to subsequent challenges with live tumor cells. Experiments are currently in progress to correlate these observations with *in vitro* assessments of cellular immunity and serological factors.

Regarding immunotherapy, we have begun studies on the efficacy of modified tumor antigens in immunotherapy of canine lymphosarcoma and human ovarian carcinoma. One large lymph node was removed from each of 4 dogs with spontaneous lymphosarcoma manifested by generalized lymphadenopathy. The tumor antigens were extracted with 3 M KCl and acetoacetylated by diketene, using a 1000-fold excess of diketene to total protein concentration of the extract. Following surgery, the dogs were maintained on combination chemotherapy (cyclophosphamide, vincristine sulfate, cytosine arabinoside, prednisone, and L-Asparaginase) for periods ranging from 1—6 months. Chemotherapy was then discontinued, a period of 2—3 weeks allowed for immunological recovery as assessed by beginning increase in lymphocyte count, and the animals were then injected, deep intramuscularly, 2 or 3 times at biweekly intervals with 3 mg of the modified extract in an emulsion of saline and Freund's complete adjuvant; the injected volume varied from 1 to 2 ml.

Of the 4 dogs so treated one remained in remission for 9 months. At time of relapse another lymph node was removed for the preparation of modified extract. After surgery the animal was kept on chemotherapy, resulting in remission. It is planned to discontinue chemotherapy, to allow a period of immune recovery and to reinstitute immunotherapy. The remaining 3 dogs are in remission but a significant period of time has not yet elapsed for evaluation.

Recently we had the opportunity to study 4 cases of human ovarian carcinoma. All had ascitic fluid positive for cancer cells and all had metastatic disease which, though of minimal extent at the time of surgery, could not be removed. Following surgery, the 4 patients were treated with chlorambucil on a continuous basis for various periods of time until the white blood cell count dropped to 2—3 $\times 10^3$. Chemotherapy was then discontinued for 2—3 weeks before instituting immunotherapy. Recovery of the immunologic competence of each patient was ascertained by the reappearance of positive skin tests with conventional antigens, and beginning of recovery of the WBC.

Cell-surface antigens of autologous tumor cells, obtained from each patient at time of surgery, were extracted with 3 M KCl and the antigens were chemically modified by acetoacetylation, using diketene at 1000-fold excess to total protein concentration of the extract. The modified extract was injected twice, 2 weeks apart, deep intramuscularly (in the buttocks) at a concentration of 1 mg in an emulsion of saline and Freund's complete adjuvant; the injected volume varied from 0.5 to 2 ml.

Of the 4 patients treated, one remained in remission for 11 months and is still in remission and clinically free of tumor at the time of writing. Another patient, considered to be *in extremis* prior to treatment, entered into remission following treatment and remained so for 9 months. At the time of relapse she was treated with chemotherapy followed by immunotherapy. However, the volume of tumor (which was large) did not regress by chemotherapy or immunotherapy. At the time of writing (15 months following initial immunotherapy) the patient is still alive but considered terminal. The other 2 patients treated are clinically well 5 months following initial immunotherapy.

Although these preliminary results are encouraging, it is premature to draw conclusions in view of the use of Freund's complete adjuvant in the immunization procedure, the limited number of patients, and the relatively short duration of observation.

From these limited trials we cannot confirm the value of tumor immunotherapy by chemically modified antigens but wish to assert the potential of the approach, which is based upon theoretical considerations and is corroborated by work with model protein systems. The proposed approach is different from previous, mainly unsuccessful attempts to augment the host's immunological response to tumors by immunization with tumor preparations chemically modified by attaching strong immunogenic groups or haptens to the "tumor antigens". The present approach advocates chemical "elimination" of tumor-specific antigenic determinants to which circulating antibodies may be directed, while leaving those determinants to which other components of the immune response are directed, notably those participating in delayed hypersensitivity. In this connection it is interesting to note recent experiments [14] on the use of chemically modified tumor cells in immunoprophylaxis. These workers have shown that cells to which strong antigenic determinant groupings have been attached failed to protect mice from subsequent challenge with tumor cells, whereas cells modified with reagents which are generally not considered good haptens afforded a high degrees of immunoprophylaxis. Their results strongly support the theoretical considerations reported here. Experiments are now in progress to evaluate the further potential of this approach for immunoprophylaxis and immunotherapy.

We would like to acknowledge the collaboration of Dr. D. ANDERSON, Dr. G. COLGROVE, Mr. S. FONG, and Drs. M. SHIFRINE, K. THOMPSON, J. TRELFORD and M. WORLEY.

References

1. BENACERRAF, B., GELL, P. G. H.: Studies on hypersensitivity. I. Delayed and Arthus-type skin reactivity to protein conjugates in guinea pigs. Immunology **2**, 53 (1959).
2. BENACERRAF, B., LEVINE, B. B.: Immunological specificity of delayed and immediate hypersensitivity reactions. J. Exp. Med. **115**, 1023 (1962).
3. BURNET, M.: Cellular immunology. Melbourne: Melbourne University Press 1969.
4. DUTTON, R. W., BULMAN, N. H.: The significance of the protein carrier in the stimulation of DNA synthesis by hapten-protein conjugates in the secondary response. Immunology **7**, 54 (1964).
5. GELL, P. G. H., BENACERRAF, B.: Delayed hypersensitivity to simple protein antigens. Advanc. Immunol. **1**, 319 (1961).
6. HELLSTRÖM, K. E., HELLSTRÖM, I.: Cellular immunity against tumor antigens. Advanc. Cancer Res. **12**, 167 (1969).
7. HELLSTRÖM, I., HELLSTRÖM, K. E., EVANS, C. A., HEPPNER, G. H., PIERCE, G. E., YANG, J. P. S.: Serum-mediated protection of neoplastic cells from inhibition by lymphocytes immune to their tumor-specific antigens. Proc. Nat. Acad. Sci. (Wash.) **62**, 362 (1969).
8. KLEIN, E.: Tumor-specific transplantation antigens. Ann. N.Y. Acad. Sci. **164**, 344 (1969).
9. KLEIN, E.: The cell surface in immune response. Europ. J. Cancer **6**, 15 (1970).
10. KOLDOVSKÝ, P.: Tumor specific transplantation antigen. In: Recent Results in Cancer Research, Vol. 22. Berlin-Heidelberg-New York: Springer 1969.
11. OPPENHEIM, J. J., WOLSTENCROFT, R. A., GELL, P. G. H.: Delayed hypersensitivity in the guinea-pig to a protein-hapten conjugate and its relationship to *in vitro* transformation of lymph node, spleen, thymus and peripheral blood lymphocytes. Immunology **12**, 89 (1967).
12. ORSINI, F., CUDKOWICZ, G.: Thymic antigen-reactive cells do not specify serological properties of antibody. Cell Immunol. **2**, 300 (1971).
13. PARISH, C. R.: Immune response to chemically modified flagellin. II. Evidence for a fundamental relationship between humoral and cell-mediated immunity. J. Exp. Med. **134**, 21 (1971).
14. PRAGER, M. D., DERR, I., SWANN, A., COTROPIA, J.: Immunization with chemically modified lymphoma cells. Cancer Res. **31**, 1488 (1971).
15. SCIBIENSKI, R., FONG, S., BENJAMINI, E.: Cross-tolerance between serological non-cross-reacting forms of egg white lysozyme. J. Exp. Med. **136**, 1308 (1972).
16. SENYK, G., BRADY-WILLIAMS, E., NITECKI, D., GOODMAN, J.: The functional dissection of an antigen molecule: Specificity of humoral and cellular immune responses to glucagon. J. exp. Med. **133**, 1294 (1971).
17. TAYLOR, R. B., IVERSON, G. M.: Hapten competition and the nature of cell-cooperation in the antibody response. Proc. Roy. Soc. B. **176**, 393 (1971).
18. THOMPSON, K., HARRIS, M., BENJAMINI, E., MITCHELL, G., NOBLE, M.: Cellular and humoral immunity: A distinction in antigenic recognition. Nature (Lond.) **238**, 20 (1972).
19. WEISS, D. W., BONHAG, R. S., LESLIE, P.: Studies on the heterologous immunogenicity of a methanol-insoluble fraction of attenuated tubercle bacilli (BCG). II. Protection against tumor isographs. J. Exp. Med. **124**, 1039 (1969).

2. Clinical

Clinical Screening of Systemic Adjuvants of Immunity*

A. Bluming, L. Vogel, and J. L. Ziegler

Solid Tumor Center of the Uganda Cancer Institute, Department of Surgery, Makerere University Medical School, Kampala, Uganda

The *in vitro* destruction of target cells by sensitized lymphocytes is believed to occur as a two-step process: 1. The lymphocytes adhere to the target cells, a step which depends upon immunologic specificity; 2. the target cells are destroyed, the extent being determined in large part by the metabolic activity of the adherent lymphocytes [5, 13].

Several investigators have suggested that in tumors containing tumor-specific transplantation antigens, nonspecific immunologic stimulation might increase the tumoricidal effects of the sensitized lymphocytes by stimulating lymphocyte metabolism, and thereby improve the prognosis of the patient [11].

Human malignant melanoma reported to be an autologous antigenic tumor [7, 8, 10, 12], appeared a reasonable choice for testing the efficacy of nonspecific immunologic stimulation in an human tumor system. Since the effectiveness of immunotherapy is believed to decline rapidly with increasing tumor mass [1, 9, 10], only patients free of objective tumor following primary tumor excision and regional node exploration and extirpation were considered evaluable for the purpose of this study. These patients have an estimated overall recurrence rate of 70%.

Before undertaking a prolonged trial of repetitive BCG vaccination in melanoma patients, we designed a pilot study to measure the nonspecific effects of this agent on cellular and humoral immunity in man. This pilot study compared the effects of 2 BCG preparations. The first, produced by Glaxo Laboratories in England, is used as an international standard; it has a moist weight of 0.15 mg/ml and is administered in doses of 0.1 ml by intradermal inoculation. The second, produced by the Pasteur Institute and reconstituted in our laboratory, had a moist weight of 300 mg/ml and was administered in doses of 0.5 ml by dermal scratching (Fig. 1). 20 fresh dermal scratches each 5 cm long constituted a single application site. Approximately 30 min was required for the BCG solution to be absorbed into this abraded area.

A total of 12 patients, 6 in each group were evaluated during the course of this pilot study. Patients were arbitrarily assigned to one of the 2 groups, depending solely upon the degree of cooperation expected from the individual patient, since application by dermal scratching requires more patient cooperation than do intra-

* Supported by contract no. PH 43-67-1343 from the National Cancer Institute, National Institutes of Health, Bethesda, Md.

dermal injections. BCG was administered every 4 days for a total of 7 vaccinations. Table 1 lists the immunologic tests performed and illustrates the chronological relationship of the individual tests to the course of BCG administration.

Cellular reactivity was tested by evaluating the response to a newly encountered skin-test antigen, picryl chloride [2]. On day 1 of BCG immunotherapy a sensitizing dose of picryl chloride was applied topically. A challenge dose was applied at day 14 and again at day 32 after sensitization. A positive response was defined as the presence of papules, vesicles or 5 mm of induration in the challenge area 48 hours

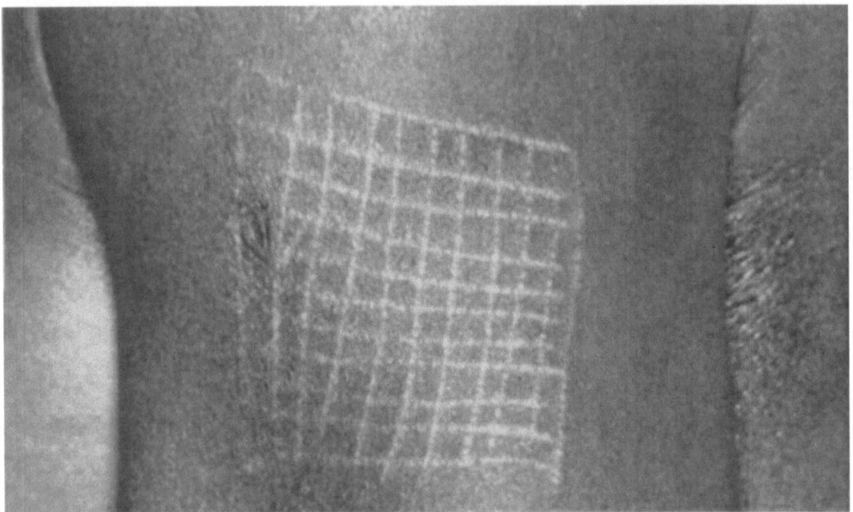

Fig. 1. Appearance of BCG scarification site 3 weeks after application

after application. Reactivity to a battery of recall antigens was tested using intermediate strength PPD, streptokinase-streptodornase (SKSD), mumps, and candidin as the recall antigens. Skin tests using these antigens were performed 2 days prior to the start of BCG immunotherapy and again 4 days after the last BCG vaccination. To insure prior exposure to at least 1 recall antigen, all patients were sensitized to 1-chloro-2,4-dinitrobenzene (DNCB) on admission, challenged before the start of immunotherapy and then rechallenged at the time of recall antigen skin testing 4 days after the last BCG vaccination. Absolute peripheral lymphocyte counts were calculated before, during, and after completion of immunotherapy as indicated in Table 1.

Circulating antibody reactivity was tested by evaluating the response to a newly encountered polysaccharide antigen from *Pasturella tularensis* [14]. Each patient was sensitized to tularemia antigen on day 1 of BCG immunotherapy, and hemagglutinating antibody titers were measured on days 1, 4, 7, 14, 28, and 32. Circulating antibody reactivity to a recall antigen (the anamnestic response) was tested using Vi antigen, an *E. coli* polysaccharide [6]. All patients were given a sensitizing dose of Vi antigen on admission and serial hemagglutinating antibody titers were measured. A second sensitizing injection of Vi antigen was administered on day one of BCG immunotherapy, and antibody titers were measured on days 1, 4, 7, 14, 28, and 32. Both tularemia and Vi antibody titers were assayed using twofold serum dilutions and all antibody-containing sera were incubated with 6-mercaptoethanol and dialyzed against iodoacetamide to measure the contribution of IgM to these titers [4]. Immunoglobulin levels were determined by quantitative immunodiffusion [3] in sera drawn on admission, on day 1 of BCG immunotherapy, and 4 days after the last BCG vaccination.

Table 1. Schedule of immunologic testing

	Admission	Prior to start	BCG immunotherapy		
			Day 1	During therapy	Day 32
Cellular reactivity					
1. Picryl chloride			+ (Sens)[a]	+ (ch)[b]	+ (ch)[b]
2. Recall antigens		+			+
3. DNCB	+ (Sens)[a]	+ (ch)[b]			+ (ch)[b]
4. Circulating lymphocyte counts			+	+[c]	+
Circulating antibody reactivity					
1. Tularemia			+ (Sens)[a]	+[c]	+
2. Vi antigen	+ (Sens)[a]		+ (Sens)[a]	+[c]	+
3. Immunoglobulins			+	+	+

[a] Sensitizing dose applied. — [b] Challenge dose applied.
[c] Determinations performed on days 4, 7, 14, and 28.

Patients served as their own controls for evaluation of reactivity to the recall skin-test antigens, including DNCB. Six normal adult African members of the hospital staff served as controls for the primary circulating antibody response to tularemia and the anamnestic response to Vi antigen inoculation. Control information on the frequency of successful primary sensitization to picryl chloride was obtained from the same 6 staff members and from 4 adult African patients hospitalized for treatment of non-malignant, non-infectious disease.

We compared the effects of Glaxo and Pasteur Institute BCG on these tests of immunologic reactivity. Only 1 of the 10 controls was successfully sensitized to picryl chloride. A single 2 mm papule constituted the positive response in this one case. None of the 6 Glaxo BCG-treated patients reacted to picryl chloride challenge either during or immediately after BCG immunotherapy. Of the 6 Pasteur Institute BCG-treated patients, 4 were successfully sensitized to pricryl chloride, responding to the challenge dose with over 20 mm of induration, and in 3 cases, with bullae formation. The effect of both modes of repetitive BCG vaccination on cutaneous reactivity to the 4 recall antigens, PPD, SKSD, mumps, and candidin, is presented in Table 2. All 6 Pasteur BCG-treated patients acquired visible reactivity to at least one antigen during the course of immunotherapy, and conversions included reactions to antigen other than PPD in all but 1 of these patients. None of the Glaxo BCG-treated patients acquired reactivity as a result of BC 6 vaccination. All of the Glaxo patients were PPD-positive prior to the start of therapy while only 2 of the Pasteur group were reactive to PPD before BCG administration. The importance of this difference in explaining these results is currently under investigation. 2 patients from each group lost reactivity to at least 1 of the 4 antigens. Three of the 6 patients in each group were successfully sensitized to DNCB before immunotherapy. After therapy, 5 of the 6 in each group were positive. The maximum change in absolute number of circulating lymphocytes during therapy and overall change in lymphocyte count from start to end of therapy showed no particular trend in either group.

Table 2. Specific and nonspecific effect of repeated BCG vaccination on cutaneous reactivity to four recall antigens

Effect	Mode of BCG administration		
	Total	Intradermal	Scarification
Conversion from neg. to pos.	6	0	6[a]
Conversion from pos. to neg.	4	2[b]	2[c]

[a] Tests included: PPD (4), mumps (3), streptokinase-streptodornase (SKSD) (1), Candida (1).
[b] Tests included: SKSD (1), mumps, candida (1).
[c] Tests included: SKSD (2).

In contrast to the differences noted between the 2 groups in both primary and anamnestic cellular reactivity, no difference was apparent in the effects of the two preparations on circulating antibody reactivity. Specifically, no difference was noted between the 2 groups after primary tularemia vaccination or after anamnestic Vi challenge, and both groups were similar to control subjects with regard to their change in titer. Incubation with 6-mercaptoethanol showed that the anamnestic response to Vi antigen, when present, resided entirely in the IgM fraction, whereas the IgM contribution to the primary response to tularemia antigen varied. Pretreatment levels of IgG, IgM, and IgA were similar for both groups. No consistent trend was observed in the effect of either mode of BCG administration on circulating levels of any of the 3 classes of immunoglobulins tested.

In summary, a potentiating effect of the Pasteur preparation on cellular reactivity to both primary sensitization and recall antigens was observed during the study; no such effect was noted with the Glaxo intradermal preparation. No significant effect on circulating antibody levels was noted in either of the 2 BCG-treated groups. The difference in administered dose may be responsible for the difference in cellular immunologic stimulation observed between the 2 preparations used in the study: 150 mg of Pasteur Institute BCG was administered for each vaccination as opposed to 0.015 mg for the Glaxo preparation. If one assumes similar absorption for both preparations, the former dose is 10,000 times larger than the latter. The Glaxo preparation has been estimated to have 1.5 to 8 times the viability of the Pasteur Institute BCG used in this study. Nevertheless, the magnitude of the difference in administered dose makes the total number of administered viable organisms approximately 1,000 times greater with the Pasteur Institute preparation used as described.

Although each course of therapy was continued for only 28 days, a significant difference in duration of remission emerged between the 2 groups (Fig. 2). All Glaxo-treated patients developed recurrent tumor by 30 weeks, whereas all but 1 of the Pateur Institute-treated patients remain free of tumor at 50 to 59 weeks from the time of surgery.

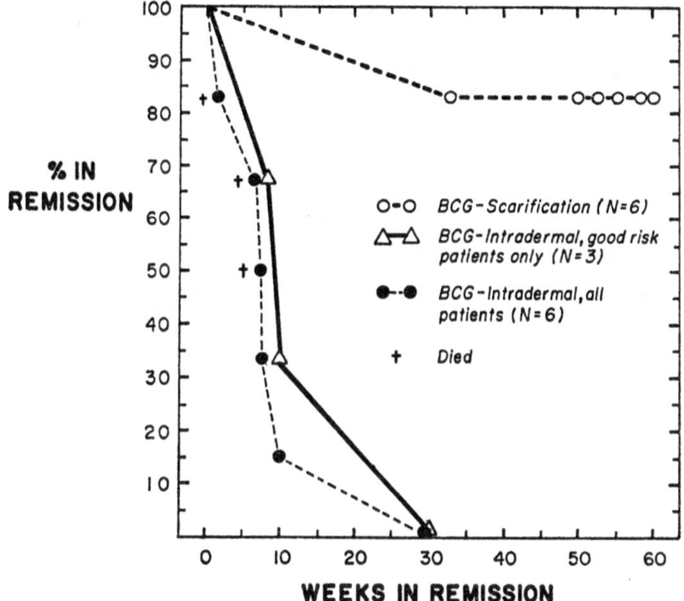

Fig. 2. Duration of remission in BCG-treated patients

To assess the value of this mode of therapy in the treatment of this disease, a randomized trial is now in progress to compare the therapeutic effectiveness of repetitive Pasteur Institute BCG vaccination with both chemotherapy and no therapy in malignant melanoma patients free of clinical tumor after wide local resection and regional node extirpation.

References

1. Alexander, P., Connell, D. I., Mikulska, Z. B.: Treatment of a murine leukemia with spleen cells or sera from allogeneic mice immunized against the tumor. Cancer Res. **26**, 1508 (1966).
2. Bullock, W. E.: Studies of immune mechanisms in leprosy. Depression of delayed allergic response to skin test antigens. New Engl. J. Med. **278**, 298 (1968).
3. Fahey, J. L., McKelvey, E. M.: Quantitative determination of serum immunoglobulins in antibody-agar plates. J. Immunol. **94**, 84 (1965).
4. Grubb, R., Swahn, B.: Destruction of some agglutinins but not of others by two sulfhydryl compounds. Acta path. microbiol. scand. **43**, 305 (1958).
5. Holm, G., Perlman, P., Werner, B.: Phytohaemagglutinin-induced cytotoxic action of normal lymphoid cells on cells in tissue culture. Nature (Lond.) **203**, 841 (1964).

6. Landy, M., Lamb, E.: Estimation of Vi antibody employing erythrocytes treated with purified Vi antigen. Proc. Soc. exp. Biol. (N.Y.) **82**, 593 (1953).
7. Lewis, M. D.: Possible immunological factors in human malignant melanoma in Uganda. Lancet **1967 II**, 921.
8. Lewis, M. D., Kiryabwire, J. W. M.: Aspects of behavior and natural history of malignant melanoma in Uganda. Cancer (Philad.) **21**, 876 (1968).
9. Mathé, G., Amiel, J. L., Schwarzenberg, L., Schneider, M., Cattan, A., Schlumberger, J. R., Hayat, M, de Vassel, F.: Active immunotherapy for acute lymphoblastic leukaemia. Lancet **1969 I**, 697.
10. Morton, D. L., Malmgren, R. A., Holmes, E. C., Ketcham, A. C.: Demonstration of antibodies against human malignant melanoma by immunofluorescence. Surgery **64**, 233 (1968).
11. Stewart, T. H. M.: The presence of delayed hypersensitivity reactions in patients toward cellular extracts of their malignant tumors. A correlation between the histologic picture of lymphocyte infiltration of the tumor stroma, the presence of such a reaction, and a discussion of the significance of this phenomenon. Cancer (Philad.) **23**, 1380 (1969).
12. Ulrich, W. J., Nathanson, L., Schwartz, R. S., Skinner, M.: *In vitro* lymphocyte stimulation by a soluble antigen from malignant melanoma. New Engl. J. Med. **283**, 329 (1970).
13. Wilson, D. B.: Quantitative studies on the behavior of sensitized lymphocytes *in vitro*. J. exp. Med. **122**, 143 (1965).
14. Wright, G. W., Feinberg, R. J.: Hemagglutination by tularemia antisera: further observations on agglutination of polysaccharide-treated erythrocytes and its inhibition by polysaccharide. J. Immunol. **68**, 65 (1952).

BCG Vaccination and Leukemia Mortality

S. R. Rosenthal, R. G. Crispen, M. G. Thorne, N. Piekarski, N. Raisys, and P. Rettig

Institution for Tuberculosis Research, Department of Preventive Medicine and Microbiology, University of Illinois at the Medical Center; Chicago Board of Health; Cook County Hospital; Research Foundation, Chicago, Ill.

In a previous publication from this laboratory [35], evidence was presented that BCG is not only effective in the treatment of cancer and leukemia in remission but also is as a vaccine against neoplasia, because BCG stimulates the lympho-reticulo-endothelial system and in this way enhances immune surveillance [6, 38].

This mechanism may account for the suppression of incipient neoplastic cell foci and thus prevent clinical manifestations of cancer. Good [12] Director of the Sloan-Kettering Institute in New York City, states that: "Cancer or potential cancer probably arises in everyone of us every day of our lives in the form of mutant cells. But they are promptly and effectively eliminated by lymphoid cells which recognize the foreignness of the mutants and act accordingly. When the policing cells are defective, however, such mutants may gain a foothold."

Spontaneous regressions of carcinoma of the breast, prostate, kidney, or lung have been observed [10] and remissions from carcinoma of the breast, prostate or lung after surgery, radiation and chemotherapy may last from 5 to 25 years followed by recurrence. It is postulated that as long as the immunological mechanism of the body is properly functioning and is not overtaxed, tumor proliferation is suppressed. Furthermore, a higher incidence of lymphomas and other neoplasms occur in persons with immunological deficiencies, such as acquired hypogammaglobulinemia and after exposure to immunosuppressive drugs [9, 26].

Studies from this laboratory have shown that BCG is a potent stimulator of the host's immunologic mechanism through the lympho-reticuloendothelial system (RES) [13, 18, 24, 27, 29, 30, 31]. Clinically BCG has been shown to be highly effective against tuberculosis [1, 4, 32] and leprosy [5] and more recently BCG has been applied with a certain degree of success in the treatment of acute leukemia in children [21, 22], a variety of cancer in adults [17, 39], in Hodgkin's disease [37], and in melano-carcinoma [3, 15, 23, 28, 36]. Experimentally, BCG can be effective when given before tumors or leukemia are transplanted in the host [13, 19, 25].

The present study compares the mortality rates from leukemia (all forms) in Chicago in infants 0 through 6 years of age, vaccinated at birth with BCG, with rates in a similar non-vaccinated population. The period surveyed was 1964 through 1969, the only one for which computerized data are available.

Material and Methods

Newborns in the maternity division at the Cook County Hospital, Chicago were vaccinated with BCG at 2 to 3 days of age. The multiple puncture method was used and the concentration of the vaccine was 2×10^8 organisms in 1 ml vials [33]. This was a service program for vaccination against tuberculosis. The number vaccinated (50—75%) depended in great measure on the personnel available. A certain percentage of the inoculated infants returned to the clinic at regular intervals for follow-up. There the reactions to the vaccine, the results of tuberculin testing and the general health of the children were determined.

The leukemia mortality (all forms) was obtained through the Department of Registration and Statistical Service of the Chicago Board of Health. Only the black population was considered in this analysis since 97% of the infants born at the hospital are black. The leukemia deaths were checked against the BCG vaccination records. The non-vaccinated population was obtained from the United States census tables for Chicago. The number in the various age groups was estimated from the 1970 census less the number vaccinated.

Results

There were 21 deaths from leukemia in 1964 through 1969 in 172,986 black, non-vaccinated infants aged 0 through 6 years: a rate of 2.02/100,000/year. In contrast, there was one death from leukemia in 54,414 infants of the same age and race, vaccinated at birth: a rate of 0.31/100,000/year. This difference is statistically significant ($p = 0.04$); p was calculated as the probability of the exact treatment of a fourfold table [11].

In the Table the results are given according to age: under 1 year of age, 1 through 3, and 4 through 6. This division corresponds to the step-like increase in mortality from leukemia. The one vaccinated infant who died of leukemia was vaccinated on April 1, 1963, and died on December 14, 1968 from acute lymphatic leukemia. This child was not seen in the clinic so that its reaction to tuberculin was not known. A positive tuberculin reaction is considered as presumptive evidence that the

Table. BCG vaccination and leukemia mortality rates — Chicago 1964 through 1969

Age (years)	Non-vaccinated			Vaccinated		
	Population [a]	Deaths	Rate/100,000/year	Population	Deaths	Rate/100,000/year
Under 1	21,901	0	—	7,820	0	—
1—3	68,824	8	1.94	26,482	0	—
4—6	82,261	13	2.64	20,112	1	0.83
Total	172,986	21	2.02	54,414	1	0.31

[a] All-negro population.

vaccination is still operative. In the assay group of children who returned to the clinic at regular intervals, more than 96% of the vaccinated children reacted to 5 TU of tuberculin 3 to 6 months after vaccination. Six years after vaccination 76% reacted. A test was considered positive by the Mantoux method when the induration was 6 mm or more in diameter and by the tine test when one or more papules were 2 mm or more in diameter.

Comment

A study of a similar nature was reported from the Institute of Microbiology of the University of Montreal [7]. It was found that death from leukemia was half as common among the BCG-vaccinated as among the non-vaccinated individuals ($p < 0.001$) under 15 years of age for each of the years 1960—1963. All were from the province of Quebec, Canada. This work was criticized because the children were not all vaccinated at birth and thus the vaccinated children were not in that group throughout their lives as they were in the control group. To overcome this criticism, a second analysis was done in the children aged 0 to 4 years 90% of whom were vaccinated at birth. In this age group the death rate from leukemia in the vaccinated group was less than one-half that in the non-vaccinated group, and similar to was the overall statistics [8]. Criticisms of the population basis of that study [16] are not applicable to the present study because of the restricted population used.

In the present study all the infants were vaccinated at birth and the vaccinated as well as the non-vaccinated were black and derived from the same rather localized areas of the city of Chicago. Thus the 2 groups are more or less homogeneous. Nonetheless, this is a retrospective study and it is not known how many of the vaccinated emigrated from Chicago nor how many of the non-vaccinated were born elsewhere. However, of 11,989 vaccinated infants included in this study who where followed intensively (clinic, etc.), 169 moved out of town and were lost to follow-up. This loss represents 1.4% of the 11,989 cases; therefore, if we extrapolate to the total group, it is unlikely that this would be a serious flaw in the statistics.

In retrospective studies of large BCG-vaccinated populations care must be exercised in evaluating the results. The ideal studies will be those where vaccination was practiced at birth and the children were followed from infancy. Depending upon the locality, the rate of infection by atypical or typical mycobacteria will vary. In a Chicago study, for example, it was found that whereas newborns did not react to the typical or atypical tuberculins, they began to become positive as early as 2 to 5 years of age (4% to PPD-S and PPD-B and 22% to PPD-G)[1] [14]. Such infection with mycobacteria may also influence resistance to leukemia.

Those vaccinated and reinfected by tubercle bacilli experience a stimulation of the RES by specific antigen; however, it does not follow that they will retain their nonspecific resistance to neoplasia. It has been shown experimentally that large amounts of specific antigen are necessary to maintain nonspecific immunity [20], and BCG has not been cultured from the organs of vaccinated hosts later than one or one

[1] PPD-S (purified protein derivative-ammonium sulfate precipitate).
PPD-B (purified protein derivative-Battey).
PPD-G (purified protein derivative-Gause).

half years after vaccination [33]. Thus if BCG vaccination against neoplasia is to be considered, relatively frequent revaccination will be necessary, possibly at yearly intervals.

Retrospective studies at best have many pitfalls. The results of statistically oriented, controlled studies must be evaluated before definite conclusions can be drawn. To expedite future controlled studies one may consider vaccinating newborns, families where there is a history of cancer in the family, and older age groups (40 and over) in whom the immune system is believed to become progressively less effective [12].

The recommended method of vaccination is multiple puncture [33], or one of its modifications, the scarification method [21]. Aerosol vaccination [34] might also be considered because it is an effective method of stimulating the RES and producing an increased resistance against specific infection [2].

References

1. ARONSON, J., ARONSON, C., TAYLOR, K.: A twenty-year appraisal of BCG vaccination in the control of tuberculosis. Arch. intern. Med. **101**, 880 (1958).
2. BARCLAY, W. R., BUSEY, W. M., DALGARD, D. W., GOOD, R. C., JANICKI, B. W., KASIK, J. E., RIBI, E., ULRICH, C. E., WALINSKY, E.: Protection of monkeys against airborne tuberculosis by aerosol vaccination with Bacillus Calmette-Guérin. Amer. Rev. resp. Dis. **107**, 351 (1973).
3. BLUMING, A. Z., VOGEL, C. L., ZIEGLER, J. L., MODY, N., KAMYA, G.: Immunological effects of BCG in malignant melanoma: Two modes of administration compared. Ann. intern. Med. **76**, 405 (1972).
4. *British Medical Research Council*: BCG and vole bacillus vaccines in the prevention of tuberculosis in adolescence and early adult life: Third report to the MRC by their tuberculosis vaccines clinical trials committee. Brit. med. J. **4**, 973 (1963).
5. BROWN, J., STONE, M., SUTHERLAND, I.: BCG vaccination of children against leprosy in Uganda: Results at end of second follow-up. Brit. med. J. **1**, 24 (1968).
6. BURNET, F.: Immunological aspects of malignant disease. Lancet **1967 I**, 1171.
7. DAVIGNON, L., ROBILLARD, P., LEMONDE, P., FRAPPIER, A.: BCG vaccination and leukemia mortality. Lancet **1970 II**, 638.
8. DAVIGNON, L., LEMONDE, P., ST. PIERRE, J., FRAPPIER, A.: BCG vaccination and leukemia mortality. Lancet **1971 I**, 80.
9. DOAK, P., MONTGOMERIE, J., NORTH, J., SMITH, F.: Reticulum cell sarcoma after renal homotransplantation and azathioprine and prednisone therapy. Brit. med. J. **12**, 746 (1968).
10. EVERSON, T.: Spontaneous regression of cancer. Ann. N.Y. Acad. Sci. **114**, 721 (1964).
11. FISCHER, R. A.: Statistical Methods for Research Workers, p. 96. New York: Hafner 1963.
12. GOOD, R. A.: Disorders of the immune system. Immunobiology. Stamford, Connect.: Sinaur Associates 1972.
13. HALPERN, B., BIOZZI, G., STIFFEL, C., MORTON, D.: Effet de la stimulation du système réticulo-endothélial par l'inoculation du bacille de Calmette-Guérin sur le développement de l'épithéliomy atypique T-S de Guérin chez le rat. C. R. Soc. Biol. (Paris) **153**, 919 (1959).
14. *Institution for Tuberculosis Research*, University of Illinois, Chicago Board of Health, Cook Counte Hospital, Research Foundation: Biennial Report **12**, 64 (1967).
15. JEHN, V. W., NATHANSON, L., SCHWARTZ, R. S., SKINNER, M.: *In vitro* lymphocyte stimulation by a soluble antigen from malignant melanoma. New Engl. J. Med. **283**, 329 (1970).
16. KINLIN, L. J., PIKE, M. C.: BCG vaccination and leukemia. Lancet **1971 II**, 398.
17. KLEIN, E.: Clinical studies with BCG in patients with various neoplasms. Conference on the Use of BCG in Therapy of Cancer, Washington, D.C., October 5—6, 1972. Nat. Cancer Inst. Monogr. **39** (1973).

18. Lamensans, A., Mollier, M. F., Laurent, M.: Action du BCG sur l'activité catalasique hépatique chez la souris. Relations avec le système réticuloendothélial et la résistance à la leucose greffée AKR. Rev. franç. Étud. clin. biol. **13**, 871 (1968).
19. Lemonde, P., Clode, M.: Effect of BCG infection and polyoma in mice and hamsters. Proc. Soc. exp. Biol. (N.Y.) **111**, 739 (1962).
20. Mackaness, G. B.: The immunological basis of acquired cellular resistance. J. exp. Med. **120**, 105 (1964).
21. Mathé, G.: Immunological treatment of leukaemias. Brit. med. J. **11**, 487 (1970).
22. Mathé, G., Amiel, J., Schwartzenberg, L., Schneider, M., Catton, A., Schlumberger, J., Hayat, M., de Vassal, F.: Acute immunotherapy for acute lymphoblastic leukemia. Lancet **1969 I**, 697.
23. Morton, D., Eilber, F., Malmgren, R., Wood, W.: Immunological factors which influence response to immunotherapy in malignant melanoma. Surgery **68**, 158 (1970).
24. Niederman, J., McCallum, R., Henle, G., Henle, W.: Infectious mononucleosis clinical manifestations in relation to EB virus antibodies. J. Amer. med. Ass. **203**, 205 (1968).
25. Old, L., Clarke, D.: Effect of bacillus Calmette-Guérin infection on transplanted tumours in the mouse. Nature (Lond.) **184**, 291 (1959).
26. Page, A., Hansen, A., Good, R.: Occurrence of leukemia and lymphoma in patients with agammaglobulinemia. Blood **21**, 197 (1963).
27. Pearl, R.: Cancer and tuberculosis. Amer. J. Hyg. **9**, 97 (1929).
28. Pinsky, C., Hirshaut, Y., Oettgen, H.: Treatment of malignant melanoma by intratumoral injection of BCG. Proc. Amer. Ass. Cancer Res. **13**, 21 (1972).
29. Rosenthal, S. R.: Focal and general tissue responses to an avirulent tubercle bacillus (BCG); intracardiac route. Arch. Path. **22**, 348 (1936).
30. Rosenthal, S. R.: Studies with BCG. IV. The focal and the general tissue response and the humoral response; the intradermal route. Amer. J. Dis. Child. **54**, 296 (1937).
31. Rosenthal, S. R.: The general tissue and humoral response to an avirulent tubercle bacillus. Illinois Medical and Dental Monographs. Urbana, (Ill.): University of Illinois Press 1938.
32. Rosenthal, S. R.: BCG Vaccination Against Tuberculosis. Boston: Little, Brown 1957.
33. Rosenthal, S. R , Loewinsohn, E., Graham, M. L., Liveright, M. G., Thorne, M. G., Johnson, V.: BCG vaccination against tuberculosis in Chicago. A twenty-year study statistically analyzed. Pediatrics **28**, 622 (1961).
34. Rosenthal, S. R., McEnery, J. T., Raisys, N.: Aerogenic BCG vaccination against tuberculosis in animal and human subjects. J. Asthma Res. **5**, 309 (1968).
35. Rosenthal, S. R.: BCG in cancer and leukemia. Bull. Inst. Pasteur **70**, 29 (1972).
36. Seigler, H. F., Shingleton, W. W., Metzgar, R. S.: Non-specific and specific immunotherapy in patients with melanoma. Surgery **72**, 162 (1972).
37. Sokal, J., Aungst, W.: Response to BCG vaccination and survival in advanced Hodgkin's disease. Cancer (Philad.) **24**, 128 (1969).
38. Thomas, L.: Discussion of Medawar, P.: Reactions to homologous tissue antigens in relation to hypersensitivity. Cellular and Humoral Aspects of Hypersensitive States, p. 529. New York: Hoeber 1959.
39. Villasor, R.: The clinical use of BCG vaccine in stimulating host resistance to cancer. Philipp. med. Ass. **41**, 619 (1965).

Immunologic Effects of BCG in Patients with Malignant Melanoma

M. R. MARDINEY, Jr., L. CHESS, G. N. BOCK, P. C. UNGARO, and D. H. BUCHHOLZ

Section of Immunology and Cell Biology, National Institutes of Health, National Cancer Institute, Baltimore Cancer Research Center, Baltimore, Md.

The utilization of BCG as an effective therapy of neoplastic disease is predicated on two major assumptions: 1. that BCG will nonspecifically activate immunologic responsiveness to a wide range of antigens, some of which are tumor-specific; 2. that this activation of immune responsiveness will enhance humoral and cell mediated cytotoxicity directed against the tumor cell itself. The present study was designed to yield experimental data in man relevant to the first of these assumptions and to further define the mechanisms of immunologic activation effected by the administration of BCG in patients with malignant melanoma.

Our protocal consisted of application by scarification of freeze-dried BCG vaccine to alternate extremities twice weekly for 4 weeks, and weekly thereafter. The dose was 15 mg of freeze-dried BCG vaccine obtained from the Research Foundation of the University of Illinois.

Prior to and during therapy, three parameters of immunologic response were assessed: 1. *in vivo* delayed hypersensitivity measured by the i.d. administration of a battery of antigens including candida, histoplasmin, mumps, and intermediate-strength PPD; 2. immunoglobulin and complement levels; 3. *in-vitro* reactivity of frozen-stored lymphocytes assayed by the incorporation of tritiated thymidine in response to PHA, allogeneic cells, and specific antigens. The last part of the study was based on earlier observations by this laboratory indicating that the inherent inability to quantitatively compare the *in vitro* responses of lymphocytes from one day to the next could be abrogated by using frozen-stored lymphocytes [2, 4].

Material and Methods

Skin Tests. 0.1 ml dermatophytin 0 (Holister Stier Laboratories, Spokane, Washington), histoplasmin (Parke-Davis Co., Detroit, Michigan), mumps skin-test antigen (E. Lilly, Indianapolis, Indiana) and intermediate strength PPD (Parke-Davis), were diluted as recommended by the manufacturer and given i.d. before and at monthly intervals following therapy. Prior to therapy, patients were sensitized with 2,000 μg 1-chloro-2,4-dinitrochlorobenzene (DNCB) (Eastman) and challenged with 50 μg after 2 weeks. All tests were assayed for erythema and induration at 24 and 48 hours: 10 mm of erythema and induration was considered a positive response to histoplasmin, mumps and PPD. 10 mm of erythema alone was considered a positive response to dermatophytin and to DNCB.

Cell-Associated Immune Function. Frozen-stored patient leukocytes were assayed for tritiated thymidine incorporation in response to a variety of antigens (PPD, tetanus, toxoid, and SKSD), phytohemagglutinin (PHA-M, Difco, Inc., Detroit, Michigan), mumps skin test antigen (E. Lilly), and allogeneic cells in the one-way mixed-lymphocyte reaction (MLR). The methods of cell freezing and storage in addition to the methods of culture and assay of tritiated thymidine incorporation have been described [1, 2, 4]. Leukocytes frozen in the presence of 10% DMSO and 0.1% EDTA were stored in the vapor phase of a liquid nitrogen freezer and later thawed, washed and resuspended in R.P.M.I. 1640 media containing 15% fresh homologous human plasma to a final concentration of 3×10^6 cells/ml. To 1 ml of cells were added 0.5 ml of a solution containing 2 μg of PPD, a 1:100 dilution of tetanus toxoid, 300 μg of SKSD, a 1:100 dilution of mumps antigen, or a 1:100 dilution of PHA. One-way mixed-leukocyte cultures contained 0.5 ml of patient responding cells and 0.5 ml of allogeneic irradiated frozen-stored leukocytes. Cells were incubated at 37 °C in a 5% CO_2-95% air, humid atmosphere. In the present protocol, cells from a given individual were obtained by leukophoresis prior to and at monthly intervals during BCG administration. On a given day, cells were thawed and cultured and tritiated thymidine incorporation compared. Results are expressed as disintegrations per minute $\pm$ standard error of triplicate cultures. Any 2 means greater than 3 average standard errors apart are statistically significant at greater than the 95% confidence level.

Immunoglobulin and H(C'3) Levels. The technique of single radial immunodiffusion on agar plates (Hyland Laboratories, Costa Mesa, Calif.), was used for immunoglobulin and complement (C'3) determinations [3].

Results

Four patients with metastatic melanoma admitted for evaluation to the Baltimore Cancer Research Center of the National Cancer Institute were studied. Pertinent clinical data are presented in Table 1. Prior therapy was limited in all patients to surgical removal of primary lesions and lymph node metastases. Patients J. L. and J. W. had no demonstrable visceral disease; patient M. R. had a small defect noted on liver scan which was stable over a prolonged period and was not associated with abnormal liver function; and patient E. D. had extensive pulmonary metastases.

Results of skin testing prior to and during BCG therapy are given in Table 2. The PPD reaction changed from negative to positive in all patients. However, PPD reaction changed to negative in patient E. D. after 3 months of therapy. The candida skin-tests also changed in 2 patients during therapy. These patients, J. L. and J. W., had no evidence of systemic or localized candida infection.

In vitro assessment of cell-mediated immunologic function utilizing frozen-stored lymphocytes will be depicted in Figs. 2 to 6. An example of the type of reproducibility obtained from the cells of a normal individual in this system is presented

Table 1

Patient	Age	Sex	Duration of Disease	Primary Site and Progression	Prioir Rx	Stage at Onset of Rx
M.R.	39	F	8 years	Pigmented mole on back; metastatic disease to left calf and inguinal nodes	Excision of lesion and metastatic lesions of calf and inguinal nodes	? lesion in liver (by liver scan) — no def. metastatic disease
E.D.	24	M	10 months	No primary found-had cervical node involvement and pulmonary metastases	Excision of cervical nodes	Pulmonary metastases
J.L.	25	M	4 years	Lesion of upper back; metastatic disease to axillary nodes	Local excision of primary and axillary nodes	No visceral metastatic disease
J.W.	41	M	9 months	Multiple skin nodules, left inguinal metastases	Resection of skin lesion, and inguinal nodes	No visceral metastatic disease

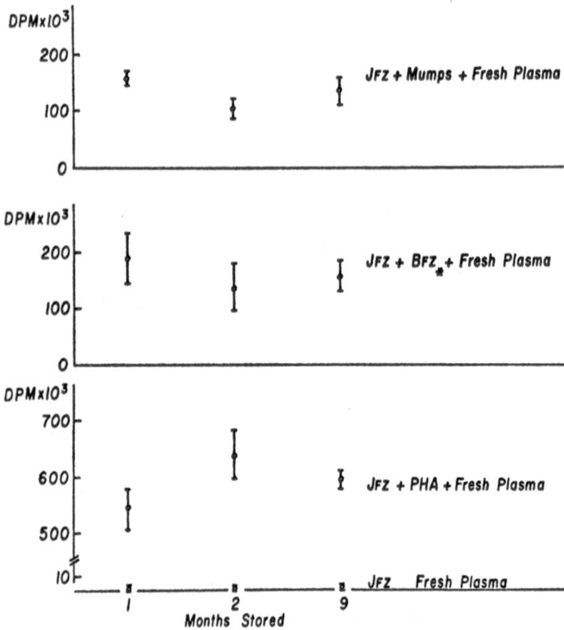

Fig. 1. *In vitro* leukocyte thymidine incorporation of normal control J: J_{fz} + mumps response to mumps antigen; J_{fz} + B_{fzx} — one-way mixed-leukocyte response to irradiated cells of individual B; J_{fz} + PHA — response to PHA; J_{fz} — control culture

Table 2. Skin tests to common antigens prior to and during BCG vaccination

Patient	PPD		Mumps		Candida		Histoplasmin	
	Before	After	Before	After	Before	After	Before	After
E.D.	—	+ → —	+	+ → —	+	+ → —	—	—
M.R.	—	++	—	—	—	—	—	—
J.L.	—	++	+	+	—	+	—	—
J.W.	—	++	+	+	—	+	—	—

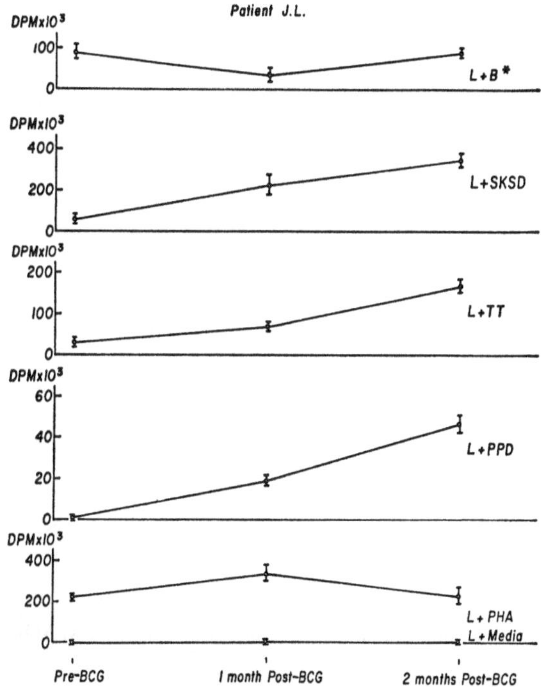

Fig. 2. *In vitro* leukocyte thymidine incorporation responses of patient J. L.: L + B — one-way mixed-leukocyte response to irradiated cells of individual B; L + SKSD — response to streptokinase-streptodornase; L + TT — response to tetanus toxoid; L + PPD — response to purified protein derivative; L + PHA — response to phytohemagglutinin; L + medium — control culture

in Fig. 1. In this experiment, cells from a normal individual J_{fz} were obtained at various periods of time and stored in the frozen state. Cells stored for 1, 2 and 9 months were thawed on the same day and reacted in the same experimental system to mumps antigen, irradiated frozen allogeneic leukocytes, and PHA. Tritiated thymidine incorporation was measured on day 4 for PHA and day 7 for the other stimuli. No statistical difference exists between the responses of the cells compared.

The responsiveness of cells from patients J. L., J. W. and E. D. (obtained prior to BCG therapy and at 1 and 2 months intervals following therapy) to irradiated allogeneic lymphocytes, SKSD, tetanus toxoid, PPD and PHA is depicted in Figs. 2

to 5. Tritiated thymidine incorporation was measured for PHA on day 4 and for the other stimuli on day 7. The changes in response to PHA were minimal and no consistent trend following therapy could be found. The only statistically significant change in PHA response is noted in patient E. D. where the PHA response, in fact, decreased.

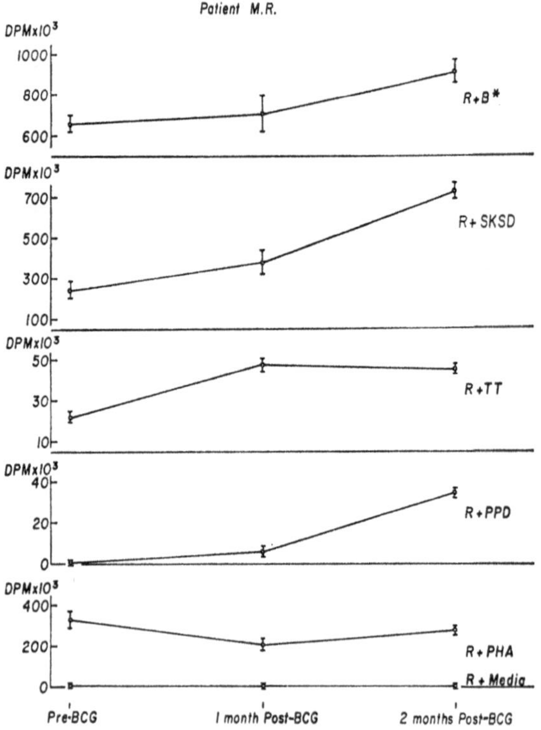

Fig. 3. *In vitro* leukocyte thymidine incorporation responses of patient M.R. Abbreviations as in Fig. 2

In contrast, 3 of 4 patients' cells underwent increased thymidine incorporation upon exposure to PPD during BCG therapy. Patient E. D. failed to respond *in vitro* to PPD despite *in vivo* conversion of his skin test. Leukocyte thymidine incorporation upon exposure to antigens unrelated to BCG, i.e., tetanus toxoid, and SKSD, was significantly augmented in patients J. L., J. W. and M. R. These patients did not receive tetanus toxoid immunization during this period of time and did not have clinically apparent streptococal infection. The data are comparable to the skin-test data, in which reactivity to an antigen (candida) unrelated to BCG occurred. Tritiated thymidine incorporation is clearly different from the responses to specific antigen. In only one patient (M. R.) was there a suggestion of augmented MLR response, but this was not statistically significant.

Fig. 6 represents the changes in IgG concentrations pre- and post-BCG in our 4 patients. 3 patients, J. L., J. W. and M. R. had significantly augmented IgG levels. Patient E. D. did not show a rise in IgG and in fact, his IgG levels fell considerably.

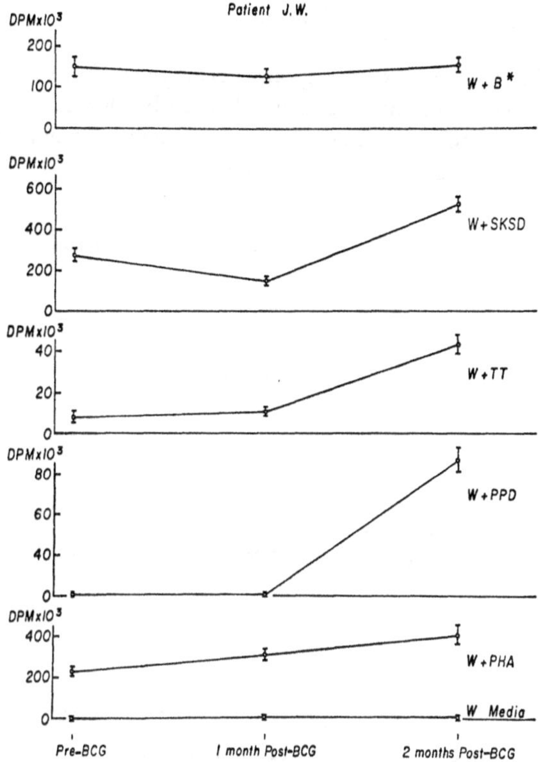

Fig. 4. *In vitro* leukocyte thymidine incorporation responses of patient J.W. Abbreviations as in Fig. 2

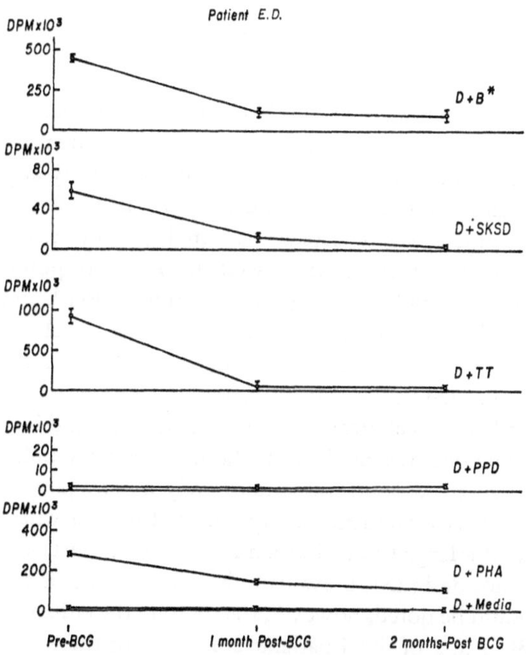

Fig. 5. *In vitro* leukocyte thymidine incorporation responses of patient E.D. Abbreviations as in Fig.2

E. D. is of special interest because his responses as judged by both IgG determinations and *in vitro* lymphocyte reactivity were not enhanced by BCG.

In contrast to the IgG responses observed, no enhancement or depression of response to IgM, IgA, or C′3 was effected by BCG.

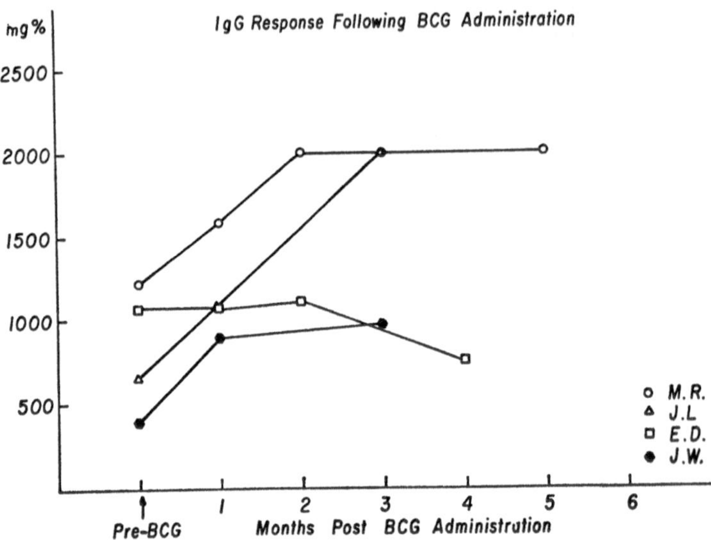

Fig. 6. IgG normal range: 1200 mg ± 319 mg/100 ml

Discussion

The data presented suggest that BCG will enhance immune function in some patients with melanoma. Cell-mediated enhancement was demonstrated *in vivo* by activation of delayed hypersensitivity responses and *in vitro* by augmented lymphocyte reactivity to antigens related and unrelated to BCG. In addition, humoral immunologic enhancement was reflected in elevated IgG levels. It is significant that the activation of immune function was selective. *In vitro* responses not dependent on previously sensitized lymphocytes (those occurring to PHA and allogeneic cells) were not significantly affected by BCG. This dichotomy would suggest that BCG has its main effect on the "secondary" response, since it appears to active lymphocytes previously committed to specific antigens.

The relationship between clinical status prior to therapy and immunologic activation is of interest. The one patient (E. D.) who had extensive pulmonary metastases prior to therapy failed to respond immunologically by any parameters tested. This observation is analogous to experience in experimental animals where the effectiveness of BCG in the face of a large tumor burden has been demonstrated.

This study was not designed to evaluate the effectiveness of BCG in the therapy of melanoma. It should be noted, however, that despite the enhancement of immunologic activity by BCG in 3 of the 4 patients studied, 2 of these 3 eventually showed progressive metastatic disease. Only patient M. R. continues to respond immunologically and to be clinically free of tumor progression 2 years after initiation of treatment. Whether the response of M. R. is related to prior tumor sensitization or to a multitude of other vectors involved in host-tumor interactions, cannot be ascertained with the present data.

The data presented do suggest, however, that if host cell-mediated and/or humoral immune function is of importance in the eventual outcome of the interaction between host and tumor, then BCG or analogous agents may become useful adjuncts to present therapeutic procedures.

References

1. Bredt, A. B., Mardiney, M. R., jr.: Effects of amantadine on the reactivity of human lymphocytes stimulated by allogeneic lymphocytes and phytohemagglutinin. Transplantation **8**, 763 (1969).
2. Chess, L., Bock, G. N., Mardiney, M. R., jr.: Reconstitution of the reactivity of frozen-stored lymphocytes in the mixed lymphocyte reaction and in response to specific antigens. Proc. of the Sixth Leukocyte Culture Conference (Schwartz, M. R., Ed.), pp. 501—514. New York: Academic Press 1971.
3. Fahey, J. L., McKelvey, E. M.: Quantitative determinations of serum immunoglobulins in antibody-agar plates. J. Immunol. **94**, 84 (1965).
4. Mangi, R. J., Mardiney, M. R., jr.: The *in vitro* transformation of frozen-stored lymphocytes in the mixed lymphocyte reaction and in culture with phytohemagglutinin and specific antigens. J. exp. Med. **132**, 401 (1970).

Attempts at Immunotherapy of 100 Acute Lymphoid Leukemia Patients: Some Factors Influencing Results

G. Mathé [1], P. Pouillart [1], L. Schwarzenberg [1], R. Weiner [1], H. Rappaport [1], M. Hayat [2], F. de Vassal [2], J. L. Amiel [2], M. Schneider [2], C. Jasmin [2], and C. Rosenfeld

Institut de Cancérologie et d' Immungénétique, Hôpital Paul-Brousse [1] and Service d'Hématologie de l'Institut Gustave-Roussy [2]

Introduction and Experimental Basis

There is an extensive literature on experimental active *immunoprevention* of cancer, which is the stimulation of immune reactions *before* the establishment of the tumor. This stimulation can be specific, consisting of the administration of irradiated neoplastic cells, which generally produces a moderate effect [10, 22] or it can be nonspecific, consisting of the application of one or several agents that we have called "systemic immunity adjuvants" (SIA) [13], the most widely used being BCG injected intravenously [2, 4, 21, 26]. A marked effect is generally achieved by a combination of both means. Though the agents are administered by different routes, the effect of combined administration is usually much greater than that of the adjuvant given alone, which is itself superior to that of the irradiated tumor cells (ITC) [21].

Our present work is concerned with *active immunotherapy* (AI), which is the stimulation of immune reactions *after* the establishment of the tumor. We are in urgent need of a weapon complementary to chemotherapy which, in disseminated tumors, is not by itself capable of eradicating "the last cell" because it obeys first-order kinetics [31, 32].

Using subcutaneously grafted L 1210 leukemia as the first model to evaluate the action of AI, we have shown that immune stimulation can be followed by regression of the grafted tumor [12, 21]. A study of the conditions in which this treatment was effective indicated that:

1. BCG given alone is rarely or only slightly effective, while ITC (irradiated tumor cell) are more frequently active, and systemic immunity adjuvants (SIA) can potentiate the effect of the cells (even when they are given in different sites and possibly at different times) in such a way that animals can be cured (Fig. 1).

---

[1] 14-16, avenue Paul-Vaillant Couturier, Villejuif

[2] 16 bis, avenue Paul-Vaillant Couturier, Villejuif

2. BCG only produces a noticeable effect if given repeatedly, whereas repeated injection of ITC is not much more effective than a single injection.

3. The effectiveness of AI is limited, and the most important limiting factor is the number of tumor cells. SIA, ITC, or a combination of both, is only effective when the number of grafted leukemic cells is 10^5 or less (Fig. 2) [12].

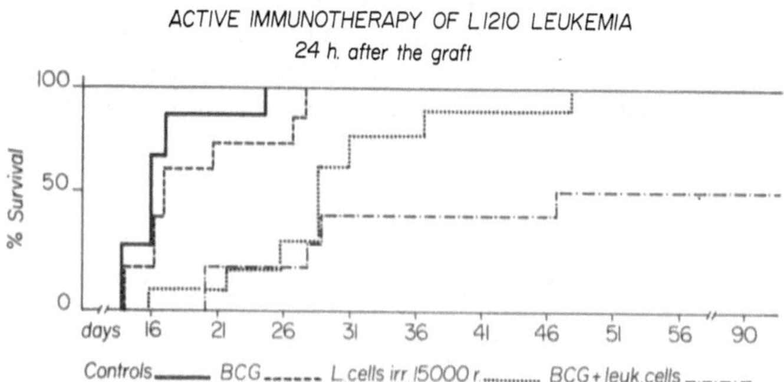

Fig. 1. Cumulative survival of mice grafted with L 1210 leukemia and not treated or treated by BCG (first injection 24 h after the graft and injections repeated every 4 days) or irradiated leukemia cells (one injection 24 h after the graft), or a combination of both [21]

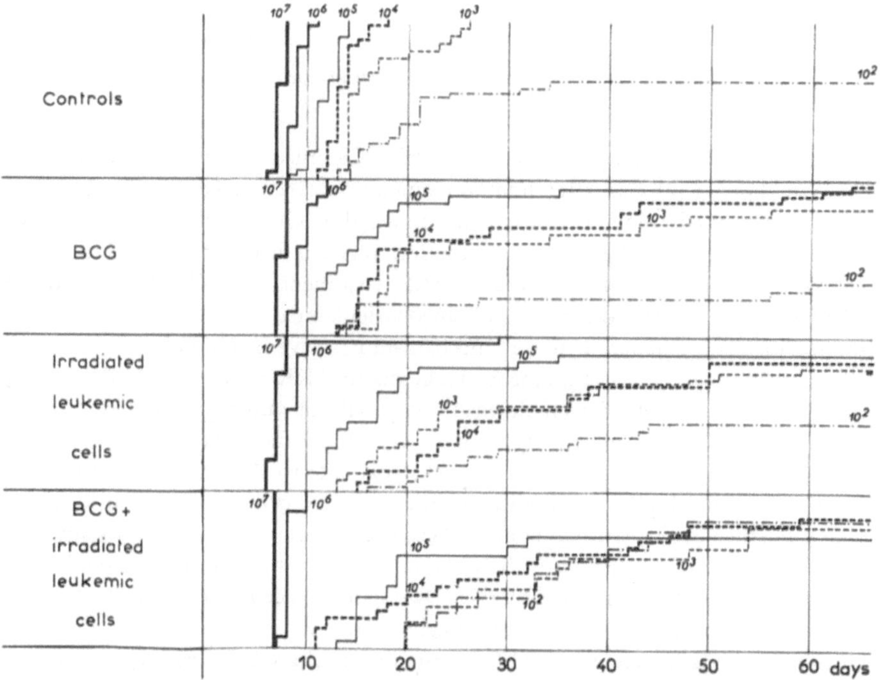

Fig. 2. Cumulative survival of mice grafted with 10^2 to 10^7 L 1210 leukemia cells, not treated or treated in the 24 h following the graft by BCG (repeated injections) or irradiated leukemic cells (one injection), or a combination of BCG and leukemic cells [12]

AI has been shown to work on other leukemias, namely Rauscher, E♀Kl, grafted intravenously [22]. It has also been shown, using L 1210 [13] and E♂G2 leukemias [3], that AI can work in systems where the number of grafted cells was higher than 10^5 but is reduced by chemotherapy. These experimental data indicate that AI is best suited for treatment of leukemias in situations where the total number of tumor cells is small, i.e. the "residual disease" following chemotherapy.

We chose for the first clinical trials of AI the residual disease in acute lymphoid leukemia (ALL) after chemotherapy. It was suspected that ALL was an unwise choice for an attempt at immune stimulation because there might be a state of immune tolerance of leukemic cells. Such a tolerant state had been conventionally

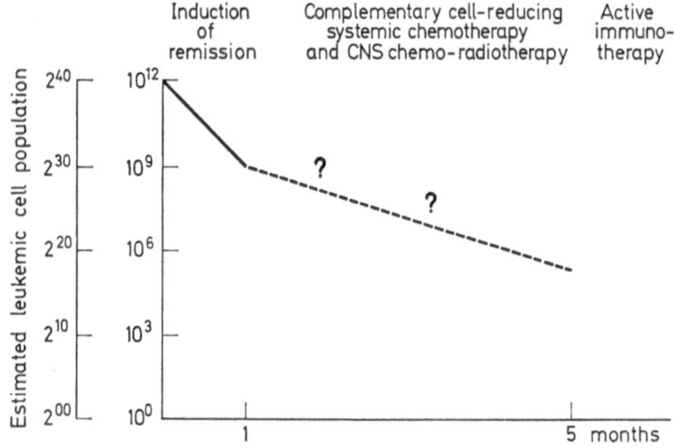

Fig. 3. Principle of the treatment protocols

assumed to exist in spontaneous leukemia of AKR mice, but turned out to be a myth. We showed [6] that after immunostimulation AKR mice are able to reject an isogeneic graft of spontaneous leukemia (induced by Gross virus), and to produce antileukemic cell antibodies. This observation was confirmed by [27]. Moreover, [1] showed that antilymphocyte serum (ALS) treatment of AKR mice shortened the latent period for the onset of spontaneous leukemia, thus confirming that an immunologically mediated "defense" mechanism is active in the host.

We have applied AI to spontaneous leukemia in AKR mice at 6 months of age, when leukemia is barely detectable macroscopically at autopsy, and have shown that AI can be efficient and can significantly reduce mortality [18].

An additional reason for submitting ALL patients to AI was the detection by [7] and [33] of autologous antibodies against leukemic cells in the serum of some patients. Further evidence for immune reactivity against tumor-associated antigens (TAA) in ALL patients has been the demonstration of the transformation *in vitro* of patient lymphocytes stimulated by their own leukemic cells [9] and of the toxicity of patient lymphocytes for their leukemic cells [11].

Further reasons for choosing ALL for the first trial are its sensitivity to chemotherapy (which must not be confused with curability [14]), and the rarity of growth enhancement of experimental leukemias by immune stimulation (a phenomenon seen frequently in solid tumor systems) [20].

Therefore, we chose ALL for the first AI trials. The experiments cited above suggested that, for optimum chance of success, the patient should have the smallest possible number of leukemic cells. To achieve this, we reduce the cell number by chemotherapy, inducing an apparently complete remission (ACR). We then try to obtain a further reduction in tumor cell load by using sequential complementary systemic chemotherapy. In addition, we give intrathecal (IT) chemotherapy and central nervous system (CNS) irradiation (Fig. 3) because of the high incidence of meningeal relapses in ALL patients and the well-known isolation of the CNS from systemic immune reactions [8]. Our available clinical data show the efficacy of both IT chemotherapy and CNS irradiation [28]. Finally, we administered AI comprising BCG, or irradiated tumor cells, or both.

In a first trial, 20 patients were given AI and 10 controls were left untreated after complementary chemoradiotherapy. While all the latter relapsed within 130 days, 7 out of the 20 immunotherapy patients have not yet relapsed, the follow-up after completion of complementary radiochemotherapy being from 4½ to about 7 years [15] (Fig. 4).

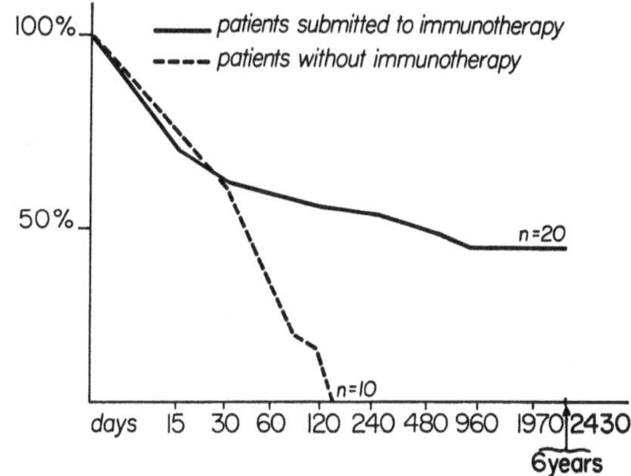

Fig. 4. Actuarial curves of patients of our first trial [15] subjected or not subjected to active immunotherapy after stopping chemotherapy. (Note that time scale is geometrical)

The objectives of the present study are 1. to evaluate the actuarial results of AI in 100 patients for whom we still have the diagnostic (pretherapy) bone marrow smears and for whom the shortest follow-up is 18 months; 2. to identify retrospectively some factors that influence the effectiveness of AI, particularly cytological variety. We have proposed four distinct varieties of ALL: "prolymphocytic" AL (PLcAL), "microlymphoblastic" AL (mLbAL), "macrolymphoblastic" AL (MLbAL) and "prolymphoblastic" AL (PLbAL) [24, 25].

Patients and Methods

1. Patients

The criteria used to select patients for this study were as follows: 1. patients were treated for ALL according to the protocol in current clinical use; 2. a pre-

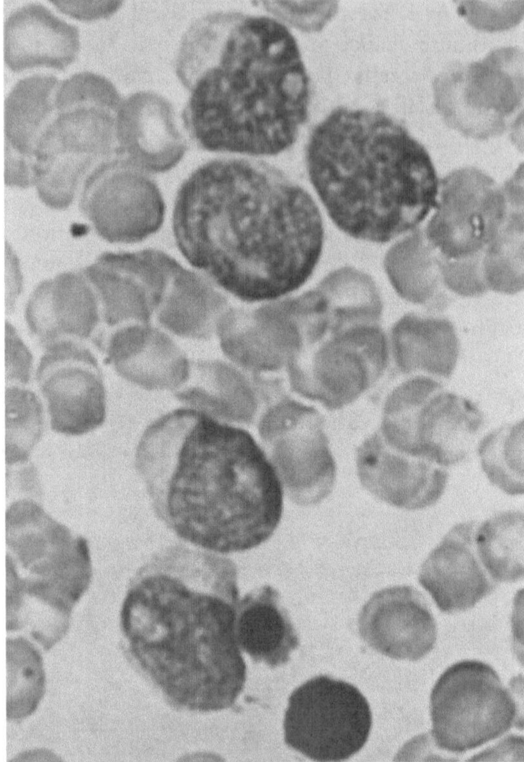

Fig. 5a—d. Morphological aspects of the 4 varieties of acute lymphoid leukemias: a) prolymphoblastic AL; b) macrolymphoblastic AL; c) microlymphoblastic AL; d) prolymphocytic AL [17, 25]

treatment bone marrow smear was available for review and retrospective cytological classification. All patients satisfying these criteria were included.

2. Classification of ALL

The classification is based on the appearance at time of diagnosis of leukemic cells stained by the May-Grunwald-Giemsa method. The criteria to differentiate the four varieties have been published [24] and are presented in color photographs in a WHO monograph [25]. Fig. 5 illustrates their characteristics as seen in black and white. The cells conventionally considered typical "lymphoblasts" have been called "microlymphoblasts" when their diameter is less than 11 μ and "macrolymphoblasts" when it is greater. Cells more differentiated than the typical lymphoblasts have been called "prolymphocytes", and those less differentiated have been called "prolymphoblasts". The leukemias are given the names of the cells which predominate (Fig. 5). The classification was made in double-blind fashion by two different cytologists and twice by the same cytologist, and reproducibility is high (86%) [23].

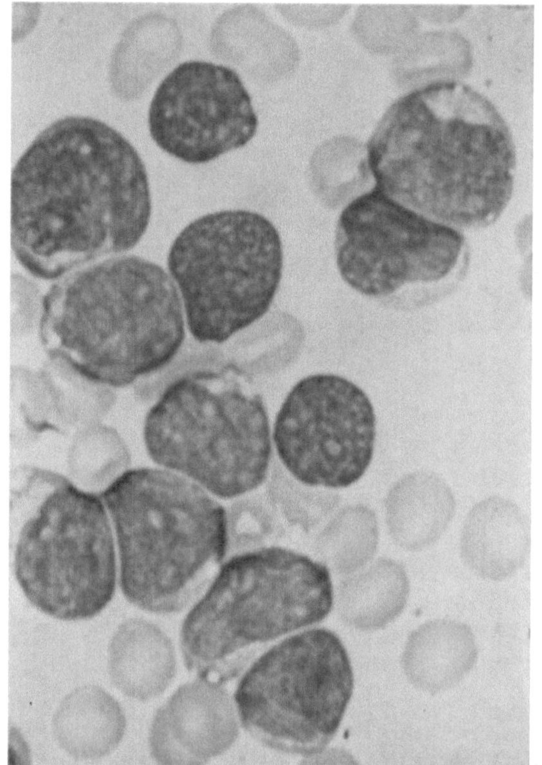

b

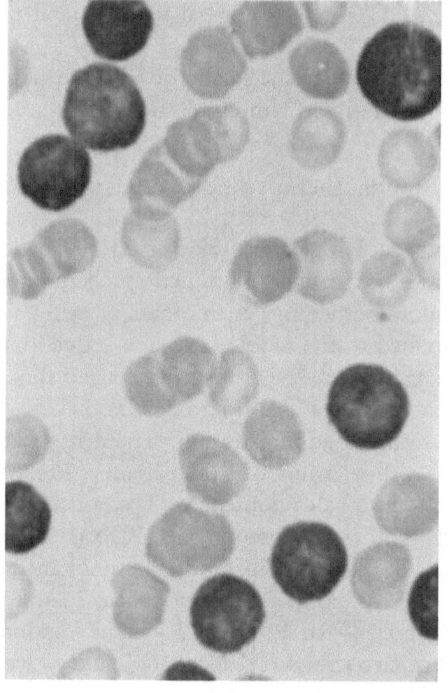

c

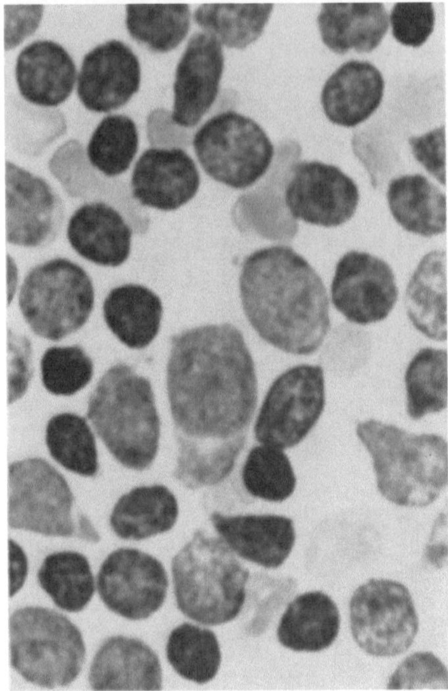

d

The age and sex of the 100 ALL patients are shown in Figs. 6 and 7. Also shown are the relative incidences of the four cytological varieties and the age and sex of the patients for each variety. The incidence peak at 5 years of age is more marked for the mLbAL than for the others, but it exists for all. One can see that the great majority of the patients with the microlymphoblastic variety are younger than 15.

3. Protocols of Active Immunotherapy and Preceding Chemoradiotherapy

The principle of the protocols was the same for all 100 patients (Fig. 3). The protocols comprise 3 phases: 1. remission-induction chemotherapy; 2. complementary cell-reducing chemoradiotherapy (chemotherapy being systemic and intrathecal, and radiotherapy applied to the whole CNS); 3. active immunotherapy.

The protocols have changed since 1964, when we started this research, in order to give our patients the benefit of new drugs and new knowledge about their value and the most efficient methods of administration. There have been two kinds of chemotherapy protocols for this group of 100 patients (Fig. 8). In Protocol 4, chemotherapy was short (2½ months) and intensive. It consisted of 3 times repeating the remission-induction chemotherapy: prednisone (PDN), vincristine (VCR) and daunorubicine (DRB). In all the other protocols, complementary cell-reducing chemotherapy was longer — 5—6 months for Protocols 6, 7 and 8; 7—8 months for Protocols 3 and 5; and 24 months for Protocol 1 — but less intensive since only one (Protocols 1, 3 and 5) or two drugs (Protocols 6, 7 and 8) were given together and at doses adapted to avoid risk of fatal toxicity.

IT chemotherapy varied from 5 injections of methotrexate (MTX) (5 mg/inj.) to 18 injections of MTX combined with cytosine arabinoside (CAR) (10 mg/inj.) [1]. Radiotherapy consisted of the application of 1000 rads (Protocols 1, 3, 4, 5 and 6) to 1500 rads (Protocols 7 and 8) to the whole CNS [2].

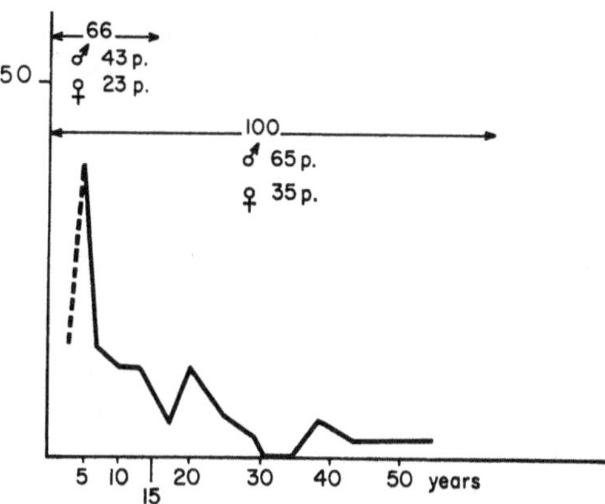

Fig. 6. Population of 100 ALL patients according to age and sex

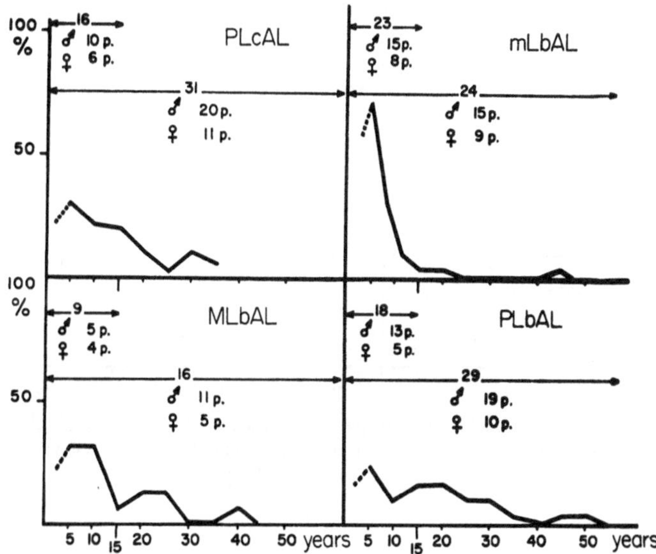

Fig. 7. Relative incidence of the 4 varieties for all patients under 15 years. Relative incidence in males and females. Incidence according to age

AI has consisted of "specific" stimulation by ITC and a non-specific stimulation by BCG applications combined for some protocols (5—8), with injections of *Corynebacterium parvum* (CP) or *C. granulosum* (CG) and, in the latest ones [30, 31], poly IC

[1] Our recent analysis has shown that this combination adds no benefit to MTX alone as far as the incidence of meningeal relapses is concerned [28].

[2] This radiotherapy has been shown to significantly enhance IT chemotherapy [28].

as a third component. The first 3 of these agents have been provided by the Institut Pasteur and poly IC by the Laboratoire Choay. Their ability to stimulate immune reactions have been verified in our screening system in mice [8, 20].

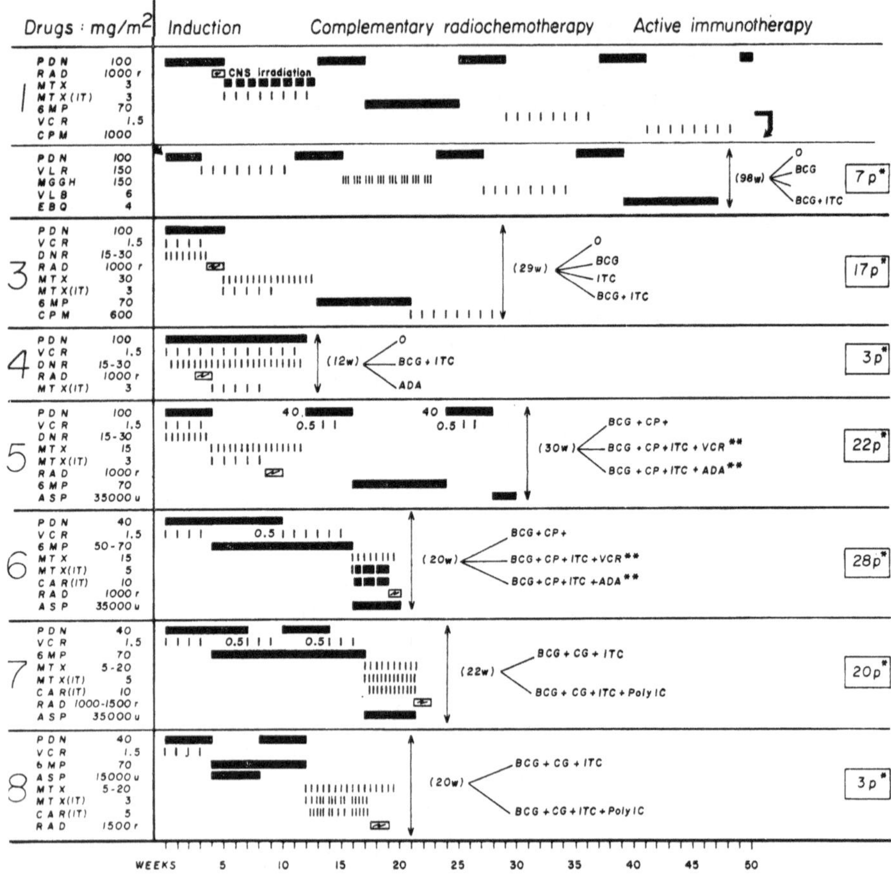

Fig. 8. The different protocols to which the 100 patients of the present study are submitted. * Number of cases in which diagnostic bone marrow smears were available to be reviewed for this study ** For doses see ref. [16]

BCG is applied by skin scarifications every 4th day, for the first month, and from then on every 8th day. 20 cutaneous scratches, each 5 cm long, are arranged in a square; 2 ml of a suspension containing 75 mg/ml of living bacteria are applied to the scarified area.

Corynebacterium parvum and *C. granulosum* are injected intramuscularly at a dose of 750 γ in children and 1,500 γ in adults once a week.

Poly IC is injected at the dose of 1 mg/m^2 by intravenous infusion daily for one month.

Irradiated tumor cells (ITC) are injected intradermally each week, during 3 months, then each month, at the dose of 4×10^7 leukemic cells taken from a pool of blood from patients with acute lymphoblastic leukemia, but excluding cells from the recipients. These cells were prepared from circulating blood by leukophoresis and stored at — 70 °C in dimethyl sulfoxide. For the first 6 injections, the cells are treated by a $4^{0}/_{00}$ solution of formaldehyde to inactivate any virus present and, for the ensuing injections, the cells are irradiated with 4000 rads *in vitro.*

Patients who relapse under immunotherapy are treated again according to the complete protocol being evaluated on the wards at the time of their relapse. In other words they are again given remission-induction chemotherapy and complementary chemoradiotherapy, and then active immunotherapy.

Actuarial Results

The results of these trials have been judged by the actuarial curve of cumulative duration of the first apparently complete remission (CDFR) and of the cumulative duration of survival (CDS). All curves are presented with the necessary *geometric time scale.*

1. Overall Results

For patients of all ages, the median duration of CDFR is 12 months, and the median length of CDS is 30 months (Fig. 9). Most interesting is the observation that these curves, after a descent, flatten out into a plateau at about the 32nd month. This plateau represents 33% of patients. This is a statistical expression of "cure expectancy".

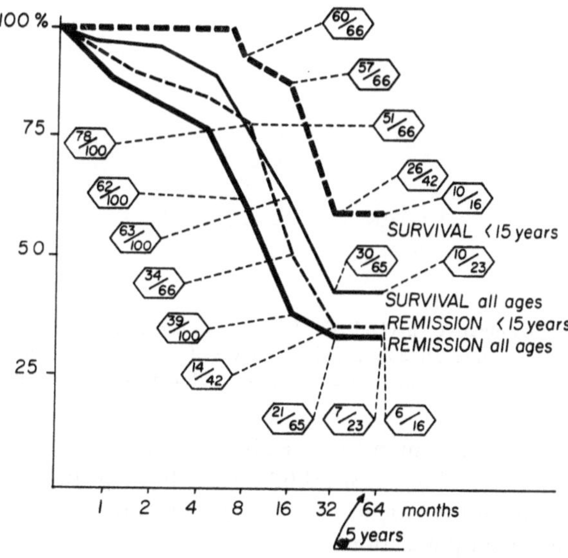

Fig. 9. Actuarial curves (1) of duration of first apparently complete remission (2) of length of survival (a) for all ages, (b) for patients under 15 years. (Note that time scale is geometrical.)

2. Results According to Age

The duration of CDFR and of CDS varies according to cytological varieties. While the CDFR curves of the PLbAL and the MLbAL patients descend regularly to a very low percentage at 16 months, those of the mLbAL and the PLcAL patients

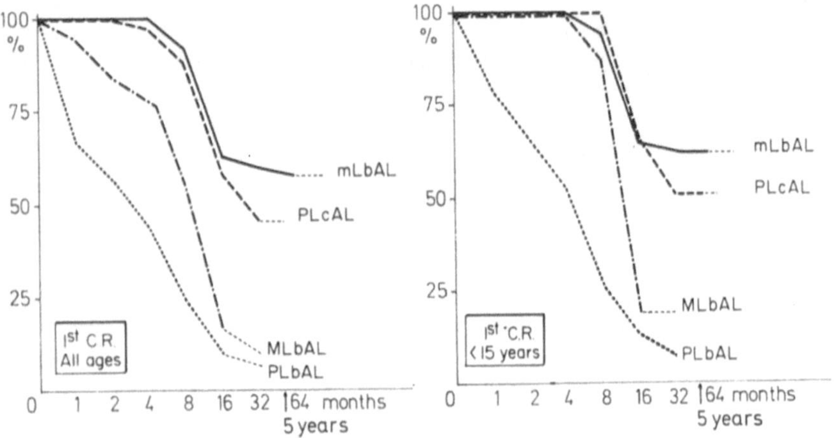

Fig. 10. Comparative cumulative total duration of first remission according to cytological varieties of ALL (all ages) (actuarial curves). Comparative cumulative total duration of first remission according to the different cytological varieties of ALL (patients under 15 years) (actuarial curves). (Note that time scale is geometrical.)

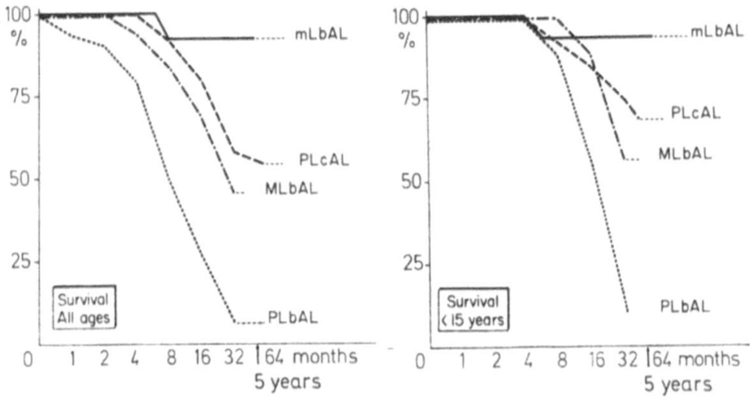

Fig. 11. Comparative cumulative survival of ALL patients according to cytological varieties (all ages) (actuarial curves). Comparative cumulative survival of ALL patients according to cytological varieties (patients under 15 years) (actuarial curves). (Note that time scale is geometrical.)

level out between 16 and 32 months to reach a plateau representing about 46% of the patients for PLcAL and 57% for mLbAL (Fig. 10). Fig. 10 also shows that this plateau is slightly higher for patients under the age of 15 (62% for the mLbAL type) than for the total patient population.

An unexpected observation is presented in Fig. 11, which shows the actuarial curves for CDS. For patients of all ages and for patients under 15 years there is a plateau representing about 50% of the population, not only for the mLbAL and PLcAL varieties, but also for the MLcAL type. This difference between CDFR and CDS under immunotherapy suggests that, while the mLbAL and the PLcAL types are sensitive to immunotherapy, MLbAL is not, but is sensitive to chemotherapy. This interpretation is supported by the observation that, when a patient who has relapsed under immunotherapy is resubmitted again to remission-induction chemotherapy, pre-immunotherapy chemotherapy, and finally immunotherapy, treatment is frequently successful.

Discussion

Before drawing conclusions from the data presented in this paper, we must critically evaluate the methodology. These 100 patients were treated successively by several protocols. Changes were made in the protocols to answer specific question(s), to introduce new agents or new modalities of administration which had been demonstrated clinically or experimentally, by us or by others, to be more effective, or to eliminate a form of therapy which had been shown to be detrimental. Our experience with each protocol, however, taught us many things about the response of ALL to therapy which we carried over to the succeeding protocols.

Protocols 1, 3 and 4, for example, in which some patients were treated with AI after sequential, long-term chemoradiotherapy while other patients, serving as controls, received no treatment after the identical chemoradiotherapy, demonstrated that AI was active in ALL [15]. Protocols 5 and 6 demonstrated that supplementary cytostatic or antiviral chemotherapy given simultaneously with AI severely reduces the effectiveness of AI [16]. In Protocol 8, the combination of asparaginase and MTX, as used in Protocols 6 and 7, was eliminated because we had shown in L 1210 leukemia that it is less active than MTX alone [17]. Some protocols were discarded before answers were obtained to their specific question(s) because we thought at the time that new information could enable us to design a potentially better protocol. We may also discard a protocol deliberately for ethical reasons.

Despite this, a retrospective study of patients treated by different protocols is possible because the same principle underlies all the protocols: use of AI to combat residual disease after complementary cell-reducing chemoradiotherapy. With regard to the correlation between therapeutic results and cytological varieties, the above objections are less important. The only cases classified were those for which we could re-evaluate the bone marrow smears taken prior to any therapy, and re-evaluation was effected by two cytologists in a strictly double-blind fashion. Finally, one of us (G.M.) reviewed each slide on two separate occasions, again in a double-blind fashion. Only then did we retrospectively analyse the response to therapy.

The following facts emerge from the data we have accumulated over the past 8 years.

1. A proportion of the ALL patients (33% for all ages, 43% for subjects under 15 years) are still in apparent complete remission. The curve of CDFR for these patients is broken at about 32 months and continues as a plateau.

2. There is a noticeable difference in the position of this plateau for the different cytological varieties we have proposed. The curves of CDFR show a plateau for a

high percentage of patients for only two cytological varieties, mLbAL and PLcAL. The percentage is especially high for the microlymphoblastic type, which is more frequent in children (Fig. 6). The fact that the curve of CDFR does not present a plateau for the MLbAL variety, while the curve of CDS for this same variety does present a plateau, strongly suggests that this variety is not sensitive to immunotherapy but is sensitive to chemotherapy.

We feel that we can draw several conclusions from these data and use the information presently available to formulate a workable basis for therapy and prognosis. The cytological correlation is very important for determining prospectively the therapeutic protocols. Since 1964 we have been treating all our ALL patients with remission-induction chemotherapy, followed by complementary cell-reducing chemoradiotherapy, and finally AI. This complementary cell-reducing chemotherapy has been moderate in intensity and duration, except for one trial. It has not itself produced a *single therapeutic death*. Other groups have been subjecting patients to very intensive and/or very prolonged "maintenance chemotherapy". The complications and deaths attributable to such vigorous chemotherapy are not rare, being 10% in some reports [29].

It seems, therefore, that the choice between protocols comprising moderate complementary chemotherapy followed by immunotherapy and protocols comprising intensive or long-term chemotherapy or both should no longer be determined by the geography of the patients or their doctors, but by the cytological variety of their disease. While it seems sound to treat the mLbAL and PLcAL types with moderate chemotherapy followed by immunotherapy, it seems reasonable to risk a more intensive and longer chemotherapy only for the other types, especially the MLbAL variety.

Weighing benefit against risk on the basis of the information we have to date, we can justify instituting intensive and long-term maintenance chemotherapy only in MLbAL and PLbAL patients. For these patients immunotherapy has not yielded the promising results indicated by the plateau feature seen in the CDFR curves for the mLbAL and PLcAL varieties. For patients with mLbAL and PLcAL varieties we maintain a pre-AI complementary cell-reducing treatment which is moderate in intensity and duration and thus minimal in risk. Further, we are justified in continuing to administer chemotherapy and radiotherapy in tandem with CNS irradiation in all patients with ALL because our data indicate that it reduces the incidence of clinical meningeal leukemic localizations in patients subsequently treated by immunotherapy [28].

These data also reveal the prognostic value of this sophisticated but technically simple classification. A predominance of microlymphoblasts in the pretherapy bone marrow smear allows us to tell the patient's family that there is about a 90% chance that he will be alive in 5 years. This type of ALL is therefore one of the most hopeful as regards prognosis of 5-year survival.

We know from BURCHENAL's study [5] that the exceptionally long-term survivor after conventional treatment may still have a relapse after 5 years. Though we have had no relapses as yet after this time, we feel it is still too early to know whether immunotherapy will prevent such very late relapses. At the present time the plateau phenomenon can only be interpreted as an expression of "curve expectancy".

References

1. ALLISON, A. C.: Potential of viral carcinogenesis by immunosuppression. Brit. med. **1970 IV**, 419.
2. AMIEL, J. L.: Immunothérapie active non spécifique par le BCG de la leucémie virale E♂ G2 chez des receveurs isogéniques. Rev. franç. Étud. clin. biol. **12**, 912 (1967).
3. AMIEL, J. L., BERARDET, M.: An experimental model of active immunotherapy preceded by cytoreductive chemotherapy. Europ. J. Cancer **6**, 557 (1970).
4. BIOZZI, G., STIFFEL, C., HALPERN, B. N., MOUTON, D.: Effet de l'inoculation du bacille Calmette-Guérin sur le développement de la tumeur ascitique d'Ehrlich chez la souris. C.R. Soc. Biol. (Paris) **153**, 987 (1959).
5. BURCHENAL, J. H.: Long-term survivors in acute leukemia. In: Advances in the treatment of acute (blastic) leukemias (MATHÉ, G., Ed.), p. 167. Recent Results in Cancer Research, Vol. 30. Berlin-Heidelberg-New York: Springer 1970.
6. DORÉ, J. F., AJURIA, E., MATHÉ, G.: Non leukaemic AkR mice are not tolerant to cells of leukaemia induced by Gross virus. Europ. J. clin. biol. Res. **15**, 81 (1970).
7. DORÉ, J. F., MOTTA, R., MARHOLEV, L., HRSAK, Y., COLAS DE LA NOUE, H., SEMAN, G., DE VASSAL, F., MATHÉ, G.: New antigens in human leukaemic cells and antibody in the serum of leukaemic patients. Lancet **1967 II**, 1396.
8. DUPLAN, J. F.: Greffes de tumeurs. In: La Greffe (MATHÉ, G., AMIEL, J. L., Eds.), p. 127. Paris: Masson 1962.
9. FRIDMAN, W. H., KOURILSKY, F. M.: Stimulation of lymphocytes by autologous leukaemic cells in acute leukaemia. Nature (Lond.) **224**, 277 (1969).
10. GLYNN, J. P., HUMPHREYS, S. R., TRIVERS, G., BIANCO, A. R., GOLDIN, A.: Studies on immunity to leukemia L 1210 in mice. Cancer Res. **23**, 1008 (1963).
11. LEVENTHAL, R. G., HALTERMAN, R. H., HERBERMAN, R. B.: In vitro and in vivo immunologic reactivity against autochthonous leukaemic cells. Abstract 203, Proceedings of the 62nd Annual Meeting of the American Association. Cancer Res. **12**, 51 (1971).
12. MATHÉ, G.: Immunothérapie active de la leucémie L 1210 appliquée après la greffe tumorale. Rev. franç. Étud. clin. biol. **13**, 881 (1968).
13. MATHÉ, G.: Active immunotherapy. Advanc. Cancer Res. **14**, 1 (1971 a).
14. MATHÉ, G.: Strategy for the treatment of acute lymphoid leukemia. Immunology. In: XIIIth International Congress of Pediatrics, Wien 1971, p. 21. Vienna: Wiener Med. Akad. 1971 b.
15. MATHÉ, G., AMIEL, J. L., SCHWARZENBERG, L., SCHNEIDER, M., CATTAN, A., SCHLUMBERGER, J. R., HAYAT, M., DE VASSAL, F.: Active immunotherapy for acute lymphoblastic leukemia. Lancet **1969 I**, 697.
16. MATHÉ, G., AMIEL, J. L., SCHWARZENBERG, L., SCHNEIDER, M., HAYAT, M., DE VASSAL, F., JASMIN, C., ROSENFELD, C., POUILLART, P.: Preliminary result of a new protocol for the active immunotherapy of acute lymphoblastic leukaemia: inhibition of the immunotherapeutic effect by vincristine or adamantadine. Europ. J. clin. biol. Res. **16**, 216 (1971 a).
17. MATHÉ, G., AMIEL, J. L., SCHWARZENBERG, L., SCHNEIDER, M., HAYAT, M., JASMIN, C., DE VASSAL, F.: Asparaginase and immune response: The place of asparaginase in a protocol envisaged to eradicate acute lymphoblastic leukaemia. In: L-Asparaginase, p. 227. Paris: CNRS 1971 b.
18. MATHÉ, G., HALLE-PANNENKO, O., BOURUT, C.: Active immunotherapy of AkR mice spontaneous leukemia. Exp. Hematol. 1,110 (1973).
19. MATHÉ, G., HAYAT, M., SAKOUHI, M., CHOAY, J.: L'action immuno-adjuvante du poly IC chez la souris et son application au traitement de la leucémie L 1210. C.R. Acad. Sci. (Paris) **272**, 170 (1971).
20. MATHÉ, G., KAMEL, M., DEZFULIAN, M., HALLE-PANNENKO, O., BOURUT, C.: An experimental screening for "systemic adjuvants of immunity" applicable in cancer immunotherapy. This volume.
21. MATHÉ, G., POUILLART, P., LAPEYRAQUE, F.: Active immunotherapy of L 1210 leukaemia applied after the graft of tumour cells. Brit. J. Cancer **23**, 814 (1969).
22. MATHÉ, G., POUILLART, P., LAPEYRAQUE, F.: Active immunotherapy of mouse RC 19 and E♀ K1 leukaemias applied after the intravenous transplantation of the tumour cells. Experientia (Basel) **27**, 446 (1971 a).

23. Mathé, G., Pouillart, P., Rappaport, H., Hayat, M., Steresco, M., Lafleur, M.: Classification and subclassification of acute leukemias correlated with clinical expression, therapeutic sensitivity and prognosis. Acute Leukemias, Nomenclature Classification, Clinical Trials, Methodology and Actuarial Results, Vol. I (Mathé, G., Pouillart, P., Schwarzenberg, L., Eds.). Berlin-Heidelberg-New York: Springer 1973.
24. Mathé, G., Pouillart, P., Steresco, M., Amiel, J. L., Schwarzenberg, L., Schneider, M., Hayat, M., de Vassal, F., Jasmin, C., Lafleur, M.: Subdivision of classical varieties of acute leukemia: correlation with prognosis and cure expectancy. Europ. J. clin. biol. Res. **16**, 554 (1971b).
25. Mathé, G., Rappaport, H.: Histocytological typing of the neoplastic diseases of the haematopoietic and lymphoid tissues. Genève: WHO 1974.
26. Old, L. J., Clarke, D. A., Benacerraf, B.: Effect of bacillus Calmette-Guérin infection of transplanted tumors in the mouse. Nature (Lond.) **184**, 291 (1959).
27. Oldstone, M. B. A., Aoki, T., Dixon, F. J.: The antibody response of mice to murine leukemia virus in spontaneous infection: absence of classic immunologic tolerance. Proc. nat. Acad. Sci. (Wash.) **69**, 134 (1972).
28. Pouillart, P., Schwarzenberg, L., Schneider, M., Amiel, J. L., Mathé, G.: Les méningites lymphoblastique. Incidence, prévention et traitement. Press Med. **1**, 387 (1972).
29. Simone, J. V., Holland, E., Johnson, W.: Fatalities during remissions of childhood leukemia. Blood **39**, 759 (1972).
30. Skipper, H. E., Schabel, F. M., Wilcox, W. S.: Experimental evaluation of potential anticancer agents. XIII. On the criteria and kinetics associated with "curability" of experimental leukemia. Cancer Chemother. Abstr. **35**, 1 (1964).
31. Skipper, H. E., Schabel, F. M., Wilcox, W. S.: XIV. Further study of certain basic concepts underlying chemotherapy of leukemia. Cancer Chemother. Abstr. **45**, 5 (1965).
32. Skipper, H. E., Schabel, F. M., Wilcox, W. S.: XXI. Schedulling of arabinosylcytosine to take advantage of its S-phase specificity against leukaemia cells. Cancer Chemother. Abstr. **51**, 125 (1967).
33. Yoshida, T. O., Imai, K.: Auto-antibody to human leukaemic cell membrane as detected by immune adherence. Europ. J. clin. biol. Res. **15**, 61 (1970).

Immunotherapy of Acute Myeloblastic Leukemia in Man*

R. Powles, T. J. McElmain, P. Alexander, D. Crowther, G. Fairley, and M. Pike

Institute of Cancer Research, Royal Marsden Hospital, Sutton, Surrey and ICRF Dept. of Medical Oncology, St. Bartholomews Hospital, London

With one notable exception [6] there is no evidence that immunological procedures are useful for the treatment of cancer in man [4, 7].

Five factors of importance considered by our group have led us to choose acute myeloblastic leukemia for a clinical study of immunotherapy. I intend to discuss these factors briefly and then present the clinical results obtained in this study.

1. Large Mass of Chemotherapy-Sensitive Tumor

Animal data have repeatedly shown the importance of using tumor cells for immunotherapy of tumor-bearing animals [8], but in man [3] studies with malignant melanoma have shown it is critical that this material should be available in large quantities and that there should be minimal residual disease before immunization. Acute leukemia in man offers this opportunity. Before treatment very large numbers of cells may be collected from the blood of these patients and often no detectable disease remains after quite short periods of chemotherapy. This is a situation ideal for immunotherapy.

2. Tumour Antigenicity

We have previously shown that stored leukemia cells from patients with acute leukemia stimulate *in vitro* DNA synthesis in autologous lymphocytes [10]. Both lymphoblastic and myeloblastic leukemia cells produce this response, suggesting that some material in the surface of these cells behaves like an antigen. This effect is not the result of the storage procedure because separate experiments show no stimulation occurs when stored remission bone marrow containing no leukemia cells is treated and tested in an identical manner.

* Supported by the Imperial Cancer Research Fund, the Leukemic Research Fund, the Joseph Frazer Strong Trust and the Medical Research Council.

3. Host Response to the Antigenic Tumour

We have previously described experiments [10] showing that human leukemia cells may be specifically immunogenic in man. This was demonstrated by the change in leukemia cell recognition by lymphocytes described above after immunization of the patients with their own stored irradiated leukemia cells

The dose of cells used to obtain this response was large (1×10^9) and in most cases the response was only transitory. This response was usually specific for the leukemia-cell antigen, but occasionally the mixed-lymphocyte reaction, if severely depressed, was also enhanced by autoimmunization.

4. Cross-Antigenicity

Interference by transplantation antigens present in the surface of leukemia cells in mixed-cell cultures prevents direct determination of individual specificity of the antigen(s) in human acute leukemia. Preliminary experiments have shown that addition to the above reactions of sera taken from the patients on the same or previous occasions frequently enables inhibiting factors to be detected [11]. These inhibit leukemia cell recognition but are not patient-specific. This suggests that the leukemia antigen in man may be common to all patients.

5. Normal Cell-Mediated Immune System in the Host

We have found that patients with acute lymphoblastic leukemia even up to 2½ years after the cessation of chemotherapy may have a defect of cell-mediated immunity giving an abnormally low mixed-lymphocyte reaction, which is not the result of previous intensive chemotherapy. This was shown by a comparison with patients "cured" of chorioepithelioma following similar chemotherapy who were found to have normal mixed-lymphocyte reactions. At present it is not possible in Britain to conduct a trial involving patients with myeloblastic leukemia with remissions not maintained by chemotherapy and so lymphocyte function in such a group cannot be determined. However, in a group of patients receiving immunotherapy with weekly s.c. BCG and allogeneic leukemia cells the mixed-lymphocyte reaction was found to revert to normal in myeloblastic leukemia but not in the lymphoblastic variety.

These five factors indicated that the remission phase of myeloblastic leukemia (unlike lymphoblastic leukemia) offered an extremely good clinical situation for detecting a possible therapeutic response following immunological procedures. The immunization should consist of frequent long-term injections of large doses of leukemia cells. It is immensely advantageous in the design of such a trial if the tumor antigen is common to all patients, and we think that this occurs in this disease. It means that allogeneic cells (carrying the common antigen) may be used for immunization instead of autologous cells. In animal experiments this situation increases therapeutic benefit, but the real advantage of using allogeneic cells is logistic. If autologous cells are used, then only patients with high initial WBC counts suitable for leukapheresis may be included in the trial. The cells from patients who do not go into remission are wasted. These factors severely limit the nature and extent of the trial. In addition, the number of immunizing doses for any one patient is clearly finite, and also there is always risk of accidently giving back to the patient viable autologous leukemia cells. However, if allogeneic cells are used, then a single suitable high-count donor (who may die without going into remission) may easily provide enough cells for the long-term immunotherapy of several other patients (i.e. from one donor as many as 1,000 ampules each containing 1×10^9 cells). A large bank of cells may be built up for use on all patients. In addition to immunizing with allogeneic cells we also give the patients frequent percutaneous BCG injections because animal data from our Institute show this increases the therapeutic response to the tumor [8].

We designed our clinical trial as follows.

Leukemia cells were collected from the peripheral blood of all suitable patients with acute myeloblastic leukemia using a NCI/IBM Cell Separator [5].

Useful quantities of cells can be obtained from patients with peripheral-blood leukemia-cell concentrations as low as $1000/mm^3$, and as many as 1×10^{12} cells may be conveniently collected from a single donor if the blood count is very high. We have treated 56 patients (including some with acute lymphoblastic leukemia) aged between 9 and 70 years in this way, and they suffer no discomfort during the 2 to 5 hours required to remove the cells. There have been no deaths associated with this procedure.

The leukemia cells are sealed in 150—1,000 glass ampules, depending upon the yield, with 10% dimethylsulfoxide, frozen slowly at 1° per minute to — 30 °C (by means of a Planer Ltd. Gas Phase-Programmed Freezer) and stored in liquid nitrogen. Each ampule contains approximately 1×10^9 cells. When required, the cells are rapidly thawed at 37 °C, washed and resuspended in Medium 199 at 4 °C. This process is found to damage only a small fraction of the cells.

All myeloblastic leukemia patients presenting at our unit (including those who have been leukapheresed) are then entered into the trial. This trial is at present in three parts (Barts I, II, III), each with a slightly different chemotherapy protocol. All patients are treated with rubidomycin and cytosine to induce remission as described in a previous report [2]. This particular protocol was deliberately designed to reduce chemotherapeutic suppression of immunological competence to a minimum, so it was neither intense nor prolonged, and we avoided the use of strongly immunosuppressive drugs. We were lucky, because there is little doubt that the regime we have chosen is a good one, between 40 and 60% of the patients passing into full remission. Of 46 patients who passed into full remission 31 were given only maintenance chemotherapy of either continuous methotrexate and 6-mercaptopurine (Barts. I) [2] or pulsed chemotherapy with cytosine plus alternatively 6-thioguanine or rubidomycin given for 5 days every month (Barts. II and III). Actuarial analysis of remission duration in patients treated with two alternative methods of maintenance chemotherapy (Fig. 1) shows that length of remission is the same for either method. The essential feature of this trial was to see whether intensive immunotherapy given to patients receiving the pulsed maintenance chemotherapy would favourably influence the course of the remission. Patients in remission were selected at random and the exact immunotherapy protocol was as follows.

Only patients in full remission were immunized. As soon as full remission was obtained, immunotherapy patients received BCG and irradiated allogeneic myeloblastic leukemia cells, in addition to the monthly maintenance chemotherapy. The cells were injected weekly into three limbs, and BCG (Glaxo Laboratories) inoculated simultaneously into the fourth limb. The cells were irradiated and injected into patients both i.d. and s.c. The total number of cells injected on each occasion was approximately 1×10^9 in a volume of 5—10 ml. The BCG was injected percutaneously with a Heaf Gun (40 punctures at 2 mm with a dose equivalent to 1×10^6 live

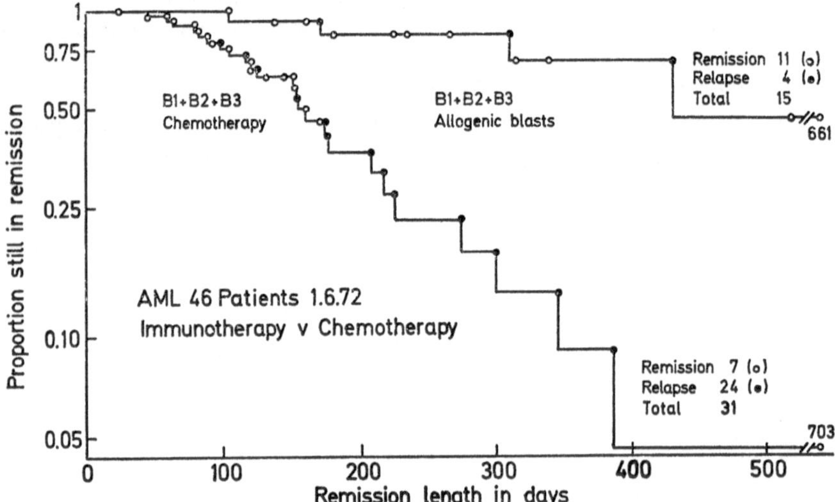

Fig. 1. Actuarial analysis of the proportion of patients remaining in remission and the expected mean duration of remission (0.50), comparing Barts. I (B 1) patients on maintenance chemotherapy with Bart. II and III (B 2 and B 3) patients on chemotherapy. The open circles are patients in remission and the black circles are patients at the time they relapsed. Barts. I maintenance chemotherapy includes 15 patients receiving methotrexate and 6-mercaptopurine; B 2 and B 3 patients received pulsed maintenance chemotherapy of five days of cytosine monthly with alternate months rubidomycin or 6-thioguanine

organisms). The limb receiving the BCG was varied from week to week in a regular rotation.

Fig. 2 shows the actuarial analysis (May 1972) of remission duration in 15 patients on chemotherapy plus allogeneic cells and BCG and compares this with 31 patients receiving chemotherapy alone (6 of these 31 patients were also given for short periods BCG, either alone or plus autologous cells, but separate analysis shows that these patients fared no differently from the chemotherapy-only group and so they have not been excluded). Of the 31 patients on chemotherapy alone, 24 have relapsed, and of the 15 receiving additional allogeneic cells 5 have relapsed. There are 2 patients, 1 in each group, still in remission after nearly 2 years of maintenance. The mean remission length for the 2 groups is 155 days for chemotherapy maintenance alone compared with 430 days for those receiving additional immunotherapy. It must be pointed out that 2 of these 15 immunotherapy patients received only immunotherapy without any maintenance chemotherapy and both did well, one relapsing at 520 days and the other remaining in full remission at 661 days. Therefore we have recently started another group of patients in remission on allogeneic cells and BCG (RMH I). So far 9 patients have been included in this trial, and separate analysis, although premature, shows the same pattern as in Fig. 2.

We believe these data demonstrate that immunological procedures used in the way we have described can favorably influence the course of some acute myeloblastic leukemia patients in remission. What we have not shown is that immuno-

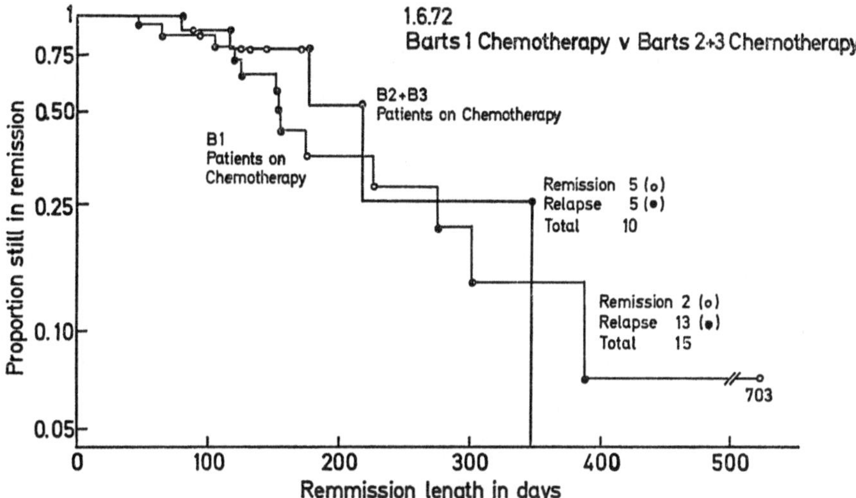

Fig. 2. Actuarial analysis of the proportion of patients remaining in remission and the expected mean duration of remission (0.50), comparing B 1 ,B 2 and B 3 patients receiving only chemotherapy with B 1, B 2 and B 3 patients also receiving irradiated allogeneic cells weekly and percutaneous BCG weekly. The open circles are patients in remission and the black circles are patients at the time they relapsed

therapy is the best form of treatment for this condition. The very favorable results of both the South-Western and Sloan-Kettering groups reported at this conference suggest that very intensive chemotherapy may ultimately control this disease, and we are now including such a program in our trial.

The immunotherapy program needs to find a parameter which can serve as a guide in deciding the optimal regime for each individual patient. We have previously described a serum factor [1] that may fulfil this role, but it will be some time before we know its relevance to the management of these patients.

Lastly, I must point out that the final assessment of the best way to manage patients with leukemia should not be in terms of mean remission length as we have presented our results today. Increases of mean remission lengths, even of many months, are not really of importance to the patient and may be a poor guide to improved methods of treatment. For example, one of the 4 immunotherapy patients in our study who relapsed while receiving only immunotherapy was treated with the same drugs used initially to induce remission and he rapidly passed into a second remission in which he has been maintained on immunotherapy for over 1 year. The duration of his first remission would be no guide to the later course of his disease. Therefore, the only true measure of success in treating this disease will be the proportion of patients who become long-term survivors.

References

1. ALEXANDER, P., POWLES, R. L.: The possible occurrence *in vivo* of the autostimulating factor for lymphocytes. Birth Defects; Original Article Series Vol. IX, No. 1, p. 111. The National Foundation — March of Dimes, 1973.
2. CROWTHER, D., *et al.*: Combination chemotherapy using L-Asparaginase, daunorubicin, and cytosine arabinoside in adults with acute myelogenous leukaemia. Brit. med. J. **1970 IV**, 513.
3. CURRIE, G. A., LEJEUNE, F., HAMILTON FAIRLEY, G. H.: Immunization with irradiated tumor cells and specific lymphocyte cytotoxicity in malignant melanoma. Brit. med. J. **1971 II**, 305.
4. CURRIE, G. A.: Eighty years of immunotherapy: A review of immunological methods used for the treatment of human cancer. Brit. J. Cancer **26**, 141 (1972).
5. FREIREICH, E. J., JUDSON, G., LEVIN, R. H.: Separation and collection of leukocytes. Cancer Res. **25**, 1516 (1965).
6. MATHÉ, G.: Approaches to the immunological treatment of cancer in man. Brit. med. J. **1969 IV**, 7.
7. *Medical Research Council, United Kingdom*: Preliminary report to the Medical Research Council by the Leukaemia Committee and the Working Party on Leukaemia in Childhood. Treatment of acute lymphoblastic leukaemia. Comparison of immunotherapy (B.C.G.), intermittent methotrexate, and no therapy after a five-months intensive cytotoxic regimen. (Concord Trial) Brit. med. J. **1971 IV**, 189.
8. PARR, I.: Treatment of the L 5178Y murine lymphoma by specific and nonspecific immunotherapy. Proceedings of the Fourth Congress on Cancer, Immunity and Tolerance in Oncogenesis. Perugia, Italy: Perugia University 1971.
9. PARR, I.: Response of syngeneic murine lymphomata to immunotherapy in relation to the antigenicity of the tumour. Brit. J. Cancer **26**, 174 (1972).
10. POWLES, R. L., BALCHIN, L. A., HAMILTON FAIRLEY, G., ALEXANDER, P.: Recognition of leukaemia cells as foreign before and after autoimmunization. Brit. med. J. **1971 I**, 486.
11. POWLES, R. L., BALCHIN, L. A., HAMILTON FAIRLEY, G., ALEXANDER, P.: Recognition of. leukaemia cells as foreign before and after autoimmunization. Year Book of Cancer, vol. 16. Chicago: Year Book Medical Publishers (in press).

Acute Myeloblastic Leukemia: Replication of Avian Influenza Virus in Human Myeloblasts and First Attempt at Clinical Application

C. SAUTER [1], J. LINDENMANN [2], A. GERBER, and G. MARTZ [1]

Division of Oncology, Department of Medicine [1] and
Division of Experimental Microbiology, Institute of Medical Microbiology [2]
University of Zurich, Zurich

Introduction

In the past 40 years many attempts have been made to destroy tumors directly with viruses (viral oncolysis) [9, 12]. Only recently was it realized that tumor cells lysed by certain viruses can be used to render animals resistant to a later challenge with the same (noninfected) tumor cells [3, 7]. The viruses used for these experiments were influenza and vesicular stomatitis, both enveloped viruses. Since these envelopes are probably derived from the cell membrane, the increased immunogenicity of the virus-infected tumor cell might be visualized in a simple way, as shown in Fig. 1.

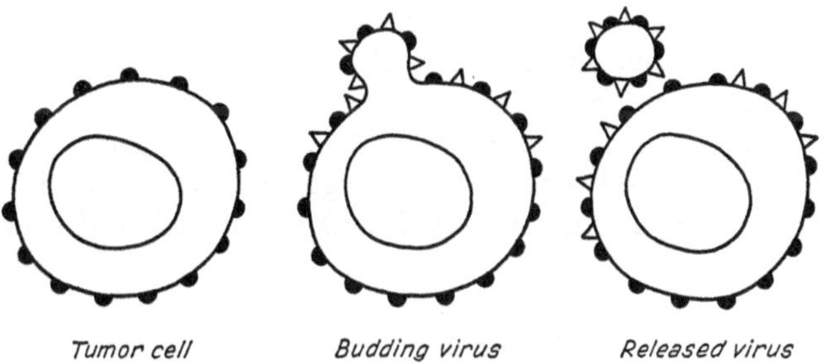

Fig. 1. Model of the hypothesis of potentiation of tumor-associated antigens by budding viruses

If tumor-associated antigens are carried in the viral envelope, they are perhaps more effectively presented to the host's immune system. Also, viral antigens present on cellular membranes could act as immunological carriers. In the case of influenza viruses, production of neuraminidase offers an additional explanation, since it was shown that neuraminidase treatment of tumor cells increases their immunogenicity [1, 8, 11].

For application of this immunizing system to man we therefore chose an influenza virus. As the disease to be treated we chose acute myeloblastic leukemia (AML) for the following reasons:

1. no curative treatment is presently available;
2. tumor cells are easily isolated;
3. tumor-associated antigens are reported to be present [4, 10, 15].

It appears impossible to obtain sufficiently large numbers of tumor cells from leukemic patients for viral oncolysis to be performed entirely *in vitro*. We therefore decided to rely, at least in part, on replication of the virus in the target tumor cells *in vivo*, i.e. in the tumor-bearing patient. This implies that the virus must be non-pathogenic for the host. For this reason we chose a strain of avian influenza virus not known to be pathogenic for man and adapted it by serial *in vitro* passages to human leukemic myeloblasts [5, 6]. This adaptation was necessary to enable the virus to go through a complete replication cycle in the tumor cell in question in order to exert its immunological helper effect.

In this report we present data on the *in vitro* replication of this adapted avian myxovirus in the myeloblasts of a 71-year-old patient suffering from AML, and the results of a first clinical application.

Material and Methods

Virus Adaptation

An avian influenza virus (Turkey/England/63, Langham strain), obtained from H. G. PEREIRA, World Influenza Center, Mill Hill, after 4 allantoic passages had the following passages in our laboratory: 3 ICR mouse kidney cell, 18 KB, 2 HeLa and 28 AML cell passages in myeloblasts from 12 different patients. The myeloblast passages were interrupted 8 times by single egg passages to avoid loss of virus. After a final egg passage the virus was used for *in vitro* infection of myeloblasts from our patients.

Myeloblast Cultures

The myeloblasts were isolated from the peripheral blood of the patients by dextran sedimentation. Sedimented cells were washed twice in Earle's balanced salt solution (EBSS). The washed cells were resuspended at a concentration of 3 to 5×10^6/ml in the following medium: Eagle minimum essential medium with 15% fetal calf serum and 0.3 mg/ml glutamine, 50 µg/ml asparagine, 400 U/ml penicillin and 400 µg/ml streptomycin. Incubation was done in stationary cultures at 37 °C in a CO_2 incubator.

Virus Titrations

Plaque assays were done in chick-embryo fibroblast monolayers.

Results of *in-vitro* Infection of the Patient's Myeloblasts by the Adapted Avian Myxovirus

On 10 September AML was diagnosed in a 71-year-old woman (see Tables 1 and 2) suffering from diabetes and cardiac insufficiency. On the same day, peripheral blood leukocytes were isolated and infected *in vitro* with the myeloblast-adapted

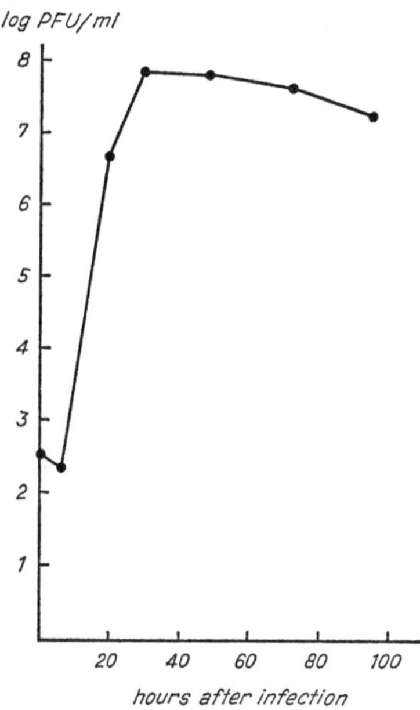

Fig. 2. *In-vitro* replication of avian influenza virus in a culture of myeloblasts isolated from the peripheral blood of a patient with AML. PFU = plaque-forming unit

myxovirus. The results of this *in-vitro* infection are shown in Fig. 2. There was definite replication of the virus, reaching a maximum infectivity titer of $10^{7.9}$ PFU/ml and a maximum HA titer of 1:64.

Therapeutic Application of the Adapted Avian Myxovirus

On 16 September 7×10^8 peripheral white blood cells were again isolated and infected *in vitro* with 8×10^7 PFU of the virus taken at 96 h from the replication curve shown in Fig. 2; this virus had therefore already successfully replicated in the myeloblasts of this patient. After 2.5 h of incubation at 36 °C, the virus-infected cells were infused into the patient by i.v. drip for 5.5 h. Four days later 10^8 PFU of the same virus, again taken from the growth curve of Fig. 2, were injected i.m. Sequelae probably due to the virus infusion were a chill of 30 min duration beginning 10 min after the start of the infusion and fever up to 39 °C during the first 3 days after the virus application.

The hematological changes in the peripheral blood are shown in Fig. 3 and Table 1.

The bone-marrow composition is shown in Table 2. All attempts to isolate the infused myxovirus from peripheral blood and throat washings of the patient failed.

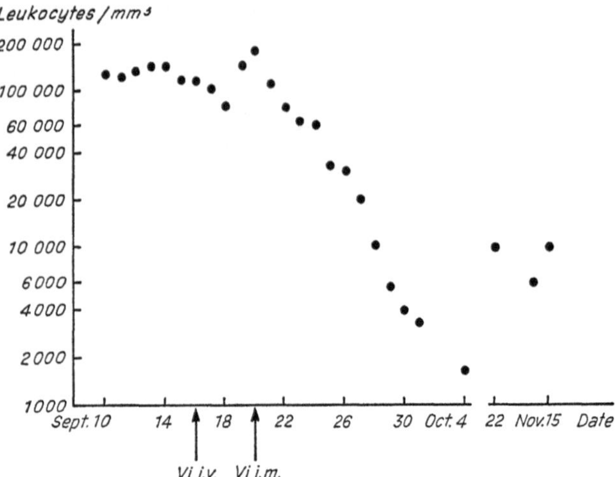

Fig. 3. Peripheral leukocytes (semilogarithmic scale). Vi i.v.: avian influenza virus infusion. — Vi i.m.: avian influenza virus intramuscularly

Table 1. Hematological data of the peripheral blood

Date	9/10/71	9/15	10/5	11/9	11/15
Leukocytes $\times 10^3$/mm³	128	117	3	6	10
Myeloblasts (%)	88	88	55	0	0
Granulocytes (%)	6	8	0	29	58
Monocytes (%)	0	1	0	51	30
Lymphocytes (%)	6	2	45	20	11
Hemoglobin (g-%)	8.6	9.7	9	9.6	8.1
Reticulocytes (%)	3.2		0.2	0.3	5.6
Platelets $\times 10^3$/mm³	136		233	210	141

Table 2. Bone-marrow composition

Date	9/10/71	10/22	11/10	11/18
Erythropoietic cells (%)	6	1.5	10	14.5
Granulopoietic cells (%)	9	1	10	39
Myeloblasts (%)	83.5	95.5	76	40.5

Intracutaneous injections of 10^8 twice frozen and thawed unifected peripheral leukocytes in 0.2 ml EBSS gave the following results: negative on day 1 after infusion of the virus-infected cells; on day 33, positive immediate reaction (at 30 min 15 mm weal and flare) and positive delayed reaction (at 24 h 5 mm induration and 8 mm redness).

Pseudomonas was isolated from the blood of the patient on 21 October, during a temporary agranulocytosis (see Table 1). After one week of treatment with antibiotics the patient became afebrile. On 18 November the patient, now in fairly good general condition, suddenly died due to bleeding from a lung abscess, from which *Pseudomonas* was again isolated. Attempts at isolating the virus from autopsy material were again negative.

Discussion

Since AML still has a very poor prognosis especially in older people, new therapeutic approaches have to be found. On the basis of viral oncolysis in animals, as outlined in the introduction, we decided to adapt an avian myxovirus to leukemic myeloblasts. This adaptation was successful as is clear from the replication curve in Fig. 2, and its clinical use induced a partial remission in a 71-year-old AML patient. The effect of viruses on malignant cells *in vivo* can be due to several mechanisms [13].

1. Direct oncolytic effect. In our patient a direct massive viral oncolysis seems improbable, since at no time was viremia detected. The slow decrease of leukemic cells (see Fig. 3) starting only 6 days after the virus infusion argues against direct lysis of the tumor cells.

2. Interferon induction. Interferon has an inhibitory effect on several tumors in the mouse [16]. The production of interferon in our patient was probably only of short duration since single virus injections [2] or natural virus infections [14] induce interferon for a few days only.

3. Postoncolytic immunity [7]. Three observations favor the explanation that this partial remission was due to postoncolytic immunity.

a) The leukemic cells started to decline between day 6 and day 8 after the virus infusion, at a time when an immune reaction could well be functioning.

b) Positive delayed reaction with uninfected leukemic cells 33 days after the virus infusion.

c) Slow decline of leukemic cells over several weeks. Sera from mice immunized with viral oncolysates can protect other animals against challenge with tumor cells. However, such sera have no direct cytotoxic effect [8] and seem to act in a protracted manner.

We believe that application of this avian myxovirus can be considered for treatment of AML, provided the following conditions are fulfilled:

1. The patient should not be in extremis, since it is several weeks before the remission can be expected.

2. The patient should not have had immunosuppressive treatment during the weeks before virus administration.

3. Isolation of large numbers of myeloblasts must be possible.

4. The clinician must have access to a competent virological laboratory.

5. Strong virus replication must be confirmed in the leukemic myeloblasts *in vitro*.

Acknowledgements

Supported by the Julius Müller Foundation for Cancer Research, Zurich, and the Hans Groeber Stiftung, Vaduz. The authors gratefully acknowledge the assistance of Mrs. S. EKENBARK, Miss E. HEROLD, Mrs. A. HALLER, Miss J. BOERSMA, Miss B. PFISTER, Miss R. LEEMANN and Miss M. SCHAICH.

References

1. BAGSHAWE, K. D., CURRIE, G. A.: Immunogenicity of L 1210 leukemia cells after treatment with neuraminidase. Nature (Lond.) **218**, 1254 (1968).
2. BARON, S., BUCKLER, C. E.: Circulating interferon in mice after intravenous injection of virus. Science **141**, 1061 (1963).
3. BOONE, C., BLACKMAN, K., BRANDCHAFT, P.: Tumor immunity induced in mice with cell-free homogenates of influenza virus-infected tumor cells. Nature (Lond.) **231**, 265 (1971).
4. DORÉ, J. F., MOTTA, R., MARHOLEV, L., HRSAK, I., COLAS DE LA NOUE, H., SEMAN, G., DE VASSAL, F., MATHÉ, G.: New antigens in human leukemic cells, and antibody in the serum of leukemic patients. Lancet **1967 II**, 1396.
5. GERBER, A., SAUTER, C., LINDENMANN, J.: Fowl plague virus adapted to human epithelial tumor cells and human myeloblasts *in vitro*. I. Characteristics and replication in monolayer cultures. Arch. ges. Virusforsch. **40**, 137 (1973a).
6. GERBER, A., SAUTER, C., LINDENMANN, J.: Fowl plague virus adapted to human epithelial tumor cells and human myeloblasts *in vitro*. II. Replication in human leukemic myeloblast cultures. Arch. ges. Virusforsch. **40**, 255 (1973b).
7. LINDENMANN, J., KLEIN, P. A.: Viral oncolysis: Increased immunogenicity of host cell antigen associated with influenza virus. J. exp. Med. **126**, 93 (1967a).
8. LINDENMANN, J., KLEIN, P. A.: Immunological aspects of viral oncolysis. Recent Results in Cancer Research, Vol. 9. Berlin-Heidelberg-New York: Springer 1967.
9. MOORE, A. E.: The oncolytic viruses. Progr. exp. Tumor Res. (Basel) **1**, 411 (1960).
10. SAUTER, C., KISTLER, G. S.: Rosette formation in white blood cell cultures from patients with acute myeloblastic leukemia. Experientia (Basel) **26**, 526 (1970).
11. SIMMONS, R. E., RIOS, A.: Immunotherapy of cancer: Immunospecific rejection of tumors in recipients of neuraminidase-treated tumor cells plus BCG. Science **174**, 591 (1971).
12. SOUTHAM, C. M.: Present status of oncolytic virus studies. Trans. N.Y. Acad. Sci., Ser. II, **22**, 657 (1960).
13. WEBB, H. E., WETHERLEY-MEIN, G., GORDON SMITH, C. E., MCMAHON, D.: Leukemia and neoplastic processes treated with Langat and Hyasanur forest disease viruses: A clinical and laboratory study of 28 patients. Brit. med. J. **1966 I**, 258.
14. WHEELOCK, E. F., SIBLEY, W. A.: Interferon in human serum during clinical viral infections. Lancet **1964 II**, 382.
15. YOSHIDA, T., IMAI, K.: Auto-antibody to human leukemic cell membrane as detected by immune adherence. Rev. europ Étud. clin. biol. **15**, 61 (1970).
16. YOUNG, C. W.: Interferon induction in cancer: With some observations of the clinical effects of poly I:C. Med. Clin. N. Amer. **55**, 721 (1971).

Preliminary Results of a Randomized Trial of BCG Immunotherapy in Burkitt's Lymphoma*

I. T. MAGRATH, J. L. ZIEGLER, and A. Z. BLUMING

Uganda Cancer Institute Kampala, Uganda

Introduction

Burkitt's lymphoma is an exceptional malignancy in that chemotherapy alone will induce complete and often sustained remissions in 90% of patients. Some patients have remained free from disease for periods in excess of 10 years [5] but more often relapse occurs (in 65%) almost always in the first year, and may or may not be responsive to further chemotherapy. Randomized trials of various chemotherapeutic regimens have not shown that multiple doses of cyclophosphamide or combinations of drugs have a significant advantage over a single dose of cyclophosphamide [6, 7, 9].

Because of the positive correlation in Burkitt's lymphoma of clinical course with cutaneous reactivity to recall [8] and autologous tumor antigens [2], we attempted to determine whether relapse could be prevented by potentiating cell-mediated immunity with BCG after inducing remission with cyclophosphamide. The present report is an account of the preliminary results of this ongoing clinical trial.

Method

All untreated patients with histologically and cytologically proven Burkitt's lymphoma are initially staged according to the extent of their tumor (Table 1) and

Table 1. Clinical staging of Burkitt's lymphoma

Stage I	Localized facial tumor
Stage II	Multiple facial tumors
Stage III	Intra-abdominal, intra-thoracic, osseous or paraspinal tumor
Stage IV	Bone marrow or meningeal tumor

* At the time of going to press there are 21 evaluable patients in the BCG treated group and 19 in the control group. Eleven relapses have occured in each group, and there are no differences in remission duration. Differences in relapse sites between the groups are still present, but these can be adequatly explained on the basis of differences in sites of presenting tumour.

then treated with i.v. cyclophosphamide (40 mg per kg) repeated after 2 weeks. Two weeks after the second dose of cyclophosphamide, patients are randomized by stage to have either BCG, or no further therapy. BCG application is made in a manner identical to the method of MATHÉ [4]. An area 5 cm × 5 cm is scarified and Pasteur Institute BCG (150 mg lyophilized vaccine equivalent to a maximum of 3×10^8 viable organisms in 0.5 ml of distilled water) applied to this area and allowed to dry. A total of 13 applications are performed in each patient, using each limb in turn, the first 7 at 4-day intervals, the last 6 at weekly intervals, giving a total of 10 weeks of immunotherapy. Skin tests using three recall antigens are performed at the time of randomization, after 7 applications and upon completion of therapy in the BCG-treated group, and at equivalent times in the control group. Serum is taken upon admission and at regular intervals thereafter for immunoglobulin levels and serological studies. Differential blood counts are performed weekly.

Results

Of 28 patients with Burkitt's lymphoma admitted to the Lymphoma Treatment Centre since Feb. 1971, 18 were admitted to the trial. Of the remainder, 4 died and 5 relapsed prior to randomization, and one defaulted after initial treatment and was lost to the study. The 9 evaluable patients in each group were comparable with regard to age, sex and clinical stage (Table 2).

Table 2. Comparison of BCG-treated and control patient groups

	BCG	Control
Total no.	9	9
Median age	7 years	6 years
Male/Female	3/6	5/4
Stage I—II	1	1
Stage III	7	7
Stage IV	1	1

All patients were followed for at least 3 months, and 5 in each group for at least 9 months. At present, 3 have relapsed in the BCG-treated group and 6 in the control group. Of the former, 2 relapses were manifested solely by malignant cells in the cerebrospinal fluid after 3 and 7 applications of BCG, respectively. In the control group, however, all patients had tumor outside the central neıvous system, whether or not there was neurological involvement (Table 3).

There was no significant difference in duration of remission between the groups (Fig. 1).

Comparison of cutaneous reactivity at the time of randomization and 10 weeks later showed that there was an increase in the total number of positive skin tests (induration greater than 5 mm diameter at 48 h) in the BCG-treated patients, but not in the control group (Table 4). All patients in the BCG group who were negative to tuberculin (PPD, 10 T.U.) prior to BCG therapy became positive, as did 3 patients

Table 3. Relapse patterns in BCG-treated patients and controls

	Number of patients	Total relapses	Extra CNS relapses
BCG	9	3	1
Control	9	6	6

CNS = Central nervous system.

Table 4. Positive skin tests to mumps, candida, and Sk-Sd in BCG patients and controls

	Number of patients	Positive skin tests prior to therapy	Positive skin tests later	Percent increase tests
BCG	9	8/27 (30%)	16/27 (60%)	30%
Control	7	11/21 (52%)	9/21 (43%)	—9%

Each patient had 3 skin tests:

1. Varidase (Sk-Sd) (diluted 1.50, i.e. each ml containing 400 U streptokinase and 100 U streptodornase).
2. Mumps skin-test antigen (Eli Lilly and Company, Indianapolis, Indian).
3. *Candida albicans* (Dermatophytin "O" 1:100 diluted 1:20 Hollister-Stier).

A positive reaction was defined as 5 mm or more of induration at 48 h.

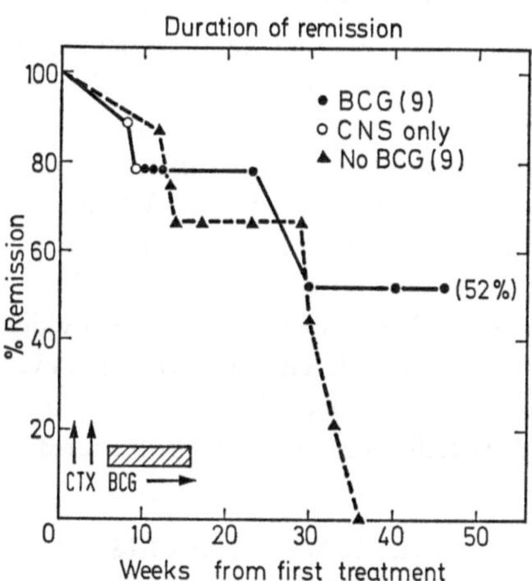

Fig. 1. Remission duration in BCG-treated patients and controls. With such small numbers, little account can be taken of the parts of the curves efter 30 weeks

Actuarial curves showing the predicted complete remission rate (i.e. percentage of patients who have relapsed) at intervals after presentation. The patients in the BCG group who relapsed with malignant CSF pleocytosis only are depicted by open circles.

There is no significant difference in these curves. Although some patients in the BCG group have not yet relapsed, they are still at risk until duration of remission is in excess of one year.

in the control group. 8 of the 9 patients in the BCG group had conversions from negative to positive reactions to one or more recall antigens (a total of 10 conversions), against only 3 patients in the control group (3 conversions).

There were no significant serial alterations in immunoglobulin levels or absolute lymphocyte counts in either of the groups. Serological studies are not yet complete.

No patient treated with BCG developed any toxic effects which could be attributed to BCG. Reactions were never florid, and no significant local discomfort was experienced apart from the scarification procedure.

Discussion

Since BCG administration has been shown to potentiate cell-mediated immunity [1] and is of value in prolonging remission in acute lymphoblastic leukemia [4], we hoped it might reduce relapse frequency in Burkitt's lymphoma patients with a minimal tumor load, i.e. after chemotherapy-induced remission.

The number of evaluable patients in this trial is small at present, and many are still at risk of relapsing so that definite conclusions cannot be drawn. Although there was no significant difference in overall relapse frequency between the two groups, relapse outside the central nervous system (CNS) occurred less often in the BCG-treated patients. Since tumor cells in the cerebrospinal fluid may not be accessible to the host immune system, it may be permissible, in assessing the efficacy of BCG, to consider only extra-CNS relapses. The results of the present study would then suggest that BCG has a protective effect.

It has been suggested that the presence of blocking antibodies in Burkitt's lymphoma may be manifested as a coating of IgG on the surface of the tumor cells [3]. It is of interest therefore that the tumor of the single patient in the BCG-treated group who relapsed with extra-CNS tumor did manifest surface IgG (demonstrated by immunofluorescent techniques) and may therefore have been immunoresistant.

The present study has served to demonstrate that BCG is safe and well tolerated; although no clear evidence of prevention of relapse has been obtained, there is also no evidence that tumor growth is enhanced. Further evidence of potentiation of delayed hypersensitivity was obtained. This suggests that, even should BCG therapy prove to be of no value when administered alone, it may be a useful adjuvant when used in conjunction with specific immunization procedures.

Acknowledgements

This study is supported by research grant no. 509431 from the Cancer Research Campaign, and contract P 43-67-1343 of the National Institutes of Health, Bethesda, Md. The help of Mrs. PAMELA MAGRATH who administered the BCG, and of physicians who referred patients is gratefully acknowledged.

References

1. BLUMING, A. Z., VOGEL, C. L., ZIEGLER, J. L., MODY, N., KAMYA, G. W. S.: Immunological effects of BCG in patients with malignant melanoma. A comparison of modes of administration. Ann. intern. Med. **76**, 405 (1972).

2. Bluming, A. Z., Ziegler, J. L., Fass, L., Herberman, R. B.: Delayed cutaneous sensitivity reactions to autologous Burkitt lymphoma protein extracts. Clin. exp. Immunol. **9**, 713 (1971).
3. Klein, G.: Dilemmas of the experimentalist. Israel J. med. Sci. **7**, 111 (1971).
4. Mathé, G.: Approaches to the immunological treatment of cancer in man. Brit. med. J. **1969 IV**, 7.
5. Morrow, R. H., Pike, M. C., Kisuule, A.: Survival of Burkitt's lymphoma patients in Mulago Hospital, Uganda. Brit. med. J. **1967 IV**, 323.
6. Ziegler, J. L.: Treatment of Burkitt's lymphoma. Cancer (Philad.) **30**, 1534 (1972).
7. Ziegler, J. L., Bluming, A. Z., Magrath, I. T., Carbone, P. P.: Intensive chemotherapy in patients with generalized Burkitt's lymphoma. Int. J. Cancer **10**, 254 (1972).
8. Ziegler, J. L., Bluming, A. Z., Fass, L., Morrow, R. H.: Relapse patterns in Burkitt's lymphoma. Cancer Res. **32**, 1267 (1972).
9. Ziegler, J. L., Morrow, R. H., Fass, L., Kyalwazi, S. K., Carbone, P. P.: Treatment of Burkitt's tumour with cyclophosphamide. Cancer (Philad.) **26**, 474 (1970).

BCG Immunotherapy in the Treatment of Inoperable Carcinoma of the Lung

A. PINES

East Herts Hospital, Herts.

Introduction

In carcinoma of the bronchus, once the condition becomes inoperable, the prognosis is virtually hopeless. The results of radical radiotherapy have been claimed to be good, but in my experience almost all the patients treated have relapsed during the succeeding 12 months.

After the initial experimental work of OLD and many others and Professor MATHÉ's work in acute lymphatic leukemia, it seemed worthwhile to see if BCG would help in maintaining improvement after cytotoxic or radiotherapeutic treatment. Since immunotherapy cannot cope with more than a small total of cancer cells in the body, indications were deliberately limited.

The *patients* selected (all men aged 50—70 years) each had tumor which was inoperable but still confined to the chest. The mediastinal glands were usually involved.

The *treatment* was begun 10 to 14 days after the end of cytotoxic treatment or of radiotherapy. It consisted of BCG (Glaxo), 25—125 million organisms per application. This was given with a multiple-puncture gun (200 needles; Heaf) weekly. The method was well tolerated by the patients. At times the effects were too strong and proceeded to ulceration, but this was quickly relieved by a cream of cortisone and neomycin. The degree of penetration of the skin was usually 2 mm, but in those with more severe reactions was reduced to 1 mm. Occasional glandular enlargement was noted. Systemic disturbance occurred sometimes especially after the end of about a year of treatment, consisting of vague malaise and slight fever for 1 or 2 days after the inoculation. The BCG was given at weekly intervals for the first year, then afterwards fortnightly.

Results

a) Six patients were given intensive cyclophosphamide treatment resulting in disappearance of lesions. BCG was given afterwards but was without effect. Similar negative results were obtained with palliative radiotherapy (3,000 rad) in another 6 patients. All relapsed soon after the end of treatment.

6 patients with undifferentiated or oat-cell carcinoma responded well to radical radiotherapy (5,000 to 7,000 rad). However, all relapsed despite BCG treatment over the next few months.

b) *Squamous-cell* carcinoma seemed to respond well after radical radiotherapy, so a randomized control trial was instituted. This was by random blind selection

Table 1. Initial data in patients with squamous carcinoma treated by radical supervoltage X-rays

		BCG	Controls
No. of patients (all male)		11	10
Age	60 years	1	1
	70 years	9	6
	72 years	1	3
Mean		62.9	66.3
Site of carcinoma			
Upper lobe	Right	6	4
	Left	2	1
Lower lobe	Right	2	3
	Left	1	2
Total X-rays			
5,000—5,900 rad		4	4
6,000—6,600 rad		7	6
Mean		5,980	5,533

Table 2. Results of BCG in squamous carcinoma treated with radical supervoltage X-rays

	BCG	Control
Alive — no evidence of carcinoma	2	1
Dead	9	9
Probable cause of death		
Respiratory infection only	3	1
Local recurrence	6	2
Metastases	0[a]	6[a, b]

[a] Difference significant at the 2% level.
[b] Sites were brain (2), liver (2), liver and skin (1) and neck glands (1).

half the patients being allotted to BCG treatment; they were amenable to classification according to age, sex, cell type, extent of disease and amount of radiotherapy. Statistical analysis showed no difference among these categories (Table 1).

Only patients whose treatment began 12 to 24 months ago have been considered. Eleven patients were given BCG and two are still alive and well with no signs of metastases. Of 10 patients not given BCG only one is still alive at the end of a year.

(Tables 2 and 3). Survival during the first 10 months of treatment favored the patients given BCG (at the 2% level of significance) but not after this period (Table 3).

Metastases were diagnosed clinically before death in 6 of the control patients and in 4 of these a post-mortem examination confirmed this. In none of the patients

Table 3. Survival after treatment. D = dead; L = living; * = metastases present

Time (months)	Control patients		BCG-treated patients	
2	DD*			
4	DDDD**			
6	D*		DD	
8				
10				
12	D*	L	DDD	
14				
16				
18	D*		DDDD	L
20				
22				
24				L

treated with BCG was there evidence of extrathoracic metastases; this was confirmed in 7 patients by post-mortem examination. In 6 of these, however, there was local recurrence of cancer, causing death in 4 patients and complicating death from coronary thrombosis in a further 2 patients. This difference is significant at the 2% level (Table 2).

Skin Testing

This was done before and after radiotherapy with Depot PPD, tuberculin (PMKO, a derivative of the cell wall of *Mycobacterium tuberculosis*), and 2 preparations of *Candida albicans*. Afterwards it was continued three-monthly in both the BCG and the control patients.

Before radiotherapy the reactions were usually depressed and remained so in most of the control patients. Afterwards the reactions were absent but soon after BCG was started they became brisk in survivors and depressed in those deteriorating, though there were exceptions. The reaction was strongest to PPD and less so to the others. The best indication was the strength of the local reaction to the BCG, which often became depressed when patients deteriorated.

Conclusions

It seems, therefore, that BCG does have some effect in certain patients with carcinoma of the bronchus, but *only* in those with squamous cancer and in whom radical radiotherapy could be given. It seems to prevent metastases, or perhaps, if they were there at the time of radiotherapy, it does not allow them to grow, and to control the small number of dividing cells present. However, if radiotherapy has not killed sufficient of the original tumor cells, it is not surprising that BCG cannot control these larger numbers of cells, allowing local recurrence in 6 out of the 11 patients. Conceivably the appearance of blocking antibodies might have accounted for later deterioration after the initial success: I have no information on this. BCG did not prevent secondary infections.

Further trials of BCG in larger numbers of patients would be worthwhile, especially with surgical removal of the tumor. For more advanced cases, some way of improving radiotherapy could be important.

Immunotherapy might be improved by the combined use of BCG and irradiated autochthonous cancer cells, but there are formidable theoretical and practical difficulties.

Addendum

The current series comprises 42 patients. In 22 treated with BCG, 18 have died on obviously determined with metastases in only one patient. Of 20 control patients, 18 have died or deteriorated with metastases in 12.

Acknowledgements

To Professor G. Mathé for his encouragement; to Dr. I. Sutherland, Medical Research Council, for statistical help; to Dr. R. Foord, Glaxo Laboratories Ltd., for BCG and generous help; to Dr. W. D. Linsell, Hertford County Hospital, for the post-mortem examinations; to Dr. Paul Strickland, Mount Vernon Hospital, and Dr. Rhona Lindup, Royal Free Hospital, for the radiotherapeutic treatment on which this work was based.

Effect of BCG Stimulation on the Growth Rate of Pulmonary Metastases in 3 Patients with Melanoma

P. Rümke [1], J. Bernheim [1], D. H. van der Vorm [1], H. A. van Peperzeel [1], and R. Looysen [2]

The Netherlands Cancer Institute [1] and Dept. of Pulmonary Diseases [2], University of Amsterdam, Amsterdam

The immunologically stimulating effect of BCG cannot be expected to lead to the eradication of a malignancy that has already spread. However, the efficacy of BCG administration can be monitored provided the rate of growth of metastases can be measured.

We used the method of [1] to measure the rate of growth of round pulmonary metastases. X-ray photographs of the chest are evaluated by means of a transparent ruler inscribed with circles of known diameter increasing by 0.5 mm steps. The size of the metastases is determined by matching circles with the circumference or with a segment of the round secondaries. Growth curves are then constructed by plotting the changes in diameter semilogarithmically against time. Straight lines are generally obtained, indicating a constant rate of growth. Different pulmonary metastases in the same patient usually have the same growth rate [2, 3].

We selected three patients with round pulmonary metastases from a malignant melanoma; they were in good clinical condition and had no other manifest metastases. The BCG used (batch P 18, kindly supplied by Dr. Cohen of the Rijks Instituut voor de Volksgezondheid) was originally derived from strain 1173 of the Institut Pasteur and contained 33.6×10^6 viable mycobacteria per ampoule before freeze-drying, and 16.8×10^6 viable mycobacteria per ampoule after freeze-drying. Dry weight was 123.6 μg per ampoule. The contents of one ampoule were dissolved in 0.5 ml water for one dermal scarification of 20 × 5 cm acording to the method of Mathé. The procedure was done once a week, on the patient's upper arms and upper legs alternately. X-ray photographs of the chest were taken on the same day.

The first patient (male, aged 52 years) developed pulmonary metastases 4 years after the excision of a melanoma of the helix of the ear with regional metastases. Since he was symptom-free, he was not treated for the lung metastases for 14 months. During this period, before BCG stimulation was started, the growth curves of the metastases (Fig. 1) showed that the volume-doubling time was 148 and 266 days. One week after the first BCG scarification, the curves already showed some regression, which continued for 3 weeks. The calculated volume decrease for metastases I, II, III, IV, and V was respectively 23, 16, 29, 24 and 24%. After 3 weeks the metastases started to grow again, initially even faster than before, despite continuation of the

BCG regime. After seven BCG scarifications, we attempted stimulation with *Corynebacterium parvum* (batch EZ 174 from the Wellcome Research Laboratories), administering weekly intradermal injections of 0.2 ml suspension, containing 1.4 mg of active material. Seven injections were given and evoked marked inflammatory reactions without any striking effect on the growth curves. Nearly 3 months later combined chemotherapy was started because of severe signs of abdominal metastases. The

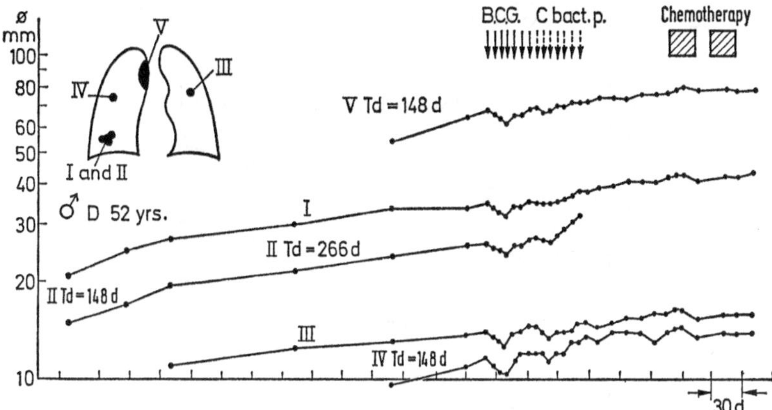

Fig. 1. Effect on growth of pulmonary metastases of stimulation with BCG and *Corynebacterium parvum*, followed by chemotherapy

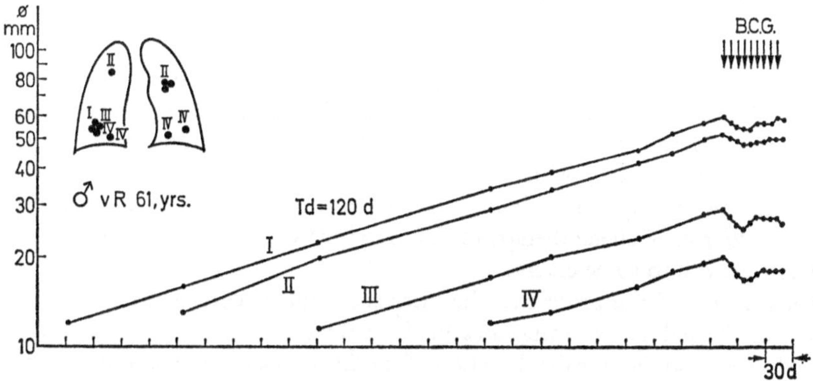

Fig. 2. Effect on growth of pulmonary metastases of BCG stimulation

abdominal symptoms completely disappeared, but there was no reduction in the size of the pulmonary metastases; however, growth may possibly have stopped. This patient had a positive tuberculin reaction before the BCG regime was started.

The second patient (male, aged 61 years) developed pulmonary metastases 4 years after the excision of a melanoma of the heel. Since he had no complaints, he received no treatment during the next 3 years. The tumor volume-doubling time was 120 days (Fig. 2). His tuberculin reaction was positive before the BCG regime of 9 weekly scarifications was started. In this patient, too, the growth curves of the 4 metastases showed a clear regression during the first 3 weeks. The calculated regression in the volume of the metastases after 3 weeks was 23, 21, 36 and 39%, after which they started to grow again. In the meantime neurological signs of brain metastases had developed, so the BCG treatment was replaced by chemotherapy. Standard X-ray photographs could no longer be taken.

The third patient (male, aged 28 years) developed pulmonary metastases 2 years after the excision of a melanoma of the neck. The BCG regime was started 4 months later. At first only one metastasis could be measured. Its volume doubled in about 71 days. The growth curves (Fig. 3) show that during the seven BCG scarifications

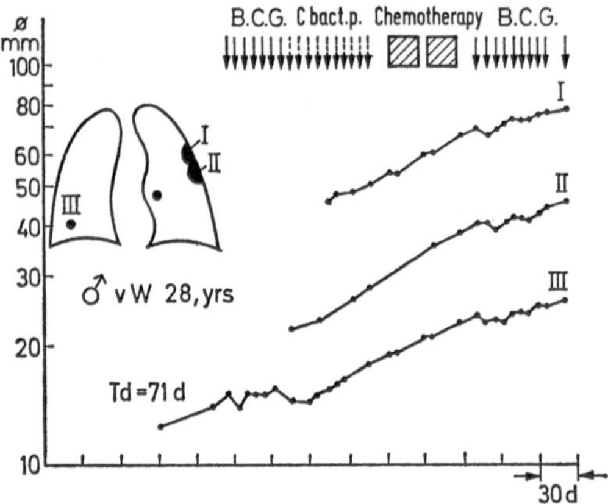

Fig. 3. Effect on growth of pulmonary metastases of BCG stimulation with BCG and *Corynebacterium parvum*, followed by chemotherapy and further BCG stimulation

this metastasis almost stopped growing. There was no progression during the first 3 weeks of treatment with *Corynebacterium parvum*, but after that the three metastases had a growth rate almost identical to the rate measured before BCG treatment. Combined chemotherapy, which was given because of the development of skin metastases, did not appear to influence the growth of the pulmonary metastases. After two courses of chemotherapy the BCG regime was restarted and again seemed to inhibit growth to some extent.

There is no definite proof that the brief and limited regression or arrest of the growth of the pulmonary metastases in these three patients was immunologically induced. *In vitro* studies for the detection of specific cellular immune reactivity would be required to determine this. It is also clear that there was not much benefit for the patients. However, studies of the kind described here may have a future role in evaluating the effectiveness of different types of immunological stimulation and other therapeutic approaches. It may even be possible to compare the effect of different regimes in the same patient.

References

1. Breur, K.: Growth rate and radiosensitivity of human tumours. Europ. J. Cancer **2**, 157 (1966).
2. Charbitt, A., Malaise, E. P., Tubiana, M.: Relation between the pathological nature and the growth rate of human tumors. Europ. J. Cancer **7**, 307 (1971).
3. Peperzeel, H. A. van: Patterns of tumor growth after irradiation. Thesis, Amsterdam: University of Amsterdam 1970.

Immunotherapy of a Solid Tumor (Melanoma) with BCG: A Comment on the Risks of Enhancement

J. L. BERNHEIM

Laboratorium voor Medische Cancerologie en Klinische Navorsing
Vrije Universiteit Brussel, Jules Bordet Institute, Brussels

The immunotherapy with BCG of established solid tumors has hitherto met with little success, either experimental or clinical. At this time, immunotherapy of metastatic melanoma cannot be undertaken instead of chemotherapy unless one can quantify the net effect on the tumor, as in the case of measurable pulmonary metastases (see preceding paper, RÜMKE *et al.*, p. 469). Such empirical work is justified because there are good reasons to believe that at least some of the following assumptions are valid.

1. Melanoma is immunogenic and patients have cell-mediated immunological cytotoxicity to tumor cells demonstrable *in vitro* [4].

2. This specific cell-mediated immunity is insufficient to reverse the progression of tumor growth *in vivo.*

3. Patients with advanced cancer have depressed cell-mediated immunity. (Our own preliminary evidence indicates that melanoma patients have a rather higher immunological competence than other metastatic cancer patients.[1])

4. BCG may either increase the total number of immunocompetent cells, or "activate" effector cells [5].

The temporary decrease in the size of pulmonary metastases of melanoma described by RÜMKE *et al.* can be interpreted as reflecting disappearance of tumor cells. The quick resumption of the original growth rate after a phase of accelerated growth resembled the effect of a single dose of radiotherapy, in which case the accelerated growth was shown by VAN PEPERZEEL (1970) to be caused by an increased growth fraction and shortened cell-cycle phases.

Alternatively, a devil's advocate's interpretation of the same curves as reflecting the reduction of a supposedly immunologically effective round-cell infiltration followed by recolonization, cannot be ruled out, of course. Such would be the result if the weak immunological reaction against the tumor antigens were suppressed by diversion of immunocompetent cells by a potent antigen like BCG.

Some experimental results indeed suggest BCG might enhance tumor growth in certain circumstances. WEISS *et al.* [15] found that high doses of the methanol-

[1] This information become available after the date when this paper was orally presented, and was included on May 15th, 1973.

insoluble fraction of BCG had this adverse effect. BCG can also enhance established DMBA induced mammary tumor in rats [10]. Finally, and most disturbingly, the appearance of blocking factors may follow BCG immunotherapy in man, as recently described by [8].

Antigen competition, i.e. a reduced immunological response to an antigen if the organism is at the same time or shortly before made to respond to another antigen, has been studied mainly on the *primary antibody response*, and by means of *closely related competing antigens*. Therefore these studies may have little bearing on the situation we are concerned with: *secondary* (*cell-mediated*) response to tumor antigens as hypothetically affected by a *totally different antigen* (BCG) administered subsequently. With this restriction it should nevertheless be mentioned that weaker antigens can be "crowded out" by more potent ones [1]. Antigenic competition may [7] or may not [2] suppress a secondary response. Moreover, antigen-stimulated T cells produce a factor which temporarily and non-specifically inactivates other immunocompetent cells, as first shown by [6].

Deleterious antigen competition may also be implied by the observation that, in mice, resistance to brucella infection induced by vaccination is reduced by a previous administration of BCG [11].

Metcalf [9] showed that more reticular tumors arise in mice subjected to repeated antigenic stimulation with *Salmonella adelaide* flagellar antigen or bovine serum albumin (BSA). Rauscher virus leukemogenesis is increased by previous immunization with BSA in adjuvant [12]. These observations caused [13], who recently reviewed the problem of antigenic competition, to suggest that this mechanism may play a role in the breakdown of immune surveillance. This author concludes from the present literature that secondary responses are generally more difficult to inhibit by antigenic competition. If this applies to the response to tumor antigens, subsequent immunological stimulation by potent antigens like BCG may have advantages that outweigh its possible immunosuppressive effects by sequential competition.

The confused situation in antigen competition was best illustrated by [3] demonstration that, with two unrelated antigens, the antibody response to one can be enhanced, depressed or modified by the presence of the other.

There is need for more empirical trials in animal systems to determine dosages, routes and time schedules of administration so as to discriminate between tumor enhancement and inhibition. Until then, the use of BCG (and other immunostimulants) in established human solid tumors will have to be restricted to exceptionally well controllable cases.

References

1. Abramoff, P., Wolfe, H. R.: Precipitin production in chickens. XIII. Quantitative study of the effect of simultaneous injection of two antigens. J. Immunol. **77** (1956).
2. Adler, F. L.: Antibody formation after injection of heterologous immune globulin. II. Competition of antigens. J. Immunol. **78**, 201 (1957).
3. Adler, F. L.: Competion of antigens. Progr. Allergy **8**, 41 (1964).
4. De Vries, J. E., Rümke, Ph., Bernheim, J. L.: Cytotoxic lymphocytes in melanoma patients. Int. J. Cancer **9**, 560 (1972).

5. Evans, R., Alexander, P.: Mechanism of immunobiologically specific killing of tumor cells by macrophages. Nature (Lond.) **236**, 168 (1972).
6. Gershon, R. K., Kondo, K.: Antigenic competition between heterologous erythrocytes. I. Thymic dependency. J. Immunol. **106**, 1524 (1971).
7. Lawrence, W., Simonsen, M.: The property of "strength" of histocompatibility antigens and their ability to produce antigenic competition. Transplantation **5**, 1304 (1967).
8. Levy, N. L., Mahaley, M. S., Day, E. D.: Serum mediated blocking to cell-mediated anti-tumour immunity in a melanoma patient: association with BCG immunotherapy and clinical deterioration. Int. J. Cancer **10**, 244—248 (1972).
9. Metcalf, D.: Recticular tumours in mice subjected to prolonged antigenic stimulation. Brit. J. Cancer **15**, 769 (1961).
10. Piessens, W. F., Lachapelle, F. L., Legros, N., Heuson, J. C.: Facilitation of rat mammary tumour growth by BCG. Nature (Lond.) **228**, 1210 (1970).
11. Renoux, G., Renoux, M.: Interférences de l'inoculation de BCG avec la résistance non spécifique ou l'immunité dans la brucellose de souris. C.R. Acad. Sci. (Paris) **272**, 156 (1971).
12. Siegel, B. V., Morton, J. I.: Depressed antibody response in the mouse infected with Rauscher leukaemia virus. Immunology **10**, 559 (1966).
13. Taussig, M. J.: Antigenic Competition. In: Current topics in microbiology and immunology **60**, 125 (1973).
14. Van Peperzeel, H. A.: Patterns of tumour growth after irradiation. Amsterdam: Thesis 1970.
15. Weiss, B. W., Bonhag, R. S., Leslie, P.: Studies on the heterologous immunogenicity of a methanol-insoluble fraction of attenuated tubercule bacilli (BCG). II. Protection against tumour isografts. J. exp. Med. **124**, 1230 (1966).

BCG Stimulation of Immune Responsiveness in Patients with Malignant Melanoma*

J. U. Gutterman, G. Mavligit, Ch. M. McBride, E. III. Frei, and E. M. Hersh

Section of Immunology, Department of Developmental Therapeutics and Department of Surgery, The University of Texas at Houston, M. D. Anderson Hospital and Tumor Institute, Houston, Texas

Introduction

The demonstration of tumor-associated cell-surface antigens, and specific immune responses to these antigens, in both animal and human tumors, has led to immunotherapeutic approaches to the control of a number of neoplasms [12]. Following the demonstration that bacillus Calmette-Guérin (BCG) vaccine is a potent non-specific immunostimulant in a variety of animal tumor models [17], clinical trials were conducted in leukemia [11] and melanoma [1]. The initial clinical results were encouraging, but they have been empirical and arbitrary in regard to dose, route, schedule, and type (strain) of BCG preparation used.

The objectives of this study were:

1. To determine the clinical efficacy of live BCG in two dose schedules as an immunostimulating agent in recurrent malignant melanoma. Recurrent melanoma was chosen because of its poor prognosis [16, 20] and because melanoma is known to have tumor-associated antigens [15].

2. In addition to evaluating the clinical course of patients, several immunological parameters were studied serially, including the primary immune response to keyhole limpet hemocyanin, established delayed hypersensitivity to a battery of established antigens, lymphocyte blastogenesis *in vitro*, immunoglobulin levels, and lymphocyte and monocyte counts.

In this report the initial and early serial immunological data are reported and are correlated with BCG dose and clinical status. Definitive analysis must await longer patient follow-up.

Patient Selection

The criteria for admission to the study were malignant melanoma with no evident disease but a high probability of relapse. They included the following clinical situations:

* Supported by: U.S. Public Health Service Contract PH 43 68 949 from the Collaborative Research Program, Transplantation-Immunology Branch, National Institutes of Allergy and Infectious Diseases, National Institutes of Health, and Grants CA 05831 and FR 05511 from the National Institutes of Health.

1. Trunk primary with 5 or more positive regional nodes; 2. recurrent melanoma which had been totally removed by surgery; 3. multiple primary melanomas; 4. chemotherapy-induced complete remission of disseminated metastatic disease. 13 melanoma patients entered the study including 6 with recurrent regional node melanoma, 5 with distant spread removed by surgery, one patient with multiple primaries, and one chemotherapy-induced remission.

Prior to immunostimulation, the patients were evaluated for metastatic disease with the following tests: complete history and physical examination, complete and differential blood count, urinalysis, blood-urea nitrogen, serum creatinine, transaminase, alkaline phosphatase, bilirubin, uric acid, calcium, LDH, PA and lateral chest X-ray, metastatic bone survey (including lumbo-sacral, thoracic, cervical spine, and skull), liver scan, electroencephalogram, brain scan, bone marrow aspirate and biopsy. In addition, the majority of patients had whole-lung tomograms. Informed consent was obtained.

Immunotherapy

Group 1 consisting of 7 patients, received high-dose BCG. BCG was applied by scarification and a high dose schedule or a low-dose schedule was given to alternate patients. The preparation used (obtained from Tice Research Laboratories, Chicago) was lyophilized at 15 mg/vial and was given in a dose of 30 mg (approximately 6×10^8 live organisms) per scarification. Scarification with a guage 18 needle was applied to the upper arms or upper legs with 20 scratches each 5 cm long as described previously by MATHÉ [11]. 5 patients are under treatment with the following schedule (Schedule A): weekly for 12 weeks, then every other week for 12 weeks, then monthly for 6 months. 2 patients are under treatment with the following schedule (Schedule B): twice weekly for 3 weeks, then monthly for 11 months. The schedules are selected on the basis of the patient's ability to get to the hospital.

Group II, consisting of 6 patients, was treated with the same preparation of BCG at a dose of 3 mg (approximately 6×10^7 organisms) per scarification. Four patients were treated by Schedule A and 2 patients by Schedule B.

Immunological Evaluation. Prior to BCG administration, skin tests with established delayed-hypersensitivity antigens were applied at least 7 days following the last surgical procedure or 30 days following the last dose of chemotherapy. The skin-test antigens included dermatophytin, dermatophytin 0 and candida antigen or monilia mixture (all from Hollister-Stier ,and all given in 0.1 ml of a 1/20 dilution of the stock), 50 U streptokinase-streptodornase in 0.1 ml (Varidase, Lederle) and 0.1 ml, 1/20 dilution of stock solution mumps antigen (Lyovac-Mumpsvax, Merck, Sharpe and Dohme), 0.1 ml PPD (tuberculin purified protein derivative with Tween 80 preservative, intermediate test strength, Parke Davis). The antigens were injected i.d. on the forearm and induration was measured at 24 and 48 h. The average of 2 perpendicular measurements were recorded in millimeters. Skin tests were repeated monthly for the first 3 months and every other month for the next 9 (Table 1).

Lymphocyte Cultures. The lymphocyte cultures were prepared as described previously [7]. Cultures contained 10^6 lymphocytes, 1 ml of autologous serum and 2 ml of Minimum Essential Medium. Cultures were stimulated with the following:

0.05 ml of Phytohemagglutinin-M (PHA, Difco), 300 μg keyhole limpet hemocyanin (KLH), 2,000 μg varidase (Lederle), 0.1 ml concanavalin A (Nutronal Biochemical Corporation), 0.05 ml pokeweed nitrogen (Grand Island Biological Corporation), and 0.1 and 0.2 ml PPD (0.25 mg/ml; Parke-Davis). All cultures were harvested at 5 days and the blastogenic response was measured by tritiated thymidine incorporation and recorded as counts per minute (cpm) per 10^6 lymphocytes. Lymphocyte cultures were done weekly during the first month and then monthly thereafter (Table 1).

Table 1. Plan of immunological studies

Immunological test	Day of test relative to start of therapy									
	−2	0	7	14	21	28	35	42	49	56
Established delayed hypersensitivity skin tests	×					×				×
Lymphocyte cultures	×		×	×	×	×		×		×
Immunoglobulins	×			×		×		×		×
WBC + differential	×		×	×	×	×		×		×
KLH immunization				×						
KLH skin test								×		
KLH antibody titer				×	×	×	×	×		×
KLH lymphocyte cultures				×	×	×	×	×		×

Keyhole Limpet Hemocyanin (KLH) Immunization. Primary immunization with KLH was performed as previously described [2]. 50 μg was given i.d. as the immunizing dose at the completion of the second week of BCG. The skin-test dose of KLH was also 50 μg. The measurements were performed as described above. Skin tests were repeated 2 weeks, 6 weeks, and 10 weeks after immunization. The lymphocyte blastogenic response to the antigen *in vitro* was determined as described above with 300 μg KLH per ml of culture. Antibody titers to KLH were measured by passive hemagglutination using chronic chloride-treated, KLH-coated red cells as the antigen [2]. IgG antibody responses were determined by the resistance to 2-mercaptoethanol (2 Me). The antibody titers were expressed as $\log_2$ of the highest positive serial 2-fold dilution. The antibodies were measured weekly after the immunization for the first 4 weeks and then every other week for the next 4 weeks, and once monthly thereafter (Table 1).

Lymphocyte and Monocyte Count. White blood-cell counts with absolute lymphocyte and monocyte counts were done weekly for the first 4 weeks of treatment every other week for the next 4 weeks, and monthly thereafter × (Table 1).

Quantitative Immunoglobulins. The immunoglobulins were determined by quantitative immunodiffusion on sera drawn prior to study, every other week during the first 2 months, and monthly thereafter (Table 1).

Statistical Analysis. Statistical analysis was done by the Wilcoxon test or Chi-square test, when appropriate.

Results

The clinical data and response to therapy are shown in Table 2a, and the overall immunological data in Tables 3—5.

7 patients were treated with high-dose BCG. 5 received Schedule A and 2 Schedule B. There were 4 males and 3 females and their median age was 50. All but one patient had recurrent melanoma in either regional nodes or lung. Patient P.R. had 3 primary melanomas in the course of a 2 year period. Two patients in this group have relapsed. Patient H.P. developed a pulmonary lung nodule and multiple

Table 2a

Patient	Age/Sex	Primary	Interval to metastasis (weeks)	Metastasis (stage)[a]
A. High dose				
1	49/M	Deltoid	336	Supraclav (III)
2	53/F	Trunk	24	Axilla, Trunk (IV)
3	45/F	Trunk	104	Axilla (III)
4	50/F	Face, Foot	—	I
5	62/M	Foot	78	Ing. Nodes (IV)
6	64/M	Ear	256	Cerv. Nodes (III)
7	33/M	Neck	96	Trunk, Lung (IV)
B. Low dose				
8	66/F	Arm	48	Knee (IV)
9	69/F	Ear	64	Neck (III)
10	34/M	Trunk	12	Axilla (III)
11	35/M	Trunk	24	Axilla (III)
12	54/M	Trunk	144	Trunk, Lung (IV)
13	63/M	Unknown	—	Lung (IV)

[a] Criteria for staging [14].

skin nodules at the site of previous node dissection after 11 weeks of weekly BCG. Patient J.T. developed 3 pulmonary nodules and partial collapse of a lumbar vertebra 13 weeks after starting BCG. Both are still living and receiving chemotherapy with imidazole carboxamide with BCG. Patient M.G. developed Jacksonian seizures 22 weeks after starting BCG therapy. Results of extensive evaluation for brain metastasis including skull X-rays, electroencephalogram, brain scan, four-vessel angiography, and pneumoencephalogram and examination of spinal fluid were negative. She was treated empirically with 6,000 rads whole-brain irradiation and Dilantin and the seizures are now under control. Because of the lack of demonstration of metastasis, she is included in the remission group at the present time. In both these groups, it is too early to assess therapeutic benefit.

6 patients were treated with low-dose BCG: 4 were treated by Schedule A and 2 by Schedule B. There were 4 males and 2 females. Their median age was 58.5 years. All of the melanoma patients had recurrent lesions treated by surgery except for patient 13 who presented as a stage IV metastatic melanoma involving the lung with

an unknown primary. He had entered complete remission after 3 drug therapy (imidazole carboxamide, BCNU and vincristine). None of these patients have relapsed.

Scarification was very well tolerated by all patients. About half of the patients experienced fever of less than 101 °F with mild malaise starting 24 h after scarification and lasting for 24—48 h. Most patients noted increased heat with edema and itching over the site of the most recent vaccination as well as other scarification sites. Focal infection at the site of scarification did not occur. Disseminated BCG disease has not been observed in any patient.

Table 2b

Patient	Previous therapy	Interval from metastasis to BCG (weeks)	Schedule	Remission duration (weeks)	Site of relapse	Current status
A. High dose						
1	Surgery	4	A	19[a]		
2	Surgery	4	A	25[a]		
3	Surgery	2	A	14[a]		
4	Surgery	—	A	12[a]		
5	Perfusion	2	A	11	Lung, skin	DIC + BCG
6	Surgery	4	B	13	Lung	DIC + BCG
B. Low dose						
8	Surgery	40	A	22[a]		
9	Surgery	4	A	24[a]		
10	Surgery	32	A	15[a]		
11	Surgery	4	A	13[a]		
12	Surgery	2	B	15[a]		
13	Chemotherapy	36	B	18[a]		

[a] DIC = Imidazole carboxamide.

Immunological response to KLH immunization is shown in Table 3. Neither of the two patients who have relapsed developed a positive skin test to KLH. In contrast, all of the 10 patients in remission who had not previously been immunized with KLH developed a positive skin test. By 4 weeks, patients receiving high-dose BCG had greater skin-test reactivity to KLH than those receiving low-dose BCG.

The *in vitro* blastogenic responses to KLH after immunization are shown in Table 3. At 28 days the overall response of the high-dose group was significantly greater than that of the low-dose group and the relapse group. However, at 42 days both the high-dose and the low-dose group were equal in response. Neither of the 2 patients who have relapsed had a detectable antibody response to KLH by day 28. On day 42 one of the patients had a minimal response. The high-dose group had a more vigorous response than the low-dose group early after immunization, but this was not significant.

Skin-test reactivity to PPD after BCG treatment is shown in Table 4. All except one patient on low-dose BCG have converted PPD skin tests.

The overall blastogenic response to PPD showed little difference in patients receiving low or high doses. By 8 weeks, the median response of the high-dose group was 15,600 cpm and of the low-dose group 11,300 cpm. However, by day 49 the response of the remission patients was significantly higher than that of the relapse patients. While the relapse group had good blastogenic response to PPD until this time, there was a sharp falling off at this point, shortly before the time the two patients relapsed. (The median response at day 49 was 1,600 cpm.)

Table 3. Immunological response to KLH immunization in BCG-treated patients

BCG group	Days after KLH immunization					
	0			28		
	S.T.[a]	BR	AB	S.T.	BR	AB
High	0	2.9	0/0	15.0	16.9	5.6/3.8
Low	0	1.0	0/0	6.0	5.1	3.8/3.4
Relapse	0	1.6	0/0	0	1.4	0/0

[a] Skin test response — median measurement in mm. Blastogenic response — Median net cpm/10^6 lymphoyates $\times 10^3$. Antibody response — Mean total/2ME resistant.

Table 4. Skin test reactivity to PPD with BCG treatment

BCG group	Weeks after BCG started		
	0	4	8
Low	2[a] (0—6)	5 (0—8)	9 (0—15)
High	2 (0—6)	12 (2—16)	18[b] (11—35)
Relapse	3 (0—6)	5 (0—10)	21.5 (8—35)

[a] Median measurement in mm with ranges in parenthesis.
[b] Difference between high and low group at eight weeks significant; $P < 0.05$ (Wilcoxin).

The overall change in diameter of skin-test reactivity to the battery of antigens is shown in Table 5. There was a striking increase in the diameter of the skin-test reactions in patients receiving high-dose BCG. By 8 weeks, the median measurement for all 5 skin tests was 10 mm in contrast to 1 mm prior to therapy. The increased overall diameter was not as great in the low-dose group. In fact, by 8 weeks the median measurement was zero for that group. The median measurement prior to therapy in the relapsing group was 7 mm, but at 8 weeks the median measurement was zero.

Patients receiving high-dose BCG had greater than 50% conversion of negative skin tests. Only 30% of negative skin tests converted to positive in the low-dose BCG group. Finally, only 30% of negative skin tests converted to positive in the relapsing group. Half of the positive skin tests in the relapsing group converted to negative during the course of therapy. In contrast, only one positive skin test converted to negative in both remission groups.

2 patients receiving low-dose BCG were anergic to the battery of 5 established antigens as well as PPD prior to therapy. Both patients converted the PPD and KLH skin tests. In addition, one patient converted the Candida skin test and the other patient converted both Candida and Dermatophytin-O and both remain free of recurrent disease.

Table 5. Delayed hypersensitivity to battery of five skin tests

Size of skin tests (mm)		1—10	11—20
BCG group	Weeks after BCG		
High	0	80[b]	20
	4	64	36
	8[a]	36	66
Low	0	89	11
	4	65	35
	8	68	32
Relapse	0	60	40
	4	67	33
	8	80	20

[a] Skin test reactivity between high and low dose BCG significant; $P < 0.05$ (Wilcoxin); skin test reactivity between high BCG group and relapse significant $P < 0.02$ (Wilcoxin).
[b] Figures shown indicate %.

There was no overall change in the *in-vitro* lymphocyte blastogenic response of remission or relapse patients to phytohemagglutinin pokeweed nitrogen or streptolysin 0. Similarly, there were no significant changes in abolute lymphocyte or monocyte counts in any of the patient groups. Finally, there was no significant change in immunoglobulin levels during therapy for any of the groups. The values prior to therapy and during therapy were within the range of a normal population.

Discussion

The initial report by Mathé *et al.* suggesting a beneficial effect with BCG vaccination in the treatment of acute lymphoblastic leukemia [10] has stimulated additional trials with nonspecific immunotherapy in human malignancies. Recently, Bluming *et al.* have presented provocative data suggesting that the Pasteur strain of BCG given by scarification may prolong disease-free intervals in malignant melanoma [1]. In contrast, i.d. vaccination with Glaxo BCG was associated with early relapse. However, as the authors point out, the latter treatment may have adversely affected those patients. The British used the Glaxo strain of BCG (administered i.a.) in doses of less than 1 mg per week and failed to confirm any therapeutic benefit of BCG in acute lymphoblastic leukemia [18]. From these studies and also from work done in animals suggesting that different strains of BCG may have different therapeutic efficacy [19], it appeared to us that a further evaluation of dose, route, schedule, and type of BCG preparation was required in order to design optimal programs of nonspecific immunotherapy in man.

This study was designed primarily to ascertain possible differences in the therapeutic and immunological effects of 2 different dose levels of a lyophilized strain of BCG. Since 4 of the patients admitted to the study could not return for weekly BCG, they were separately randomized to Schedule B.

Since all evidence in animal models has suggested that immunotherapy is effective only if a low tumor burden (less than 10^5 cells) is present [11] immunostimulation was used only in patients in whom clinical disease was not detectable.

A clear difference in immunological reactivity between the remission and relapse groups of patients was observed. From this preliminary analysis, the best prognostic indicator was the primary immune response to KLH. The inability of patients who subsequently relapsed to develop delayed hypersensitivity to KLH corresponds to previous observations by Eilber and Morton [3]. In their study the inability to develop delayed hypersensitivity to DNCB was associated with a high relapse rate in a series of cancer patients following surgery.

In addition to a deficiency in developing delayed hypersensitivity to a primary antigen, the present study demonstrates a striking deficiency in primary antibody response in the relapse group of patients compared to remission patients. This impairment in primary antibody response has been previously reported in patients with lymphoma [6] and other solid tumors [9]. It will be of interest to follow further those patients in remission who have not been able to mount a primary antibody response.

The serial evaluation of skin-test reactivity revealed quite different changes in the relapse group compared with the remission group. In particular, the loss of established delayed hypersensitivity seemed to be a poor prognostic indicator However, in the present study the ability to convert PPD after BCG treatment has not been of much prognostic importance.

The pretherapy evaluation of delayed hypersensitivity was not a good prognostic indicator. In fact, both anergic patients are still in remission. The conversion of at least 2 skin tests in both of the anergic patients is of considerable interest. Despite the risk of disseminated BCG disease, we felt that the poor prognosis in these patients justified immunotherapy with the live vaccine. We have also observed positive conversion of skin tests in two other anergic patients (one with acute leukemia and one with histiocytic lymphoma) treated with liquid form Pasteur strain BCG in another immunotherapy trial now in progress (unpublished observations).

Lymphocyte blastogenic responses to mitogens and antigens other than KLH were not significantly different between the relapse patients and the remission patients. Jones *et al.* [8] recently showed no change in lymphocyte reactivity to PHA with BCG treatment in a group of patients with acute leukemia. Perhaps using lower doses of nitrogens, such as reported recently by Faguet *et al.* [4] will reveal changes in lymphocyte reactivity *in vitro*. As in the report by Bluming *et al.* [1], there was no change in the lymphocyte counts or immunoglobulin levels during this study.

This study suggests that high doses of BCG may be associated with heightened immune reactivity as compared to lower doses. This is particularly suggestive in the analysis of skin-test reactivity. The high-dose BCG group had a greater skin-test reactivity in 8 weeks than the low-dose group. This was also true for the skin-test reactivity to the primary antigen KLH.

It is too early to assess the clinical results of these two groups of BCG patients. Our previous experience has shown that 51% of patients with Stage III trunk melanoma are dead within one year of recurrence, and that 83% of patients with Stage IV distant recurrence are dead within one year. We have not used an untreated control group in this trial, since we felt a Phase I study in regard to dose and schedule was of critical importance. The prognosis of these patients was sufficiently poor that we felt that randomizing between treatment groups was justified. One of the patients on the less intensive schedule has relapsed, and the only relapse of the intensive schedule has been one patient receiving high doses.

However, further follow-up will be necessary for any definitive clinical conclusions.

Acknowledgements

The authors wish to acknowledge the fine technical assistance of Mrs. ANNETTE MATTHEWS and Miss SARAH DYRE. We also wish to thank Misses MARY LOU BUDDE, KATHY DANDRIDGE, and JUDY GRANT for administering the BCG.

References

1. BLUMING, A. Z., VOGEL, C. L., ZIEGLER, J. L., MODY, N., KAMYA, G.: Immunological effects of BCG in malignant melanoma: Two modes of administration compared. Ann. intern. Med. **76**, 405 (1972).
2. CURTIS, J. E., HERSH, E. M., HARRIS, J. E., MCBRIDE, C. E., FREIREICH, E. J.: Immune response to keyhole limpet haemocyanin: Inter-relationships of delayed hypersensitivity, antibody response and *in vitro* blast transformation. Clin. exp. Immunol. **6**, 473 (1970).
3. EILBER, F. R., MORTON, D. L.: Impaired immunologic reactivity and recurrence following cancer surgery. Cancer (Philad.) **25**, 362 (1969).
4. FAGUET, G. B., BALCERZAK, S. P., LOBUGLIO, A. F.: A new phytohemagglutinin (PHA) assay for detecting defective cellular immunity in neoplasia. (Abstract No. 113). American Society of Hematology **66**, (1971).
5. GATTI, R. A., HARRIOCH, D. B., GOOD, R. A.: Depressed PHA responses in patients with non-lymphoid malignancies. In: Proceedings of the Fifth Leukocyte Culture Conference (HARRIS, J. E., Ed.), p. 339. New York: Academic Press 1970.
6. HERSH, E. M., CURTIS, J. E., HARRIS, J. E., MCBRIDE, C., ALEXANIAN, R., ROSSEN, R.: Host defense mechanisms in lymphoma and leukemia. In: Leukemia-Lymphoma, p. 146. 1970.
7. HERSH, E. M.: Blastogenic responses of human lymphocytes to Xenogeneic cells *in vitro*. Transplantation **12**, 287 (1971).
8. JONES, I. H., HARDISTY, R. M., WELLS, D. G., KAY, H. E. M.: Lymphocyte transformation in patients with acute lymphoblastic leukemia. Brit. med. J. **1971 IV**, 329.
9. LEE, A. K. Y., ROWLEY, M., MACKAY, I. R.: Antibody-producing capacity in human cancer. Brit. J. Cancer **24**, 454 (1970).
10. MATHÉ, G., AMIEL, J. L., SCHWARZENBERG, L., SCHNEIDER, M., CATTAN, A., SCHLUMBERGER, J. R., HAYAT, M., DE VASSAL, F.: Active immunotherapy for acute lymphoblastic leukemia. Lancet **1969 II**, 697.
11. MATHÉ, G., POUILLART, P., LAPEYRAQUE, F.: Active immunotherapy of L 1210 leukemia applied after the graft of tumor cells. Brit. J. Cancer **23**, 814 (1969).
12. MATHÉ, G.: Active immunotherapy. Advances Cancer Res. **14**, 1 (1971).

13. Mathé, G., Amiel, J. L., Schwarzenberg, L.: Preliminary result of a new protocol for the active immunotherapy of acute lymphoblastic leukemia: Inhibition of the immunotherapeutic effect by vincristine or adamatadine. Rev. Europ. Étud. clin. biol. **16**, 216 (1971).
14. McBride, C. M.: Advanced melanoma of the extremities. Arch. Surg. **101**, 122 (1970).
15. Morton, D. L.: Immunological studies with human neoplasms. J. reticuloenthoth. Soc. **10**, 137 (1971).
16. Nathanson, L., Hall, T. C., Vawter, G. F., Farber, S.: Melanoma as a medical problem. Arch. intern. Med. **119**, 479 (1967).
17. Old, L. J., Benacerraf, B., Clarke, D. A., Carswell, E. A., Stockerte: The role of the reticuloendothelial system in the host reaction to neoplasia. Cancer Res. **21**, 1281 (1961).
18. Preliminary report of working part on Leukemia in Childhood: Treatment of acute lymphoblastic leukemia. Comparison of Immunotherapy (BCG), intermittent methotrexate, and no therapy after a five-month intensive cytotoxic regimen (Concord Trial). Brit. med. J. **1971 IV**, 189.
19. Reif, A. E., Kim, C. A. H.: Leukemia L 1210 therapy trials with antileukemia serum and bacillus Calmette Guerin. Cancer Res. **31**, 1606 (1971).
20. Stehlin, J. S., Hills, W. J., Rufino, C.: Disseminated melanoma. Arch. Surg. **94**, 495 (1967).

Clinical Results with Corynebacteria

L. Israel

C.H.U. Lariboisière, Paris

The putative effectiveness of corynebacteria in treating human cancer has now been under trial for 5 years. Our results may be summarized as follows:

1. In a first trial, 141 patients with advanced metastatic cancer, all receiving combination chemotherapy, were randomly allocated to either a control group or to a group receiving 4 mg of heat-killed *C. parvum* s.c. once a week in addition to combination chemotherapy. Mean survival from the start of therapy was 6 months for the control group and 10.5 months for the treated group ($p < 0.001$). For the main subgroup of bronchogenic squamous-cell carcinoma, mean survival was 9.25 months for 20 treated patients and 5.85 months for 27 controls ($p = 0.07$).

The effect of *C. parvum* treatment was also assessed as a function of cell-mediated immunity status as assayed by a PPD skin test. Mean survival in PPD-positive patients treated with *C. parvum* was 13 months as compared to 3.6 months for PPD-negative untreated patients ($p < 10^{-9}$).

2. In a second trial, *C. parvum* and *C. granulosum* were administered not only to patients treated with myelotoxic chemotherapy, but also to patients receiving no other therapy. A third category of patients was given the same chemotherapy without immunotherapy. After 4 months of treatment, these 3 groups were compared for changes in 5 delayed-hypersensitivity reactions, i.e. PPD, mumps, candidin, C.C.B. Pasteur and DNCB. The results of this trial are shown in the Table.

3. A randomized trial is at present under way to compare the relapse-free interval in a control group and in a group treated weekly with corynebacteria after adequate tresection of primary melanoma. As yet, it is too early to draw any conclusions from the results obtained.

4. In a few clinical cases, results with *C. parvum* alone have been impressive: objective regression of the size of disseminated lymph nodes in one case of lympho-

Table. Changes in delayed hypersensitivity reactions of 5 antigens in 3 groups of patients after 4 months of therapy

Group	% converted to negative (at least one test)	% no change	% converted to positive (at least one test)
Chemotherapy alone	45%	40%	15%
C. parvum alone	20%	40%	40%
C. parvum plus chemotherapy	8%	33%	59%

sarcoma and one case of Hodgkin's disease; disappearance of ascites in one case of disseminated germinative carcinoma of the ovary.

From these trials it may be concluded that:

a) treatment with corynebacteria is safe;

b) after 4 months of treatment, delayed hypersensitivity reactions in cancer patients treated with immunosuppressive chemotherapy change to positive in 59% of cases when *C. parvum* is administered concomitantly, whereas conversion to positive is seen in only 15% of patients treated with chemotherapy alone;

c) in advanced cases treated with chemotherapy and *C. parvum*, survival is positively and significantly influenced;

d) many more trials must be performed in order to determine the doses, schedules and clinical situations in which corynebacteria give the best results in cancer patients.

References

1. Fischer, J. C., William, R., Mannick, G.: The effect of nonspecific immune stimulation with *Corynebacterium parvum* on patterns of tumor growth. Cancer (Philad.) **26**, 1379 (1970).
2. Halpern, B., Prevot, A. R., Biozzi, G., Stiffel, C., Mouton, D., Morard, J. C., Bouthillier, Y., Decreusefond, C.: Stimulation de l'activité phagocytaire du système réticulo-endothélial provoquée par *Corynebacterium parvum*. J. reticuloendoth. Soc. **1**, 77 (1964).
3. Israel, L., Halpern, B.: Le *Corynebacterium parvum* dans les cancers avancés. Première evaluation de l'activité thérapeutique de cette immuno-stimuline. Nouv. Presse méd. **1**, 19 (1972).
4. Lamensans, A., Stiffel, C., Mollier, M. F., Laurent, M., Mouton, D., Biozzi, G.: Effet protecteur de *Corynebacterium parvum* contre la leucémie greffée AKR. Relations avec l'activité catalasique hépatique et la fonction phagocytaire du système réticuloendothélial. Rev. franç. Étud. clin. biol. **13**, 773 (1968).
5. Woodruff, M. F. A., Boak, J. L.: Inhibitary effect of injection of *Corynebacterium parvum* on the growth of tumour transplants in isogenic host. Brit. J. Cancer **20**, 345 (1966).

A Clinical Trial of Autogenous Vaccines in the Treatment of Osteogenic Sarcoma

R. C. Marcove

Bone Service, Department of Surgery, Sloan-Kettering Memorial Center, New York, N.Y.

In June 1963, a lyophilized homogenous vaccine prepared from the primary tumor tissue was given to a child with osteogenic sarcoma and pulmonary metastasis. During the 15-day course of injections the child gained 7 pounds; following treatment the disease progressed and the patient died. However, the temporary improvement suggested that immunotherapy may have inhibited tumor growth. A more formal controlled trial of immunotherapy in less advanced disease, designed by the author, was begun in April 1966. At first, the vaccine was prepared in the laboratory of Dr. C. Southam and later by the immunological team of Dr. R. A. Good, L. Old, H. Oettgen and Y. Hirshaut. Patients under the age of 25 with osteogenic sarcoma of the long bones but no evidence of spread beyond the primary site and who had been treated by amputation were included in the study. The autogenous vaccine was given in the postoperative period following amputation. If multiple metastasis (usually pulmonary) appeared, the vaccine was judged a failure. If there was subsequent pulmonary resection for multiple metastases, any observed beneficial effect was credited to this surgical treatment [1]. A preliminary report is presented on the patients who received vaccine treatment through April 1973 (Fig. 1).

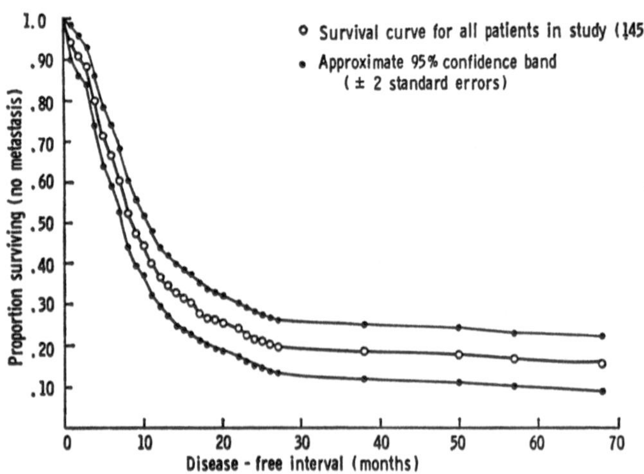

Fig. 1. Control series: Survival curve for 145 patients with osteogenic sarcoma [10]

Diagnosis of Osteogenic Sarcoma

(Figs. 2 and 3)

Several months of dull, low-grade pain and gradual swelling are the most common clinical signs of osteogenic sarcoma. If the pain is more intense or the swelling more sudden than expected, and if the radiological diagnosis is equivocal,

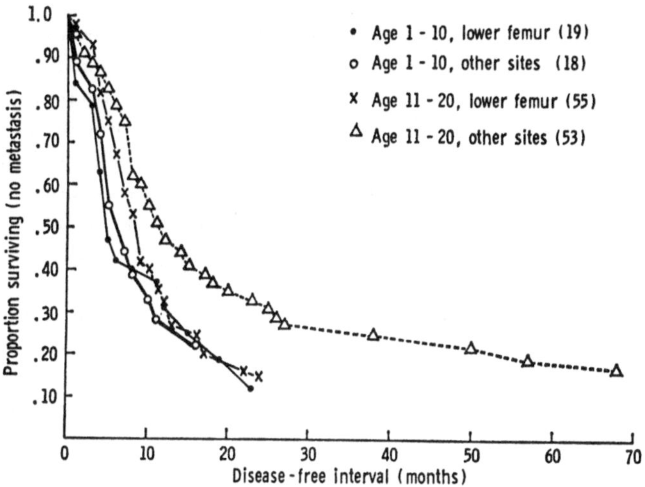

Fig. 2. Breakdown of cases of osteogenic sarcoma under age 21 yields four survival curves

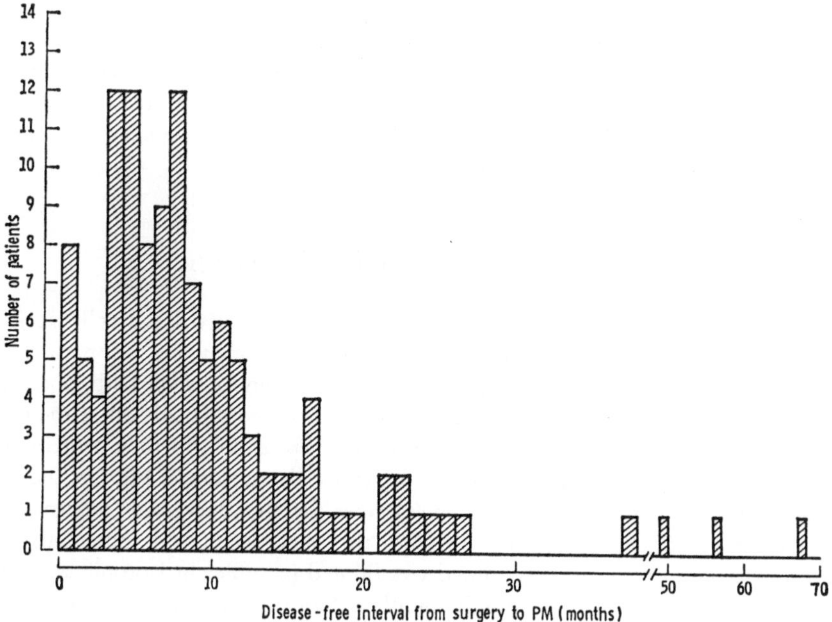

Fig. 3. Disease-free interval after surgery in osteogenic sarcoma to development of pulmonary metastases

other possibilities, such as osteomyelitis, eosinophilic granuloma or aneurysmal bone cyst should be considered.

The radiologic appearance of osteogenic sarcoma usually shows an osteolytic, osteoblastic or mixed picture. An adjacent soft tissue mass can often be identified with productive radiologic densities consistent with ossification, calcification or both. Skipped areas of tumor up and down the involved bone shaft are generally so small that they are not found on the initial X-ray. Medullary extension of the sarcoma is usually distal to the soft tissue mass.

The histopathology of osteogenic sarcoma is variegated. The essential finding, however, is a malignant spindle-cell stroma forming osteoid or immature bone which is neither reactive nor periosteal. As the bone production becomes denser, the osteocytes become more mature (Phemister's normalization process) [2, 3].

Large areas of spindle cells or cartilage formation may be present, including bone formation due to endochondral ossification [4]. This process of bone formation is also seen in chondrosarcoma and therefore is not in itself diagnostic for osteogenic sarcoma [5, 6, 7]. Also, a small biopsy specimen, especially from a needle aspiration, may show only a few spindle cells which can be seen in reticulum-cell sarcoma or fibrosarcoma, making a false diagnosis a real possibility. Likewise, a limited biopsy may show only cartilage, mimicking a diagnosis of a chondrosarcoma or giant cells, or it may show large angiomatous formations, mimicking a giant-cell tumor or angiosarcoma [8]. For these reasons, large, adequate, open biopsy specimens are necessary for accurate diagnosis.

Materials and Methods — Controls

A series of 145 consecutive patients with osteogenic sarcoma under the age of 21, treated between January 1949 and December 1965, has been previously reported in the literature [9, 10]. Nine patients, between the ages of 21 to 25, treated routinely (without vaccine) during this same period, were added to the present series (1966 to 1973) as a control group for the vaccine study.

Preparation of the Lysed-Cell Vaccine

The trial began with the administration of a UV-irradiated lysed cell vaccine. This vaccine was prepared by putting the tumor specimen and approximately 4 times its weight of saline into a Viritis homogenizer in an ice water bath, operated at maximum speed for 15 minutes. This procedure ruptured virtually all of the cells and large proportion of the nuclei. The resulting suspension was then centrifuged for 15 minutes at 8,000 g which sedimented intact cells and nuclei but left the cell sap, microsomes, mitochondria and membranes in the harvested supernatant. Transmission of 253.7 mμ UV light through this supernatant was measured in a Beckman DU Photometer; the specimen was diluted in sufficient isotonic saline to allow at least 50% transmission through a depth of 2 mm. If the preparation contained large amounts of hemoglobin, a considerable dilution was necessary. The preparation was then placed in open Petri dishes to a depth of 2 mm and irradiated from a "germicidal" UV lamp to provide a dose of 50,000 ergs/mm^2 at the bottom of the fluid layer. The material was ampuled aseptically in volumes of from 1 to 5 ml. Concentrations of these extracts and the total dosage given to the patients varied widely. We have no data on actual concentration or the amount of tissue solids which were administered, but the irradiated supernatants represented the yield from as much as 200 mg of tumor per ml to as little as 31 mg per ml. The total dosage administered per patient was the yield from as much as 14 gm of tumor tissue to as little as 1.8 gm. Vials were stored in a "Revco" freezer at approximately — 60 °C.

Preparation of the Whole-Cell Vaccine

A gamma-irradiated whole-cell suspension was prepared by mincing the tumor with scissors and scalpels; fragments were eliminated by sedimentation or by filtration through surgical gauze. The resulting suspension, which consisted predominantly of single cells, was then centrifuged and the cells were resuspended in Solution A (15) at a concentration of 10^7 cells/ml. The suspensions were irradiated from a Cobalt-60 source to a dose of 10,000 rads, ampuled in 1 ml aliquots and stored at — 60 °C. Immediately before administration, a vial of vaccine was allowed to thaw at room temperature. The contents were mixed by twice drawing up a syringe out of the vial and then administered by s.c. or i.m. injection into the gluteal or deltoid region.

The injections were usually started between 7 and 10 days after surgery (never later than 28 days) and continued at approximately 2-week intervals for as many doses as were available. Patients who lived outside the commuting area of this hospital received at least the first dose of vaccine while hospitalized and thereafter

Table 1. Osteogenic sarcoma. Whole-cell vaccine trials (discontinued)

No.	Initials	Vaccine type	Sex	Age (years)	Site of tumor	Pre-op. radiation (1000 R)	Date amputation	Time from amp to met (most)
				Patients with pulmonary metastasis				
1.	P.M.	whole cell	F	15	upper tibia	0	5-1-68	20.0
2.	J.S.	whole cell	F	10	upper femur	0	5-16-68	16.1
3.	C.P.	whole cell	F	16	upper humerus	0	7-22-68	0.7
4.	E.M.	whole cell	M	11	upper tibia	0	8-16-68	3.8
5.	K.G.	whole cell	F	12	lower femur	0	9-3-68	5.0
6.	S.G.	whole cell	F	10	upper tibia	0	10-2-68	11.2
7.	R.B.	whole cell	F	14	upper fibula	0	10-7-68	6.5
8.	D.S.	whole cell	M	16	upper tibia	0	10-30-68	4.8
9.	C.R.	whole cell	F	15	lower femur	0	12-10-68	4.2
10.	E.W.	whole cell	M	19	lower femur	0	1-24-68	3.3
11.	G.P.	whole cell	M	14	lower femur	0	8-22-69	4.3
12.	M.B.	whole cell	F	20	lower femur	0	9-23-69	5.4
				Patients with no evidence of disease				
13.	K.K.	whole cell	F	11	upper tibia	0	10-4-68	37.0

Table 2. Osteogenic sarcoma. Patients with pulmonary metastasis, multiple, clinical and at surgery lysed cell trials

No.	Initials	Vaccine type	Sex	Age (years)	Site of tumor	Pre-op. radiation (1000 R)	Date amputation	Time from amp to met (mos)
1.	J.R.	lysed cell	M	17	upper fibula	12	7-1-66	7.7
2.	G.K.	lysed cell	M	15	upper tibia	12	10-10-66	5.7
3.	K.W.	lysed cell	M	8	lower femur	12	2-9-67	4.9
4.	L.J.	lysed cell	F	10	upper humerus	0	2-23-67	10.3
5.	R.F.	lysed cell	M	16	upper tibia	0	8-9-67	20.0
6.	M.C.	lysed cell	M	11	lower femur	0	12-13-67	5.5
7.	N.H.	lysed cell	F	16	upper humerus	0	12-19-67	7.2
8.	R.S.	H_2O lysed	M	12	upper humerus	0	9-5-69	4.5
9.	J.J.	lysed cell	M	16	upper humerus	0	1-29-71	14.9
10.	M.C.	lysed cell	F	9	upper tibia	0	9-15-71	5.7
11.	A.C.	lysed cell	M	18	upper humerus	0	11-8-71	4.3
12.	C.K.	lysed cell	M	23	lower femur	0	1-13-72	5.0

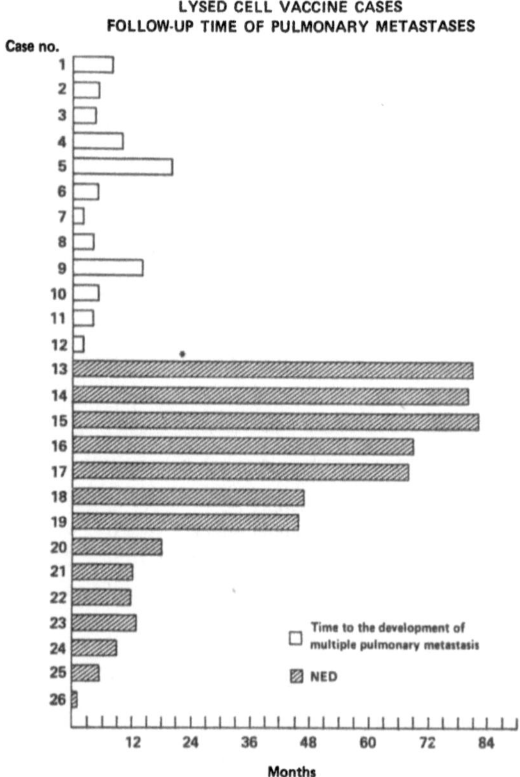

Fig. 4. Follow-up time of pulmonary metastases in patients treated with lysed-cell autogenous vaccine

Table 3. Osteogenic sarcoma. Patients with no evidence of disease or single patient with solitary metastasis at surgery lysed cell trials

No.	Initials	Vaccine type	Sex	Age (years)	Site of tumor	Pre-op. radiation (1000 R)	Date amputation	Length of follow-up (mos)
13.	J.R.	lysed cell	F	15	lower femur	0	4-27-66	81
14.	K.P.	lysed cell	F	4	upper tibia	12	5-16-66	80
15.	C.N.	lysed cell	M	18	upper tibia	12	6-3-66	82
16.	J.R.	lysed cell	M	15	upper tibia	0	4-10-67	69
17.	P.D.	lysed cell	M	7	upper humerus	0	7-20-67	68
18.	W.M.	H_2O lysed	M	24	lower femur	0	2-14-69	47
19.	J.C.	H_2O lysed	M	20	lower femur	0	3-3-69	46
20.	R.B.	lysed cell	F	17	upper tibia	0	11-9-71	18
21.	E.V.	lysed cell	M	16	upper humerus	0	2-17-72	12
22.	V.R.	lysed cell	M	36	distal femur	0	2-22-72	13
23.	K.M.	lysed cell	M	52	distal femur	0	3-31-72	13
24.	M.S.	lysed cell	M	21	upper humerus	0	6-9-72	9
25.	M.L.	lysed cell	M	14	upper humerus	0	10-2-72	5
26.	J.B.	lysed cell	M	15	upper tibia	0	3-1-72	1

LYSED CELL VACCINE CASES FOLLOW-UP TIME

% of cure all cases done 1 or more years ago:

$$\frac{11}{23} = 43\%$$

(all cases studied have been treated before 4/72)

% of cure all cases done 2 or more years ago:

$$\frac{7}{16} = 44\%$$

(all cases studied have been treated before 4/71)

% of cure all cases done 3 or more years ago:

$$\frac{7}{15} = 46.6\%$$

(all cases studied have been treated before 4/70)

% of cure all cases done 5 or more years ago:

$$\frac{5}{12} = 41.6\%$$

(all cases studied have been treated before 4/67)

Fig. 5. Analysis of survival of treated patients receiving lysed-cell autogenous vaccine

through the cooperation of their local physicians who received shipments of the vaccine packed in dry ice and stored it in a household-type deep freezer at temperatures around — 10 °C.

The gamma-irradiated whole cell suspension was given to patients during 1968 and 1969. Of the 13 patients who received the whole-cell preparation, listed in Table 1, only one is still free of disease at this time. The whole-cell vaccine has been abandoned as ineffective. The lysed cell series includes, however, 3 patients who received an H_2O osmotically lysed cell preparation in 1969. Figs. 4 and 5 and Tables 2 and 3 illustrate the survival time of patients who received the lysed-cell vaccine.

Results

The race, sex, age, site of tumor, preoperative duration of symptoms and/or signs, amount of preoperative radiation (if given) and the date of amputation were recorded for each patient in the control and vaccine group (whole-cell and lysed-cell vaccines). The date of latest follow-up was noted for patients with no evidence of disease; the time from amputation to last negative and first positive chest X-ray was noted for those patients with pulmonary metastases. If the chest X-ray was positive for multiple metastases, the vaccine was judged a failure in that patient.

An historical control, including 145 patients under the age of 21 (later increased to age 25 — with a similar cure rate) treated before the vaccine trials were begun, was employed, as the scarcity of patients with osteogenic sarcoma did not permit randomization. However, the control group consisted of a consecutive series of cases from this hospital and all slides were reviewed by the same pathologist.

The distribution of patients by race, sex, age, site and preoperative duration was similar in the control and the vaccine series. Some patients in the control and lysed-cell series had received preoperative radiation therapy, while none in the whole-cell series was irradiated prior to surgery. However, analysis of the control series showed that preoperative radiation therapy had no effect on the course of the disease [10].

The length of the disease-free interval from surgery (surgery entailed amputation, except in one case) to the onset of demonstrable pulmonary metastasis (the date of the first positive X-ray) was felt to be the most suitable criterion for evaluating the effect of the vaccine. It is important to note, however, that X-rays were not taken on as regular a basis in the control series as in the vaccine series. Thus, metastases in the control group tended to be diagnosed at a later date, making the disease-free interval in the control series appear longer. The median interval from the last negative to the first positive chest film was 7 months for the control series. For 28 patients in the control series the closest available date for the onset of pulmonary metastases was the date of death, since there was no follow-up X-ray examination.

Taking into consideration the lack of regular follow-up for patients in the control series (which causes the control series curve to be higher than if pulmonary metastases had been diagnosed more promptly), it might be conjectured that the whole-cell vaccine group is perhaps similar in effect to the control, that is, the whole-cell vaccine group performs more successfully in relation to the control than appears here.

As mentioned, use of the whole-cell vaccine has been abandoned. Continuation of the trial using the lysed cell preparation is indicated, however, because of the strong favorable trend evident in our results to date.

References

1. Martini, N., Huvos, A. G., Miké, V., Marcove, R. C., Beattie, E. J., jr.: Multiple pulmonary resections in the treatment of osteogenic sarcoma. Ann. thorac. Surg. **12**, 271 (1971).
2. Phemister, D. B.: A study of the ossifications in bone sarcoma. Radiology **7**, 17 (1926).
3. Phemister, D. B.: Chondrosarcoma of bone. Surg. Gynec. Obstet. **50**, 216 (1930).
4. Marcove, R. C., Huvos, A. G.: Cartilaginous tumors of the ribs. Cancer (Philad.) **27**, 794 (1971).
5. Copeland, M. M., Geschickter, C. F.: Malignant bone tumors, Primary and Metastic. A Monograph for the Physician.: American Cancer Society 1963.
6. Dahlin, D. C., Coventry, M. B.: Osteogenic sarcoma. A study of six hundred cases. J. Bone Jt Surg. **49**, 101 (1967).
7. McKenna, R. J., Schwinn, C. P., Soong, K. Y., Higinbotham, N. L.: Sarcomata of the osteogenic series (osteosarcoma, fibrosarcoma, chondrosarcoma, parosteal osteogenic sarcoma and sarcomata arising in abnormal bone). An analysis of 552 cases. J. Bone Jt Surg. **48**, 1 (1966).
8. Farr, G. H., Huvos, A. G., Marcove, R. C., Higinbotham, N. L., Foote, F. W., jr.: Telangiectatic osteogenic sarcoma. In preparation.
9. Marcove, R. C., Miké, V., Hajek, J. V., Levin, A. G., Hutter, R. V. P.: Osteogenic sarcoma in childhood. N.Y. St. J. Med. **71**, 855 (1971).
10. Marcove, R. C., Miké, V., Hajek, J. V., Levin, A. G., Hutter, R. V. P.: Osteogenic sarcoma under the age of twenty-one. A review of one hundred and forty-five operative cases. J. Bone Jt Surg. **52**, 411 (1970).
11. Cutler, S. J., Ederer, F.: Maximum utilization of the life table method in analyzing survival. J. chron. Dis. **8**, 699 (1958).
12. Marcove, R. C., Miké, V., Huvos, A. G., Southam, C. M., Levin, A. G.: Vaccine trial for osteogenic sarcoma. A preliminary report. Ca-A Cancer Journal for Clinicians **23**, 74 (1973).

Immunization with Cultured Cell-BCG Mixtures*

J. E. Sokal and C. W. Aungst

Department of Medicine B, Roswell Park Memorial Institute,
New York State Department of Health, Buffalo, N.Y.

In 1965, [5] initiated exploratory trials of immunotherapy for chronic myeloid leukemia. Patients with leukemia under satisfactory control were immunized with cultured cells, believed to be myeloblasts, in the hope that this would prevent or delay myeloblastic transformation. There was some evidence that this line of cultured cells possessed an antigen in common with the buffy coat of patients with myeloid leukemia, but not with leukocytes from normal individuals. The goal of immunization was to induce strong delayed hypersensitivity against antigens of these cultured cells. The first trial was with irradiated cells injected i.m. This resulted in antibody production, but not delayed hypersensitivity to the target cells. Our present immunization technique was then adopted. This uses living BCG organisms as adjuvant, and i.d. vaccination.

More recently, we have used a second cultured cell line in our antileukemic vaccinations. We have also immunized 3 patients with osteogenic sarcoma with mixtures of BCG and cultured allogeneic osteosarcoma cells after potentially curative amputation.

Clinical Material and Methods

24 patients with myeloid leukemia have received 3 or more vaccinations with mixtures of BCG and cultured cells. All patients continued to receive antileukemic chemotherapy, as indicated by their hematologic status. 16 of these patients had uncomplicated Philadelphia chromosome-positive leukemia under good chemotherapeutic control. 8 were poor-risk patients whose clinical status ranged from good to preterminal. 3 of the latter were Philadelphia chromosome-negative; of these one was in partially controlled blastic status. 1 Philadelphia chromosome-positive patient was drug-resistant, but not blastic. 4 Philadelphia chromosome-positive patients were first vaccinated after myeloblastic transformation; in 2 of these, full reversal of early blastic crisis was achieved with combination chemotherapy and splenectomy, and immunization was started thereafter; in the other 2, remission was not obtained and immunization was started after the white blood cell count was reduced to low normal levels, even though peripheral blood or marrow still

* Supported in part by United States Public Health Service Grant CA-12243.

showed 50% or more of blasts plus promyelocytes. These patients were immunized with one or both of the following cell lines:

1. RPMI 6410. This line was established from the peripheral blood of a patient with fulminating acute myeloblastic leukemia, Philadelphia chromosome-negative. The cells were originally believed to be myeloblasts [2], but studies 1—2 years later demonstrated that the cells then being grown produced immunoglobulins and therefore, were probably lymphoid cells.

2. RPMB 7642. This line was established from the peripheral blood of a patient with Philadelphia chromosome-positive leukemia who was in advanced blastic crisis. These cultured cells were originally myeloblasts; they were Philadelphia chromosome-positive and immunoglobulin-negative. However, after a few months in culture, the Philadelphia chromosome could no longer be demonstrated and the cells were immunoglobulin-positive. We believe that the originally predominating myeloblasts were overgrown by lymphoid cells which also became established.

The 3 patients with osteogenic sarcoma were first vaccinated 1—3 days after amputation of the involved extremity. One of these patients was in good clinical status at the time of immunization; the other 2 were in fair status, having lost weight, and were anemic. Initial immunization of these 3 patients was with irradiated autologous tumor cells mixed with BCG organisms. Subsequently, they were vaccinated with RPMI 5959-T cells. This cultured line was established at our Institute several years ago by Dr. G. E. Moore from a metastatic tumor of a patient with osteogenic sarcoma.

Individual vaccinations consisted of 50—350 million cultured cells mixed with BCG organisms (Research Foundation, Chicago) and injected i.d. in a volume of 0.5 ml. The usual dose of this BCG preparation is 60 μg dry weight for vaccination against tuberculosis. The doses of BCG used for the first few vaccinations were usually 120—240 μg. Subsequently, after patients exhibited sensitization to these organisms, the doses of organisms in the vaccine were reduced to 20—90 μg.

The first three vaccinations were administered at 3—6 week intervals. Subsequently, the interval between vaccinations was gradually extended to a maintenance schedule of 3—4 vaccinations per year.

Results

Immunologic Responses

Delayed hypersensitivity responses to a battery of antigens were determined periodically in these patients. This battery included "specific" antigens (tuberculin PPD; irradiated or homogenized cultured cells of the line used for immunization; and fetal calf serum, a constituent of the culture medium which adsorbs to the cells) and antigens unrelated to any component of the vaccine mixture (mumps, Varidase, monilia and trichophyton). Increase in reactivity to the latter antigens is evidence that general stimulation of cellular immune responses has been achieved.

We observed progressive increases in both specific and nonspecific responses with successive immunizations, usually reaching a plateau after 6—10 vaccinations. The degree of immunologic stimulation achieved is shown in Table 1, which

Table 1. Changes in the distribution of delayed skin test responses to a battery of specific and non-specific antigens, after repeated vaccination with cultured cell-BCG mixtures

No. of vaccinations	% of all skin test responses				
	Negative	a	b	c	d
None	38	40	17	5	0
3	14	20	46	14	6
6 or more	8	9	32	35	16

[a] Erythema 1.0 cm without induration or induration 0.5—0.9 cm.
[b] Induration, 1.0—2.0 cm.
[c] Induration, 2.1—4.0 cm.
[d] Induration, more than 4.0 cm.

summarizes the changes in the patterns of delayed skin-test responses of 15 patients in good clinical status (14 with chronic myelocytic leukemia and one with osteogenic sarcoma) who received 6 or more vaccinations. None of these patients was initially anergic and most had positive responses to at least 2 antigens. However, 78% of all the initial skin-test responses were negative or weak, and none were very strong (++++). After 3 vaccinations, there was a rather symmetrical distribution of skin-test responses with a sharp mode at moderate response (++). After 6 or more vaccinations, negative and weak responses decreased further, the mode shifted to strong response (+++), and there were a significant number of very strong responses. This progressive increase in the strength of delayed skin-test responses was observed both for specific antigens and for antigens unrelated to components of the vaccine mixtures. However, the strongest individual responses of most patients were to antigens of the target cells.

Table 2. *In vitro* lymphocyte response to irradiated RPMI 5959-T cells after vaccination with mixtures of these cells and BCG. Mixed-cell cultures were harvested at 7 or 8 days, after a 24-hour labeling period with 1.0 μc of ^{3}H-thymidine. Each experiment included control cultures of irradiated target cells alone and leukocytes alone

Patient and vaccination status (5959-T cells + BCG)		Blastogenic response ratio[a]
T.D.	6 weeks after 1st vaccination	<1
	7 weeks after 3rd vaccination	8
	5 weeks after 4th vaccination	9
	17 weeks after 4th vaccination	10
B.B.	5 weeks after 1st vaccination	<1
	3 weeks after 3rd vaccination	10
	6 weeks after 4th vaccination	16
	13 weeks after 4th vaccination	7
R.M.	4 weeks after 1st vaccination	<1
	4 weeks after 2nd vaccination	2
	7 weeks after 2nd vaccination	4

[a] $\frac{\text{cpm, mixed-cell cultures} - \text{cpm, target cells only}}{\text{cpm, leukocytes only}}$.

We also studied *in vitro* blastogenic response of patients' lymphocytes to the target cells, in the 3 cases of osteogenic sarcoma. None of these patients showed evidence of lymphocyte reactivity to the cultured osteosarcoma cells after their first vaccination with these cells. After the second or third vaccination, however, all 3 patients exhibited an unequivocal blastogenic response *in vitro*. Table 2 presents results of serial studies of these patients.

The patients immunized with mixtures of BCG and cultured cells have not shown any changes in serum electrophoretic patterns attributable to repeated vaccination, nor any increases in circulating immunoglobulin levels. Particularly interesting is the fact that these patients developed only traces of precipitating antibody to fetal calf serum. In contrast, patients receiving cultured cells by other routes develop strong precipitins to fetal calf globulins [4]. These data suggest that the technique of immunization we have used principally stimulates cellular immune responses rather than antibody production.

Clinical Response

One of the patients with osteogenic sarcoma, who developed pulmonary metastases 2 months after his third vaccination, had a transient partial response to adriamycin therapy, and died of his neoplastic disease 9 months after amputation (8 months after his first vaccination with cultured cells). The other 2 patients have received no other treatment and are in good health, apparently free of disease, 18 and 13 months after amputation.

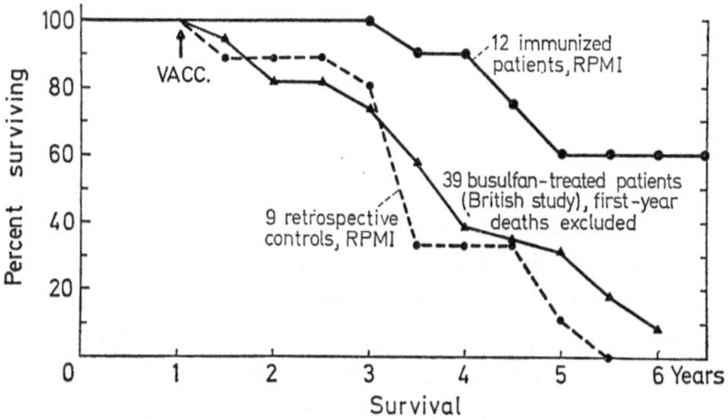

Fig. 1. Survival curves for immunized patients with uncomplicated Ph′-positive myeloid leukemia (date of diagnosis assumed to be one year prior to first vaccination), retrospectively selected Ph′-positive Roswell Park controls, and busulfan-treated British patients (karyotypes unknown; first-year deaths excluded)

12 of the patients with uncomplicated Philadelphia chromosome-positive leukemia were first immunized more than a year ago. In order to prepare a survival plot for these patients, who entered our program at different times in the course of their disease (averaging a little more than a year after diagnosis), we have arbitrarily assigned all patients a hypothetical date of diagnosis, one year before their first vaccination. Fig. 1 shows life-table survival plots for these immunized patients,

9 retrospectively selected Roswell Park controls (Philadelphia chromosome-positive patients, diagnosed during the same time period, who were doing well after one year of chemotherapy) and a recent series of busulfan-treated patients from England. First-year deaths have been excluded from the British series, in order to make the data comparable. The difference in survival between the immunized patients and the control groups is statistically significant ($p < 0.01$).

6 of the poor-risk patients can be evaluated at this time. The 2 patients whose blastic crisis could not be reversed died within 6 months of their first vaccination; there was no evidence of significant benefit from immunotherapy.

The Philadelphia chromosome-negative patient in incompletely controlled blastic status (subacute myeloblastic leukemia) died 17 months after his first vaccination (2 years after diagnosis). The busulfan-resistant, Philadelphia chromosome-positive patient is alive 21 months after her first vaccination and 57 months after diagnosis, but her leukemia is proving increasingly difficult to control with alternative drugs, and her functional status has deteriorated. We believe that these 2 patients probably benefited from immunotherapy, but it is quite possible that they might have done equally well without immunization.

The 2 patients first immunized after reversal of early blastic crisis have had survivals substantially in excess of any we had previously observed in comparably treated patients not receiving immunotherapy. In the first case, immunizations were discontinued after 2 years; he did well for an additional year, but then developed recurrent blastic crisis and died 40 months after his first vaccination. The second patient is doing well 21 months after his first vaccination, and will be continued indefinitely on immunotherapy.

Discussion

Our program of immunotherapy, both in myeloid leukemia and osteogenic sarcoma, is based on several assumptions: 1. that these diseases are virus-induced, 2. that tumor cells in different patients have common virus-determined antigens, and 3. that the cultured cells used for immunization carry such tumor-associated antigens and thus stimulate an immune response which is useful in protecting the host against autologous neoplastic cells. It is possible that myeloid leukemia may prove to be a virus-induced disease, and circumstantial evidence has been presented by [3], that osteogenic sarcoma is virus-induced and that tumors of different patients have common antigens. However, we have no evidence that the cultured cells used in our vaccines do, in fact, share common antigens with leukemic myeloblasts or native osteosarcoma cells. We hope to undertake appropriate studies to resolve these points in the near future.

The technique of immunization used in this study induced general stimulation of cellular immune reactivity, and specific delayed hypersensitivity to antigens of the target cells, with relatively little stimulation of antibody production. These features are now generally recognized as desirable for antitumor immunotherapy. Presumably, there would be less danger of stimulating the production of blocking antibodies [1] with this technique than with methods which stimulate considerable antibody production.

The course of the patients with myeloid leukemia who entered our immunotherapy program at a time when their disease was under good control, has been substantially better than would have been expected with conventional therapy alone (Fig. 1). These immunized patients did not differ from other patients with myeloid leukemia, treated by us or by others, and we conclude that their improved survival is attributable to immunotherapy. Of particular interest to us has been the course of the 2 patients first immunized after reversal of early blastic crisis. Their survival has been far in excess of what we have been able to accomplish with combination chemotherapy alone.

Since our immunized patients developed both strong delayed hypersensitivity to antigens of the target cells in vaccines, and substantial general increase of cellular immune reactivity, the increased survival we have recorded could be due either to specific immunization against leukemic myeloblasts or to general stimulation of immunological reactivity. The course of patients with a variety of malignant neoplasms correlates with the status of their cellular immune reactivity, and there is no reason to believe that chronic myeloid leukemia should be an exception to this rule. Thus, it is not clear at present whether we are observing the results of specific antitumor immunization, or of nonspecific immunologic stimulation. We expect to answer this question during the next few years.

References

1. Hellström, I., Sjogren, H. O., Warner, G., Hellström, K. E.: Blocking of cell-mediated tumor immunity by sera from patients with growing neoplasms. Int. J. Cancer **7**, 226 (1971).
2. Iwakata, S., Grace, J. T., jr.: Cultivation in vitro of myeloblasts from human leukemia. N.Y. St. J. Med. **64**, 2279 (1964).
3. Morton, D. L., Malmgren, R. A.: Human osteosarcomas: Immunologic evidence suggesting an associated infectious agent. Science **162**, 1279 (1968).
4. Sokal, J. E., Aungst, C. W., Han, T.: Use of BCG as adjuvant in human cell vaccines. Cancer Res. **32**, 1584 (1972).
5. Sokal, J. E., Grace, J. T.: An attempt to protect patients with chronic myelocytic leukemia (CML) against blastic transformation. Proc. Amer. Ass. Cancer Res. **10**, 85 (1969).

The course of the patients with myeloid leukemia who entered our immunotherapy program at a time when their disease was under good control has been [illegible] better than would have been expected with conventional therapy alone [illegible]. These immunized patients did not differ from other patients [illegible] [illegible] their improved survival [illegible] [illegible] after reversal of early blastic crisis. Their survival [illegible] [illegible]

[illegible]

Recent Results in Cancer Research

Sponsored by the Swiss League against Cancer. Editor in chief: P. Rentchnick, Genève

1 SCHINDLER, R.: Die tierische Zelle in Zellkultur. Geb. DM 19,80; US $ 8.10
2 Neuroblastomas — Biochemical Studies. Edited by C. BOHUON, (Symposium). Cloth DM 19,80; US $ 8.10
3 HUEPER, W. C.: Occupational and Environmental Cancers of the Respiratory System. Cloth DM 41,00; US $ 16.80
4 GOLDMAN, L.: Laser Cancer Research. Cloth DM 19,80; US $ 8.10
5 METCALF, D.: The Thymus. Its Role in Immune Responses, Leukaemia Development and Carcinogenesis. Cloth DM 29,00; US $ 11.90
6 Malignant Transformation by Viruses. Edited by W. H. KIRSTEN, (Symposium). Cloth DM 39,00; US $ 16.00
7 MOERTEL, CH. G.: Multiple Primary Malignant Neoplasms. Their Incidence and Significance. Cloth DM 22,00; US $ 9.00
8 New Trends in the Treatment of Cancer. Edited by L. MANUILA, S. MOLES, and P. RENTCHNICK. Cloth DM 39,00; US $ 16.00
9 LINDENMANN, J., and P. A. KLEIN: Immunological Aspects of Viral Oncolysis. Cloth DM 22,00; US $ 9.00
10 NELSON, R. S.: Radioactive Phosphorus in the Diagnosis of Gastrointestinal Cancer. Cloth DM 19,00; US $ 7.80
11 FREEMAN, R. G., and J. M. KNOX: Treatment of Skin Cancer. Cloth DM 19,00; US $ 7.80
12 LYNCH, H. T.: Hereditary Factors in Carcinoma. Cloth DM 29,00; US $ 11.90
13 Tumours in Children. Edited by H. B. MARSDEN and J. K. STEWARD. Cloth DM 87,00; US $ 35.50
14 ODARTCHENKO, N.: Production Cellulaire Erythropoiétique. Relié DM 34,00; US $ 13.90
15 SOKOLOFF, B.: Carcinoid and Serotonin. Cloth DM 29,00; US $ 11.90
16 JACOBS, M. L.: Malignant Lymphomas and Their Management. Cloth DM 22,00; US $ 9.00
17 Normal and Malignant Cell Growth. Edited by R. J. M. FRY, M. L. GRIEM, and W. H. KIRSTEN (Symposium). Cloth DM 63,00; US $ 25.70
18 ANGLESIO, E.: The Treatment of Hodgkin's Disease. Cloth DM 26,50; US $ 10.90
19 BANNASCH, P.: The Cytoplasm of Hepatocytes during Carcinogenesis. Electron- and Lightmicroscopical Investigations of the Nitrosomorpholine-intoxicated Rat Liver. Cloth DM 35,50; US $ 14.50
20 Rubidomycin. A new Agent against Cancer. Edited by J. BERNARD, R. PAUL, M. BOIRON, C. JACQUILLAT, and R. MARAL. Cloth DM 53,00; US $ 21.70
21 Scientific Basis of Cancer Chemotherapy. Edited by G. MATHÉ (Symposium). Cloth DM 31,00; US $ 12.70
22 KOLDOVSKÝ, P.: Tumor Specific Transplantation Antigen. Cloth DM 26,50; US $ 10.90
23 FUCHS, W. A., J. W. DAVIDSON, and H. W. FISCHER: Lymphography in Cancer. With contributions by G. JANTET and H. RÖSLER. Cloth DM 84,00; US $ 34.30
24 HAYWARD, J. L.: Hormones and Human Breast Cancer. An Account of 15 Years Study. Cloth DM 37,50; US $ 15.30
25 ROY-BURMAN, P.: Analogues of Nucleic Acid Components. Mechanisms of Action. Cloth DM 31,00; US $ 12.70
26 Tumors of the Liver. Edited by G. T. PACK and A. H. ISLAMI. Cloth DM 62,00; US $ 25.30
27 SZYMENDERA, J.: Bone Mineral Metabolism in Cancer. Cloth DM 35,50; US $ 14.50
28 MEEK, E. S.: Antitumour and Antiviral Substances of Natural Origin. Cloth DM 18,00; US $ 7.40
29 Aseptic Environments and Cancer Treatment. Edited by G. MATHÉ (Symposium). Cloth DM 24,50; US $ 10.00
30 Advances in the Treatment of Acute (Blastic) Leukemias. Edited by G. MATHÉ (Symposium). Cloth DM 42,00; US $ 17.20
31 DENOIX, P.: Treatment of Malignant Breast Tumors. Indications and Results. Cloth DM 53,00; US $ 21.70

32 NELSON, R. S.: Endoscopy in Gastric Cancer. Cloth DM 53,00; US $ 21.70

33 Experimental and Clinical Effects of L-Asparaginase. Edited by E. GRUNDMANN and H. F. OETTGEN (Symposium). Cloth DM 64,00; US $ 26.20

34 Chemistry and Biological Actions of 4-Nitroquinoline 1-Oxide. Edited by H. ENDO, T. ONO, and T. SUGIMURA. Cloth DM 36,—; US $ 14.70

35 PENN, I.: Malignant Tumors in Organ Transplant Recipients. Cloth DM 26,50; US $ 10.90

36 Current Concepts in the Management of Lymphoma and Leukemia. Edited by J. E. ULTMANN, M. L. GRIEM, W. H. KIRSTEN, and R. W. WISSLER (Symposium). Cloth DM 48,—; US $ 19.60

37 CHIAPPA, S., R. MUSUMECI, and C. USLENGHI: Endolymphatic Radiotherapy in Malignant Lymphomas. With contributions by G. BONADONNA, B. DAMASCELLI, G. FAVA, F. PIZZETTI, U. VERONESI. Cloth DM 48,—; US $ 19.60

38 KOLLER, P. C.: The Role of Chromosomes in Cancer Biology. Cloth DM 48,—; US $ 19.60

39 Current Problems in the Epidemiology of Cancer and Lymphomas. Edited by E. GRUNDMANN and H. TULINIUS (Symposium). Cloth DM 58,—; US $ 23.70

40 LANGLEY, F. A., A. C. CROMPTON: Epithelial Abnormalities of the Cervix Uteri. Cloth DM 58,—; US $ 23.70

41 Tumours in a Tropical Country. A Survey of Uganda (1964—1968). Edited by A. C. TEMPLETON. Cloth DM 72,—; US $ 29.40

42 Breast Cancer: A Challenging Problem. Edited by M. L. GRIEM, E. V. JENSEN, J. E. ULTMANN, and R. W. WISSLER (Symposium). Cloth DM 48,—; US $ 19.60

43 Nomenclature, Methodology and Results of Clinical Trials in Acute Leukemias. Edited by G. MATHÉ, P. POUILLART, and L. SCHWARZENBERG (Symposium). Cloth DM 58,—; US $ 23.70

44 Special Topics in Carcinogenesis. Edited by E. GRUNDMANN (Symposium). Cloth DM 58,—; US $ 23.70

45 KOLDOVSKÝ, P.: Carcinoembryonic Antigens. Cloth DM 38,—; US $ 15.50

46 Diagnosis and Therapy of Malignant Lymphoma. Edited by K. MUSSHOFF (Symposium). Cloth DM 62,—; US $ 25.30

47 Investigation and Stimulation of Immunity in Cancer Patients. Edited by G. MATHÉ and R. WEINER (Symposium). Cloth DM 96,—; US $ 39.20

Special Supplement: Biology of Amphibian Tumors. Edited by M. MIZELL. Cloth DM 96,00; US $ 39.20

In Production

48 Platinum Compounds in Cancer Chemotherapy. Edited by T. A. CONNORS and J. J. ROBERTS (Symposium)

49 Complications of Cancer Chemotherapy. Edited by G. MATHÉ and R. K. OLDHAM (Symposium).

Prices are Subject to change without notice